# Textbook of
# Dental Materials

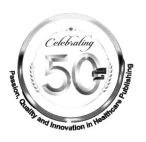

# Textbook of
# Dental Materials

**Vijay Prakash** MDS (Manipal)
Professor
Department of Prosthodontics and Implantology
Divya Jyoti College of Dental Sciences and Research
Modinagar, Uttar Pradesh, India

**Ruchi Gupta** MDS (Rohtak)
Professor
Department of Conservative Dentistry and Endodontics
Divya Jyoti College of Dental Sciences and Research
Modinagar, Uttar Pradesh, India

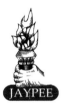

JAYPEE
**JAYPEE BROTHERS MEDICAL PUBLISHERS**
*The Health Sciences Publisher*
New Delhi | London | Panama

**Jaypee Brothers Medical Publishers (P) Ltd**

**Headquarters**
Jaypee Brothers Medical Publishers (P) Ltd
4838/24, Ansari Road, Daryaganj
New Delhi 110 002, India
Phone: +91-11-43574357
Fax: +91-11-43574314
Email: jaypee@jaypeebrothers.com

**Overseas offices**

J.P. Medical Ltd
83, Victoria Street, London
SW1H 0HW (UK)
Phone: +44 20 3170 8910
Fax: +44 (0)20 3008 618
Email: info@jpmedpub.com

Jaypee Brothers Medical Publishers (P) Ltd
17/1-B Babar Road, Block-B, Shyamoli
Mohammadpur, Dhaka-1207
Bangladesh
Mobile: +08801912003485
Email: jaypeedhaka@gmail.com

Jaypee-Highlights Medical Publishers Inc
City of Knowledge, Bld. 235, 2nd Floor,
Clayton, Panama City, Panama
Phone: +1 507-301-0496
Fax: +1 507-301-0499
Email: cservice@jphmedical.com

Jaypee Brothers Medical Publishers (P) Ltd
Bhotahity, Kathmandu, Nepal
Phone: +977-9741283608
Email: kathmandu@jaypeebrothers.com

Website: www.jaypeebrothers.com
Website: www.jaypeedigital.com

*Textbook of Dental Materials*

*First Edition*: **2019**

ISBN: 978-93-5270-266-4

*Printed at* Sanat Printers

## Dedicated to

*My father late Shri CP Gupta who has always been my inspiration*
*Dhaanvi and Keshav for bringing immense joy in my life*
*All students who will continue to innovate, inspire and*
*practice in right spirit for the betterment of humanity.*

**—Vijay Prakash**

*My parents, children, teachers and students*
*who have inspired me in the journey of life.*

**—Ruchi Gupta**

The practice of dentistry is incomplete without thorough knowledge of dental materials. Being in the age of information, it is important for health professionals, clinicians or students in dentistry to keep themselves updated. Success in clinical practice demands not only intimate knowledge of dental materials but also the recent advances in this field. The study of dental materials involves basic sciences, applied aspect, manipulation, techniques and methods of testing.

*Textbook of Dental Materials* is inspired during teaching of dental materials for more than a decade to a number of students. During our interactions with students, we realized that there is a need for a simple, concise textbook on this subject. Hence, we tried to write this book in simple, short format which is easy to understand, comprehensive and at the same time covers the entire syllabus laid down by the Dental Council of India (DCI). The basic aim was to introduce and simplify the complex subject of dental materials to young graduate students. There are numerous line diagrams, flowcharts, tables and high quality illustrations to assist the students for better grasping of the subject.

This book contains 30 chapters which are written sequentially and divided into eight sections based on the purpose of each material. Section 1 is on the General Properties of Dental Materials which includes three chapters, one chapter on biocompatibility of dental materials. Section 2 contains five chapters which includes the Auxiliary Dental Materials such as Gypsum products, Dental waxes, Casting investments, Die and die materials and finishing and polishing materials. Section 3 is dedicated to various Impression materials covered in four chapters. Special focus is on the chapter Elastomeric impression materials. Section 4 is based on Denture Base Materials with a chapter each on Dental polymers and Denture base resins including the recent developments.

Next six chapters are covered in Section 5 under the broad heading of Direct Restorative Materials. This section starts with a chapter on Dental Amalgam, its properties, mercury toxicity and hygiene. Next chapter is on Enamel and dentin bonding agents focusing on different generations of bonding. Aesthetic restorative materials such as composite resins is covered in detail in this chapter. Different composite restorative materials are discussed at length including methods of polymerization. The chapter also includes recent topics such as indirect composites, flowable, packable, nanocomposites among others. The next two chapters in this section are on Dental cements and Pulp protective agents. The chapter on dental cements includes various cements used in dentistry, their uses, composition, classification, properties, manipulation and recent advances. Pulp protecting agents are materials which are used in approximation of pulp. Focus here is on direct and indirect pulp capping agents. The last chapter in this section is on Direct filling gold, although this material is not commonly used in dentistry now but still students should learn about various aspects of this material.

Section 6 of the book discusses various Indirect Restorative Materials such as Dental Ceramics, casting alloys and wrought alloys. The chapter on dental ceramics includes metal ceramic restorations and all ceramic restorations in detail. This chapter also highlights recent materials such as CAD–CAM ceramics and 3D printing. The next three chapters in this section are dedicated to nature of alloys, casting alloys, casting procedures and its defects. Casting alloys such as gold alloys, metal ceramic alloys and base metal alloys are discussed in detail in these chapters. A section of titanium and its casting is also included. Casting procedures and defects are sequentially explained with the help of numerous line diagrams and illustrations. Another chapter in this section is on Wrought alloys and its uses in dentistry. The last chapter is on Soldering and welding procedure and techniques.

Section 7 is based on Endodontic and Preventive Materials. The chapter on Endodontic materials explores various materials which are used in the field of endodontics. There is a wide array of materials with recent developments discussed in this chapter. The chapter on preventive materials focuses on various materials dedicated to prevention of dental diseases. In this chapter, a complete section is on Bleaching materials which are widely used in the practice of dentistry.

Section 8 includes the Recent Trends in Dental Materials with a chapter each on Dental implant materials and the latest trends in material science. The chapter on dental implant materials describes various implant materials, graft materials and special focus on bioceramics. One of the highlights of this book is the inclusion of this chapter which focuses on the materials which will be the future of dental practice. This chapter includes various materials such as smart materials, biomimetics, zirconia-based material, use of lasers, nanotechnology, tissue regeneration techniques, and oral cancer detection tests amongst various other materials.

In each chapter, 'clinical significance of various materials' are highlighted to assist students in understanding the clinical application of that material. At the end of each chapter, a section is dedicated to 'Test Yourself' which includes multiple choice questions, long questions and short notes. This section aims to help students to prepare for various competitive examinations and university examination. Another highlight of the book is 'Quick Revision Chart' which includes various materials which are commonly asked in examination for quick revision before the final examination. Additionally, online resources for both students and instructors are provided along with this book in the form of multiple choice questions including image-based questions, and power point presentations, respectively.

This book will not only help graduate students but also dental hygienists and dental technicians. It will be a quick reference book for the postgraduates and clinicians. In the long run, successful practice of dentistry will involve thorough knowledge of various materials, their correct manipulation and appropriate selection of material in a given clinical situation. Also, mutual understanding and respect between clinicians, dental hygienists, dental technicians, and patients will result in successful treatment outcome. We sincerely hope that young students will improve, innovate and practice dentistry and help in taking our profession to greater heights. We wish you all success in your career.

'A journey of a thousand miles begins with a single step'.

**Vijay Prakash**
**Ruchi Gupta**

# ACKNOWLEDGMENTS

First of all we bow down to the Almighty God for blessing us with his kindness and wisdom to accomplish this work. Any book written has contributions from a number of people directly or indirectly and this work is no different. We extend our sincere and heartfelt gratitude to our teachers, who have always encouraged us to perform at the highest level and have shaped our careers. It will always be a privilege to be associated with them. Our deepest gratitude goes to our friends and our colleagues who have made learning a fun experience. We sincerely thank all our students over more than a decade who have always inspired us to excel in our field.

Our love, gratitude and respect to our parents, who have always been there during the test of time. They have been our pillars of strength and have always motivated us. Our deep appreciation goes to our family especially our brothers and sister, for their unconditional love and support. Lots of love to our children, who have adjusted to our work time in completing this book.

We are very grateful to the whole team of M/s Jaypee Brothers Medical Publishers (P) Ltd, who helped and guided us, especially Shri Jitendar P Vij (Group Chairman), Mr Ankit Vij (Managing Director), Mr MS Mani (Group President), Ms Ritu Sharma (Director–Content Strategy), Ms Sunita Katla (Executive Assistant to Group Chairman and Publishing Manager), Ms Pooja Bhandari (Production Head), Ms Samina Khan (Executive Assistant to Director–Content Strategy), Dr Ambika Kapoor (Development Editor), Ms Seema Dogra (Cover Visualizer), Mr Deep Kumar (DTP Operator), Mr Amit Mathur (Graphic Designer), Ms Geeta Rani (Proofreader), and their team members, for all their support and work on, this project and make it a success. Without their cooperation, we could not have completed this project.

# CONTENTS

## Section 5: Direct Restorative Materials

# Section

# 1

# General Properties of Dental Materials

# Introduction to Dental Materials

*'The way to get started is to quit talking and start doing.'*

—*Walt Disney*

## INTRODUCTION

Throughout the history of human civilization, replacement of lost body parts has challenged mankind and replacement of tooth and adjacent structures is no exception. Dental practitioners have always sought for an ideal material which will replace the lost tooth and adjacent tissues thus, restoring esthetics and function. The quest for an ideal material will continue to be focused by the clinicians worldwide. The practice of dentistry is largely dependent on material, its manipulation and techniques of use. Material science will keep on evolving with newer innovations and techniques and dental practitioners will have to keep updated with latest information which would be highly valuable for treating the patient more efficiently and effectively.

## DEFINITION

The science of dental material is dealing with the development, properties, manipulation, care, evolution, and evaluation of materials used in the treatment and prevention of dental diseases.

Dental materials can be broadly categorized as metals, ceramics, composites and polymers.

Metals in pure form are rarely used in dentistry except pure titanium and gold foils. Pure titanium finds application in fabrication of dental implants, inlays, onlays, crowns and fixed dental prosthesis. Pure gold in form of gold foils is used as directly filling material, which is rare currently.

Dental ceramic is widely used to fabricate inlays, onlays, crowns and fixed dental prosthesis. Metal ceramic and all ceramic restorations are commonly used because of improved strength and higher esthetics. Yttria Stabilized Zirconia (YSZ) can also be used for endodontic post and core and manufacturing implant body.

Dental composites, cements and polymers are commonly used as preventive as well as restorative material. Some of these materials are capable of releasing sustained and controlled agents capable of preventing dental disease such as dental caries.

However, despite massive strides in technology in dentistry still there is a search for ideal restorative material.

## HISTORICAL BACKGROUND

Timeline for history of dental materials is as follows:
- *4500–4000 BC:* Babylonians, Assyrians and Egyptians were familiar with silver, gold, copper and lead
- *990 BC:* Iron was used by Phoenicians
- *700–500 BC:* Gold crowns and bridges were commonly used by Etruscans
- *About 100 AD:* Celsus advocated the use of lint and lead for filling large cavities
- *1480: Johannes Arculanus* used gold leaf to fill cavities to restore teeth
- *1460–1520: Giovanni de Vigo* described the removal of caries before using gold leaf for filling the cavities
- *1562: Ambroise Pare* prepared artificial teeth from bone and ivory **(Fig. 1.1)**
- *1728: Pierre Fauchard* called Father of Modern Dentistry **(Fig. 1.2)**, described materials and practices in dentistry in his book Le chirurgien dentiste, ou Traite des dents
- *1746: Claude Mouton* introduced the gold shell crowns which were swaged from one piece of metal
- *1756: Philip Pfaff* first used plaster models prepared from sectional wax impressions

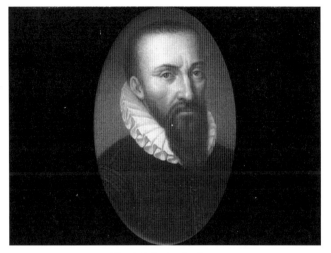

**Fig. 1.1:** Ambroise Pare.

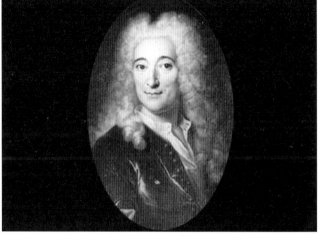

**Fig. 1.2:** Pierre Fauchard, father of modern dentistry.

- *1789: Dr John* Greenwood made dentures for US President George Washington **(Fig. 1.3)**
- *1801:* First American book on dentistry published by RC Skinner titled as 'Treatise on the Human teeth'
- *1812:* Gold foil produced by Marcus Bull
- *1832: James Snell* introduced the zinc oxychloride cement
- *1833:* Silver paste which was amalgam of silver and mercury was introduced in the United States by *Crawcour brothers*
- *1838:* Ash tube tooth was first marketed **(Fig. 1.4)**
- *1840:* First dental school called the Baltimore College of Dental Surgery established in the United States
- *1864: Rubber dam* introduced to isolate teeth by Barnum
- *1870:* Zinc phosphate cement was first used
- *1878: Richmond Crown* was introduced
- *1878:* Silicate cement developed by *Fletcher*
- *1885: Davis Crown* was introduced
- *1889: Charles Land* introduced porcelain jacket crowns and high fusing inlays
- *1907: WH Taggart* introduced Lost wax technique for casting
- *1930:* Unfilled resins as PMMA (poly methyl methacrylate) were first used as denture base resins
- *1938:* First nylon toothbrush introduced with synthetic bristles
- *1942:* Diamond abrasive instruments introduced for dental use
- *1949: Oskar Hagger* first bonded acrylic resin with the tooth dentin
- *1951:* Inorganic fillers were added to the direct filling materials
- *1955: Michael Buonocore* first introduced the acid etch technique for bonding to tooth enamel

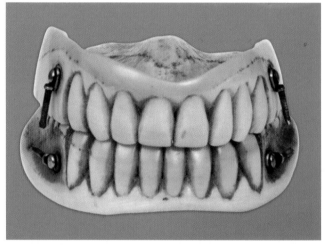

**Fig. 1.3:** Dentures for American President George Washington made with ivory, wood and metal fasteners.

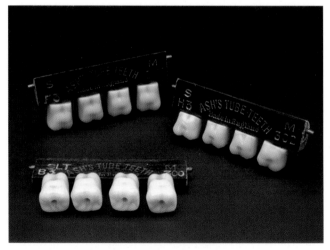

**Fig. 1.4:** Ash's tube teeth.

- *1956: RL Bowen* developed the first generation dentin adhesive
- *1962: Bowen* developed Bis-GMA which was used as composite resins for restorations
- *1965: PI Branemark* first placed dental implant in human jaw
- *1968: Smith* introduced the zinc polycarboxylate cement
- *1971: Dr Francois Duret* (France)—First developed dental CAD-CAM system
- *1972:* Glass ionomer cement was introduced by *A Wilson* and *Kent*
- *1977:* Light cure composites first introduced in the market
- *1980s:* Introduction of lasers in dentistry
- *1985: Dr Werner Mormann* and *Dr Marco Brandestini* (Switzerland)—developed the first commercial CAD-CAM system (CEREC)
- *1996:* Chemical vapor deposition (CVD) burs were introduced for efficient cutting
- *1997: Swift–Ferrari–Goracci* introduced the self-etching adhesives
- *1997:* Erbium YAG laser was first used on dentin to treat tooth decay
- *2007:* Seventh generation bonding agents were introduced
- *2009:* CEREC AC powered by *BlueCam* was introduced to make impressions and create crowns or veneers chairside.

# IDEAL REQUIREMENTS FOR DENTAL MATERIALS

Although currently no single dental material meets all the ideal requirements.
*The requirements for an ideal dental material is given below:*
- Should be biocompatible, nonirritating, nontoxic and inert
- Should have adequate strength to resist masticatory load
- Should be tarnish and corrosion resistant
- Should be dimensionally stable
- Should be esthetic
- Should be easy to manipulate and should be easily available
- Should be odorless and tasteless
- Should have good bonding to the tooth and other restorative materials
- Should be easily repairable
- Should be economical.

## Classification of Dental Materials

- *According to their use*
  - **Preventive materials:** Those materials which help in preventing or inhibiting the progression of dental caries. These materials have antibacterial properties and can prevent leakage. For example, pit and fissure sealants, liners, bases, cements releasing fluoride, chlorhexidine, etc.
  - **Restorative materials:** Those materials which are used to repair or replace tooth structure. For example, amalgams, composites, compomers, cast metals, metal ceramics, ceramics and denture polymers
  - **Auxiliary materials:** Those materials which are used in the process of fabricating dental prosthesis but are not part of the prosthesis. For example, acid etchant, dental waxes, gypsum products, bleaching trays, impression materials, acrylic resin used for fabricating mouth guards or occlusal splints.
- *According to their location of fabrication*
  - **Direct restorative materials:** Those materials which are used to restore prepared cavity directly in the mouth. For example, amalgam, composite materials, glass ionomers, etc.
- *According to the duration of their use*
  - **Temporary restorations:** Those restorative materials which are used for short period of time such as few days to few weeks. For example, temporary cements
  - **Permanent restorations:** Those restorative materials which are used for long-term applications. For example, inlays, onlays, crowns, partial dentures, fixed partial dentures.
- *According to the chemical nature of the materials*
  - **Metals:** These materials solidify with their atoms in a regular or crystalline arrangements. They have high strength and hardness. They are good conductors of heat and electricity
  - **Ceramics:** It is a compound which is formed by the union of metallic and nonmetallic elements. These materials have high strength and hardness which are chemically inert
  - **Polymers:** These are long-chain organic molecules which are characterized by covalent bonds between each molecule. They are poor conductors of heat and electricity
  - **Ceramics:** These materials are combination of basic metallic, ceramic and polymeric materials. They can be metal-polymer composite such as die.

# EVALUATION OF DENTAL MATERIALS

In 1919, the US Army approached the National Bureau of Standards to set up specifications for the evaluation and selection of dental amalgam to be used for Federal services. The research was carried out under the leadership of Wilmer Souder and was published in 1920. Later in the year 1928, American Dental Association (ADA) was established. ADA laid down specifications for each dental material to be used clinically. In this year ADA took over the dental research section at the National Bureau of Standards.

## ADA Acceptance Program

ADA developed the ADA acceptance program **(Fig. 1.5)** to identify the physical and chemical properties of the material that ensures satisfactory performance of the material when properly manipulated.

The products launched by the manufacturer are tested to comply with the required specifications. If the material clears the required specification it is given seal of acceptance. This can be provisional or complete acceptance depending on the extensiveness of the clinical and laboratory results. In the year 1993, ADA published the report Clinical Products in Dentistry—A Desktop Reference which listed all the accepted, certified dental materials, instruments, equipment and therapeutics. This served as quick reference guide to update dentists about new products and helped in selection of various materials.

In 1976, Medical Devices Amendments were signed into the law to protect the human population from hazardous and ineffective devices used in medical or dental field.

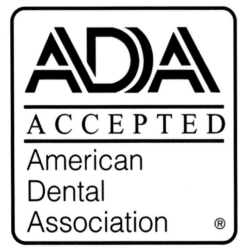

**Fig. 1.5:** ADA seal of acceptance.

A dental device classification panel developed to classify devices used in dentistry based on the relative risk, is as follows:

### Classification of Dental Devices

- *Class I devices*: These devices are considered to be of low risk and are subjected to general controls, which include registration of manufacturer's registration, practices followed and record keeping
- *Class II devices*: If the devices are not adequate to ensure safety and effectiveness. These devices are required to meet the performance standards established by the Food and Drug Administration
- *Class III devices*: The most stringent category. It desires that material or device should be approved for safety and effectiveness before given permission for marketing.

All dental products or devices should adhere to appropriate specification or standards. The manufacturer is responsible to comply with these specifications solely. It is important for a product to display the following information:
- Serial number
- Composition
- Physical properties as obtained after standard test
- Biocompatibility data if needed
- Information about every provision of official specification about that product.

## International Standards

With the increase in demand for dental devices around the world, the tests for safety and effectiveness should confirm to the international standards. There are two organizations namely FDI (Fédération Dentaire Internationale) and the ISO (International Organization for Standardization) which work toward establishing international specification for dental materials. Initially, FDI formulated international specifications for dental materials and later ISO which is a nongovernment international organization developed international standards.

The specifications are highly beneficial for dentist worldwide to select materials based on criteria which are impartial and reliable. On request from the FDI, the ISO organization established a technical committee (TC) for dentistry called as TC 106. This committee is involved in standardizing and testing methods to develop specifications for dental materials, equipments, appliances and instruments.

ISO technical committee—TC 106 Dentistry was established based on the FDI specification and ISO standards. Later subcommittees were formed to cover all the dental products. For example, TC 106/SC 1 restorative and filling materials.

# INTERNATIONAL ORGANIZATION FOR STANDARDIZATION (ISO), SUBCOMMITTEES AND WORKING GROUPS

In 2011, TC 106 Dentistry formed 7 subcommittees and 58 working groups to develop specifications for testing the safety and efficacy of dental products. Out of the 7 committees, 3 are involved and cover most of the dental restorative materials listed by the ISO standard program under the guidance of TC 106.

The three subcommittees are given below:

- **TC 106/SC 1: Filling and Restorative Materials**
  Under this category, 10 working groups (WG) are included:
  – TC 106/SC 1/WG 1: Zinc oxide eugenol cements and non-eugenol cements
  – TC 106/SC 1/WG 2: Endodontic materials
  – TC 106/SC 1/WG 5: Pit and fissure sealants
  – TC 106/SC 1/ WG 7: Amalgam or mercury
  – TC 106/SC 1/WG 9: Resin-based filling materials
  – TC 106/SC 1/WG 10: Dental luting cements, bases and liners
  – TC 106/SC 1/WG 11: Adhesion test methods
  – TC 106/SC 1/WG 13: Orthodontic products
  – TC 106/SC 1/WG 14: Orthodontic elastics
  – TC 106/SC 1/WG 15: Adhesive components.
- **TC 106/SC 2: Prosthodontics Materials**
  Under this category, 16 WG are included:
  – TC 106/SC 2/WG 1: Dental ceramics
  – TC 106/SC 2/WG 2: Dental base alloys
  – TC 106/SC 2/WG 6: Color stability test methods
  – TC 106/SC 2/WG 7: Impression materials
  – TC 106/SC 2/WG 8: Noble metal casting alloys
  – TC 106/SC 2/WG 10: Resilient lining materials
  – TC 106/SC 2/WG 11: Denture base polymers
  – TC 106/SC 2/WG 12: Corrosion test methods
  – TC 106/SC 2/WG 13: Investments
  – TC 106/SC 2/WG 14: Dental brazing materials
  – TC 106/SC 2/WG 16: Polymer veneering and die materials
  – TC 106/SC 2/WG 18: Dental waxes and baseplate waxes
  – TC 106/SC 2/WG 19: Wear test methods
  – TC 106/SC 2/WG 20: Artificial teeth
  – TC 106/SC 2/WG 21: Metallic materials
  – TC 106/SC 2/WG 22: Magnetic attachments.

- **TC 106/SC 8: Dental Implants**
  Under this category, 5 WG are included:
  – TC 106/SC 8/WG 1: Implantable materials
  – TC 106/SC 8/WG 2: Preclinical biological evaluation and testing
  – TC 106/SC 8/WG 3: Content of technical files
  – TC 106/SC 8/WG 4: Mechanical testing
  – TC 106/SC 8/WG 5: Dental implants—terminology.

# DEVELOPMENT PROCESS OF ISO STANDARDS

In the first phase, the working group of a particular product are involved and the technical experts of interested countries. An agreement is established between them and then in the second phase, the countries involved determine the detailed specifications within the standard. The last and final phase involves drafting of the final approval called Draft International Standard (DIS) by at least 75% of all voting members. After this, it is published in the ISO International Standard.

Most of these standards require periodic revision due to technological advancement, new materials and methods and safety requirements. All ISO standards require revision at the interval of not more than 5 years. Some of these standards may require revision earlier than that.

# OTHER DENTAL STANDARD ORGANIZATIONS

Other dental standard organizations are:

- *Australian Dental Standards laboratory*: Established in 1936
- *NIOM (Nordiska Institutet for Odontologisk Material provning)*: It was established for Scandinavian countries (Denmark, Finland, Iceland, Norway and Sweden) in 1969, for testing, certifying and research regarding dental materials and equipments. This institute became functional in 1973
- *CEN (Comite Europeen de Normalisation)*: It established the Task Group 55 to develop European standards. CE denotes the mark of conformity with the Essential Requirements in the Medical Device Directive. CEN describes dental materials, implants and equipment in Europe as 'medical devices used in dentistry'. All the medical devices used in dentistry marketed in Europe should have the seal of CE mark of conformity.

The field of research in dentistry is expanding in areas of metallurgy, material science, mechanical engineering, engineering mechanics, ceramics and polymer science.

These fields suggest interdisciplinary approach when examining a material. Ultimate test of material is the function and longevity in the patient's mouth. Also, clinical reviews of specifications of various dental materials become more essential with the increased focus on "evidence-based dentistry".

## SAFETY OF RESTORATIVE MATERIALS

There is no dental material which can be considered absolutely safe. The term *safety* is relatively based on the assumption that advantage of using a material far outweighs the drawbacks of using it. The two main biological effects are allergic and toxic reactions.

A Swiss based alchemist named Paracelsus (1493–1541 AD) formulated a principle on which the current field of toxicology exists. He stated that, *All substances are, poisons; there is none which is not a poison. The right dose differentiates a poison from a remedy.*

A component in a dental material is capable of producing an allergic reaction in an individual. A chemical agent can induce an antigen–antibody reaction and patient can show signs and symptoms of allergy. Although allergy and side effects in dental treatment is extremely low which is reported as 0.14% in the general population.

## CONCLUSION

There has been marked increase in newer materials, equipment and techniques in dentistry. A professional is expected to have an update on these materials because of the change in demands of modern dental practice. There will be greater restorative needs in future because of more emphasis on preventive treatment. Research in dental materials is no longer confined to only material science but has an interdisciplinary approach also because of interaction of materials at cellular and molecular levels. Also studies on tissue regeneration will continue and can, in future, totally change the concept of current use of materials.

## TEST YOURSELF

### Essay Questions

1. Classify dental materials? Write the ideal requirements of dental materials? Add a note on evaluation of dental materials?
2. Describe various international standards for evaluating safety of dental materials?

### Short Notes

1. ADA acceptance program.
2. Auxillary materials.

### Multiple Choice Questions

1. An ideal restorative material should be all, *except*
   A. Compatible with natural tissues
   B. Should match adjacent tooth structure
   C. Should bond mechanically to the tooth
   D. Should initiate repair of tissues
2. Auxillary dental materials:
   A. Helps in preventing caries
   B. Helps in restoring decayed tooth
   C. Facilitate in fabrication of dental prosthesis
   D. Helps in repairing damaged tooth

## ANSWERS

1. C          2. C

## BIBLIOGRAPHY

1. American Dental Association: Clinical Products in Dentistry: A Desktop Reference. Chicago; 1983.
2. American Dental Association: Dentist's Desk Reference: Materials, Instruments and Equipment, 2nd edition. Chicago; 1983.
3. American Dental Association: Guide to Dental Materials and Devices, 8th edition. Chicago; 1976.
4. Anusavice KJ. Phillip's Science of Dental Materials, 11th edition. Saunders St. Louis; 2003.
5. Craig RG, Powers JM. Restorative Dental Materials, 11th edition. St. Louis, Mosby; 2001.
6. Lufkin AW. A History of Dentistry, 3rd edition. Philadelphia, Lea and Febiger; 1948.
7. O' Brien, William J. Dental Materials and Their Selection, 2nd edition. Chicago, Quintessence; 1997.
8. Ring ME. John Greenwood, Dentist to President Washington. J Calif Dent Assoc. 2010;38(12):846-51.
9. Weinberger BW. An Introduction to the History of Dentistry in America: Volume Two, 1st edition. St. Louis, Mosby, 1948. p. 408.

# Structure of Matter and Properties of Dental Materials

*'Run when you can, walk if you have to, crawl if you must; just never give up.'*

—*Dean Karnazes*

## INTRODUCTION

It is important to understand various properties of dental materials which help in their selection. The knowledge of their atomic structure determines the performance of these materials whether they are ceramic, polymeric or metallic. Therefore, it is essential to have the basic understanding of the atomic structures of dental materials and their interaction.

## STATES OF MATTER

Matter mainly occurs in the form of three states namely, solid, liquid and gas. It is essentially made of large number of atoms belonging to a particular structure.

The term atom is derived from a Greek word '*atomos*' which means '*uncuttable*'. It is believed that around 460 B.C. *Democritus* a Greek philosopher proposed that all matter is made up of invisible particles which he named as atomos.

Atom is composed of nucleus which is surrounded by negatively charged electrons called the '*electron cloud*'. The nucleus is a mixture of positively charged protons and electrically neutral neutrons except in a hydrogen atom there is no neutrons. The electrons which surrounds the nucleus exists in different clouds at various energy levels. An atom if it gains electrons is called as *negative ion* and if it looses electrons it is called as *positive ion*.

The combination of two or more atoms form a molecule which is an electrically neutral entity. For example, Water ($H_2O$) is composed of two hydrogen atoms and one oxygen atom. It is the attraction between atoms and molecules which forms a structure which are visible and can be felt.

Atoms and molecules are held together by atomic interactions forming crystalline, semi-crystalline and amorphous solid structures below their melting temperatures. When a liquid is heated, energy is required to convert liquid into vapor. The amount of energy required for this conversion is called as *latent heat of vaporization*. For example, to boil 1 g of water at 100°C and 1 atmospheric pressure it requires 540 calories of heat.

Similarly, if kinetic energy of a liquid is reduced sufficiently when its temperature is reduced a second transformation occurs, i.e. conversion from liquid to solid. This energy is called *latent heat of fusion*. It is the amount of energy required to convert 1 g of liquid into solid at a given temperature and pressure. For example, 80 calories of heat is released when 1 g of water freezes.

Some solids can directly transform into a gaseous state through a process of *sublimation, e.g. formation of dry ice*. However, this phenomenon is of little use in dentistry.

## INTERATOMIC BONDING

An atom is considered electronically stable if it has eight electrons in the outermost valence shell, e.g. noble gases except helium which has only two electrons in the outermost shell. When one atom shares, loses or gains electrons from other atoms to form eight electrons in outermost shell then it achieves a stable configuration. This process between atoms form a strong or a *primary bond*. Likewise bonding also occurs between atoms and molecules but with much weaker forces called as the *secondary bonds*.

Interatomic bonds that hold atoms together can be classified as primary and secondary.

### Classification of Interatomic Bonds

- *Types of primary interatomic bonds:*
  - Ionic
  - Covalent
  - Metallic.
- *Types of secondary interatomic bonds:*
  - Hydrogen bonds
  - Van der Waals forces.

### Primary Interatomic Bonds

#### Ionic Bonds

It occurs between positive and negative charges by strong electrostatic forces of attraction, e.g. NaCl sodium chloride, in this the sodium atom donates its single electron of outermost shell to chlorine to completely fill its outermost shell resulting in a stable compound **(Fig. 2.1)**.

In dentistry ionic bonding occurs in crystalline phases of some dental materials such as gypsum products and phosphate-based cements.

#### Covalent Bonds

This type of bonding is due to sharing of one or more electrons of the outermost orbit of the atoms.

One characteristic feature of covalent bonding is their directional orientation **(Fig. 2.2)**.

For example, hydrogen molecule is a classic example of covalent bonding. In a molecule of $H_2$, one valence electron of each hydrogen atom is shared with another combining atom to result in a covalent bonding.

In dentistry it occurs in many organic compounds such as dental resins.

#### Metallic Bonds

This type of bonding occurs in metals such as pure gold. In this the valence electrons in the outermost shell are loosely bound to the nuclei and easily removed by even low thermal energies to form a 'cloud' of free electrons **(Fig. 2.3)**. These free electrons form positive ions which are neutralized by acquiring new valence electrons from adjacent atoms. They are responsible for excellent electrical and thermal conductivity of metals and their ability to deform plastically. The ease of flow of these free electrons controls the electrical and thermal conductivities of metals. Deformability is however, associated with the slip of atoms along the crystal planes. The electrons during slip deformation can easily regroup to retain the cohesive nature of the metal. For example, gold, platinum, silver, palladium.

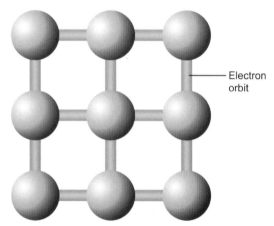

**Fig. 2.2:** Covalent bonding.

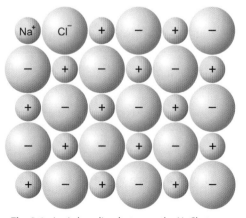

**Fig. 2.1:** Ionic bonding between the NaCl atoms.

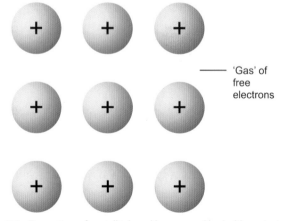

**Fig. 2.3:** Formation of metallic bond by gas or cloud of free electrons binding atoms together in a lattice structure.

## Secondary Interatomic Bonds

The secondary bonds unlike the primary bonds do not share electrons but they induce dipole forces which are capable of attracting adjacent molecules or part of a large molecule.

### Hydrogen Bonding

This type of bonding occurs because of induction of polar forces due to variation of charges among the molecules. Hydrogen bond formation occurs between water molecules. The electric charge distribution in water molecules is asymmetric. The proton side of the water molecule is positively charged, i.e. the side which is pointing away from the oxygen atom whereas the opposite side is negatively charged. This leads to formation of a *permanent dipole* which represents an asymmetric molecule. The intermolecular reactions which occurs between various organic compounds can be understood when a positive portion of one molecule is attracted to the negative portion of the adjacent molecule it results in the formation of *hydrogen bridges*.

For example, sorption of water by synthetic resins.

### Van der Waals Forces

These are weak short range forces which occur due to dipole moments between the molecules having asymmetric charge distribution. This fluctuating dipole attracts other similar dipoles. Generally electrons of the atoms are equally distributed around the nucleus and produces electrostatic field around them which has a tendency of fluctuating, i.e. charge becoming either negative or positive **(Fig. 2.4)**.

For example, chemisorption of gases by alloy liquids, attraction of inert gas molecules.

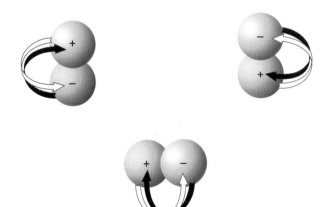

**Fig. 2.4:** Fluctuating dipole in inert gas molecules where the charges become positive and negative momentarily.

## THERMAL ENERGY

It is the amount of kinetic energy of the atoms or molecules at a given temperature. Higher the temperature, greater will be vibration of atoms resulting in increase of mean interatomic spacing as well as the internal energy. The overall effect is known as *thermal expansion.*

As the temperature of the crystal continues, the interatomic spacing will continue to increase eventually resulting in a change of state. A solid state changes to liquid and the liquid state changes to vapor. Linear coefficient of thermal expansion of materials with similar atomic or molecular structures tends to be inversely proportional to the melting temperature.

*Thermal conductivity* depends on the number of free electrons in the material. In a metallic structures such as casting alloys, dental amalgam, number of free electrons are available making them good conductors of heat and electricity whereas nonmetallic structures such as acrylic resins, resin-based composites have very less free electrons making them poor conductors of heat and electricity.

## CRYSTALLINE STRUCTURE

In crystalline solid atoms are arranged symmetrically in a space lattice by either primary or secondary forces ensuring they have minimum internal energies. Space lattice is defined as any arrangement of atoms in space in which every atom is situated similarly to every other atom.

In all there are 14 possible lattice types or forms, but most of the crystalline solids used in dentistry have cubic arrangements.

For example, dental amalgam, cast alloys, wrought metals, gold foil, pure ceramics such as zirconia, alumina.

*Types of cubic arrangements (Figs. 2.5A to C):*
- *Simple cubic*: It has 8 atoms positioned at the corners of a cube, e.g. NaCl
- *Body-centered cubic*: It has one atom at the center of each cube, e.g. Na, K, Ba, Li, Mo.
- *Face-centered cubic*: It has one atom at the center of each face in addition to those at the corners, e.g. Au, Ag, Cu, Pt, Pd.

Body-centered cubic and face-centered cubic are important in dentistry. No real material has simple cubic structure.

## NONCRYSTALLINE OR AMORPHOUS STRUCTURES

Noncrystalline solids are those structures which have randomly arranged molecules unlike the crystalline solids, e.g. certain waxes, glass, resin-based composites, glass

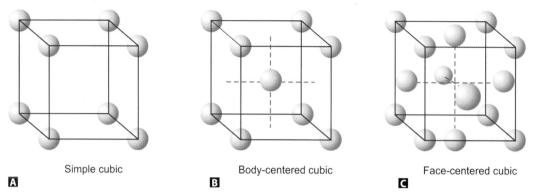

Simple cubic              Body-centered cubic              Face-centered cubic

**A**                          **B**                          **C**

**Figs. 2.5A to C:**  Diagram showing cubic arrangements: (A) Simple cubic; (B) Body-centered cubic; (C) Face-centered cubic.

ceramics, etc. The atoms in these structures have short range attractive forces. They are called as *supercooled liquids or vitreous solids* as they solidify without any arrangement like molecules in a liquid state **(Figs. 2.6A to C)**.

*Properties of noncrystalline structures:*
- Poor conductors of heat and electricity
- Do not have melting point
- These materials gradually soften on increasing the temperature. The temperature at which this change occurs is called the glass transition temperature (Tg) and is characterized by a glassy structure.
- Below (Tg) the material becomes less flowly and has greater resistance to shear deformation.

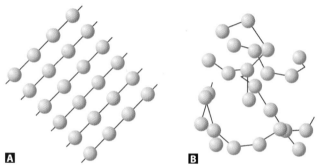

**A**                          **B**

**Figs. 2.6A and B:**  Atomic structural arrangements: (A) Crystalline; (B) Noncrystalline.

# DIFFUSION

Diffusion of molecules occurs not only in liquids and gases but also in solids. Diffusion rates of various substances depend on temperature and chemical potential gradient. The higher the temperature, the greater will be the rate of diffusion. Each alloy, crystal or compound is uniquely characterized by a diffusion coefficient. Diffusion coefficient of most of the crystalline solids at room temperature is very low. Therefore, diffusion is very slow at room temperature. However, at higher temperature, properties of metal changes rapidly by atomic diffusion.

In noncrystalline solids, diffusion occurs more rapidly and may occur at room temperature. Some metals such as mercury and gallium melt even below room temperature.

# VISCOSITY

The resistance of a fluid to flow is termed as *viscosity*.

Viscosity of some dental materials is important to understand in order to manipulate materials to get successful clinical results. Materials like cements, impression materials, gypsum products, waxes, and resins undergo liquid to solid transformation and the manner these products behave to stress is important to understand.

These materials when placed in fluid state are easy to manipulate and shaped as desired. This state of material then transforms to solid state and then removed from the mouth (like impression material) or they perform their function in the mouth (like cements). The value of viscosity is proportional to the type of the fluid. The thicker fluids show greater viscosity as compared to thin fluids which have less viscosity.

**CLINICAL SIGNIFICANCE**
- Dental materials of different viscosities are selected based on their intended clinical use. Some materials such as impression materials required to flow easily and wet the surface whereas other materials are more preferred in more viscous form such as restorative materials
- Clinical success of a dental materials is dependent on its viscosity. For example, Dental cements and impression materials undergo liquid to solid transformation in oral cavity whereas Gypsum products undergo transformation from slurry state to solid extraorally.

*Rheology refers to study of deformation and flow characteristics of materials.* Most of the liquids in motion tend to resists imposed forces that cause them to move, but usually at rest a liquid cannot support a shear stress. This resistance to fluid flow is proportional to the frictional forces within the liquid. This resistance to motion is called viscosity. Greater the viscosity of the liquid lesser is its flow. For example, honey flows slowly as compared to water or glycerin. Viscosity can be explained quantitatively in **Figure 2.7**.

In this model, a liquid say honey is allowed to flow between two plates. A shear force F is required to move the upper plate over a fixed lower plate with a velocity of V over the area A. This force F should be greater than the viscosity of the liquid in order to produce movement. Therefore, shear stress for honey can be calculated as:

$$\text{Shear stress } (\tau) = F/A \text{ and}$$

Similarly, Shear strain rate or rate of change of deformation can be calculated as:

$$(\varepsilon) = V/d,$$

where,

V = velocity of liquid

d = distance between 2 plates

Viscosity of the liquid = shear stress/shear strain.

Measured in terms of centipoise or Mpa/sec.

*Factors influencing viscosity:*
- Viscosity decreases on increasing temperature of non setting liquids such as water
- Viscosity increases with time and temperature of chemically set materials such as cements
- Viscosity is dependent on shear rate, composition, filler content, impurities etc.

## Rheological Behavior of Different Liquids (Fig. 2.8)

*Newtonian behavior:* Such type of liquids are ideal liquids where the shear stress is proportional to the strain rate. On the stress-strain plot it is a straight line. It exhibits a constant viscosity and has a constant slope. The viscosity of Newtonian liquids is constant and is independent of shear rate. For example, some dental cements and impression materials.

*Pseudoplastic behavior:* The viscosity of such liquids decrease with the increase of strain rate until it achieves a constant value. Such a fluid if spatulated faster or forced through a syringe like light body elastomer then it becomes less viscous and more flowly. For example, monophasic elastomeric impression materials, endodontic cements.

**CLINICAL SIGNIFICANCE**

Elastomeric impression material when loaded into a tray, shows a higher viscosity, whereas the same material when extruded under pressure through a syringe tip shows more fluidity. This increase in flow with increased shear rate is called as shear thinning.

*Dilatant liquids:* Such liquids demonstrate a higher viscosity with the increase in strain rate, they become more rigid as the shear strain rate increases. This behavior is opposite to that of pseudoplastic liquids, e.g. fluid denture base resins. Denture base resins become more viscous when greater pressure is applied.

*Plastic behavior:* These type of liquids behave as a rigid material until a minimum amount of shear stress is applied to attain a constant viscosity. Such materials exhibit plastic behavior. One classic example is of a ketchup bottle. To initiate flow of the ketchup, a sharp blow or thrust is required. Such liquid shows Bingham plastic behavior.

### Thixotropic Gels

Such type of materials or liquids show greater flow and reduced viscosity on repeated application of pressure. These liquids flow easily under mechanical stress.

For example, dental plaster, prophylaxis paste, resin cements, some impression materials, and fluoride gels.

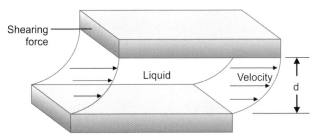

**Fig. 2.7:** Viscosity of the liquid.

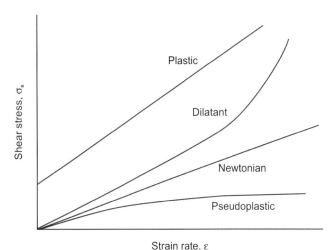

**Fig. 2.8:** Rheological behavior of different types of liquid.

Because of thixotropic nature of prophylaxis paste the material does not flow from the rubber cup until rubbed against the tooth surface.

Fluoride gels exhibit thixotropic properties such as when these materials are loaded into the trays they do not drip out. But when this tray is placed in the patient's mouth and he is instructed to bite then the viscosity of the material decreases and it flows interproximally and into deep pits and fissures of the teeth.

### Viscoelastic Behavior

When a material undergoes full elastic recovery immediately after removal of an applied load, it is called as elastic, but if the recovery takes place slowly, or if there is a degree of permanent deformation, then such materials are called as viscoelastic.

The viscoelastic deformation is a combination of elastic and plastic strain. Once the applied load is removed the recovery is only of the elastic strain and not of the plastic strain. At the same time, the recovery is not instantaneous and it takes place over a period of time.

For example, dental polymers and elastomeric impression materials exhibit viscoelastic properties.

Two properties which are important to understand using viscoelastic models are stress relaxation and creep.

#### Stress Relaxation

It is a phenomenon which occurs when an applied stress on viscoelastic material is removed it tends to recover to come to its equilibrium state. Because of this there is movement of atoms or molecules in the solid leading to its change in shape. Such rearrangement of the atoms results in relief of stress called as stress relaxation.

Change of temperature influences stress relaxation of the material. More the temperature greater is the rate of relaxation. For example, a bent orthodontic wire tends to come to its original state when heated to a high temperature.

Similarly some amorphous materials which are commonly used in dentistry such as modeling wax, baseplate wax, resins, etc. can undergo stress relaxation when manipulated and cooled leading to inaccuracy in the fit of the prosthesis.

## CREEP

*It is defined as time-dependent plastic deformation of a body under constant static load.*

It occurs when a material is heated near its melting point and is subjected to constant applied load, resulting in an increasing strain over a period of time.

Another term which is similar to creep is *sag*. It is a permanent deformation which occurs in the long span fixed partial denture under its own weight when it is heated at porcelain firing temperature. The internal strength of the metal alloy to resist such deformation is called as *sag resistance*.

Likewise the term 'flow' is used to refer to the rheology of amorphous materials such as wax. Creep is distinguished from the *flow* by the *extent of deformation* and the *rate* at which it occurs. The term creep implies to a relatively *small* deformation produced by a relatively *large* stress over a *longer* period of time. Whereas flow implies to a *greater* deformation produced more rapidly with a *smaller* applied stress or even under its own weight.

## COLOR AND COLOR PERCEPTION

The primary goal in dentistry is to obtain esthetically acceptable restorations. Today the challenge is to search direct and indirect tooth colored material which can fulfill this goal appropriately. For a restoration to simulate a natural tooth or adjacent structure, it is important to understand the factors responsible for visual perception of these structures **(Fig. 2.9)**.

*The existence of color is only possible, if three conditions are satisfied:*
1. Object or modifier since it interacts with the light source
2. Light source
3. Observer or preceptor.

Light source gives light which is important condition in color perception. Light is an electromagnetic radiation which is readily detected by naked human eye. Only the visible spectrum with wavelengths between 400 nm (violet) and 700 nm (red) are detected by the eye. The visibility of an object is only possible if the light incident on it from the light source is reflected. The reflected light is weaker in magnitude than the incident light as the latter is selectively absorbed. The signals for various colors are sent to human brain through receptors in the retina called as *cones*. These cones are sensitive to red, blue and green color.

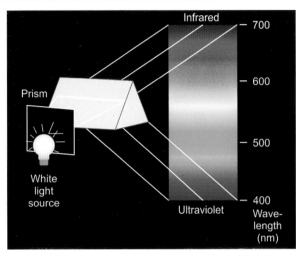

**Fig. 2.9:** Visible light spectrum.

*Factors influencing the perception of color are:*
- Intensity of light
- Age of patient
- Sex of patient
- Memory
- Fatigue of color receptor
- Cultural background.

When there is low light level, rods are more dominant than the cones and the perception of color is lost. But as the brightness of the object becomes more intense, there is a change in color. This phenomenon is called as *Bezold–Brucke effect*. If an observer looks at the red object for a fairly long time and then looks at the white background then a green hue appears because of the receptor fatigue. During shade selection if a clinician selects a shade against the dark background then it is likely that the selected shade will be shifted to complementary color of the background. For example, for orange background the selected shade shifts towards blue–green whereas for blue background it shifts towards yellow.

*Perception of color under light source (Figs. 2.10A to D)*
The type of restorative material or object will determine the appearance of that object. For excellent esthetic restorations the interaction of light with the restorative material should be similar to that of the tooth structure.

The light when it interacts with the object can:
- Reflect from its surface
- Can be absorbed
  - Can refract or
  - Can be transmitted, i.e can pass out unchanged.

This interaction determines opacity, translucency or transparency of an object. If light falls on a rough tooth restoration then it scatters in multiple directions as it is reflected at many angles by the uneven surface.

Likewise, if light falls on a smooth tooth restoration it gives a mirror like finish called as *Specular reflectance*. If light falls on a flat surface it gives a dull appearance called as *diffuse reflectance*.

If very little light passes through the object then it is termed as *opaque* (i.e. most of it get absorbed or scattered). If object allows most of the light to pass through it then it is called as *translucent*. Similarly, if an object allows 100% of light to pass through it without absorbing or scattering any light then it is called as *transparent material*.

Enamel has more translucency than dentine. It has refractive index of 1.65.

## Color Blindness

It is a condition in which a patient cannot differentiate red from green color because of the lack of either green sensitive or red sensitive cones. However, color blindness does not affect the shade selection of natural teeth.

## Metamerism

This is a phenomenon in which objects are color matched in one type of light source but appear different under another type of light source. Therefore, during color matching two or

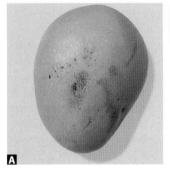
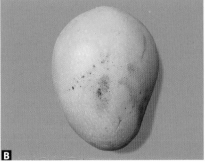
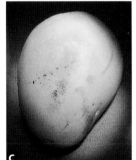
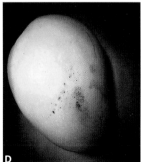

**Figs. 2.10A to D:** Appearance of Object when viewed under different light sources: (A) Mango viewed under broad daylight with white background; (B) Mango viewed under broad daylight with green background; (C) Mango viewed under halogen light of the dental chair; (D) The same mango when viewed under LED light of the Dental Chair.

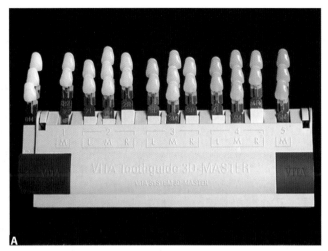 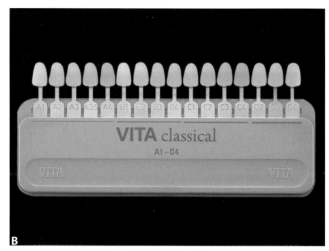

**Figs. 2.11A and B:** Shade guide for shade selection of teeth.

more type of light sources should be used. One of this light source should be natural light source to get better results.

## Shade Matching

Natural daylight is the best source of light for shade selection. Although other sources such as incandescent and fluorescent lamps can be used for shade selection using shade guide **(Figs. 2.11A and B).**

### General Principles of Shade Matching

- Shade selection should be done under good lighting condition, natural light being the best source
- Tooth to be matched should be cleaned
- Teeth to be matched are viewed at eye level
- Bright clothing should be draped and lip cosmetics should be removed before shade matching
- If unable to accurately match, select the shade with lower chroma and higher value
- Shade matching should be done quickly to avoid eye fatigue factor. In order to rest eyes focus on gray-blue surface immediately before comparison
- Shade matching should be compared under varying conditions like wet lips and dry lips
- Shade matching should be done with wet tooth surface because dry surface results in increase in value.

## Fluorescence

The energy that the tooth absorbs is converted into light with longer wavelength such that the tooth itself becomes a light source. This phenomenon of absorption of radiation of a particular wavelength and its re-emission as a radiation of a longer wavelength is called as *fluorescence.*

## Opalescence

This optical property is seen in translucent materials such as tooth enamel giving a milky white appearance when light passes through them. Such materials allow only longer wavelength to pass through them and reflect shorter wavelength giving them bluish white appearance (opalescent). But at the junction of enamel and dentin longer wavelengths are also reflected which gives an orangish glaze. This process is called as counter - opalescence. Both these phenomenon are reproduced in ceramics and composite restorations.

## Three Dimensions of Color

There are three variables which are measured to describe color namely, hue, value and chroma.

1. *Hues can be of two types:* Primary and secondary. Primary hues are those colors which cannot be formed on mixing other colors such as red, blue and green whereas secondary hues are those colors formed by mixing two primary colors such as yellow, cyan and magenta.
2. *Value:* It is the darkness or lightness of a color. Natural teeth have high value. On a scale of 1–10 where 1 = black and 10 = white. The value of most of the patients will be in the range 6–8. This lightness can be measured independent of the color hue.
3. *Chroma:* It measures the intensity of the color or degree of saturation of the hue. The term 'chroma' was coined by Munsell in 1905. Chroma is measured on the scale of 1 to 10 where 10 = saturated and 1 = least saturated. Eg. yellow color of the sunflower is more saturated than that of lemon. Usually natural teeth are low in chroma ranging between 1 and 3.

## Color Measuring Systems

- *Munsell system (Visual system)* **(Fig. 2.12)**: This system is based on the visual technique. It is based

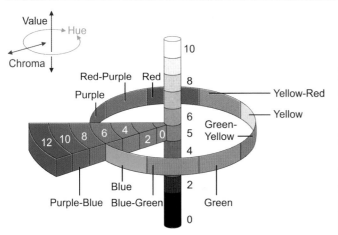

**Fig. 2.12:** Munsell color system.

on a well-defined series of color tabs. The three color parameters namely, hue, value, chroma are presented in three dimensional system.

– The *hue* of 10 colors is painted with continuous change on the circular strip with 0, 2.5, 5, 7.5 gradations for each color. The 10 colors are represented by P, PB, B, BG, G, GY, Y, YR, R, and RP

– The *value* of color is presented by 10 tabs with varying brightness from lowest to highest darkness along the vertical axial cylinder

– The *chroma* of color is presented along the radial axis with increasing saturation from /2, /4, /6,...............//16 for each hue and values.

• *CIE L a, b system (spectrophotometric system)* **(Fig. 2.13)**: This is instrument-based system. It involves systematic matching of the tristimuli values (R,G,B) of the light reflected from the surface, and comparing them with those of the standard gas filled light source and the average natural daylight. The CIE denotes Commission Internationale de I'Eclairage. The ratio of each tristimulus value of color to their sum is called as

Chromaticity coordinates. The value (black to white) is denoted as L, and chroma is denoted as red (+a), green (-a), yellow (+b), and blue (-b).

## THERMAL CONDUCTIVITY

*It is the rate at which heat passes through a material of given thickness when the temperature difference is 1°C* **(Table 2.1)**. SI Unit is $j/sec/cm^2$ or $cal/sec/cm^2$.

All metals are good conductors of heat and electricity whereas most nonmetals, polymers, ceramics, liquids and gases are good insulators.

| Table 2.1: Thermal conductivities of common dental materials. | | |
|---|---|---|
| *Material* | *Cal/sec/cm²* | *j/sec/cm²* |
| Gold | 0.710 | 2.97 |
| Dental amalgam | 0.055 | 0.23 |
| Silver | 1.006 | 4.21 |
| Gypsum products | 0.0031 | 0.013 |
| Zinc phosphate cement | 0.0028 | 0.012 |
| Resin composite | 0.0026 | 0.011 |
| Dental ceramic | 0.0025 | 0.010 |
| Tooth enamel | 0.0022 | 0.0092 |
| Tooth dentin | 0.0015 | 0.0063 |
| Zinc oxide eugenol cement | 0.0011 | 0.0046 |
| Acrylic resin | 0.0005 | 0.0021 |

### CLINICAL SIGNIFICANCE

More heat is conducted through metals and alloys than through polymer such as acrylic resin.

High value of conductivity for *dental amalgam* indicates that this material could not provide satisfactory *insulation* of the pulp. Therefore, *Cavity base* of cement is used such as *zinc phosphate* which has a lower thermal conductivity value and it insulates the pulp from thermal insult.

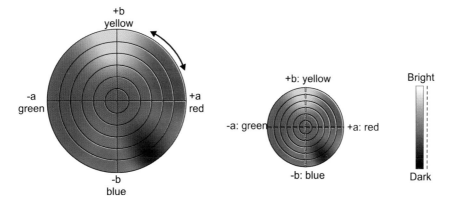

**Fig. 2.13:** CIE L a, b system.

Ideally, impression materials should be good conductors of heat such that thermoplastic materials can be manipulated uniformly and sets uniformly to minimize the distortion due to relaxation of the internal stresses. But all impression materials are not good conductors of heat and therefore, adequate precautions should be taken at the time of use.

The common denture-base material PMMA is very poor conductor of heat. The patient often complains of not so pleasant taste of the food.

## THERMAL DIFFUSIVITY

*It is a measure of the rate at which a body with a nonuniform temperature reaches a state of thermal equilibrium* **(Table 2.2)**.

Restorative materials should have low thermal conductivities and low thermal diffusivities. Although materials like direct filling gold, amalgam have high thermal conductivity and diffusivity. Therefore, cavity base is required to protect the pulp from thermal insult.

Tooth enamel and dentin are effective thermal insulators. If the remaining thickness of dentin during cavity preparation is too thin, i.e less than 0.5 – 1 mm then it should be protected with appropriate insulating base material to prevent thermal injury to the pulp.

The thermal conductivity and thermal diffusivity of different cementing materials are comparable to the natural tooth structure in contrast to the metallic tooth restorative materials.

Thermal diffusivity (D)

$D = k/c_p\rho$

where,

$k$ = Thermal conductivity
$C_p$ = Temperature-dependent specific heat
$\rho$ = Density
Units = $m^2/sec$ or $cm^2/sec$.

**Table 2.2:** Thermal diffusivity of common dental materials.

| Material | Thermal diffusivity $10^{-4}$ cm²/sec |
| --- | --- |
| Gold | 11800 |
| Dental amalgam | 960 |
| Composite resin | 19–73 |
| Zinc phosphate cement | 30 |
| Glass ionomer cement | 22 |
| Tooth dentin | 18–26 |
| Tooth enamel | 47 |

## COEFFICIENTS OF THERMAL EXPANSION

*It is defined as the change in length per unit length of a material for a change of 1°C temperature* **(Table 2.3)**. The unit is expressed as ppm/K.

**Table 2.3:** Linear coefficient of thermal expansion of common dental materials.

| Material | Coefficient of thermal expansion $10^{-6}$/°C |
| --- | --- |
| Inlay wax | 350–450 |
| Acrylic resin | 76 |
| Composite resin | 14–50 |
| Zinc oxide eugenol cement | 35 |
| Dental amalgam | 22–28 |
| Gold | 14.4 |
| Dental ceramic | 12 |
| Tooth structure | 11.4 |
| Glass ionomer cement | 10.2–11.4 |

### CLINICAL SIGNIFICANCE

In the maxillary complete denture, base covers most of the hard palate. As denture base resins are poor conductor of heat, denture patient often complains of reduced sensation of cold and hot food during eating.

- Inlay waxes have high expansion coefficient that is why it is highly susceptible to temperature changes. An accurate wax pattern that fits on a prepared tooth contracts significantly when it is removed from the tooth or from a die in a hot area and then stored in a cooler area. This dimensional change is transferred to a cast restoration which is made from that wax pattern.
- Ideally all impression materials should have coefficient of thermal expansion (CTE) as 0 to reduce dimensional changes of impression materials from thermal changes. Although none of the material currently available has CTE as 0. Therefore, adequate precautions and modifications are used during its manipulation to get desired result.
- CTE of restorative material should be as close to that of enamel and dentine as possible. Greater the difference between the CTE greater will be chances of microleakage and sensitivity to the tooth.
- The soldering or brazing material should have CTE same as that of substrate to avoid separation when cooled.
- The ceramometal bond is enhanced by mismatching the coefficient of thermal expansion.

# TARNISH AND CORROSION

## Tarnish

*Tarnish is surface discoloration of the metal surface or slight loss of surface finish or luster due to the formation of chemical film of sulfide, oxide or chloride.* It is a reversible process.

## Corrosion

*Corrosion is a process of actual, active deterioration of a metal due to the chemical or electrochemical reaction with its environment.* It is an irreversible process.

For example, rusting of iron nail in the presence of water and oxygen.

### Causes of Tarnish and Corrosion

- Tarnish is caused by soft and hard deposits such as plaque and calculus
- Stains or discoloration arises from pigment-producing bacteria, drugs-containing chemicals such as iron and mercury
- Corrosion is caused by actual deterioration of metal by reaction with its environment
- Action of moisture, acid or alkaline solutions and certain chemicals
- Water, oxygen and chloride ions present in the saliva contributes to the corrosion attack.

### Corrosion of iron can be prevented by:
- Coating the surface with oil or paint so that air and water cannot reach it
- Coating the surface with zinc
- Electroplating the surface
- Alloying the surface with chromium to form a passivating layer which is chemically resistant to corrosion. This process is called as *passivation.*

## Classification of Corrosion

- Chemical or dry corrosion
- Electrochemical or wet corrosion.

### Chemical or Dry Corrosion

Dry corrosion involves a direct combination of metallic and nonmetallic elements. This type is exemplified by oxidation, halogenation or sulfurization. There is no electrolyte or water involved in this process therefore the name dry corrosion.

For example, formation of $Ag_2S$ in dental alloys containing silver, oxidation of alloy particles in dental amalgam.

### Electrochemical or Wet Corrosion

This type of corrosion involves an oxidation-reduction reaction in the presence of an electrolyte. It consists of two different materials with the presence of water or other fluid electrolytes. It forms an electrochemical corrosion cells which involves flow of free electrons and the electrolyte provides the pathway for the transport of these electrons (**Fig. 2.14**).

An electrochemical cell consists of anode, cathode, an electrolyte and an ammeter. The anode is the surface where the positive ions are formed. This metal surface corrodes since there is loss of electrons. This reaction is called the *oxidation reaction.*

$$A^0 \rightarrow A^+ + e^-$$

At the cathode a reaction must occur that consumes the free electrons produced at the anode. The reactions at the cathode are called as *reduction reaction.* Hence, the anode loses electrons and corrodes.

$$A^+ + e^- \rightarrow A^0$$

The electrolytic solution provides the electrons to the cathode and helps in transferring the corrosion products to the anode. The external circuit completes the path through which the electrons from the anode are conducted to the cathode. The electrical potential difference or the electromotive force (EMF) is the voltage measured by this difference and is of clinical importance. For example, if two dissimilar metal restorations contact they may generate physiological response in the form of pain.

If electrochemical corrosion needs to be a continuous process the loss of electrons at the anode (oxidation reaction) should be balanced by the gain of electrons at the cathode (reduction reaction). The reduction reaction (cathodic) is found to be a primary driving force which brings about electrochemical reaction. If this is controlled the corrosion process can be minimized or eliminated.

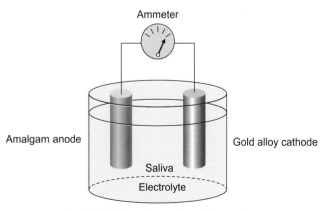

**Fig. 2.14:** Wet or electrochemical corrosion.

**Table 2.4:** Electromotive force (EMF) series of metals.

| Metal | Electrode potential |
| --- | --- |
| Gold | +1.5 |
| Silver | +0.80 |
| Copper | +0.47 |
| Hydrogen | 0.00 |
| Tin | −0.14 |
| Nickel | −0.23 |
| Iron | −0.44 |
| Chromium | −0.56 |
| Zinc | −0.76 |
| Aluminum | −1.7 |
| Sodium | −2.71 |

*Electromotive Series*

This series is the classification of elements in the order of their dissolution tendencies in water based on their equilibrium values of electrode potential. If two metals are immersed in an electrolyte and are connected by an electrical conductor, an electric couple is formed. The metal that gives up the electrons and ionizes is called the *anode*.

Hydrogen is used as the standard electrode to which other metals are compared. It is given a value of zero **(Table 2.4)**. Similarly different metals have different electrode potential (V) measured in volts or millivolts based on different electronic structure. If the electrode potential of the metal is more positive, it has less tendency to corrode whereas if a metal has electrode potential in negative it shows greater tendency to corrode. For e.g. Noble metals have very high electrode potential because its outer valence orbit has eight electrons which are stable and do not easily lose or gain electrons. Due to this they are highly resistant to corrosion.

## Types of Electrolytic Corrosion

### Galvanic Corrosion

This type of corrosion occurs when two dissimilar metals are in direct physical contact with each other.

For example, when gold restoration comes in contact with an amalgam restoration in the mouth, saliva on both restorations act as electrolyte and the difference in potential between the two restorations causes sudden short circuit resulting in a sharp pain. This sharp pain experienced by the patient is called as *galvanic shock*. If a restoration is coated with a varnish it can eliminate galvanic shock **(Fig. 2.15)**.

An electric circuit exists even when the teeth with dissimilar restorations are not in contact due to the difference in electrical potential or EMF. The current generated is less in intensity as compared to when the

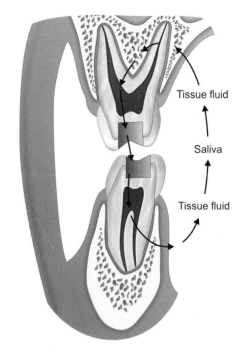

**Fig. 2.15:** Galvanic shock.

teeth are in direct physical contact. The saliva acts as an electrolyte and the hard and soft tissues constitute the external circuit.

A current can also exist in single isolated metallic restorations because of difference in electrical potential between two electrolytes namely, saliva and the tissue fluids. The tissue fluids include the dentinal fluids, soft tissue fluid, or blood which help in completing the external circuit. This current generated is of much lesser intensity than that with contacting dissimilar metallic restorations. The magnitude of this current reduces with time as the restoration becomes older but can remain indefinitely.

## Heterogeneous Compositions

This type of corrosion is based on heterogeneous composition of the surfaces of the dental alloy.

Example of this type is eutectic and peritectic alloys. When an alloy containing eutectic is immersed in an electrolyte the metallic grains with the lower potential are attacked and corrosion results.

*Cored structures* are more susceptible to corrosion than homogenized structure. This is due to difference in composition between different elements having different electrode potential. Although even homogenized structure is susceptible to corrosion because of the difference in structure between the grains and their boundaries.

In metal or alloy, the grain boundaries may act as anodes and the interior of the grain as the cathode. Impurities in any alloy enhance corrosion.

- Corrosion resistance of multiphase alloys is generally less than that of a single phase solid solution because when two phase alloy is immersed in an electrolyte, the lamellae with lower electrode potential acts as anode and corrodes
- Impurities in alloys increase corrosion and they are typically segregated at the grain boundaries
- In single phase solid solution any core structure has less corrosion resistance than homogenized solid solution because of the difference in electrode potential
- In homogenized solid solution the grain boundaries are susceptible to corrosion because these grain boundaries acts as anode and the grain interiors acts as cathode
- Solder joints between the dental alloy can corrode due to difference in composition of the alloy and the solder
- Pure metals corrodes at much slower rates than the alloys because they do not contain any significant quantity of impurities.

## Stress Corrosion

A metal which has been stressed by cold working becomes more reactive at the site of maximum stress. If stressed and unstressed metal are in contact in an electrolyte, the stressed metal will become the anode of a galvanic cell and will corrode.

## Concentration Cell Corrosion

*Crevice corrosion* occurs whenever there is variation in the electrolytes or in the composition of the given electrolytes within the system.

Differences in oxygen tension in between parts of the same restoration cause corrosion of the restoration. Greater corrosion occurs in the part of the restoration having lower concentration of oxygen.

## Protection Against Corrosion

### Passivation

It is a process by which the surface of the metal or alloy are treated to produce a thin stable inert oxide layer thus, making it corrosion resistant. This process is also called as *passive corrosion conditioning*.

### Methods of Passivation

- Electroplating surface of iron, steel and other alloys with chromium to form a passivating layer of chromium oxide. However, chromium coated metal structure are susceptible for pitting and stress corrosion. Patients should be instructed not to use bleaching agents or other abrasives to clean partial dentures
- Increasing the noble metal content increases the resistance to corrosion because their EMF is positive with regard to any common reduction reactions found in the oral cavity
- Polishing metallic restoration to high luster reduces corrosion.
  Dissimilar metal restoration should be avoided
- Use of high mercury containing alloy should be avoided
- Titanium and its alloys produces a passivating layer of titanium oxide which makes it highly biocompatible and corrosion resistant. However corrosion can occur due to formation of corrosion products at the implant abutment interface or within implant body. This can lead to eventual failure because of stress corrosion and microorganisms such as bacteria.

## MECHANICAL PROPERTIES

Mechanical properties are those properties that measure the resistance of the material to deformation or fracture under an applied load. These properties are expressed in units of stress and strain. They are important to understand and predict the behavior of the material under applied load.

### Stress

*Stress can be defined as force acting per unit area within a body subjected to external pressure or force.*

If an external force is applied to a body, an internal force equal in magnitude but opposite in direction is set-up in the body. The stress produced in the body is equal to the applied force divided by the area over which it acts.

For example, if a wire of $0.000002$ $m^2$ is stretched with 200 N force. Then the stress will be *Stress = Force/Area =* $200/0.000002$.

The unit of stress is 'Pascal'. Depending on the nature of the applied stress and the shape of the object, stresses are of three types namely, tensile, compressive and shear.

### Strain

It is the change in length $(\Delta l)$ per unit original length $(L_o)$.

Strain $(\varepsilon) = \Delta l/L_o$

The application of an external force to a body results in a change in dimension of that body.

If the wire is 0.1 m long, and if it stretches to 0.001 m under the load, the strain $(\varepsilon)$ will be:

$\varepsilon = \Delta l/l_o = 0.001$ m$/0.1$ m $= 0.0001$ m/m
$= 0.0001 = 0.01\%$.

## Types of Strain (Fig. 2.16)

### Elastic Strain

*It is reversible type of strain in which the object fully recovers its original shape when the applied force is removed.*

### Plastic Strain

*It is an irreversible type of strain in which object undergoes plastic deformation and it does not recovers its original shape when the force is removed.*

## Types of Stress (Fig. 2.17)

- *Tensile stress*: The tensile (pulling type) force produces tensile stress. This type of force tends to pull the object from both sides. It is associated with tensile strain.
  For example, a sticky candy is used to remove a crown when the patient is asked to open the mouth with the help of tensile stress (**Fig. 2.18**).
- *Compressive stress:* Compressive type of force produces compressive stress. This type of force tends to push the object from both sides or shortens it. Compressive stress is accompanied by compressive strain.
- *Shear stress:* Shear type of force tends to slide the top portion of the object over the bottom portion. The internal resistance to such force is called as shear stress. This type of stress is also always accompanied with shear strain.
  For example, orthodontic bracket is removed from the tooth enamel by applying force along the surface of enamel by a sharp instrument to initiate shear stress failure (**Fig. 2.19**).

- *Flexural (bending) stress:* This type of stress can produce all the three types of stresses in a structure. In a flexural stress mostly the structure fractures. The tensile and compressive stresses are the principal axial stresses whereas as shear stress is combination of tensile and compressive components. It is, however, the tensile stress component which causes fracture of the material.

*Flexural stresses can be produced in the following situations:*
- By subjecting a structure such as a fixed partial denture to three point loading, whereby the end points are fixed and a force is applied between these end points.
- By subjecting a cantilevered bridge that is supported at one end only with a load at the unsupported portion.
- When a patient bites into an object say an apple, forces are applied at an angle to the long-axis of the anterior teeth thereby creating flexural stresses within the teeth.

### Stress-Strain Relationship

Stress and strain are closely related and may be seen as an example of *cause and effect.*

A plot of the corresponding values of stress and strain is referred to as a *stress-strain curve.* Such a curve may be obtained in compression, tension, or shear.

For example, stress-strain curve for stainless steel orthodontic wire (**Fig. 2.20**).

The *shape and magnitude* of the *stress-strain curve* are important in the selection of dental materials.

### Proportional Limit

It is the greatest stress that a material will sustain without deviating from the linear proportionality of stress to strain.

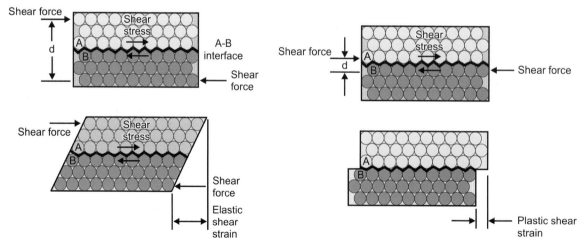

**Fig. 2.16:** Diagram to illustrate types of strain on application of force.

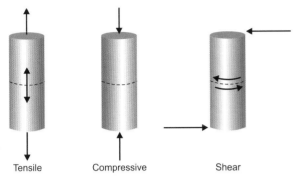

**Fig. 2.17:** Types of stresses.

Tensile    Compressive    Shear

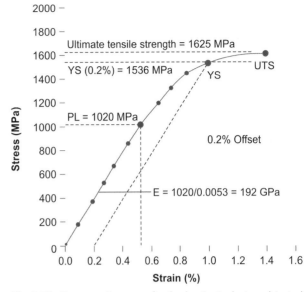

**Fig. 2.20:** Stress-strain curve of orthodontic steel wire subjected under tension.

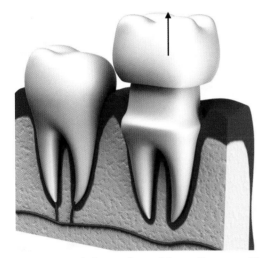

**Fig. 2.18:** Removal of crown by applying pulling type of force (Tensile stress).

Till the proportional limit, the material will obey the Hooke's law, i.e. the elastic stress is directly proportional to the elastic strain. On a stress-strain graph it appears as a straight line. If a material is stressed to a value below the proportional limit it will show reversible or elastic strain. On removal of this stress the material will return to its original shape. Likewise if a material is stressed beyond the proportional limit it will show plastic strain represented by a nonlinear curve on the stress- strain graph **(Fig. 2.21)**.

### Elastic Limit

*It is the maximum stress that a material can withstand without permanent deformation.*

It describes the elastic behavior of the material. Although the term elastic limit can be used interchangeably with the proportional limit as they describe the same stress.

### Elastic Modulus

*It refers to the relative rigidity or stiffness of a material.* It is measured by the slope of elastic region of the stress-strain graph. It has a constant value which is represented by the ratio of elastic stress to the elastic strain. For a given stress if the strain is less, then the elastic modulus is higher. It is expressed in units of force per unit area, i.e. $GN/m^2$ (giganewtons per square meter) or GPa (gigapascals).

Elastic modulus of the tensile test specimen is calculated as:

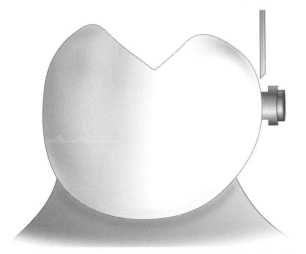

**Fig. 2.19:** Debonding of orthodontic bracket by applying shear force.

$$E = \frac{Stress}{Strain} = \frac{P/A}{\Delta l/l_o}$$

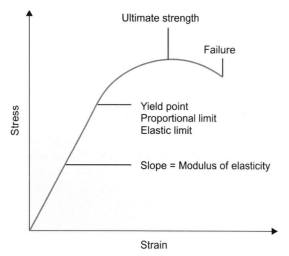

**Fig. 2.21:** Stress-strain diagram.

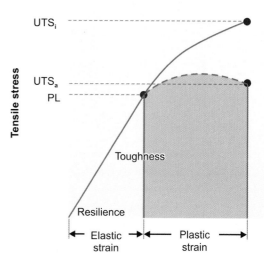

**Fig. 2.23:** Diagram to show resilience and toughness in a stress-strain graph.

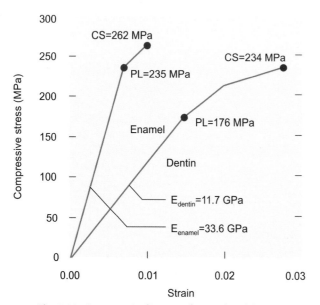

**Fig. 2.22:** Stress-strain diagram of enamel and dentin.

For example, among the elastomeric impression material, polyether impression material has the highest rigidity or elastic modulus.

Elastic modulus of dental enamel is three times more than that of dentin. Enamel is more brittle and stiff whereas dentin is more flexible and tougher **(Fig. 2.22)**.

Orthodontic wire with greater elastic modulus will be more difficult to bend than wire of same thickness and size of lower elastic modulus.

### Flexibility

*Flexibility is defined as the flexural strain which occurs when the material is stressed to its proportional limit.*

For example, an impression material should have high flexibility so that they can be removed easily from the severe undercuts.

### Resilience

The internal energy of material is increased if the interatomic distance between the atoms is increased. If the stress applied is within the proportional limit then this energy is called as *resilience*. The term resilience is associated with 'springiness'. It refers to the amount of energy absorbed when an object is stressed to its proportional limit.

In the **Figure 2.23**, the area measuring the elastic region is referred as resilience whereas the total area measuring the elastic and plastic strains denotes the toughness of an object.

For example, elastomeric impression material, resilient liners.

---

**CLINICAL SIGNIFICANCE**

- During orthodontic treatment, the movement of teeth is brought about by the energy stored in the wire which is released slowly. The energy stored and released subsequently indicates the potential springiness of the wire
- Denture liners are resilient materials which are applied on the hard denture base. These materials are capable of absorbing considerable energy without being permanently distorted
- Elastomeric impression material should not be poured immediately because it has high value of resilience.

## Poisson's Ratio

*Poisson's ratio is a ratio between the lateral and axial strain within the elastic limit.* It is required to monitor the way in which the stress changes with the alterations in specimen shape. It will give the ratio between strain occurring at 90° to the direction of the applied force and strain occurring in the direction of force.

The strain may be recoverable, non-recoverable, and partially recoverable or the recovery may be time-dependent. The extent of recovery and/or rate of recovery is a function of the *elastic properties of the material.*

When a material is subjected to axial loading in tension or compression, there is simultaneous generation of axial and lateral strain. Under tensile loading, the material elongates with the reduction in diameter or cross-section of the material, likewise under compressive loading the material shortens and there is increase in diameter or cross section of the material.

The Poisson's ratio of material represents that under say tensile loading the reduction in cross section of the material will be proportional to the elongation of the material in the elastic range. This process will continue till the material fractures in tension.

Poisson's ratio of most of the dental materials is around 0.3.

## Strength Properties

### Yield Strength

It is also called as *proof stress. It is the amount of stress at which an object exhibits a specific amount of plastic strain.*

It is used in cases where it is not possible to determine proportional limit with accuracy.

Yield strength or proof stress is often a stress at which a small amount of plastic strain in the range of 0.1–0.2% occurs. This small value of plastic strain of 0.1% or 0.2% is called as *percent offset.* The value of yield strength for 0.2% offset is greater than that of 0.1%.

Likewise if yield strengths of two materials are to be compared using similar conditions then same offset should be applied to get true values. In case of brittle materials, there is no plastic strain and therefore, determining yield strength for such materials at 0.1% or 0.2% offset will not be possible. It should be noted that the value of yield strength is always more than the proportional limit. This property is important in evaluating a material as it gives the stress at which permanent deformation of material begins. If the force of mastication is more than this stress then material will fracture and may not produce the desired results.

### Toughness

*It is the internal ability of an object to withstand stresses and strains without fracturing or breaking.*

In other words, it is the total amount of elastic and plastic deformation energy which is required to fracture or break an object. The *total area* under stress-strain graph gives an indication of toughness. Many prostheses are subjected to *intermittent stresses* over a long period of time. This results in formation of a microcrack, possibly due to stress concentration at the surface of the prosthesis. This crack slowly propagates until fracture occurs.

### Fatigue Strength

When an object is subjected to repeated stress over a period of time, it leads to initiation of crack and subsequently to propagation of crack until a sudden, unexpected fracture occurs. This type of fracture occurs because of fatigue. *The internal resistance of the material to such a fracture is called fatigue strength.*

The fracture of the material due to fatigue is called fatigue failure. This property is one of the most important properties which predicts clinical longevity of the material. Fatigue in materials can be prevented by proper designing and selection of appropriate material.

### Impact Strength

*It is defined as the energy required to fracture a material under an impact force.*

The term *"impact"* denotes the reaction of the stationary object when it collides with the moving object.

*It can be measured by:*
- *Charpy type impact tester*: This type of tester is commonly used to measure the impact strength. It has a pendulum which when released swings down to fracture a rod which is supported at both the ends. The comparison is made between the length of the spring before and after the impact to determine the loss of energy
- *Izod impact tester*: This is another type of tester which is used to determine the impact strength of a material. In this device the object to be tested is clamped vertically at one end and the impact is made near this end.

**CLINICAL SIGNIFICANCE**

- A blow by a fist or an object say during road traffic accident to the lower jaw relates to an impact force
- In an impact situation the external forces and the resulting stresses change rapidly. In such situation the static mechanical property such as proportional limit will not be useful in predicting the amount of deformity
- When a moving object with known amount of kinetic energy collides with stationary object it can either permanently deform this object or it can store the energy of collision in an elastic manner depending on the resilience of that object
- An object with high tensile strength and low elastic modulus is more resistant to impact forces than an object with low tensile strength and high elastic modulus.

The elastic modulus and tensile strengths of some of the dental materials are given below **(Table 2.5)**:

**Table 2.5:** Elastic modulus and tensile strength of dental materials.

| Type of material | Elastic modulus | Tensile strength |
|---|---|---|
| Dental porcelain | 40 GPa | 50–100 MPa |
| Alumina ceramic | 350–418 GPa | 120 MPa |
| Resin based composites | 17 GPa | 30–90 MPa |
| Poly (methamethacrylate) | 3.5 GPa | 60 MPa |
| Dental amalgam | 21 GPa | 27–55 MPa |

*Ultimate Strength*

*The ultimate strength is the maximum stress that the material can withstand before it fractures under tension or compression.*

The ultimate strength is calculated by dividing the maximum load in tension or compression by the original cross–sectional area of the test specimen. It is used in dentistry to determine the thickness or cross-section of the material required to bear the masticatory forces without fracture.

*Fracture Strength*

*Fracture strength or fracture stress is the value of stress at which the material fractures.* Flaws or defects in a material greatly influences the fracture strength of the material. For example, Identical ceramic ingots can have varying strength depending on the amount of flaws (defects) in them.

The fracture strength is inversely proportional to the square root of the flaw depth within the surface.

*Fracture Toughness*

*It is the resistance of brittle materials to the catastrophic propagation of flaws under an applied stress.* It is also called as critical stress intensity.

It is represented by $K_{Ic}$ in units of stress times the square root of crack length or $MPa \cdot m^{1/2}$ or $MN \cdot m^{-3/2}$.

**Brittleness**

The materials which are brittle, fractures at or below the proportional limit, i.e. such materials are unable to sustain any plastic strain. For example, ceramics, amalgam, gypsum material, composites, cements and some base metal alloys **(Fig. 2.24)**. The failure of these materials are usually attributed to the presence of flaws and low tensile strengths.

*Brittleness of the material is relative inability of the material to sustain plastic deformation before fracture of material occurs.* These materials in short fractures at or near proportional limit, i.e. they have little or no sustainability of plastic strain.

**CLINICAL SIGNIFICANCE**

- Brittle materials are not weak materials as most of the dental restorative materials are brittle in nature. For example, Zirconia crowns have high tensile strength but 0% elongation. A cobalt chromium partial denture have tensile strength of 870 MPa but percent elongation of only 1.5%
- Since brittle materials such as amalgam, composites, ceramics have very low or no ductility (0% elongation potential) they have very low burnishability.

**Young's Modulus**

*Modulus of elasticity (Young's modulus or elastic modulus) represents stiffness or rigidity of the material within the elastic range.* Elastic modulus represents the ratio of the

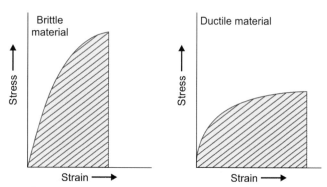

**Fig. 2.24:** Stress-strain curve for brittle and ductile materials.

elastic stress to the elastic strain. It follows, that the lower the strain for a given stress, the greater the value of the modulus.

Modulus of elasticity (E) = Stress ($\sigma$)/Strain ($\varepsilon$).

Elastic modulus is measured in MPa or GPa. It is dependent on the composition of the material.

On a stress-strain curve, the linear region of the curve determines the elastic modulus. A *steep* slope, giving a high modulus value, indicates a *rigid material*, whilst a *shallow* slope, giving a low modulus value, indicates *flexible* material.

Elastic modulus of enamel is much higher than dentin. As enamel has greater rigidity, it is more brittle than dentin which is more flexible and tougher. Because of its greater resilience dentin is capable of withstanding greater plastic deformation under compressive loading **(Table 2.6)**.

For example, if wire (a) of same shape and size as wire (b) is more difficult to bend then the other wire. Then wire (a) has greater modulus of elasticity than wire (b).

Since elastic modulus is constant it is therefore independent of the amount of elastic or plastic stress induced in a material. Also, it is independent of the ductility or strength of a material as it is measured in the straight line of stress-strain plot. A material with high modulus of elasticity can have high or low strength value. The value of modulus of elasticity can be measured by both compression as well as tensile tests.

### Dynamic Young's Modulus

There are two methods of measuring elastic modulus, i.e. static and dynamic. In the dynamic method the velocity of sound travelling through solid is measured by ultrasonic longitudinal and transverse wave trasducers and receivers. Velocity of sound and density of material helps in determining the dynamic elastic modulus and Poisson's ratio of the material. The values obtained from this method are slightly higher than those obtained from static methods but are acceptable.

**Table 2.6:** Elastic modulus of certain dental materials.

| Dental material | Elastic modulus (GPa) |
|---|---|
| Co- Cr alloy | 218 |
| Tooth enamel | 84 |
| Feldspathic porcelain | 69 |
| Dental amalgam | 28 |
| Tooth dentin | 18 |
| Composite resin | 16 |
| Acrylic denture base resins | 2.65 |

A shear modulus (G) of a material is calculated when a material is subjected to shear stress and is accompanied by shear strain. The shear modulus is calculated by formula –
$$G = E/\ 2\ (1 + \nu) = E/2\ (1 + 0.3) = 0.38E$$

### Ductility

*It is the ability of the material to sustain a large permanent deformation under a tensile load before it fractures.*

Ductility of a material is its ability to be drawn into wire under tensile load. It represents the workability of the material in the mouth. The ease of burnishability of the margins of the casting is represented by ductility of the casting alloy, e.g. a metal is considered as ductile if it is readily drawn into long thin wires.

Gold is the most ductile material followed by silver, platinum, iron, nickel, copper, aluminum, zinc and tin.

### Measurement of Ductility

*Methods of measuring ductility of a material are as follows*:
- Percent elongation after fracture
- Reduction in area of tensile test specimens
- Maximum number of bends performed in a cold bend test.

### Percent Elongation after Fracture

Among them the most common method used to determine ductility is a method in which the length of the wire is compared between the increased length under tension after fracture to that of original length before fracture. For this two marks are made on the wire and the measured distance is called as *gauge length*. This gauge length is usually 51mm. This length of wire is pulled under tensile load till it fracture. After fracture, both the fractured ends are joined and the gauge length is again measured. The ratio of increased length after fracture to the original gauge length is measured as *percent elongation* of that material. The value gives the quantitative value of ductility of the material.

### Reduction in Area of Tensile Test Dpecimens

In this method reduction in cross-sectional area of the metal wire under tensile load until it is fractured to that of the original cross-sectional area of the wire is helpful in determining the ductility of the wire.

### Maximum Number of Bends in Cold Bend Test

In this method the testing specimen (wire) is clamped in a vise and is bent around the mandrel of a specific radius. The wire is bent around the mandrel until it fractures. Greater the number of bend more is the ductility of a material. The first bend is made at 90° from vertical to horizontal and then subsequently 180° bends are given.

## Malleability

*It is the ability of a material to withstand permanent deformation without rupturing under compression such as hammering or rolling into thin sheets.*

The property of malleability increases with rise of temperature.

The most ductile and malleable metal is gold which is followed by silver. Following gold and silver, platinum is most ductile and copper is most malleable material.

Both ductility and malleability of the material reduces by increasing the *slip resistance.*

*Methods to increase slip resistance are:*
- Work hardening
- Age hardening heat treatment
- Precipitation heat treatment
- Solution hardening.

### CLINICAL SIGNIFICANCE
- Marginal adaptation of the restorations is improved by increasing the ductility and malleability of the material
- Since gold is the most ductile and malleable metal in pure form. Direct filling gold in form of gold foil can be used as restorative material in very thin sections to allow excellent compaction
- Thin platinum foils are used for fabricating porcelain jacket crowns
- Orthodontic wires are manufactured from cast ingots into wires of varying thickness
- Thin tin foils are used as separating medium in the denture fabrication procedure.

## Hardness

*Resistance offered by the surface of a material to scratching, abrasion, indentation or penetrations.*

The value of hardness is often referred to as the hardness number, depending on the method used for the evaluation. High values of hardness number indicate a hard material and vice versa. Hardness of a material can influence compressive strength, proportional limit and ductility of a material.

There are various surface hardness tests which are useful in understanding the utility of the material. Most of these hardness tests measure the material surface's ability to resist indentation or penetration by an object such as diamond point or steel under a specified load.

### Classification of Hardness Tests

- Macrohardness test—Brinell and Rockwell test: Macrohardness tests employ loads much greater than 9.8 N to determine the hardness of the material
- Microhardness test—Knoop and Vickers test: Microhardness test employ load less than 9.8 N to produce indentations to a depth of less than 19 µm.

### Methods of Measuring Surface Hardness

- *Mohs scratch test*
- *Indentation methods*
  - Brinell hardness test
  - Rockwell hardness test
  - Vickers hardness test
  - Knoop hardness test
- *Penetration*: Penetration methods: shore A and Barcol test.

#### Mohs Scratch Tests

In this test, hardness of various *raw metals* is compared by scratching one metal by another. This method is inaccurate and could not be used for many dental materials.

#### Indentation Methods

- *Brinell hardness test*: This is one of the earliest tests used to measure the hardness of the metal. This test was introduced by JA Brinell, a Swedish engineer in 1900. The indenter in this test is in the form of hardened steel ball of diameter 1.6 mm which is used to penetrate the surface of the material to be tested with a force of 123 N for 30 seconds. The diameter of the indentation is measured after removing the indenter. This diameter of the indentation measures the hardness of the material **(Fig. 2.25)**.
  - *Hardness value:* The specified load is divided by the area of the indentation. The quotient gives the

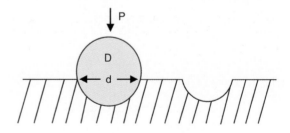

**Fig. 2.25:** Brinell hardness testing.

Brinell hardness number (BHN). The unit of BHN is kg/mm$^2$. Larger the indentation, smaller the number and softer the material likewise for harder materials smaller will be the indentation and larger will be the number. Brinell hardness number for certain dental casting alloys are given below in **Table 2.7**.

**Table 2.7:** Brinell hardness number for different casting alloys.

| Material | BHN (kg/mm²) |
| --- | --- |
| Direct filling gold | 46–69 |
| Type I gold alloy | 45 |
| Type II gold alloy | 95 |
| Type III gold alloy | 120 |
| Type IV gold alloy | 220 |
| Au–Ag–Cu alloy | 252 |

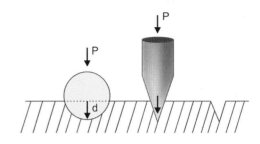

**Fig. 2.26:** Rockwell hardness testing.

- *Uses:*
    ◊ To determine hardness of the metals and dental casting alloys
    ◊ It is related to proportional limit and ultimate tensile strength of dental gold alloys
    ◊ Because of its simplicity it is used as index of properties involving more complex methods
    ◊ This method cannot be used for *Brittle materials* like ceramics, gypsum products.

- *Rockwell's hardness test*: It was developed by *Stanley P. Rockwell,* as the rapid method for determining hardness of the material. This type of test is similar to the Brinell test where a conical diamond point or steel ball is used as an indenter. In this test, depth of penetration rather than the diameter is measured by a dial gauge on the instrument. The indenter cones or balls are available in different diameters with different load applications. A superficial Rockwell method is used to test plastic material in dentistry.

This method uses a large diameter ball (12.7 mm) with a load of 30 kg for 10 minutes before measuring the depth of penetration. The test is done first by applying a preload of 3 kg **(Fig. 2.26)**.

- *Uses:* It is used to determine hardness of viscoelastic materials.
- *Advantages:*
    ◊ Hardness value obtained directly
    ◊ Simple to use.
- *Disadvantages:*
    ◊ Preload is required
    ◊ Greater time is needed

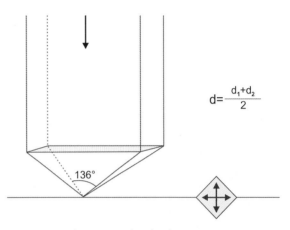

**Fig. 2.27:** Vickers hardness testing.

◊ Indentation may disappear immediately after removal of load.

- *Vickers hardness test*: This test was devised in the United Kingdom in 1925 and was formally called as Diamond pyramid hardness test. The method of indentation resembles the Brinell test except the indenter used is in the shape of square pyramid diamond. The Vickers hardness number (VHN) is calculated by dividing load with the area of indentation. The measurement is based on values of the lengths of diagonal (sides of the diamond) of the indenter after taking an average **(Fig. 2.27)**.
- *Uses*
    ◊ Used to measure the hardness of brittle material
    ◊ Hardness of dental casting gold
    ◊ Hardness of tooth structure.

To compare the *VHN* and *BHN*, the following relationship is used.

$$VHN = 1.05 \times BHN$$

*VHN* values for some of the materials are given in **Table 2.8**.

**Table 2.8:** Vickers hardness number for different dental materials.

| Material | VHN |
|---|---|
| Tooth enamel | 350 |
| Tooth dentin | 60 |
| Dental amalgam | 120 |
| Dental ceramics | 450 |
| Gold alloys | 55–250 |
| Acrylic resins | 20 |
| Cobalt chromium alloys | 420 |

- *Knoop hardness test (Fig. 2.28):* Knoop hardness test was developed as a microindentation method. The indenter used for this test is a diamond with a pyramidal shape.
  - *Hardness value:* A desired load is applied at the diamond indenting tool and the length of the diagonal of the resulting indentation is measured. The length of the largest diagonal is measured. Once the indentation is made and the indenter is removed, there is elastic recovery of the projected impression along the shorter diagonal. Knoop hardness number (KHN) is measured as the ratio of the load applied to the area of the indentation. The units for KHN is kg/mm$^2$ **(Fig. 2.29)**.
  - *Advantages:*
    ◊ Wide range of materials can be tested for hardness by varying the load
    ◊ Can be used with very light load application.
  - *Disadvantages:*
    ◊ Highly polished and flat test specimens are required
    ◊ Greater time needed to test the specimen.
  - *Uses:* Both soft and hard materials can be tested by this method.

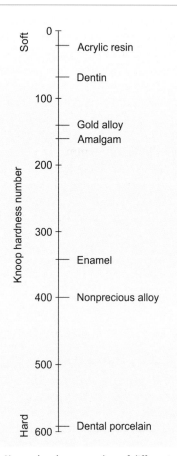

**Fig. 2.29:** Knoop hardness number of different materials.

  - *Hardness number:* It is a spring-loaded needle with a diameter of 1 mm that is pressed against the surface to be tested. If the needle does not at all press into the surface than the reading of Barcol tester is 100. As the indenter penetrated into the surface the reading of the scale is decreased.

Knoop hardness numbers of various dental materials are given in **Table 2.9**.

**Table 2.9:** Knoop hardness numbers of various dental materials

| Materials | KHN |
|---|---|
| Tooth enamel | 343 |
| Tooth dentin | 68 |
| Cementum | 40 |
| Silicon carbide abrasive | 2480 |
| Feldspathic porcelain | 460 |
| Co-Cr partial denture | 391 |
| Denture acrylic | 21 |

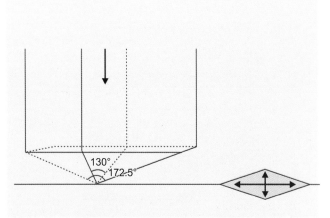

**Fig. 2.28:** Knoop hardness testing.

- *Barcol hardness test:* This test is used to measure the depth of the cure of the resin composites.
  - *Uses:*
    - ◊ Depth of cure of the resin composites
    - ◊ Depth of cure of acrylic denture resin.
- *Shore a hardness test:* This type of tester is used to measure the hardness of rubber and soft plastics. It consists of a blunt indenter of 0.8 mm in diameter which tapers to a cylinder of 1.6 mm.

  If the indenter completely penetrates the specimen than the value obtained on scale is 0 and if it does not penetrate at all then the reading is 100. Since elastomers are viscoelastic in nature an accurate reading is difficult to obtain with this method.

- *Uses:*
  - ◊ To test the hardness of soft denture liners
  - ◊ Maxillofacial elastomers
  - ◊ Elastomeric impression materials
  - ◊ Mouth protectors.

## SUMMARY

Physical and mechanical properties are the backbone of applied dental material science. The failure potential of the dental prosthesis under applied force is related to the physical and mechanical properties of the material used. Thorough knowledge of these properties is useful because it helps us in best understanding and application of the materials in different clinical situations.

## TEST YOURSELF

### Essay Questions

1. Discuss the optical properties which influences shade selection.
2. Define tarnish and corrosion. Discuss wet corrosion in detail.
3. Describe various physical and chemical properties which influences restorative materials.
4. What is flow? Describe importance of wettability in restorative dentistry.
5. Enumerate various mechanical properties. Describe importance of each in dental material science.
6. Differentiate between ductility and malleability.
7. Define hardness. Describe various hardness tests in detail.

### Short Notes

1. Galvanic corrosion.
2. Thixotrophic and pseudoplastic behavior.
3. Creep and its types.
4. Impact strength.
5. Resilience and toughness.
6. Pitting and stress corrosion.
7. Metamerism and fluorescence.
8. Fatigue strength.

### Multiple Choice Questions

1. Modulus of elasticity is defined as:
   A. Stress/strain ratio
   B. Stiffness/sponginess
   C. Force/area
   D. Sponginess/stiffness ratio

2. The most stable primary bonds are:
   A. Have random forms
   B. Have regular crystalline structures
   C. Are amorphous
   D. Have mixed physical structure

3. If a material is permanently deformed it has exceeded:
   A. Ultimate tensile strength
   B. Stiffness
   C. Proportional limit
   D. Toughness

4. Thixotropic gels:
   A. Have poor viscosity
   B. Flow under mechanical forces
   C. Flow at higher temperatures
   D. Flow at lower temperatures

5. Brinnell hardness number (BHN) of dental gold alloy is directly related to:
   A. Tensile strength
   B. Modulus of elasticity
   C. Percent elongation
   D. Resilience

6. The point at which the plastic strain develops:
   A. Elastic limit, modulus of elasticity, breaking strength
   B. Elastic limit, yield strength, proportional limit
   C. Yield strength, breaking strength, toughness
   D. Toughness, rigidity, resiliency

7. In comparison to amorphous material the crystalline materials have:
   A. No space lattice
   B. Less stability
   C. Well-defined melting point
   D. All of the following

8. If a material recovers and do not plastically gets deformed then it has good:
   A. Toughness
   B. Elasticity
   C. Malleability
   D. Ductility

9. Materials used for the restoration of tooth enamel needs high:
   A. Opacity
   B. Chroma
   C. Vitality
   D. Translucency

10. Microleakage can cause:
    A. Recurrent caries
    B. Marginal staining
    C. Postoperative sensitivity
    D. All the above

11. Area under complete stress and strain curve gives:
    A. Modulus of elasticity
    B. Toughness
    C. Resilience
    D. Proportional limit

12. Which of the following uses diamond as the reference material:
    A. Moh's scale
    B. Knoop hardness number
    C. Vicker hardness number
    D. Brinell hardness number

13. Ductility of material is expressed in terms of:
    A. Force per unit area
    B. Percentage elongation
    C. Surface hardness
    D. Stress/strain ratio

14. Marginal gap between composite restorations and tooth could be due to:
    A. Differences in thermal conductivity
    B. Pulpal pressure
    C. Differences in thermal expansion coefficient
    D. Inadequate adhesion

15. When amalgam restoration contacts with gold onlay a galvanic cell is established in which the amalgam:
    A. Oxidizes
    B. Releases metallic ions
    C. Serves as the anode
    D. All of the above

16. Which type of bonding in a material associates with high thermal and electrical conductivities:
    A. Ionic bond
    B. Metallic bond
    C. Covalent bond
    D. van der Waals

17. Elastic modulus of material refers to its:
    A. Hardness
    B. Toughness
    C. Percent elongation
    D. Stiffness

18. The ability of the elastomeric impression material to be removed from the teeth without getting permanently deformed is due to:
    A. Maximum flexibility
    B. Percent elongation
    C. Elastic modulus
    D. Ductility

19. For adherence of pit and fissure sealant to the tooth enamel the surface should be:
    A. Low in surface energy
    B. Wettable
    C. Smooth and non-porous
    D. Covered with saliva

20. Hardness determines the ability of the material to:
    A. Deform
    B. Break
    C. Get easily compressed
    D. Resist wear

## ANSWERS

| | | | |
|---|---|---|---|
| 1. A | 2. B | 3. A | 4. B |
| 5. A | 6. B | 7. C | 8. B |
| 9. D | 10. D | 11. B | 12. A |
| 13. B | 14. C | 15. D | 16. B |
| 17. D | 18. A | 19. B | 20. D |

## BIBLIOGRAPHY

1. Academy of denture prosthetics: Glossary of prosthodontics terms, 8th edn. J Prosthet Dent. 1999;81:41-126.
2. Antonson SA, Anusavice KJ. ContrasT ratio of veneering and core ceramics as a function of thickness. Int J Proshtodont 2001;14:316-20.
3. Anusavice KJ. Phillip's Science of Dental Materials, 11th edition. Elsevier, St Louis, Missouri; 2003. pp. 21-101.
4. Bergman M, Ginstrup O, Nilner K. Potential and polarization measurements in vivo of oral galvanism. Scand J Dent Res. 1978;86:135.
5. Braden M, Clarke RL. Dielectric properties of zinc oxide eugenol type cements. J Dent Res. 1974;53:1263.
6. Braden M, Clark RL. Viscoelastic properties of Elastic impression. J Dent Res. 1972;51:1525-8.
7. Braden M, Wilon AD. Relation between stress relaxation and viscoelastic properties of dental materials. J Dent. 1982;10:181-6.
8. Calamia JR, Wolff MS, Simonsen RJ. Dental clinics of North America: Successful esthetic and Cosmetic dentistry for the Modern Dental Practice, Elsevier Saunders Inc., 2007.

9. Callister WD, Rethwisch DG. Materials Science and Engineering : An Introduction, Hoboken, NJ, 2009, John Wiley & Sons.

10. Chaturvedi TP. An overview of the corrosion aspect of dental implants (Titanium and its Alloys). Ind J Dent Res. 2009;20:91-8.

11. Chu S, Devigus A, Mieleszko A. The Fundamentals of Color: Shade Matching and Communication in Esthetic Dentistry, Carol Stream, IL, 2004, Quintessence.

12. Craig RG, Peyton FA. Thermal conductivity of tooth structure, dental cements and amalgam. J Dent Res. 1961;40:411.

13. Craig RG. Restorative Dental Materials, 8th edition. St Louis: CV Mosby Co.; 1989.

14. Glantz P. On wettability and adhesiveness. Odont Rev. 1969;20:1.

15. Johnston WM, Kao EC. Assessment of appearance by visual observation and clinical colorimetry. J Dent Res. 1989;68:819-22.

16. McCabe JF, Wilson HJ. The use of differential scanning calorimetry for the evaluation of Dental Materials. II. Denture base matErials. J Oral Rehabil. 1980;7:235.

17. McCane JF. Applied Dental Materials, 8th edition. Canada CV Elsevier Science; 2003.

18. Mc Lean JW. The Science and Art of Dental Ceramics. The Nature of Dental Ceramics and their Clinical Use, Vol. 1,CA, 1979, Quintessence.

19. Metathananda IM, Parker S, Patel MP. Relationship between hardness of elastomeric impression material and Young's modulus. Dent Mater. 1996;12:74-82.

20. Meyer JM, Reclaru L. Electro chemical determination of the corrosion resistance of noble casting alloys. J Mater Sci: Mater Med. 1995;6:534-40.

21. Miller LL. Shade matching. J Esthet Dent. 1993;5:143.

22. Mumford JM. Electrolytic action in the mouth and its relationship to pain. J Dent Res. 1957;36:632.

23. O'Brien WJ, Nelson D, Lorey RE. The assessment of chroma sensitivity to porcelain pigments. J Prosthet Dent. 1983;49:63-6.

24. O'Brien WJ. Dental materials and Their Selection, 3rd edn. Quintessence Publishing Co Inc, Carol Stream; 2002.

25. Parker RM. Shade matching for indirect restorations in the esthetic zone. J Cosmet Dent. 2008;23:98-104.

26. Powers JM, Dennison JB, Koran A. Color stability of restorative resins under accelerated aging. J Dent Res. 1978;57:964.

27. Prem P, Filip K, Moustafa MN. Fracture strength and fatigue resistance of dental resin based composites. Dent Mater. 2009;25:956-9.

28. Sarkar NK, Fuys RA Jr, Stanford JW. The chloride corrosion of low gold casting alloys. J Dent Res. 1979;58:568-75.

29. Sturdevant JR, Sturdevant CM, Taylor DF, Bayne SC. The 8 year clinical performance of 15 low gold casting alloys. Dent Mater. 1987;3:347-52.

30. Upadhyay D, Panchal MA, Dbey RS, et al. Corrosion of alloys used in dentistry: A review. Mater Sci Eng A. 2006;432;1-11.

31. Walker RS, Wade AG, Iazzetti G, et al. Galvanic interaction between gold and amalgam: effect of zinc, time and surface treatments. J Am Dent Assoc. 2003;134:1463-7.

32. Yeh CL, Miyagawa Y, Powers JM. Optical properties of composites of selected shades. J Dent Res. 1982;61:797.

33. Yeh CL, Powers JM, Miyagawa Y. Color of selected shades of composites by reflection spectrophotometry. J Dent Res. 1982;61:1176.

34. Yuan JC – C, Brewer JD, Monaco EA, et al. Defining a natural tooth color space based on a 3 dimensional shade system. J Prosthet Dent. 2007;98:110-9.

# Biocompatibility of Dental Materials

## CHAPTER OUTLINE

- Biocompatibility Challenges to Oral and Maxillofacial Materials
- Factors Influencing Biocompatibility of a Material
- Adverse Effects due to Exposure of Dental Materials
- Role of ADA in Biocompatibility Testing
- Measuring of Biocompatibility
- Types of Tests
- Types of Test Programs for Biocompatibility Testing

- Correlation Between In Vitro, Animal and Usage Tests
- Biocompatibility Issues in Dentistry
- Clinical Tips for Using Dental Materials Safely and Effectively
- Guidelines to Minimize Chemical Exposure in the Dental Clinic
- Clinical Tips to Manage Aerosols in Dental Clinic

*'I have not failed. I've just found 10,000 ways that don't work.'*

*—Thomas Edison*

## INTRODUCTION

Since the prehistoric times, human beings have tried to use a number of materials and devices in the oral cavity in order to improve function and esthetics. Initially, healthcare providers experimented with lots of material and devices to repair or replace teeth. But it was realized that some materials were more successful than other materials when used in contact with the oral tissues. Many researchers in dental field found that some of the materials have greater favorable tissue response than other materials. Thus, concept of biocompatibility was studied with greater interest.

## DEFINITION

*Biocompatibility is defined as an ability of the material to elicit an appropriate biological response in a given application in the body.*

According to *Murray* et al (2007), biocompatibility is an ability of a restorative material to induce an appropriate and advantageous host response during its intended clinical usage.

## BIOCOMPATIBILITY CHALLENGES TO ORAL AND MAXILLOFACIAL MATERIALS

The oral environment is complex and varied and provides a challenge to the use of various dental materials. A dental material or device is subjected to exposure to saliva, food items, bacteria and other products. Exposure to environment such as extreme of temperature changes, pH and chemical composition of the food items demands severe requirements of material to perform. The temperature in the oral cavity can vary between 0°C and 90°C which may alter the mechanical properties of the material or subject to thermal expansion which may lead to biocompatibility issues. The pH of the oral cavity can vary depending on the oral status or medical condition of the patient like bulimia or patient with problem of gastric regurgitation or patient with high caries index. Such patient can present with special biocompatibility challenge that is not a normal physiologic condition.

After caries removal when restorative material is placed into the prepared cavity, the chemical components may migrate and cause irritation to the pulp tissues. This can be prevented by proper isolation of the restorative material by using cavity liners.

Biocompatibility depends on the host condition, material properties and where it is used. The interaction between the host and the material should not elicit any harmful effect on the host. The types of possible interactions taking place are:

- Between material and oral tissues
- Between material and pulp through the dentinal tubules
- Between the material and the periodontium, and
- Between the material and the periapical region.

The interaction between the host and the materials is influenced by the properties of material, its duration of use in the mouth, its location, i.e. where it is used and health of the host tissues. When a material is placed or implanted into the host tissues an interface is created which is dynamic in nature and it should be structurally and biologically stable. This stability depends on factors such as shape, size, location, properties, composition, duration and stress created during function of the material. Various international organizations over the world strongly recommend the use of biocompatible materials, which are free of any risks. However, there is no dental material which is absolutely free from potential risks of adverse reaction from the material to the host tissues. *There is a challenge, therefore, to select and use biomaterials whose benefits greatly outweigh the known risks from a material.* There are a number of tests to evaluate the biocompatibility of the dental materials before a recommendation is made for its use clinically. These tests include compositional analysis, surface degradation tests, cell culture tests, clinical testing in animals and finally tested in humans.

## FACTORS INFLUENCING BIOCOMPATIBILITY OF A MATERIAL

The biocompatibility of the material is influenced by following factors:
- Physical and chemical composition of the material
- Type and location of the host tissues
- Duration of exposure
- Surface characteristics of the material.

Consideration of above factors as well as cell biology, patient risk factors, clinical experience and material science, helps in determining the biocompatibility of the material.

Careful evaluation of the benefits and the associated risks of the materials, make biocompatibility a complex topic.

## ADVERSE EFFECTS DUE TO EXPOSURE OF DENTAL MATERIALS

Any material used in the oral cavity is capable of inducing local or systemic effect when in contact with the oral tissues. The effect is dependent on the products or toxins released from that material and the host response. The amount and distribution of the released substance determines the nature, severity and location of these effects.

### Classification of Adverse Effects of Dental Materials

- Systemic toxicity **(Fig. 3.1)**:
- Local toxicity
- Allergic and inflammatory reactions:
  - Cross-reactive allergy
  - Concurrent allergy
- Other reactions:
  - Genotoxicity
  - Mutagenicity
  - Carcinogenicity
  - Teratogenicity

### Systemic Toxicity

It is the type of toxicity in which the signs of adverse reactions appear in an area away or distant from the source of application. The systemic effects depend on the distribution of the released substances from the dental materials.

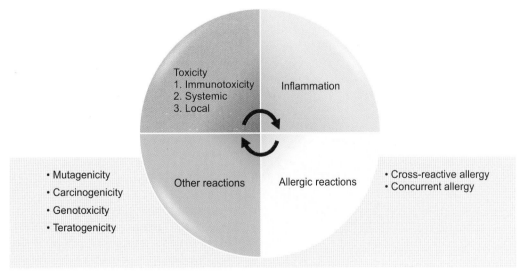

**Fig. 3.1:** Adverse effects of dental materials.

- The systemic effects depend on the following:
  - Concentration of the released substances
  - Duration of exposure
  - Excretion rate of the substance—slower the excretion rate, faster the toxicity reaches the critical level
  - Site of exposure
- The possible routes of entry into the body are through:
  - Inhalation of vapor
  - Ingestion
  - Absorption through oral mucosa
  - Leakage through root apex
- The released toxins are carried from the entry site to the site where it appears through these channels:
  - Diffusion through the tissues
  - Lymphatic vessels
  - Blood vessels.

### Local Toxicity

In such type of toxicity, the response is elicit in the vicinity or at the site of exposure of the material. The local effects of toxicity due to dental materials can occur in the pulpal tissues, in the periodontium, at the root apex or in adjacent tissues such as buccal mucosa **(Fig. 3.2)**.

*The factors influencing the local effects are:*
- Ability of substances to be distributed in these sites
- Duration of exposure
- Intensity or concentration.

### Allergic or Inflammatory Reactions

When a body is exposed to foreign substance, it responds in form of different biological response such as allergic, inflammatory, toxic or mutagenic reactions. Mostly with the exposure of dental materials, two responses are important, i.e. allergic and inflammatory.

The inflammatory response occurs because of the activation of immune system to counter the foreign body. It can occur in response to trauma, allergy or toxicity. It involves infiltration of neutrophils initially followed by action of monocytes and lymphocytic cells in later stage.

An allergic reaction is an abnormal antigen–antibody reaction which occurs to a body which is usually harmless to most individuals. It involves recognition of a substance as foreign and reacts either quickly as in anaphylaxis or slowly as in contact dermatitis. There are four types of allergic reactions according to Gell and Coombs classification of immune responses. The types I, II and III occur quickly and are modulated by antibody producing: eosinophils, mast cells and B lymphocytes, whereas type IV is delayed type reaction which is modulated by monocytes and T cells.

*Rajan* (2002) added another type called type V which is a stimulating–antibody reaction, which is rarely found and can also be subcategorized in type II allergic reaction.

### *Concurrent Allergy*

Concurrent allergy or sensitization occurs when two allergens are present in a material at the same time. In this type both allergens can induce positive response. For example, HEMA (hydroxyethyl methacrylate) and EGDMA (ethylene glycol dimethacrylate) are compounds present in composite resin which are capable of producing concurrent allergy.

---

**Classification of Immune Responses (Gell and Coomb)**

*Types of reactions*
- *Type I:* Immediate atopic or anaphylaxis reaction-mediated by IgE or IgG
- *Type II:* Cytotoxic hypersensitivity reaction
- *Type III:* Immune complex hypersensitivity reaction
- *Type IV:* Delayed type reaction, nodulated by monocytes and T cells.

---

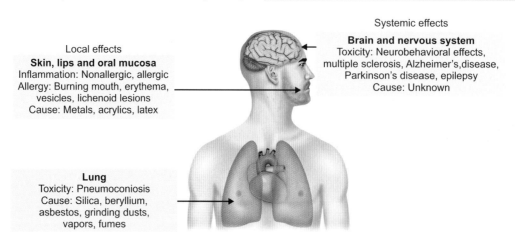

Systemic effects

**Local effects**

**Skin, lips and oral mucosa**
Inflammation: Nonallergic, allergic
Allergy: Burning mouth, erythema, vesicles, lichenoid lesions
Cause: Metals, acrylics, latex

**Brain and nervous system**
Toxicity: Neurobehavioral effects, multiple sclerosis, Alzheimer's, disease, Parkinson's disease, epilepsy
Cause: Unknown

**Lung**
Toxicity: Pneumoconiosis
Cause: Silica, beryllium, asbestos, grinding dusts, vapors, fumes

**Fig. 3.2:** Systemic and local effects due to toxicity of dental materials.

## Cross-reactive Allergy

If an individual is allergic to a particular element, then he is most likely considered to be allergic to other elements which are chemically similar and are present in the same group of periodic table. For example, patient sensitive to Ni (nickel) is most likely also sensitive to Pd (palladium).

## Other Reactions

### Genotoxicity

In genotoxicity, the substances released from the material are capable of altering the genome DNA. Genotoxic effects are reported in beryllium and gallium salts.

### Mutagenicity

It refers to the ability of the material to transfer genetic damage to the next generations of cells. This type of reaction occurs when a physical or chemical agent changes the genetic material of an organism. This genetic material is usually the DNA, i.e. the sequencing of the base pair is changed thereby leading to increased frequency of mutations in an organism. The most common causes of mutations in humans are radiations, chemicals and genetic errors in DNA replication process. In dentistry Be (beryllium), Cu (copper) and Ni (nickel) are known mutagens. Some resins have been identified to have mutagenic potential.

### Carcinogenicity

It refers to ability of the material (carcinogens) to form malignant tumors. There has been no dental material which is shown to be carcinogenic in dental patients.

### Teratogenicity

It refers to ability of some substances to cause malformations during embryonic development.

## ROLE OF ADA IN BIOCOMPATIBILITY TESTING

American Dental Association (ADA) was established in 1930 to evaluate the dental products. In the same year, ADA started the ADA's Seal of Acceptance program to promote safety and effectiveness of dental products. Although, this seal of acceptance was phased out in 2005 and the safety and effectiveness of products were published in Professional Product review. ADA/ANSI developed the specification No. 41 for biological evaluation of dental materials for standard

practices. This specification lays down biological tests for evaluation of dental materials.

In 1976, Medical Device Amendments (MDA) was formed to regulate medical devices and dental devices. It recommended that all medical devices be categorized into three classes according to the risk. Currently, the Dental Devices Branch of the Centre for Devices and Radiological Health regulates premarket clearance of the dental devices **(Table 3.1)**.

## MEASURING OF BIOCOMPATIBILITY

Biocompatibility measurement of the material depends on the actual site of use and the duration of exposure. Historically, newer materials were tried in patient's mouth to determine whether they were biocompatible. But this practice is not accepted for long now and the current materials should be extensively screened for biocompatibility.

In 1970, *Autian* described a structured approach to test biocompatibility of materials. He advocated the following approach:
- *Nonspecific approach* (cell cultures or small laboratory animals): These tests are carried out on materials which are not used clinically
- *Specific approach* (usage test, e.g. in monkeys, rabbits): Unlike the nonspecific tests, these are conducted in specimens that simulate the clinical usage of materials in the oral environment
- *Clinical testing in humans.*

In 1984, *Langeland* advocated another approach to test biocompatibility of materials. This approach was later adopted by ISO Technical Report 7405:
- Initial test (cytotoxicity, mutagenicity)
- Secondary test (sensitization, implantation tests, mucosal irritation)
- Usage tests.

The above mentioned tests are widely used to ensure that the materials used are biologically acceptable. These tests are in vitro, animal and usage tests.

**Table 3.1:** Classification of medical and dental devices based on risk.

| Type of class | About |
|---|---|
| Class I – Low risk | General controls [generally exempt from 510 (k)] |
| Class II – Moderate risk | General controls and specific controls 510 (k) generally required |
| Class III – High risk | General controls and Premarket Approval (PMA) Application (PMA required; must demonstrate safety and effectiveness without relying on a predicate device) |

# TYPES OF TESTS (FIGS. 3.3 AND 3.4)

- In vitro tests
- Animal tests
- Usage tests.

## In Vitro Test

In vitro tests are done in a test tube, cell culture dish or outside of the living organisms. They are used as the *first screening test* to evaluate a new material. The in vitro tests are subdivided into those that measure:

- Cytotoxicity or cell growth
- Metabolic or some cell function
- The effect on the genetic material in the cell (Mutagenesis assays).

In these tests, the materials are placed in contact with the cell, enzyme or an isolated biological system. The contact with these media can be either direct or indirect. In a direct contact, the materials contact the cells directly without using any barrier and in indirect contact barriers such as agar, membrane filter or dentin is used between the material and the cell system. Direct tests can be subdivided into those materials which are physically present in the cell or those materials in which some kind of extracts contact the cell system. For in vitro type of tests, two types of cell are used—*primary cells* and the *continuous cells*. Primary cells are those cells which are directly taken from the animal into the cell culture whereas continuous cells are those cells which are transformed to permit indefinite growth in the cell culture.

## Types of In Vitro Testing *(Table 3.2)*

*Cell culture testing:* This is the most common initial step in evaluating the new material by placing it or its extract into the suitable cell culture by observing any change in the cells over a period of hours or days. These cells are in the form of fibroblasts, macrophages or any other types of cells which are manufactured. The cells are placed into the culture dish or multiwell culture array which are allowed to grow and reproduce in a controlled environment. The samples of the new material or fluid extract are added to the culture and kept in the incubator for 3 days. The cultures are then examined under the microscope and are graded to evaluate its biocompatibility. The results of these tests are evaluated on the basis of the intended use of the new material.

*Direct cell culture:* In such tests, cells like mouse fibroblasts (L-929) or human epithelial cells (HeLa) are directly grown in monolayer in culture plates. A monolayer culture consists of a single, closely packed layer of cells. Then a component of the test specimen is placed directly onto the surface of cells and its toxicity is evaluated usually for short time period, i.e. less than 24 hours.

*Agar diffusion testing:* This type of testing is useful in evaluating the cytotoxicity of leachable component of the test specimen. Here also monolayer cell cultures are used which are stained with neutral red vital stain dye. Over these cells, a layer of agar is placed on which material to be tested is placed. This assembly is then incubated for 24 hours. The loss of dye within the cells indicates the presence of leachable toxic substance.

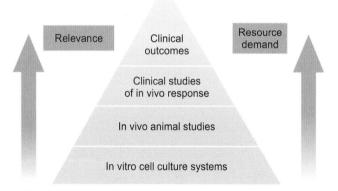

**Fig. 3.3:** Hierarchical representation of biocompatibility testing.

| Table 3.2: Different types of in vitro tests used in testing biocompatibility of the material. | |
|---|---|
| *Type of reaction* | *In vitro tests* |
| Systemic reactions | Direct cell culture |
| Local reactions | • Direct cell culture<br>• Dentin barrier testing<br>• Filter diffusion testing<br>• Agar diffusion testing |
| Allergic reactions | • Cell culture models are developed |
| Other reactions | • Ames test<br>• Micronucleus test |

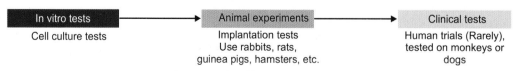

**Fig. 3.4:** Order of biocompatibility test.

*Dentin barrier testing:* A type of testing which simulates oral conditions by placing bovine dentin disc between pulpal fibroblasts and the test specimen. Cultures are kept vital for several weeks by permanently perfusing with the growth medium. This type of test is useful in identifying specific components which could be responsible for pulpal effects by crossing through dentin. It is also helpful in identifying compounds that suppress or intensify the cytotoxic effect of a substance by increasing or reducing permeability in dentin.

*Filter diffusion testing:* This type of test uses a cellulose acetate filter having pores of 0.45 µm dimension. On one side of the filter, cells are cultured, whereas on the opposite side of filter test, specimen is placed. Any leachable material in the test specimen should pass through the pores to have cytotoxicity effect on the cells. The amount and frequency of release is noted to classify the cytotoxic effect on the test specimen.

*Mutagenicity test:* Any new material is tested to rule out the possibility of causing neoplastic changes in the cells on long-term exposure. As newer materials are developed with different formulations, this type of testing is important. It is done to evaluate any changes in the cells and the cellular DNA in the forward or reverse directions. In the *forward mutation studies*, normal cells are exposed to the new material and the resultant cells are tested for any signs of mutation. Detection of changes in even small numbers of cells can lead to false results and, therefore, reverse mutation testing is frequently used. In a *reverse mutation studies*, the studies are performed on abnormal cells in the presence or absence of vital chemical, if growth occurs without the presence of chemical then DNA is repaired because of the exposure to new material. Changes in the cellular DNA in either reverse or forward direction indicate the mutagenic potential of the material. The most common short-term mutagenesis test is the *Ames test.* Other in vitro mutagenesis tests are sister chromatid exchange test (SCE), mouse lymphoma assay test (MOLY) and chromosome aberrations test (ABS).

*Advantages of In Vitro Tests*
- Relatively quick to use
- Inexpensive
- Can be standardized easily
- Suitable for large scale screening
- Has good experimental control.

*Disadvantages of In Vitro Tests*
- Questionable relevance
- Lack of inflammatory or tissue protective mechanisms
- Cannot be used to predict overall biocompatibility of the material.

## Animal Test

In this type of test, new material is placed into an intact organism such as mice, rats, ferrets, guinea pigs or hamsters. Other types of animals which can be used are monkeys, rabbits, pigs, cats or dogs. Animal tests usually differ from usage tests as the material is not directly exposed in the animal with regard to its final use. The animal test provides with a number of complex interactions between the material and the functioning biological system. This type of testing is more comprehensive and relevant as compared to the *in vitro* testing. There are a number of types of animal tests which are used for assessing the biocompatibility of the material, i.e. mucous membrane irritation test, skin sensitization test, implantation test and mutagenicity test **(Table 3.3)**.

### $LD_{50}$ Median Lethal Dose

This dose consists of chemical substance which is capable of killing 50% of experimental animals. Prior to 1980s, it was used as standard procedure to determine acute toxicity in a material, but thereafter it is no more in use because of ethical and legal issues.

### Limit Test

In this type of test, the experimental animal is administered with fixed and calibrated dose (e.g. 3 g of material/kg body weight). The experimental animals are observed for period of two weeks for any signs of toxicity. If no animal dies because of the dose, then further tests are not done and this dose is considered as upper limit for the amount of material to be administered. If any animal dies during the observation period, then a lower dose is administered in next set of animals and results are evaluated as described above.

### Implantation Test

In such test, the material to be tested is implanted in the experimental animal either intramuscularly,

**Table 3.3:** Types of animal tests.

| Type of reaction | Animal tests |
| --- | --- |
| Systemic reactions | • $LD_{50}$<br>• Limit test |
| Local reactions | Implantation tests |
| Allergic reactions | • Maximization test<br>• Buehler test |
| Other reactions | Micronucleus test |

subcutaneously or in the bone. The adjacent tissues to the implanted site are evaluated macroscopically and microscopically for any adverse reaction. The evaluation is done at different time intervals varying from one week to several months.

### Maximization Test

In this type of test, a material to be tested is injected intradermally along with an immunopotentiator such as Freund's complete adjuvants (FCA) for a period of one week. After this, the test material is applied topically to the same site for 2 days in order to amplify the immunological effect by Freund's complete adjuvants to increase the sensitivity of the test. Again after two weeks, the test material is applied to a different site on the body to assess the skin reaction after appropriate exposure time.

### Buehler Test

This test is less sensitive than the maximization tests as FCA is not injected intradermally along with the test material. It is considered more protected to the animals than the maximization test.

### Micronucleus Test

This test is considered as one of the most reliable test to determine genotoxic carcinogens. It is particularly carried out on bone marrow of rats (rodent) or in their peripheral blood.

### Advantages of Animal Tests

- Provides intact biological system
- Permits complex systemic interactions
- Provides more comprehensive response as compared to in vitro tests
- Are more relevant than in vitro tests.

### Disadvantages of Animal Tests

- Expensive
- Difficult to control
- Time consuming
- Ethical issues
- Relevance of the tests are questionable
- Difficult to interpret and quantify.

## Usage Test

These tests are done in animals or in human beings. This test requires the material to be placed in an environment which is clinically relevant to the final use of the material. If this test is done in humans it is referred to as *clinical trials*. The animals which can be used for usage tests are those that resembles more closely to the humans such as dogs or monkeys. The relevance of this test is very high as it can test the biocompatibility of the material in every regard, including the exposure time, location, environment or technique of placement. The human clinical trials are often referred to as *gold standard* of tests as biocompatibility is best judged by these tests. However, the ultimate relevance of the usage test depends on the quality with which the test simulates the clinical situation in terms of time, location, area or environment **(Table 3.4)**.

### Pulp/Dentin Test

Any material used in the proximity to pulp needs to have compatibility to the vital tissue (pulp). The material to be tested is either placed in the teeth of experimental animals or in human teeth which are extracted for orthodontic reason. In the human teeth, class V cavity is prepared as atraumatically as possible and the test material is filled. After period of few days, weeks or months, the teeth are extracted and prepared histologically to microscopically study the signs of acute or chronic inflammation.

### Endodontic Usage Test

In this type of test the material to be tested is placed in the root canals after doing endodontic treatment in experimental animals. The biocompatibility of the material is evaluated by histologically studying the apical tissues.

### Intraosseous Implant Test

Such test involves the material to be tested for dental implant is inserted into the jaws of the experimental animal. Histological evaluation of the tissues in contact with the implant surface is done.

### Clinical Trials

This test is the Gold standard of testing biocompatibility of a material as the material is directly tested in human beings. But any material cannot be directly tested in humans because of legal and ethical issues. The material to be tested

| Table 3.4: Different types of usage tests. | |
|---|---|
| Type of reaction | Usage tests |
| Local reaction | • Pulp/dentin test<br>• Endodontic test<br>• Intraosseous implant test |

should first clear the in vitro tests, animal test and usage test (in animals) before trying in human subjects. The Food and Drug Administration (FDA) clearance is necessary before any trial in human beings.

A test material should first clear the in vitro and animal tests then an IND (Investigational New Drug) application (Notice of claimed investigational exemption for new drug) is submitted to the FDA for approval. The IND should include the following points:

- Novelty of the test material or drug, its composition and the manufacture
- All results of in vitro and animal tests conducted using the test material
- Application of the proposed material, its availability and its method of use
- Method to determine the safety of the drug and its outcome in humans.

Once the FDA satisfactorily approves the test material, it can be tried in human subjects in three phases:

1. *Phase I trial*: The test material is administered or applied in few healthy individuals after obtaining informed consent. The material is given in increment till a desired effect is observed or any adverse effect is noted. This determines the *safe dose* of the test material.
2. *Phase II trial*: In this phase, the test material is given to small group of patients in order to determine the therapeutic dose of the material.
3. *Phase III trial*: In this phase, large scale testing is done after dividing into the control and test groups. The test groups should have other materials with which the new test material can be compared. The phase helps in determining the *safe and effective dose* for the new material.

    All the data obtained from the three phases is compiled and submitted to the FDA in NDA category (New Drug Application). After evaluation, the FDA designates the new material (drug) as complete or incomplete. A *complete* material is allowed by FDA to be marketed whereas the *incomplete* material is sent for further tests before its final acceptance.

4. *Phase IV trial*: After use of new material any report on allergic reactions or drug interactions or other abnormality should be brought to the notice of FDA at timely interval. This will help in recognizing delayed effect of the material with prolonged use.

### Advantages of Usage Test

- Very high relevance
- Superior to any in vitro or animal tests.

### Disadvantages of Usage Test

- Highly expensive
- Extremely complex
- Time consuming
- Major legal and ethical issues
- Often difficult to control
- Difficult to quantify and interpret.

*Ryge criteria or the United States Public Health Services (USPHS) criteria* are used to clinically test the restorative material. According to this criteria, the test material is placed in the patient's mouth after obtaining permission from the Institutional Review Board and informed patient consent. The new material is evaluated clinically for a period of 1 year. If the success rate is less than 90%, then the new test material is withdrawn from the market. The Ryge or USPHS criteria are given in the **Table 3.5**.

The criteria assessment of the new restorative material is done by two independent examiners. The criteria use a grading system based on the subjective observations of the parameters such as color of restoration, secondary caries, recurrent caries, etc. Each parameter is graded using scoring system where following grades are given:

- *Alpha*: Perfect
- *Beta*: Clinically acceptable
- *Charlie*: Restoration requires placement
- *Delta*: Failure.

## TYPES OF TEST PROGRAMS FOR BIOCOMPATIBILITY TESTING

The test programs refer to the sequence or approach in which the tests are done.

The tests are done following the three basic phases:

1. *Primary phase*: In vitro tests
2. *Secondary phase*: Animal tests, and
3. Usage or tertiary phase: Usage test.

The test programs are of two types:

1. Linear progression of tests
2. Nonlinear progression of tests.

### Linear Progression of Tests

In this approach, the tests are done progressively from primary phase to the usage phase. First the test material is subjected to in vitro testing. If the test material is successfully tested in primary phase, then it goes for secondary phase testing. Likewise if the material is successfully tested in secondary phase, then it goes for usage phase testing. When a material successfully tested in all three phases, then it is considered safe for clinical trials (**Fig. 3.5**).

**Table 3.5:** Ryge criteria or USPHS criteria for evaluating restorative material.

| Criteria | Test procedure | USPHS score | |
|---|---|---|---|
| Retention | Visual inspection with mirror at 18 inches | • Complete retention of the restoration<br>• Mobilization of the restoration, still present<br>• Loss of the restoration | Alpha<br>Bravo<br>Charlie |
| Color match | Visual inspection with the mirror at 18 inches | • Restoration is perfectly matched for the color shade<br>• Restoration is not perfectly matched<br>• Restoration is unacceptable | Alpha<br>Bravo<br>Charlie |
| Marginal integrity | Visual inspection with explorer and mirror, if needed | • Absence of discrepancy at probing<br>• Presence of discrepancy at probing, without dentin exposure<br>• Probe penetrates in the discrepancy at probing, with dentin exposure | Alpha<br>Bravo<br>Charlie |
| Marginal discoloration | Visual inspection with mirror at 18 inches | • Absence of marginal discoloration<br>• Presence of marginal discoloration, limited and not extended<br>• Evident marginal discoloration, penetrated toward the pulp chamber | Alpha<br>Bravo<br>Charlie |
| Surface texture | Visual inspection with explorer and mirror, if needed | • Surface is not rough<br>• Surface is slightly rough<br>• Surface is highly rough | Alpha<br>Bravo<br>Charlie |
| Surface staining | Visual inspection with explorer and mirror, if needed | • Surface is not staining<br>• Surface is slightly staining<br>• Surface is highly staining | Alpha<br>Bravo<br>Charlie |
| Postoperative sensitivity | Ask patients | • Absence of dentinal hypersensitivity<br>• Presence of mild and transparent hypersensitivity<br>• Presence of strong and intolerable hypersensitivity | Alpha<br>Bravo<br>Charlie |
| Gingival bleeding | Visual inspection with explorer and mirror, if needed | • Gingival tissues are perfect<br>• Gingival tissues are slightly hyperemic<br>• Gingival tissues are inflamed | Alpha<br>Bravo<br>Charlie |
| Secondary caries | Visual inspection with explorer and mirror, if needed | • No evidence of caries<br>• Evidence of caries along the margin of the restoration | Alpha<br>Bravo |

*Drawbacks*

- As the tests are done sequentially, this approach is time consuming
- Sometimes, in vitro tests and animal tests may not predict the results of the usage tests. For example, zinc oxide eugenol cement when subjected to in vitro testing, destroys all cells in the culture medium whereas it has been successfully used in clinical practice for several years without showing any signs of pulp damage.

### Nonlinear Progression of Tests

In such tests, the approach is different from the linear program. Here, all the tests are conducted simultaneously. As time progresses, usage phase of testing predominates. Secondly, any test can be conducted any time during the development of the material (**Fig. 3.6**).

## CORRELATION BETWEEN IN VITRO, ANIMAL AND USAGE TESTS

All the three tests namely in vitro, animal and usage tests are used together as no single test is used to evaluate

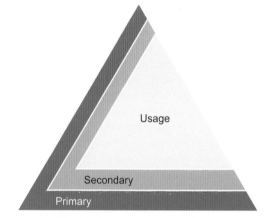

**Fig. 3.5:** Linear progression of tests.

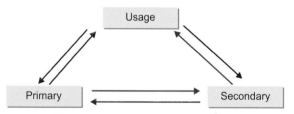

**Fig. 3.6:** Nonlinear progression of tests.

biocompatibility of new material. However, the method of using these tests together is controversial and is still evolving. When testing a new biomaterial three phases are usually used. These phases are primary, secondary and usage.

- *Primary tests* are performed initially in the testing of new material and these tests are in vitro in nature. These tests may also include some animal tests to determine the systemic toxicity of the material.
- *Secondary tests* are conducted after primary tests to explore chronic biological response such as allergy, inflammation, estrogenicity, surface effects and osteoinduction.
- Next is the *usage test* as the new biomaterial is now tested in clinically relevant situations.

The testing of the new material follows the *linear paradigm* from the primary to the usage tests. This paradigm is depicted in the form of triangle with the bottom of the triangle formed by primary tests and the apex formed by the usage tests. The quantity of material tested is represented by the width of the triangle. The majority of the materials are tested in the primary phase and those materials which pass this phase are subjected to the secondary test. The fewer materials which pass the secondary tests are finally subjected to the usage tests. This linear paradigm is the most efficient and cost-effective way of testing biocompatibility of newer materials currently, although it is also challenged over the years.

The studies by *Major* et al (1977) have challenged the linear testing paradigm. Therefore, several newer schemes are developed to test the biocompatibility of the material although the basic linear paradigm is preserved. *Nonlinear paradigm* is proposed and will form the basic standard of testing in the future. In this, all the three tests are done initially but as the testing progresses the usage tests predominate. The common progression is from primary to secondary to the usage tests but any of these tests can be done at any time of development of the material.

## Standardization

In an attempt to make testing of the materials for biocompatibility, more uniform American Dental Association/American National Standards Institute approved the Document No. 41 for recommended standard practices for biological evaluation of dental materials in 1972. This original document was updated in 1982 to include mutagenicity tests. It follows the linear paradigm for screening and testing using initial, secondary and usage tests. The initial test includes in vitro assays for cytotoxicity, red blood cell membrane lysis, mutagenesis and carcinogenesis at the cellular level. Materials which pass this test are tested by one or more secondary tests in

small animals and finally when they are through this test. They are then subjected to one or more *in vivo* usage tests.

Another agency is the International Organization for Standards (ISO) in 2002 considered different areas of biological testing. This is the ISO standard 10993, which includes genotoxicity, carcinogenicity, reproductive toxicity and interaction with blood testing. These tests are broadly divided into initial and supplementary tests. The initial tests include the in vitro and the animal tests whereas the supplementary tests include the animal and the usage tests. Sometimes, specialized tests may also be included.

Some ISO 10993 parts which include biological testing are given below in **Table 3.6**.

The standardization of the biocompatibility testing has broadened the understanding of various materials. As biologic testing involves numerous variables, the standardization of the testing is critical. Each of the testing standards divides the materials based on the type of tissue contact and the site of contact. The selection of the appropriate test methodology depends on the area of implantation of material or use, the tissues with which the material is contacting and the duration of its contact. Although standardization provides with a number of benefits, they still have a number of drawbacks such as standardization methodology cannot keep pace with the newer scientific development, may be arbitrary in nature and may have economic impact on the manufacturer, clinician and the patients.

## BIOCOMPATIBILITY ISSUES IN DENTISTRY

### Amalgam

Biocompatibility of amalgam has always been subject of controversy since its inception about 150 years ago. There are concerns about the possibility of leaching out of mercury from the restoration and dissolve in saliva. Mercury can exist in inorganic or organic form. The organic form (methyl mercury) is the most toxic form as it is responsible for toxic reactions in the environmental disasters, seafood consumption and leather industry. Mercury is easily

| **Table 3.6:** Some ISO 10993 parts which include biological testing. | |
|---|---|
| ISO 10993-3:1992 | Tests for genotoxicity, carcinogenicity and reproductive toxicity |
| ISO 10993-4:1992 | Tests for materials that interact with blood |
| ISO 10993-5:1992 | Tests for cytotoxicity: in vitro methods |
| ISO 10993-6:1994 | Tests for local effects after implantation |
| ISO 10993-10:1994 | Tests for irritation and sensitization |
| ISO 10993-11:1993 | Tests for systemic toxicity |

absorbed in the body in the vapor form, but in amalgam, it exists in the metallic form which forms an alloy. The US Public Health Service and Food and Drug Administration (2006) reviewed various studies and concluded that there is no proof of any mercury toxicity from dental amalgam to the patient except for allergy **(Table 3.7)**.

## Resin-based Materials

Resin-based materials are commonly used as restorative materials and as cements. These materials consist of monomers, fillers, initiators, accelerators and additives which are combined by some type of curing mechanism (self or light curing). If the composition of resin material is altered or if complete curing is not carried out, then some of the components can leach into the saliva and pass into the tubules through the pulp chamber. In vitro test of freshly set self-cured or light-cured composites are capable of causing moderate cytotoxicity in cultured cells in 24–72 hours of exposure. The cytotoxicity is significantly reduced 24–48 hours after setting and in the presence of dentin barrier. The chances of moderate cytotoxicity are reduced in recently introduced resins. Studies show that light cured composite resins are less cytotoxic than self-cured composite resins. If remaining dentin thickness is < 0.5 mm then a protective liner or bonding agent is used to minimize the reaction of pulp to resin materials **(Table 3.8)**.

## Dentin Bonding Agents

Long-term in vitro studies on components of dentin bonding agents conclude that they have ability to permeate up to 0.5 mm into the dentin up to 4 weeks from the application. Many of these components are cytotoxic in nature if tested alone. Hydroxyethyl methacrylate (HEMA) which is component of most of the bonding agents shows at least 100 times less cytotoxicity than Bis-GMA. The cytotoxic effect of dentin bonding agents is significantly reduced if dentin barrier is present or remaining dentin thickness is > 0.5 mm. If the remaining dentin thickness is < 0.1 mm, then HEMA may cause cytotoxicity in vivo.

## Latex

In dentistry, latex is commonly used as rubber dam and gloves. The incidence of latex hypersensitivity is reported in the literature. According to FDI in 1991, the incidence of latex hypersensitivity in surgical personnel can be between 6–7%. Both dentists and patients are exposed to latex hypersensitivity **(Fig. 3.7)**. Adverse reaction because of hypersensitivity can be in the form of localized rashes, swelling, sometimes, serious wheezing and anaphylaxis.

**Table 3.7:** Biocompatibility issues in dental amalgam.

| | |
|---|---|
| Systemic toxicity | • Elemental mercury can lead to systemic toxicity<br>• Inhalation of mercury vapors is the most common route of entry into the body<br>• Other routes are ingestion, skin<br>• Exposure to mercury can occur due to improper storage of mercury, during trituration, insertion and condensation of amalgam or during removal of old amalgam restoration<br>• Safe level of mercury exposure in dental clinic is 50 µg Hg/m³/day<br>• Average permissible mercury level in urine is 6.1 µg Hg/ L |
| Local toxicity | Pulp reaction<br>• Reduced number of odontoblasts, dilated capillaries and inflammation is observed if deep amalgam restoration done with direct condensation<br>• Hg, Ag, Zn and Sn may be detected in dentinal tubules of deep cavities<br>• Oral mucosal reaction<br>• Hg exposure can lead to gingivitis, bleeding gums, bone loss around the teeth<br>• Amalgam tattoos can occur due to unintended spillage of amalgam in periapical region |
| Allergic reaction | *Type IV:* Delayed allergic type of reaction may occur |
| Other reaction | No evidence of mutagenic or carcinogenic reaction |

**Table 3.8:** Biocompatibility issues with resin-based composites.

| | |
|---|---|
| Systemic toxicity | • There is no evidence of systemic toxicity<br>• Bisphenol A which is a precursor of bisphenol A glycidyl methacrylate can act as xenoestrogen and can cause reproductive anomalies. But research shows that this effect is highly nonsignificant in context of dental composites |
| Local toxicity | • HEMA (hydroxyethyl methacrylate) and TEGDMA (triethylene glycol dimethacrylate) can release cytotoxic substance from uncured or partially cured composites<br>• Curing shrinkage of composites can lead to marginal leakage |
| Allergic reaction | • Bis-GMA, TEGDMA, and MMA act like allergens and can produce type IV delayed hypersensitivity reaction<br>• Clinician should wear gloves while handling composite resins. Monomers can penetrate latex or nitrile gloves, therefore, *neoprene* (polychloroprene gloves) should be used |
| Other reaction | Some components of composite resins such as TEGDMA and glutaraldehyde can show mutagenic potential |

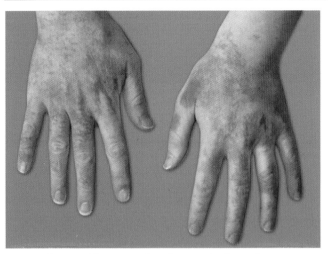

**Fig. 3.7:** Allergic reaction after wearing latex gloves.

The contact of latex containing products to oral mucous membrane can lead to serious systemic allergic reaction such as angioneurotic edema, chest pain, rash on neck and chest. Patient with history of eczema and allergies are more prone with such hypersensitive reactions.

## Casting Alloys

Metals and alloys used in dentistry except for the noble metal alloys are biocompatible because of the formation of a protective passivating film on the surface. This passivating film helps in providing corrosion resistance. If this protective film is not formed or interrupted, then either repassivation occurs or this film is not formed and the underlying metal surface is prone for corrosion.

Among the metals and alloys used in dentistry, nickel is one of the most common causes of allergic reaction. Nickel containing alloys are widely used to fabricate crowns, fixed partial dentures, removable partial dentures and certain orthodontic appliances. An allergic reaction to nickel containing alloys is well reported in the literature. Cross-reactivity between nickel and palladium allergy is well-known. Patient who are allergic to palladium has 100% chances to be allergic to nickel whereas patients with known allergy to nickel have 33% chances to be allergic to palladium. Patients with known sensitivity to nickel are contraindicated to receive nickel chromium restorations.

Another component of concern is beryllium. Beryllium is used in Ni-Cr alloys in the concentration of 1–2% by weight to increase the castability of these alloys and to reduce their melting range. It also forms thin adherent oxide film which helps in improving chemical bonding of porcelain.

Beryllium containing particles when inhaled can reach the alveoli of the lungs to cause chronic inflammatory reaction called as berylliosis. It is potentially harmful for laboratory personnel who may inhale beryllium dust during grinding and polishing of the alloys. Beryllium is also identified as potential carcinogen and acidic environment enhances beryllium release from Ni-Cr alloys.

Titanium and titanium alloys are frequently used in implant dentistry because of its excellent biocompatibility. It is capable of rapidly forming a thin, inert oxide layer when exposed to the air. This biocompatible film of titanium dioxide aids in direct attachment of bone to the metal surface without any intervening soft tissue capsule. It has been reported recently that under certain chemical condition and exposure to high pH in the oral environment, titanium and its alloys may not exhibit high corrosion resistance **(Table 3.9)**.

## Dental Ceramics

Two types of ceramic materials are used in dentistry:
1. Hard ceramics which are used to fabricate crowns, fixed partial dentures, inlays and onlays
2. Ceramics which are intended to react with the surrounding tissues.

| Table 3.9: Biocompatibility issues in casting alloys. | |
|---|---|
| Systemic toxicity | • No studies to prove systemic toxicity due to dental alloys |
| Local toxicity | • Nickel and copper can cause gingival inflammation<br>• Chromium, nickel and cobalt can show cytotoxic potential<br>• Casting alloys in intimate contact with the soft tissue creates *microenvironment* The soft tissue is the gingival sulcus where microenvironment forms. The release of elements forms the alloy is likely to get deposited into this microenvironment. |
| Allergic reaction | • Among elements in dental casting alloys, nickel has greatest allergic potential followed by cobalt and chromium<br>• Cross-reactive allergic can occur for Pd and Ni<br>• Lichenoid type reaction can occur in oral mucosa adjacent to the casting alloys |
| Other reaction | • Berrylium has mutagenic potential<br>• Nickel sulfide has carcinogenic potential<br>• Oxidative state of chromium determines its mutagenicity $Cr^{3+}$ is not mutagenic but $Cr^{6+}$ is mutagenic |

Hard ceramics are usually insoluble and have little concern with the biocompatibility. Second type of ceramic interacts with the surrounding tissues. These materials are compounds that contain calcium and phosphorus, e.g. Bioglass, calcium phosphate ceramics. These materials interact with the surrounding bone to form a bond between the material and the tissue to become stronger than the bone or the material itself. These materials are reactive with bone and become either integrated with bone or be part of the healed bone. In this process, some of them may be resorbed or dissolved and replaced by a new bone (**Table 3.10**).

**Table 3.10:** Biocompatibility issues in dental ceramics.

| | |
|---|---|
| Systemic toxicity | • Inhalation of ceramic dust during finishing can lead to silicosis. It is a lung disease which is characterized by fever, cough and breathing problems |
| Local toxicity | • Lithium and aluminum oxide ceramic containing lanthanum glass shows a very low degree of cytotoxicity |
| Allergic reaction | • No reports |
| Other reaction | • Zirconium oxide ceramic contains small amount of radioactivity due to contamination of thorium and uranium. Although the radioactivity is not significant |

## Zinc Oxide Eugenol Cement (Table 3.11)

**Table 3.11:** Biocompatibility issues in Zinc oxide eugenol cement.

| | |
|---|---|
| Systemic toxicity | No reports on systemic reaction |
| Local toxicity | • ZOE cement can produce cytotoxic reaction, if directly applied to the pulp<br>• If dentin layer is in between the cement and pulp then no inflammatory reaction takes place<br>• It has obtundent effect when used in deep cavities as eugenol is capable of blocking transmission of action potentials |
| Allergic reaction | • Eugenol can be allergic to some individuals<br>• Some clinicians can develop allergic contact dermatitis |
| Other reaction | No evidence of mutagenicity |

## Zinc Phosphate Cement (Table 3.12)

**Table 3.12:** Biocompatibility issues in zinc phosphate cement.

| | |
|---|---|
| Systemic toxicity | No evidence |
| Local toxicity | • Pulpal reaction—initially mixed cement has very high pH because of the presence of phosphoric acid (about 2), then it subsequently increases to 5.5. If remaining dentin thickness is less, there is high chance of pulp irritation<br>• If remaining dentin thickness is more, there is less chance of acid penetration<br>• Again thin consistency of the mix initiates greater pulp reaction because of the presence of greater amount of acid. This is called as *phosphoric acid sting*.<br>Precautions:<br>• The powder-liquid ratio of cement should never be altered as it increases the acid content<br>• Cavity liner or varnish is applied on the dentin to prevent acid penetration |
| Allergic reaction | No evidence |
| Other reaction | No evidence of mutagenicity or carcinogenic reactions |

## Calcium Hydroxide (Table 3.13)

**Table 3.13:** Biocompatibility issues in calcium hydroxide cement.

| | |
|---|---|
| Systemic toxicity | No evidence |
| Local toxicity | • In some cultures, calcium hydroxide was found to be highly cytotoxic; but in others, they were nontoxic<br>• *Direct pulp capping*: When calcium hydroxide is applied directly on the exposed pulp, it causes superficial coagulation necrosis. This acts as a stimulus for the differentiation of secondary odontoblasts that initiates the formation of secondary dentin<br>• *Indirect pulp capping*: If calcium hydroxide is applied in close proximity to the pulp, it exerts antimicrobial effect and reduces the permeability of dentin. If the remaining dentin thickness is < 5–10 μm, it initiates tertiary dentin formation |
| Allergic reaction | No evidence |
| Other reactions | No evidence of mutagenicity or carcinogenesis |

## Glass Ionomer Cement (GIC) (Table 3.14)

| **Table 3.14:** Biocompatibility issues in glass ionomer cement. | |
|---|---|
| Systemic toxicity | No evidence |
| Local toxicity | • Unset glass ionomer cement is cytotoxic to the pulp. It is due to the presence of acid and release of fluoride ions<br>• Humidity is required for hydration and completion of setting reaction. If less humidity is there, it can cause incomplete setting of the cement<br>• Dentin should be moist and not dry or desiccated before placement of the cement<br>• Resin modified GIC is cytotoxic when left uncured and after curing it is nonsignificant |
| Allergic reaction | • No evidence in case of conventional GIC<br>• Release of HEMA (hydroxyethyl methacrylate) from resin- modified GIC can cause reaction in some individuals |
| Other reaction | No evidence of mutagenicity or carcinogenicity |

## Denture Base Resins (Table 3.15)

| **Table 3.15:** Biocompatibility issues in denture base resins. | |
|---|---|
| Systemic toxicity | No evidence of systemic toxicity. If accidently some monomers enter the body through blood vessel, it is rapidly converted to methacrylic acid and excreted from the body |
| Local toxicity | • Self-cure acrylic resins are most cytotoxic and light cure resins are least<br>• Components of acrylic resins such as methyl methacrylate, ethylene glycol dimethacrylate (EGDMA) and dibenzoyl peroxide contribute to cytotoxic effect<br>• UDMA (urethane dimethacrylate) present in light polymerizing resins is highly cytotoxic<br>• N,N-dimethyl-p-toluidine causes reversible cell damage |
| Allergic reaction | • Denture base resins can cause allergic reaction in some individuals<br>• Components in resin which can cause allergy are methyl methacrylate, dibenzoyl peroxide, EGDMA and hydroquinone |
| Other reaction | No evidence of mutagenicity or carcinogenicity |

## Impression Materials (Table 3.16)

| **Table 3.16:** Biocompatibility issues in impression materials. | |
|---|---|
| Systemic toxicity | • Wide variety of impression materials used in dentistry such elastomers, agar, alginate, impression compound, etc.<br>• Dibutyl phthalate present in polysulfide elastomer contains component which when used in high concentration is cytotoxic in nature. But in impression material, since it is used in very small quantity, it is nonsignificant |
| Local toxicity | • Addition polysilicones are nontoxic but some condensation silicone may show cytotoxic potential<br>• Polysulfide impression shows very small amount of cytotoxicity whereas polyether impression material may show greater amount of cytotoxicity. It is, therefore, recommended to remove the remnants of impression material after the completion of impression procedure |
| Allergic reaction | Few individuals may report allergic reaction such as contact dermatitis |
| Other reaction | No evidence of mutagenicity or carcinogenicity |

## CLINICAL TIPS FOR USING DENTAL MATERIALS SAFELY AND EFFECTIVELY

• *Follow manufacturer's instructions:* Since the manufacturer has determined the best method for better storage and safety use. It is always advisable to carefully read and follow the instruction manual for storage, manipulation and protection of a particular dental material

• *Expiry date:* The expiry date of the material should always be noted and the material use should be discontinued after that. The expired products should be disposed off and replaced by newer products

• *Exposure to heat, light and air:* Most of the dental materials are sensitive to heat, light and air. Therefore, the materials should be properly stored in a cool dry place. Any exposure leads to deterioration in the properties of the material.

## GUIDELINES TO MINIMIZE CHEMICAL EXPOSURE IN THE DENTAL CLINIC

- Minimize the use of hazardous chemicals in the dental clinic
- Carefully read and follow the instructions manual
- Store as per the manufacturer's instructions
- Wash hand immediately after use
- Avoid direct skin contact with the chemicals
- If chemical contact happens accidently, wash immediately
- Maintain good ventilation in the dental clinic
- Do not eat, drink, smoke or use cosmetics in area where chemicals are used
- Always keep away vaporizing chemicals from heat sources or alcohol flame
- Always keep fire extinguisher in the dental clinic for safety
- Do not handle chemical if not trained to do so
- Keep neutralizing agents for strong acids and alkaline solutions
- Dispose of chemicals following the instructions carefully.

## CLINICAL TIPS TO MANAGE AEROSOLS IN DENTAL CLINIC

- Always use high vacuum suction in procedures involving aerosols
- Use rubber dams
- Avoid spraying of chemicals
- Frequently clean air and vacuum filters
- Always cover ultrasonic cleansers and chemical containers
- Use powder free gloves
- Use vacuum dust cleaning system involving dust during laboratory procedures
- Always use protective barriers such as mouth mask, gloves and eye wear.

## TEST YOURSELF

### Essay Questions

1. Define Biocompatiblity? Describe various tests used to determine Biocompatibility of dental materials?
2. Describe various factors influencing biocompatibility of dental materials?
3. Discuss various Biocompatibility issues in dentistry?

### Short Notes

1. Usage test
2. Mutagenicity and carcinogenicity
3. Mercury toxicity
4. Estrogenicity
5. Latex allergy

### Multiple Choice Questions

1. Concurrent allergens are:
   A. Two allergens present in a material at the same time
   B. Two allergens present in a material at different times
   C. Two or more allergens present in the material at the same time
   D. Two or more allergens present in the material at different times
2. Malformations occurring during embryonic development is called as:
   A. Mutagenicity
   B. Genotoxicity
   C. Tetrogenicity
   D. Carcinogenicity
3. Ability of the material to transfer genetic damage to next generation of cells is called as:
   A. Mutagenicity
   B. Genotoxicity
   C. Carcinogenicity
   D. Tetrogenicity
4. All of the following are in vitro tests, *except:*
   A. Agar diffusion testing
   B. Dentin barrier testing
   C. Implantation testing
   D. Filter diffusion testing
5. All are true about animal tests, *except:*
   A. Provide intact biological system
   B. Provide complex system interaction
   C. Have ethical issues
   D. Can be standardized easily
6. Biocompatibility of dental materials is not tested through:
   A. Invitro tests
   B. Animal tests
   C. Genotoxicity test
   D. Usage test

7. Which of the following tests is gold standard for testing biocompatibility of a material:
   A. In vitro tests
   B. Animal tests
   C. Genotoxic tests
   D. Usage tests

## ANSWERS

| | | | |
|---|---|---|---|
| 1. A | 2. C | 3. A | 4. C |
| 5. D | 6. C | 7. D | |

## BIBLIOGRAPHY

1. Amin A, Palenik CJ, Cheung SW, Burke FJ. Latex exposure and allergy: a survey of general dental practitioners and dental students. Int Dent J. 1998;48:77-83.
2. Bergman M. Side-effects of dental materials reported in Scandinavian countries. Dent Mater J. 2000;19(1):1-9.
3. Demirci M, Hiller KA, Bosl C, Galler K, Schmalz G, Schweikl H. The induction of oxidative stress, cytotoxicity and genotoxicity by dental adhesives. Dent Mater. 2008;24:362-71.
4. Dodes JE. The amalgam controversy. An evidence-based analysis. J Am Dent Assoc. 2001;132:348-56.
5. Hanks CT, Wataha JC, Sun Z. In vitro models of biocompatibility: a review. Dent Mater. 1996;12(3):186-93.
6. Hume WR, Gerzina TM. Bioavailability of components of resin-based materials which are applied to teeth. Crit Rev Oral Biol Med. 1996;7:172-9.
7. International Organization for Standardization. (2003). Biological evaluation of medical devices. Part 1: Evaluation and testing within a risk management process. [online]. Available from http://www.iso.org/standard/44908.html [Accessed April, 2017].
8. Kovarik RE, Haubenreich JE, Gore D. Glass ionomer cements: a review of composition, chemistry and biocompatibility as a dental and medical implant material. J Long Term Eff Med Implants. 2005;15(6):655-71.
9. Lautenschlager EP, Monaghan P. Titanium and titanium alloys as dental materials. Int Dent J. 1993;43:245-53.
10. LeGeros RZ. Properties of osteoconductive biomaterials: calcium phosphates. Clin Orthop Relat Res. 2002;395:81-98.
11. Lygre H. Prosthodontic biomaterials and adverse reactions: a critical review of the clinical and research literature. Acta Odontol Scand. 2002; 60:1-9.
12. Mackert JR. Dental amalgam and mercury. J Am Dent Assoc. 1991;122:54-61.
13. Messer RL, Lockwood PE, Wataha JC, Lewis JB, Norris S, Bouillaguet S. In vitro cytotoxicity of traditional versus contemporary dental ceramics. J Prosthet Dent. 2003;90:452-8.
14. Mjor IA, Hensten-Pettersen A, Skogedal O. Biologic evaluation of filling materials. A comparison of results using cell culture techniques, implantation tests and pulp studies. Int Dent J. 1977;27:124-9.
15. Polyzois GL. In vitro evaluation of dental materials. Clin Mater. 1994;16(1):21-60.
16. Powell D, Lawrence WH, Turner J, Autian J. Development of a toxicity evaluation program for dental materials and products. I. Screening for irritant responses. J Biomed Mater Res. 1970;4: 583-96.
17. Rankin KV, Jones DL, Rees TD. Latex glove reactions found in a dental school. J Am Dent Assoc. 1993;124:67-71.
18. Schafer TE, Lapp CA, Hanes CM, Lewis JB, Wataha JC, Schuster GS. Estrogenicity of bisphenol A and bisphenol A dimethacrylate in vitro. J Biomed Mater Res. 1999;45:192-7.
19. Schmalz G, Garhammer P. Biological interactions of dental cast alloys with oral tissues. Dent Mater. 2002;18:396-406.
20. Schweikl H, Hiller KA, Bolay C, Kreissl M, Kreismann W, Nusser A, et al. Cytotoxic and mutagenic effects of dental composite materials. Biomaterials. 2005;26:1713-9.
21. Wataha JC, Hanks CT. Biological effects of palladium and risk of using palladium in dental casting alloys. J Oral Rehabil. 1996;23:309-20.
22. Wataha JC. Biocompatibility of dental casting alloys. A review. J Prosthet Dent. 2000;83:223-34.
23. Wataha JC. Biocompatibility of dental materials. In: Craig RG, Powers JM (Eds). Restorative Dental Materials, 11th edition. Philadelphia: Mosby; 2002. pp. 125-62.
24. Wataha JC. Predicting clinical biological responses to dental materials. Dent Mater. 2012;28:23-40.
25. Wataha JC. Principles of biocompatibility for dental practitioners. J Prosthet Dent. 2001;86:203-9.

# Section 2

# Auxiliary Dental Materials

*'The only way to do great work is to love what you do. If you have'nt found it yet, keep looking. Don't settle.'*
—***Steve Jobs***

## INTRODUCTION

Gypsum is a naturally occurring white mineral which is available in many parts of the world. It usually occurs below the earth's surface. It can also be synthesized artificially by calcining the byproduct during the manufacturing of phosphoric acid. Gypsum products used for dental use are almost pure calcium sulfate dihydrate ($CaSO_4.2H_2O$). Various products of gypsum have been used over different centuries for construction purposes.

## GYPSUM

It is defined as the natural hydrated form of calcium sulfonate, *$CaSO_4.2H_2O$ gypsum dihydrate.*

The term 'gypsum' is derived from the Greek word called 'Gypsos' which means chalk or plaster.

## HISTORICAL BACKGROUND

- In ancient times, gypsum was mixed with lime and water to join stone blocks to build Egyptian pyramids

- Assyrians have referred in their script as 'Gypsum Rock'
- Natural gypsum is available as selenite, satin spar and alabaster
- *Philipp Pfaff* first introduced gypsum to dentistry
- One form of gypsum is called plaster of Paris (POP). It is so named as first it was obtained by burning deposits near Paris
- Alabaster was one of the first products of gypsum to be widely used to make sculptures
- It is one of the most widely used minerals in the world.

## USES

### Dental Applications

- Used to make study casts for planning treatment **(Fig. 4.1)**
- Used for mounting casts on articulators
- Used for making impressions of edentulous jaws if there are no undercuts
- Used for making positive reproductions or replicas of the oral structures

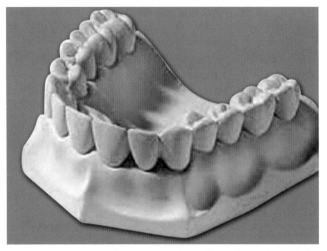

**Fig. 4.1:** Gypsum products commonly used to make study models.

- Used for making molds for casting dental restorations if the dental plaster is mixed with fillers such as silica
- Used in soldering procedures
- Used as one of the components in toothpaste.

## Orthopedic Application

Used to make casts to immobilize fractured bone.

## Industrial Applications

- Used in home and building constructions to form walls of plaster
- Used to make casting molds for cups, saucers and plates
- Used to add in Portland cement to prevent flash setting of concrete mix
- Used to make drywall finish for walls and ceiling with gypsum boards
- Used as fertilizer for soil conditioning
- Transparent gypsum (selenite) used for windows when glass was not available
- It gives some fire protection to the walls as it contains large quantity of water in them
- Widely used to make sculptures
- It is added in paint as fillers.

## MANUFACTURE OF DENTAL STONE AND PLASTER

Gypsum is commercially grinded into fine powder and is heated to drive off water of crystallization that is chemically bound to the calcium sulfate dihydrate. The reaction is as under:

$$CaSO_4 \cdot 2H_2O \xrightarrow{110-130°C} CaSO_4 \cdot \frac{1}{2}H_2O$$
Cacium sulfate dihydrate      Calcium sulfate hemihydrate

The product formed is called as plaster of Paris or dental plaster which is fibrous aggregate of fine crystals. On heating the product further, it forms hexagonal anhydrite of $CaSO_4$. This process of dehydration is called as calcination. Calcination can occur either in presence or absence of water, i.e. wet or dry calcination. If this product is heated between 200 and 1000°C, then orthorhombic anhydrite crystals of $CaSO_4$ is formed. The reaction is summed up as:

$$CaSO_4 \cdot \frac{1}{2}H_2O \xrightarrow{100-200°C} CaSO_4 \xrightarrow{200-1000°C} CaSO_4$$
(Calcium sulfate hemihydrates)    (Hexagonal anhydrite)    (Orthorhombic anhydrite)

## METHODS OF CALCINATION

### Dry Calcination

In this process, the calcium sulfate dihydrate crystals are heated in an open vat or rotary kiln at temperatures varying between 120° and 200°C. At this temperature, water of crystallization is driven off and the dihydrate crystals are converted into the hemihydrate crystals. The resulting crystals are called as β-*hemihydrate* crystals. They consist of large, irregularly-shaped orthorhombic crystal particles with capillary pores. They have low density, high relative surface area and large packing ability. The β-hemihydrate crystals are called as *dental plaster*.

### Wet Calcination

The dihydrate crystals in this process are heated in an autoclave to result in smaller, regularly-shaped crystalline particles in the form of rods or prisms. Autoclaving of the particles is done in superheated steam at a pressure of 117 kPa and temperature of 123°C for 5–7 hours. These particles are relatively stronger and denser. The resulting crystals are called as α-*hemihydrates*. During wet calcination, adequate water is present to allow complete solution conversion, therefore, undergoing recrystallization. The α-hemihydrates are called as dental stone, die stone or improved stone **(Table 4.1)**.

### Improved Stone

This is also called as α-modified hemihydrates. These particles are produced under increased pressure and are finely ground to be denser. The gypsum material is boiled in a solution of 30% calcium chloride and magnesium chloride in presence of small amounts (≤1%) of sodium succinate. These two chlorides act as deflocculants which help to segregate each particles which otherwise would have agglomerated. This type of gypsum is smoother and denser than the other hemihydrates. These particles have better

**Table 4.1:** Comparison between the α-hemihydrates and β-hemihydrates.

| Features | α-hemihydrates | β-hemihydrates |
|---|---|---|
| Particle size | Small | Large |
| Particle shape | Regular shape crystals in the form of rods and prism | Irregular shape crystals which are rough and fibrous aggregates |
| Strength | High | Low |
| Density | More dense | Less dense |
| Crystal structure | Prismatic | Orthorhombic |
| Water/Powder (W/P) ratio | Less (0.22–0.24) | Greater (0.45–50) |
| Manufacture | Wet calcination | Dry calcination |
| Uses | Casts for denture constructions, dies for crowns and bridges, inlays | Study models and for mounting casts |
| Manufacturing method | Gypsum heated in presence of crystal modifier in autoclave under steam pressure | Gypsum heated in open containers |
| Examples | Dental stone, die stone | Dental plaster |

packing ability and thus require less water for mixing. They are called as improved stone and are mainly used for dies. Type IV stone is example of improved stone.

# TYPES

According to ADA/ANSI specification No. 25 gypsum products are classified into five types. These types vary according to their use, properties and handling characteristics **(Table 4.2)**.

## Type I—Impression Plaster

- Impression plaster is used to make impression of the edentulous jaws provided undercuts are not present
- They are hard and brittle with very low strength. They are not suitable for making impression of the dentulous jaws because of the undercuts of teeth and adjacent structures
- They have short setting time of approximately $4 \pm 1$ minutes. Short setting time is advantageous as longer setting time will be uncomfortable to the patients during impression making

- They have relatively low setting expansion of 0.13% and, therefore, have better accuracy
- They have highest W/P ratio, i.e. 0.50–0.75. High water content reduces the heat build-up during setting. Therefore, chances of any damage to the mucosal tissues are minimal
- They have least strength among the gypsum types. This property is useful if the set impression material is difficult to remove from the undercut then it can be broken in the mouth and then rejoined outside the mouth
- It absorbs the palatal secretions during setting
- It is easy to manipulate and handle
- Impression plasters are rarely used as impression materials nowadays as less rigid materials such as hydrocolloids and elastomers are available **(Fig. 4.2)**.

## Type II—Model Plaster

- Model plaster also called as laboratory type II plaster
- Primarily used to make study casts **(Fig. 4.3)**
- Used to mount casts on the articulators
- Used to fill flask for denture fabrication

**Table 4.2:** Properties of different types of gypsum products.

| Types | Water/Powder (W/P) | Setting time | Setting expansion (2 hours) | Compressive strength (1 hour) | Porosity |
|---|---|---|---|---|---|
| Type I | 0.50–0.75 | 4 ± 1 | 0.00–0.15 | 4 MPa | - |
| Type II | 0.45–0.50 | 12 ± 4 | 0.00–0.30 | 9 MPa | 35% |
| Type III | 0.28–0.30 | 12 ± 4 | 0.00–0.20 | 20.7 MPa | 20% |
| Type IV | 0.22–0.24 | 12 ± 4 | 0.00–0.10 | 34.5 MPa | 10% |
| Type V | 0.18–0.22 | 12 ± 4 | 0.10–0.30 | 48.3 MPa | - |

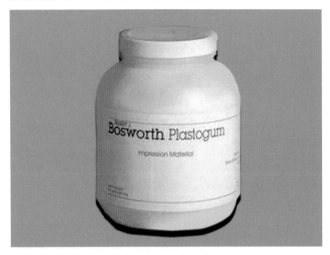

**Fig. 4.2:** Impression plaster.

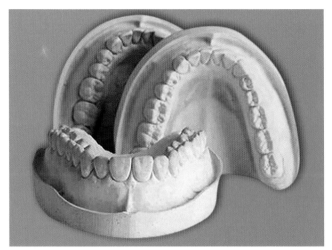

**Fig. 4.4:** Casts made with dental stone.

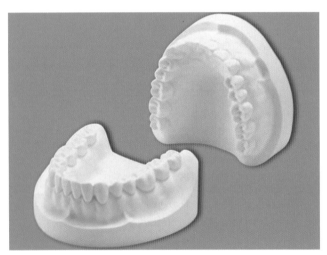

**Fig. 4.3:** Plaster models.

- Primarily composed of β-hemihydrates and modifiers
- It is usually available as natural white color to contrast with the colored dental stone
- Model plasters have low compressive strength of 9 MPa and tensile strength of 0.6 MPa. Although it has greater strength than impression plaster
- W/P ratio of model plaster is 0.45–0.5 and has higher setting expansion than impression plaster
- One special type of model plaster is called the orthodontic plaster which has faster setting time of 2–3 minutes.

*Uses of Plaster Models*

- Help in studying occlusal relationship of dental arches
- Help in studying tooth size, position, tooth shape and arch relationship

- Help in studying hard and soft tissues from the lingual side when teeth are in occlusion
- Provide three dimensional pictures of patient's hard and soft tissues
- Helpful in patient education
- Helpful in keeping records for legal purposes
- Provides preoperative record and helps in assessing the final treatment outcome.

## Type III—Dental Stone

- These are called α-hemihydrates which have improved hardness as compared to model plaster
- Type III stone has minimum 1 hour compressive strength of 20.7 MPa and maximum up to 62 MPa
- Dental stone is used to make casts which is used to process dentures because they have adequate strength and hardness and also it is easier to remove dentures after processing **(Fig. 4.4)**
- Primarily composed of α-hemihydrates, 2–3% coloring agent, accelerators–potassium sulfate, retarder–borax
- Water powder ratio of type III dental stone is 0.28–0.30
- Setting expansion after 2 hours is about 0.20%. Slight setting expansion is tolerated in casts that reproduce soft tissues but not when tooth is present
- The minimum setting time allowed for setting varies between 30 minutes and 60 minutes depending on the setting rate of the stone and type of impression material. For stiffer impression material such as polyether, greater setting time is required.

## Type IV—Die Stone

- This type of gypsum product is having *high strength, high abrasion resistance and low expansion*

- It is primarily used as die material on which wax patterns of inlays, onlays, crowns and bridges are fabricated **(Fig. 4.5)**
- Primary requirements of die material are high strength, hardness, abrasion resistance and minimum setting expansion
- Type of gypsum product is α-hemihydrates which are cuboidal-shaped particles and have better properties than other hemihydrates
- The surface of die stone dries more rapidly and therefore surface hardness increases faster than the compressive strength
- The W/P ratio of die stone is 0.22–0.24
- The surface hardness is 92 RHN and that of type III stone is 82 RHN
- It has low expansion of 0.08% and has high strength of 79 MPa.

### Type V—High Strength and High Expansion Die Stone

- This type of die stone has greater compressive strength than the type IV die stone
- The improved strength is due to reduced W/P ratio (0.18–0.22)
- They have greater setting expansion than die stone, i.e. 0.10–0.30%
- It is indicated when greater expansion is required during the fabrication of cast crowns
- Greater setting expansion is helpful in compensating casting shrinkage of high melting metal alloys
- Its use in fabrication for dies for inlays should be avoided as higher expansion produces tightly fitting inlays which are unacceptable for use **(Fig. 4.6)**.

## SYNTHETIC GYPSUM

- The products of gypsum such as α and β hemihydrates can be produced from the byproducts of phosphoric acid production
- Synthetic gypsum is costlier than natural gypsum
- If produced properly, synthetic gypsum has showed superior properties than natural gypsum.

## IDEAL REQUIREMENTS

- Should be dimensionally stable
- Should reproduce finer details accurately
- Should have adequate strength, hardness and abrasion resistance
- Should be compatible with different impression materials
- Should be biocompatible
- Should be easy to manipulate and easily available
- Should provide good color contrast with various waxes, which are used to fabricate wax patterns
- Should easily flow at the time of pouring the impression to record the finer details.

## PROPERTIES

### Setting Reaction

It is a hydration reaction in which calcium sulfate hemihydrates dissolves in water to form dihydrate which has reduced solubility than hemihydrates. It is an exothermic reaction where heat is liberated on setting. This reaction is reverse of that which occurred during calcining

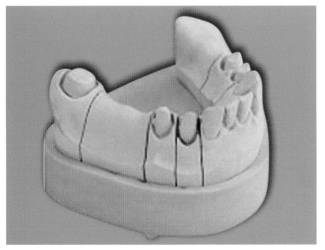

**Fig. 4.5:** Die stone used to make dies for wax pattern fabrication.

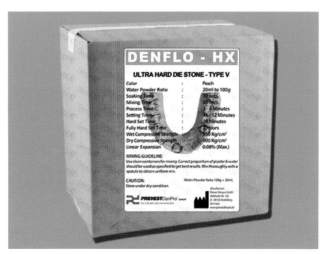

**Fig. 4.6:** Type V dental stone.

or autoclaving process. During setting, following reaction takes place:

$$(CaSO_4)_2 \cdot H_2O + 3H_2O \rightarrow 2\,CaSO_4 \cdot 2H_2O$$

Calcium sulfate<br>hemihydrate           Calcium sulfate dihydrate

$$+ \text{Unreacted } (CaSO_4)_2 \cdot 1/2H_2O + \text{Heat}$$

The amount of heat liberated during setting reaction is 3900 calories per gram mole. Complete conversion of hemihydrates to dihydrates is not possibly achieved unless it is exposed to high humidity for long duration. The setting reaction of hexagonal anhydrite is faster than the orthorhombic anhydrite because the particles of the latter are more closely packed and stable. The crystallization of calcium sulfate dihydrate occurs while most of the hemihydrates crystals are dissolved. Weaker the set material, greater the conversion of hemihydrates to dihydrates.

### Theories of Setting Reaction

*Colloidal theory:* This theory was proposed by Mahaelis in 1893. According to this theory, when powder is mixed with water, plaster attains the colloidal state through sol–gel mechanism. The hemihydrate crystals forms dihydrates in the sol state and once the entire measured quantity of water is consumed, it gets converted into solid gel.

Hemihydrate + water → hemihydrate sol + water → dihydrate sol + remaining water → dihydrate gel

*Hydration theory:* This theory advocates that hemihydrates are converted to dihydrates by joining together the sulfate groups with the help of hydrogen bonding to form set material.

*Crystallization theory or Dissolution-precipitation theory:* This is the most accepted theory which was first proposed by Henry Louis Le Chatelier in 1887 and was supported by Dutch chemist Jacobus Henricus van't Hoff in 1907. According to this theory, difference in solubilities of calcium

sulfate dihydrate and hemihydrate are responsible for setting. The solubility of hemihydrates is four times more in water than the dihydrate at room temperature. In a setting of plaster, dissolution centers are located around calcium sulfate hemihydrates and precipitation centers are located around calcium sulfate dihydrate. The concentration of the calcium sulfate is highest around dissolution center and lowest around the precipitation center. The calcium and sulfate ions move by means of diffusion from higher concentration to the lower concentration.

The setting is explained on the basis of difference in solubility of hemihydrate and dihydrate. When the hemihydrate is mixed with water, it forms a suspension which is fluid and workable.

This hemihydrate dissolves until it forms a saturated solution which is supersaturated with dihydrate, such that the dihydrate precipitates out.

As the dihydrate precipitates, the solution is no longer saturated with the hemihydrate, so it continues to dissolve. Thus, this process of dissolution and precipitation continues, as either new crystals form or further growth occurs on those already present. This reaction is continuous and proceeds until no further dihydrate precipitates out of solution **(Figs. 4.7A and B)**. The crystals of dihydrate are called as "Spherulites" because of their needle-like appearance.

### Microstructure of Set Gypsum

The microstructure of set gypsum contains entangled mass of monoclinic gypsum crystals with lengths varying between 5 µm and 10 µm. This set mass shows inherent porosity on the microscopic level which can be of two types:

1. Microporosity due to the presence of residual unreacted water. These porosities can be roughly spherical and can be found between clumps of gypsum crystals.
2. Another form of microporosity is due to the growth of gypsum crystals. This can be associated with the setting expansion and are smaller in size as compared to the

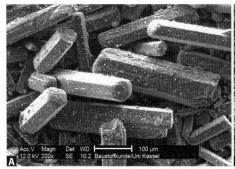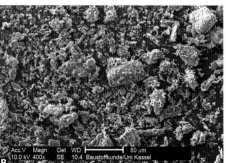

**Figs. 4.7A and B:** Scanning electronmicroscope images of: (A) α-hemihydrate; (B) β-hemihydrate crystals.

first type. They are observed as angular spaces between individual crystals in the set mass.

## Water/Powder Ratio

It is a ratio of water to the amount of hemihydrate powder which is expressed as water/powder (W/P) ratio. The ratio is obtained when volume of water in milliliters is divided by the weight of powder in grams. The amount of water and powder should be taken accurately according to the prescribed ratio of the gypsum products. The W/P ratio is a very important factor in deciding the physical and chemical properties of the final product.

Theoretically, 100 g of gypsum product (calcium sulfate hemihydrate) requires only 18.6 mL of water for chemical reaction to form calcium sulfate dihydrate. But actually different gypsum products require variable amount of water for manipulation, depending on the shape, size and density of powder particles. Like less dense, irregularly-shaped porous powder particles (beta hemihydrates) require more water for manipulation than more dense, regular particles (alpha hemihydrates). Gauging water is the amount of water that is required to mix different gypsum products. It includes the reaction water (18.6 mL) and the extra water which is added to form a workable mass **(Table 4.3)**.

For example, if the ratio is 0.28, then it means that 28 mL of water is taken and 100 g of dental stone is taken.

### Recommended W/P Ratio

*Type I-Impression plaster:* 0.50–0.75.

*Type II-Dental plaster:* 0.45–0.50.

*Type III-Dental stone:* 0.28–0.30.

*Type IV-Improved stone:* 0.22–0.24.

*Type V-High strength, high expansion:* 0.18–0.22.

### Mixing Time

It is defined as the time from the addition of powder to the water until mixing is completed. Mechanical mixing of stone and plasters is completed in 20–30 seconds. Hand manipulation takes place about one minute to obtain a smooth mix.

### Working Time

It is a time which is available to use the workable mass which maintains a uniform consistency during its usage. This time is measured from the start of mixing till the material is no longer acceptable for its intended use. Usually, 3 minutes of working time is adequate to pour an impression and to clean the mixing bowl.

## SETTING REACTION

Setting of gypsum occurs soon after mixing the powder and water in correct ratio and continues till the setting reaction is complete. During the setting, the mixed gypsum undergoes following physical stages which are discussed below:

### Fluid Stage

In this stage, the mixed gypsum is flowy which exhibits pseudoplasticity. This mix readily flows under vibration and shows a glossy surface. The impression should be poured at this stage with gypsum. The mix should be poured slowly and should be kept on vibrator such that it pushes air ahead of itself. The pouring is done from the posterior tooth and one tooth at a time. This will prevent air bubble incorporation in the cast.

### Plastic Stage

As the setting reaction continues, the gypsum crystals keep growing at the expense of aqueous phase and the viscosity of the mix increases. The mix starts to become plastic and does not readily flow under vibration. At this stage, the glossiness disappears as the aqueous phase is drawn into pores formed when the gypsum crystals are thrust apart. If the impression is attempted to pour at the stage, it will not flow completely and will not wet the impression surface. This will trap air bubbles and the poured cast will be weak in strength.

### Friable Stage

As there is continuous growth of crystals, the plastic mix is now converted to rigid solid. This solid mass is initially weak and friable. At this stage, the set mass attains its minimum

| **Table 4.3:** Amount of gauging water needed for various gypsum products. | | | |
|---|---|---|---|
| | *Type II–Dental plaster* | *Type III–Dental stone* | *Type IV–Die stone* |
| Reaction water | 18 mL | 18 mL | 18 mL |
| Extra water | 32 mL | 12 mL | 6 mL |
| Gauging water | 50 mL | 30 mL | 24 mL |
| Powder | 100 g | 100 g | 100 g |
| W/P ratio | 0.50 | 0.30 | 0.24 |

strength called the wet strength and it feels warm to touch because of the exothermic reaction.

## Carvable Stage

Gradually, the continuous growth of crystals converts the friable mix into a solid mass which can be carved but cannot be further molded. Strength at this stage gradually increases till the final strength is achieved. Once the impression is poured, it should be left undisturbed for 45–60 minutes before the impression is separated from the cast. The cast, thereafter, is disinfected with appropriate disinfectant.

## SETTING TIME

*It is defined as the time that starts from the beginning of mixing until the material hardens is known as setting time.* The freshly mixed mass is semifluid in consistency and flows freely which can be poured into the mold of any shape.

### Types of Setting Time

#### Initial Setting Time

As the reaction continues, more hemihydrate crystals react to form dihydrate crystals. The mixed material becomes rigid but is not hard. It can be carved but not molded. This is known as *initial setting time.* The mix appears dull and non-glossy because the excess water is drawn into pores formed by growing crystals which are thrust apart. The initial setting time is measured by loss of gloss and initial Gillmore test.

#### CLINICAL SIGNIFICANCE
Gypsum at the stage should not be manipulated as it is still weak and can fracture.

#### Final Setting Time

It is the time at which the material can be separated from the impression without distortion or fracture. Technically, it is considered as the time when the compressive strength is at least 80% that is attained in 1 hour. Final setting time of most modern gypsum products is 30 minutes **(Fig. 4.8)**.

#### CLINICAL SIGNIFICANCE
This stage indicates the minimal state of hardness and abrasion resistance. The set mass appears dry and weighs less than the initial set mass because of loss of water from the pores due to evaporation. Although the mass reduces but its strength is doubled. It is advisable that impression should be removed from the cast after this stage. Final setting time of gypsum is measured by Gillmore and Vicat tests.

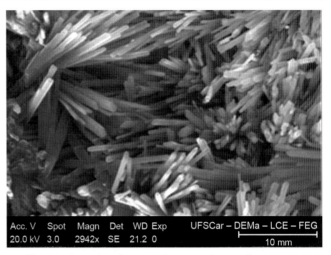

| Acc. V | Spot | Magn | Det | WD | Exp | UFSCar – DEMa – LCE – FEG |
| 20.0 kV | 3.0 | 2942x | SE | 21.2 | 0 | 10 mm |

**Fig. 4.8:** Scanning electron microscope image of set gypsum showing needle-shaped crystals.

#### CLINICAL SIGNIFICANCE
- Before impression is removed from the cast, make sure that no part of impression tray is contacting the cast
- To avoid fracture of cast during removal, do not pry or rock in one direction too far.
- If alginate impression has dried before cast removal, it is advised to soak the impression and cast in water for 15 minutes. The alginate material will soften and then can be easily removed.

### Tests for Determining Setting Time

#### Loss of Gloss Test for Initial Set

During the setting of gypsum, some of the excess water is taken to form the dihydrate resulting in the loss of gloss from the surface of plaster mix. This loss of gloss occurs in about 9 minutes and during this time, the mass does not have any comparable strength.

#### Exothermic Reaction

The temperature rise of the mass may also be used for measurement of setting time, as the setting reaction is exothermic. Till the initial set of the gypsum, the excess water present in mix absorbs heat and there is no appreciable rise in temperature. It is after the loss of gloss from the mix that an appreciable increase in heat is noted. This is seen at the end of the initial set stage.

#### Penetration Tests

By using penetrometers. Two types of penetrometers are available namely; vicat needle and gillmore needles
- Vicat needle
- Gillmore needles.

1. *Vicat needle:* This apparatus is used to measure the initial setting time of gypsum products **(Fig. 4.9)**. It consists of rod which weighs 300 g and a needle with a diameter of 1 mm. The ring container is filled with freshly mixed gypsum whose setting time is to be measured. The needle with a weighted plunger rod is supported and held just in contact with the mix and soon released after loss of gloss. Once the needle is released, it penetrates the mix till it cannot further penetrate the material. This time is called the final setting time. The setting time measured from this method varies between 20 minutes and 30 minutes. After 30 minutes, the set mix achieves almost 80% of compressive strength which is to be attained after one hour. This is called as "ready-to-use–criterion."

2. *Gillmore needles:* Gillmore needles are of two types—small and large **(Fig. 4.10)**.

   The *small Gillmore needle* has 1/4 lb weight and diameter of 1/12" while the *large Gillmore* needle weighs 1 lb weight and has diameter of 1/24". The smaller needle is used to measure the setting time of dental cements and occasionally used for gypsum products.

*Initial Gillmore test:* The mixture is spread out and the smaller needle is allowed to penetrate the surface. The initial setting time is calculated till the needle no longer penetrates the surface. The initial Gillmore test is about 13 minutes.

*Final Gillmore test:* The heavier Gillmore needle is used for the next stage in the setting process. The time elapsed at which the needle makes a barely visible mark on the surface is called as the final setting time. The final setting time is about 20 minutes by this method.

## SETTING OF GYPSUM

The setting of gypsum includes:

- *Mixing time—1 minute:* The powder is mixed with water such that the powder particles are completely wetted with water molecules
- *Working time—4 minutes:* The water for reaction is replenished from the gauging water to make pliable mix. In this stage, the mix is used to pour impression or investing or mounting of articulator
- *Loss of gloss—9 minutes:* It indicates that reaction water is exhausted in forming the dihydrate crystals. These crystals intermesh and this causes an outward thrust. Due to this outward thrust, numerous pores are created into which excess water is drawn. The loss of gloss indicates the starting of the setting process in gypsum **(Fig. 4.11)**.

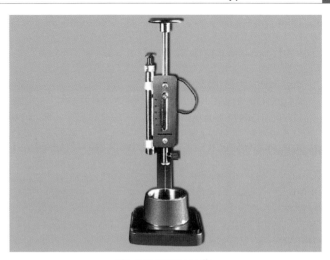

**Fig. 4.9:** Vicat needle.

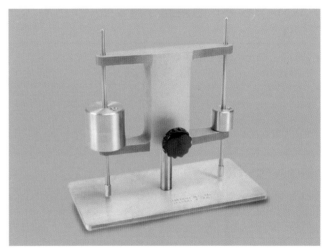

**Fig. 4.10:** Gillmore needle.

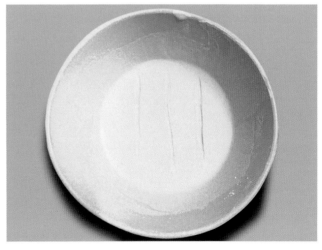

**Fig. 4.11:** Loss of gloss.

- *Initial setting time—13 minutes:* During the initial setting time, the crystals should not be disturbed as it would lead to weakening of the final product
- *Final setting time—20 minutes:* The final product of gypsum becomes hard but it should not be used at this stage. The gypsum should be allowed to set and gain strength for at least one hour.

## Ready for Use Criterion

It is the time till which the set gypsum product can be handled with safety in a usual manner. It is determined by the ability to judge which improves with experience. A set material can be used when it attains at least 80% of its compressive strength. Most of the modern gypsum products reach the ready-to-use state in about 30 minutes.

## FACTORS INFLUENCING SETTING TIME

- Manufacturing process
- Mixing and spatulation (time and rate)
- Water/powder (W/P) ratio
- Temperature
- Accelerators and retarders
- Viscosity.

## Manufacturing Process

Three methods to control the setting time that have been incorporated into the commercial products available:
1. By increasing or decreasing the solubility of the hemihydrates
2. By increasing or decreasing the nuclei of crystallization
3. By accelerating or retarding the setting time by increasing or decreasing the rate of crystal growth.

### Fineness

Finer the particle size, the faster the set, because hemihydrate dissolves faster and the gypsum nuclei will be more numerous and, therefore, more rapid rate of crystallization occurs.

### Impurities

During manufacturing process if the calcination is incomplete and gypsum particles are present or if they are added in the plaster or stone, the setting time will be reduced because of increase in nuclei of crystallization.

## Mixing and Spatulation

Within practical limits, the longer and faster the plaster is mixed, the faster it will set because nuclei of crystallization are broken and well distributed within the mass.

## Water/Powder Ratio

Greater the amount of water used for mixing, the fewer the nuclei per unit volume. Thus, setting time will be prolonged. It also results in a product which is less dense and having reduced strength. Likewise, reducing the water-powder ratio results in decreased setting time by increasing the number of crystals per unit volume.

## Temperature

There is little change between 0°C and 50°C but if the temperature of the plaster water mixture exceeds 50°C, a gradual retardation occurs. At 100°C, the solubilities of hemihydrate and dihydrate are equal, and, in that case; no reaction can occur and the gypsum will not set. At higher temperature range (50°–100°C), the tendency is for any gypsum crystals formed are converted back to the hemihydrate form.

## Modifiers (Accelerators and Retarders)

Modifiers are chemicals added in order to alter some of the properties and make it more acceptable. If the chemical added, reduces the setting time, it is called an accelerator; whereas if it increases the setting time, it is called a retarder.

### Accelerators

Accelerators decrease the setting time of gypsum. The most commonly used accelerators are potassium sulfate. Its effectiveness increases if its concentration is greater than 2%. This is also called as Syngenite.

Another accelerator is *finely powdered gypsum* (terra alba 1%) which accelerates the setting rate by acting as nuclei of crystallization. In low concentrations, salts like sodium sulfate (up to 3.4%), potassium sulfate (2 to 3%) and sodium chloride (up to 2%), are accelerators. They act by making the hemihydrates more soluble. If sodium sulfate and sodium chloride are used with higher concentrations than mentioned, they act as retarders.

Other accelerators are lime (0.1%), gum arabic 1% and potassium sodium tartrate (Rochelle salt).

### Retarders

Retarders form an adsorbed layer on the surface of the hemihydrates to reduce its solubility and on the dihydrates to inhibit its growth. Acetates, borates, citrates, tartrates, and inorganic salts like ferric sulfate, chromic sulfate and aluminum sulfate are retarders. In higher concentrations sodium chloride and sodium sulfate (above 3.4%) also act as retarders by poisoning the nuclei of crystallization.

Borax (1–2%) is the most effective retarder. During setting, it forms a coating of calcium borate around the hemihydrate. Thus, the water cannot come in contact with the hemihydrate.

Colloids such as gelatin, glue, agar, coagulated blood, etc. are effective retarders, presumably which act by nuclei poisoning.

### Viscosity

Impression plaster is used infrequently, but its low viscosity makes it possible to make impressions with a minimum of force on the soft tissues (mucostatic technique).

It has been observed that greater amount of voids are there in the cast made from stone with higher viscosities.

## STRENGTH

Strength of gypsum increases rapidly as the material hardens after the initial setting time. Compressive strength is inversely related to the water/powder ratio of the mix. The greater the amount of water used for the mix, less is the strength of the gypsum. The amount of water used depends on type of gypsum. For example, dental plaster (type II) requires more water than die stone (type IV) and has less strength. There are two types of strength of gypsum depending on the amount of free water content. These two strengths are *wet strength* and *the dry strength.*

### Types of Strength

#### Wet Strength or Green Strength

It is the strength which is obtained when excess water other than that required for hydration of hemihydrates is present in the test specimen. The wet strength (compressive), for dental plaster is 9 MPa and for improved dental stone is 35 MPa.

#### Dry Strength

When this excess water is removed by low temperature drying procedure, the strength obtained thereafter is called dry strength. This type of strength is 2–3 times greater than the wet strength. The strength of gypsum is calculated once it is completely set within approximately 24 hours. As the water evaporates on setting, space or void is formed which is filled by air. These voids negatively influence the strength of the gypsum. Thus correlation exists between the amount of excess water and the final degree of porosity due to voids. That is the reason why plaster is weaker than stone and stone is weaker than die stone. If the W/P ratio of gypsum is increased both its strength and hardness will be reduced. Recent studies have concluded that microwave drying of type IV high strength stone is acceptable at 490W for 60 seconds.

### Factors Affecting Strength

*Following are the factors affecting strength:*

- *Free water content:* The greater the amount of free water in the set stone, the lesser is the strength
- *Temperature:* Gypsum is stable at or below 40°C. Drying the gypsum at higher temperature should be carefully controlled. At 100°C or more there is faster loss of water of crystallization which can cause shrinkage and a reduction in strength
- *Effect of drying:* When gypsum loses 7% of free water on drying there is no appreciable change in the compressive strength but as soon as 7.5% of free water is lost, the strength increases sharply. And if all of the free water which is about 8.8% is lost, the compressive strength of gypsum increases by 55 MPa. The reason for this increase in strength is that the finer dihydrate crystals reinforce the larger dihydrate crystals as the water evaporates. The greatest increase in strength is when final 2% of water is evaporated. The process of drying takes about a week at normal room temperature and humidity. It can be enhanced by increasing the temperature but not beyond 60°C. If the cast is heated above this temperature, then water of hydration is driven off and the strength of the cast is reduced
- *Water/powder ratio:* The more the water, the greater will be the porosity and lesser is the strength
- *Spatulation:* Within limits, the strength increases with increased spatulation
- *Incorporation of accelerators and retarders:* Lowers both the wet and the dry strengths
- *Vacuum mixing:* The compressive strength of high strength dental stone is slightly improved with vacuum mixing.

### Tensile Strength

The tensile strength of gypsum is one fifth the compressive strength under the similar condition because of its brittleness. The one hour wet tensile strength of model plaster is 2.3 MPa as against 4.1 MPa at dry condition after 40 hours. Because of the brittle nature of gypsum, the teeth on the cast tend to fracture and do not bend when it is removed from the impression.

Gypsum when mixed at higher W/P ratio has tensile strength as low as 25% of the corresponding compressive strength when mixed at lower W/P ratio.

## DIMENSIONAL STABILITY

There is very less or nonsignificant change in cast after it has completely set. The cast should not be heated or stored at high temperature above 90°C. In this situation, the dihydrate loses water of crystallization and is converted back to hemihydrate. The changes are more significant in cast made of dental plaster as compared to dental stone or die stone as it contains more water content. The strength of the cast is reduced significantly.

## SURFACE HARDNESS AND ABRASION RESISTANCE

The surface hardness of gypsum is related to its compressive strength. The higher the compressive strength of the gypsum, higher will be its surface hardness. Once the gypsum attains its final setting its surface hardness remains constant till the time it loses most of the excess water through evaporation. Thereafter, the surface hardness increases similar to the compressive strength. Although the surface hardness increases at the faster rate than the compressive strength as the surface reaches the dry state faster than the inner portion.

Recent studies show that on application of the die hardeners on gypsum die, there is slight change in the surface hardness. However, application of die hardener helps in preventing brittle fracture of the die margins.

### Factors Influencing Surface Hardness and Abrasion Resistance

They include:
- *Application of epoxy resin or light-cured dimethacrylate resin:* If the set gypsum is impregnated with epoxy resin or light-cured dimethacrylate resin, its abrasion resistance is increased but the surface hardness and compressive strength is decreased
- *Soaking gypsum casts in glycerin or oils:* Does not improve surface hardness but the surface of the cast or dies becomes smooth
- *Application of hardening solution containing colloidal silica:* Gypsum products improves its surface hardness and abrasion resistance
- *Use of disinfectants:* Certain use of disinfectants can erode the surface of the gypsum casts or dies.

## REPRODUCTION OF DETAIL

Gypsum die does not reproduce surface detail as well as electroformed or epoxy dies because the surface of the set gypsum is porous on a microscopic level. According to ADA specification No. 25—Types I and II gypsum should reproduce a groove of 75 μm in width and type III, IV and V should reproduce groove of 50 μm in width.

Since freshly mixed gypsum is not able to wet the surface of some rubber base impression materials that well, there are chances of air bubble incorporation during pouring.

### Factors Influencing Reproduction of Detail

- *Use of surfactant:* Improves wetting of the rubber base impression with freshly mixed gypsum **(Fig. 4.12)**
- *Use of vibration:* Use of vibration during pouring of the cast reduces the presence of air bubbles
- *Presence of saliva or blood:* On the impression when poured, can result in loss of detail
- *Rising the impression and blowing of excess water:* Can improve the detail recorded by the gypsum die material.

## SETTING EXPANSION

When a gypsum product changes from hemihydrates to dihydrate, there is some kind of setting expansion which occurs. This linear expansion depends on the type of gypsum products and can vary between 0.06–0.5% **(Fig. 4.13)**.

Although, if the equivalent volumes of hemihydrates and water are compared with that of the reaction product (dihydrates), it is found that dihydrates have less volume and density than the hemihydrates which represents a linear change of 2–4%. However, this linear change is

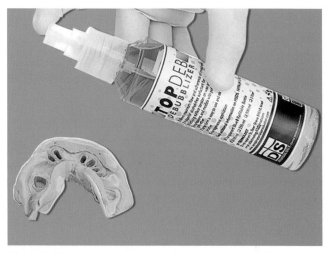

**Fig. 4.12:** Surfactant used on rubber base impression before pouring with gypsum.

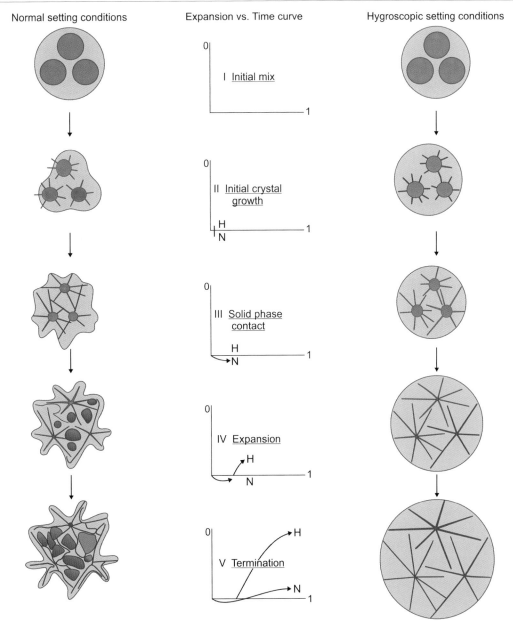

Normal setting conditions        Expansion vs. Time curve        Hygroscopic setting conditions

I  Initial mix

II  Initial crystal
   growth

III  Solid phase
    contact

IV  Expansion

V  Termination

**Fig. 4.13:** Setting expansion in gypsum products
H: hygroscopic setting condition; N: normal setting conditions.

not volumetric contraction but it is setting expansion. This phenomenon is explained on the basis of crystalline theory. The linear expansion can range from 0.06% to 0.5% depending on the type of gypsum product. This expansion is because of crystallization process due to outgrowth of crystals from nuclei of crystallization. The crystals growing from the nuclei enlarge and intermesh with each other. This growth tends to obstruct the growth of adjacent crystals. There are a number of crystals which grow like this resulting in expansion of the entire mass. This helps in setting expansion in the gypsum although the true volume of the mass is less.

$$(CaSO_4)_2\,H_2O + 3H_2O \longrightarrow 2CaSO_4 \cdot 2H_2O$$

| | | |
|---|---|---|
| Equivalent | 105.55  54.21 | 148.405 |
| volume | 159.76 | 148.405 |

The net change in volume is = –7.11%.

## Types of Setting Expansion

### Normal Setting Expansion

This type of setting expansion occurs without water immersion. This expansion occurs because of the growth of the crystals which apply outward thrust or stress which produces the expansion of the entire mass. This crystal impingement and movement result in the production of micropores. The structure immediately after setting is composed of interlocking crystals containing micropores and pores with excess water. Once this excess water is dried during setting, voids are increased.

Under normal conditions, the setting expansion is of following types:
- *Dental plaster:* 0.2–0.3%
- *Dental stone:* 0.15–0.25%
- *Die stone (high strength):* 0.08–0.10%
- *Die stone (high strength and high expansion):* 0.10–0.20%.

### Hygroscopic Setting Expansion

This type of setting expansion occurs under water and it is more than double than the normal setting expansion in air. It is because of the additional crystal growth which occurs under water as they are allowed to grow freely without constraint by the surface tension.

The most accepted theory to explain this procedure is given below:

*Stage I—Initial mix:* The initial mix is represented by the three round particles of hemihydrate surrounded by water.

*Stage II—Initial crystal growth:* The reaction starts and the crystals of the dihydrate start forming. As the setting is occurring under water, the distance between the particles remains unchanged, unlike in normal setting expansion, where particles are drawn closer to each other because of surface tension of water.

*Stage III—Solid phase contact:* In normal expansion, the water around the particles are decreased which allows the particles to be drawn further but are prevented by the outward force of the growing crystal, structures. Whereas in hygroscopic expansion crystals grow freely since water is available.

*Stages IV—Expansion and stage V—termination:* In the normal setting expansion, the crystals intermesh and entangle much faster as compared to those under hygroscopic conditions which grow more freely before the intermeshing and finally prevent further expansion.

### Importance of Setting Expansion in Dentistry

It is undesirable in impression plaster dental plaster and stone, as it will result in an inaccurate cast or change in the occlusal relation if used for mounting.

Increased setting expansion is *desired* in case of investment materials as it helps to compensate the shrinkage of the metal during casting.

### Control of Setting Expansion

It includes:
- *Water/powder ratio:* Lower W/P ratio results in increased setting expansion
- *Spatulation:* Increased spatulation increases setting expansion
- *Addition of chemical modifiers:* Modifiers generally reduce the setting expansion.

Potassium sulfate 4% solution and borax–reduces the setting expansion.

Sodium chloride and ground gypsum increases setting expansion.

## MANIPULATION

The manipulation of gypsum should be done correctly to produce an optimum restoration. The impression surface should be dried of excess water. The rubber base impression is air dried using compressed air whereas the hydrocolloid impression is dried using towel or tissue.

### Proportioning

To achieve optimum properties, the water and the powder should be accurately measured following the manufacturer's instructions. Water is measured by using a graduated cylinder and the powder is measured by using a weighing balance. Preweighed envelopes are also available which help in greater accuracy, reduce material wastage and saves time.

### Addition of Powder to Water

The preferred method is to take measured amount of water in the bowl and the weighed powder is then sifted into the water (**Fig. 4.14**).

### Mixing

#### Hand Mixing

Hand mixing is usually done when powder is sifted into the water. Preweighed amount of water is taken in a flexible, parabolic rubber bowl. A stiff blade spatula with handle is used to accomplish mixing. As the powder is sifted into water, initially hand mixing is done to ensure proper wetting

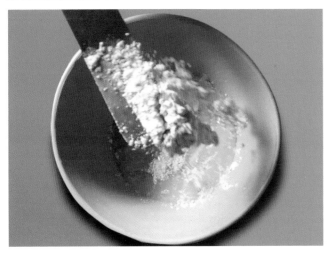

**Fig. 4.14:** Powder is sifted into the water.

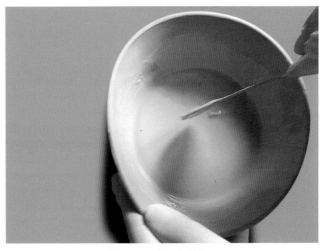

**Fig. 4.15:** Hand mixing.

of powder particles. Then the mix is stirred more vigorously with periodic wiping the inside of the bowl to ensure complete wetting of the powder particles. The mixing is continued to achieve a mix which is smooth, homogeneous and workable. Mixing should be completed within 1 minute. Longer spatulation will reduce the working time and may compromise the property of mixed gypsum (**Fig. 4.15**).

### Vacuum Mixing

This type of mechanical mixing under vacuum is initiated after 15 seconds of hand mixing. It is followed for 20–30 seconds to obtain a smooth, homogeneous mix. Mixing done mechanically under vacuum provides a gypsum mix that is free of air bubbles and homogeneous in consistency (**Fig. 4.16**).

*Advantages of vacuum mixing are:*
- Provides a stronger and denser cast
- Reduces incorporation of air.

Disadvantage of vacuum mixing is its equipment is expensive.

### Pouring of Impression

The mixed gypsum is poured immediately into the rinsed impression under vibration to avoid entrapment of air bubbles (**Fig. 4.17**). The process of pouring should be done slowly in such a manner so that it pushes air ahead of itself as it fills the impressions of the teeth. Usually, the teeth of the cast are poured in dental stone or die stone and the base is poured with model plaster for ease of trimming.

After pouring of the impression, gypsum should be allowed to set for 45–60 minutes before separating the cast

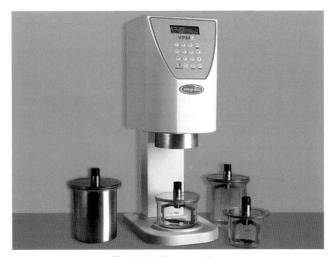

**Fig. 4.16:** Vacuum mixer.

from the impression. After separation the cast should be disinfected.

> **CLINICAL SIGNIFICANCE**
> - Excess gypsum material which is left unused should be collected in the trash and not rinsed down the drain where it can clog the waste pipes
> - Sinks in plaster room should have plaster traps
> - All equipment used for gypsum manipulation should be thoroughly rinsed under running water.

## INFECTION CONTROL

It is important to disinfect the cast if the impression was not disinfected before pouring. Disinfection is necessary to avoid cross-contamination to dental personnel

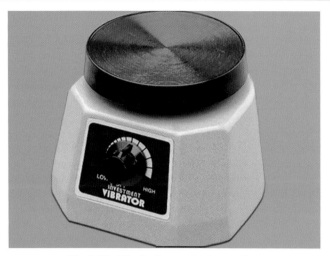

**Fig. 4.17:** Vibrator for pouring impression.

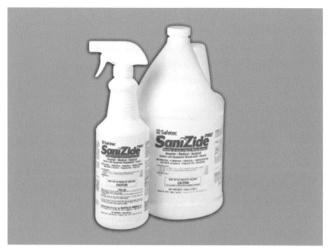

**Fig. 4.18:** Disinfectant used for casts.

by microorganisms with hepatitis B virus, HIV virus, etc. Commonly disinfectants used for stone casts are hypochlorites, iodophors and glutaraldehyde. None of these materials have shown any undesirable effect on the surface accuracy or strength of the gypsum. Recently, some stone materials are marketed which contain disinfectant. These materials are found to be as accurate as the conventional gypsum materials.

Casts are disinfected by immersing in 1:10 dilution of sodium hypochlorite for 30 minutes or using iodophor spray following manufacturer's instructions. Recently, casts are disinfected effectively by using microwave irradiation for 5 minutes at 900W **(Fig. 4.18)**.

## STORAGE OF GYPSUM PRODUCTS

All gypsum products need to be stored in airtight and moisture-proof containers. They should be stored in a dry place because they can absorb moisture from the environment. Hemihydrate powder, if left open, absorbs moisture from the atmosphere and this causes gradual deterioration. In early part of deterioration, the surface particles get hydrated forming a fine coating of gypsum crystals which shorten the setting time. If deterioration proceeds further, the mix will not set properly because insufficient hemihydrate remains to form a coherent set mass. Also, the properties of the gypsum products are compromised.

## CARE FOR THE CAST

The cast should be removed from the impression once its setting reaction is completed. The retrieved casts have relatively constant dimensions at room temperature and

humidity. If the gypsum cast has to be soaked in water, it must be placed in a water bath in which plaster debris is allowed to remain constantly on the bottom of the container to provide a saturated solution of calcium sulfate at all times. This is known as *slurry water*. The slurry water solution is the saturated solution of calcium sulfate. It is usually prepared by placing a broken cast in the water undisturbed for at least 12 hours.

The casts should not be immersed in ordinary water because in this the linear dimension reduces by 0.1% after every 20 minutes. On the other, hand the cast immersed in slurry water shows negligible expansion.

## DISPOSAL OF THE GYPSUM PRODUCTS

The waste gypsum products should be disposed in proper manner. The finer gypsum products can cause respiratory problems. The waste gypsum should be stored in containers or special polythene packs before disposal. The waste gypsum can be sent to industrial recycling plants where dihydrate is converted back to hemihydrate. The recycled gypsum can be used in power plants, in agriculture and in manufacturing of Portland cement.

## SPECIAL GYPSUM PRODUCTS

### Orthodontic Stone or Plaster

Orthodontists usually prefer using white stone or plaster for making study models. This type of gypsum has longer working time to ease in trimming. Sometimes, the models are treated with soap solution to increase the sheen **(Fig. 4.19)**.

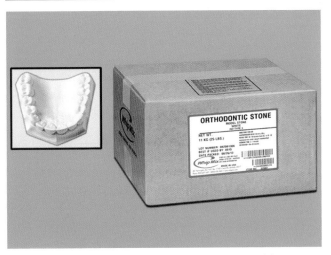

**Fig. 4.19:** Orthodontic stone used to pour models.

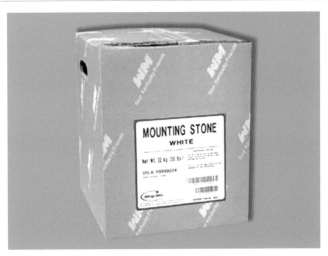

**Fig. 4.20:** Mounting stone.

## Mounting Stone or Plaster

This type of gypsum products are fast setting and have low setting expansion. They are commonly used for mounting casts on the articulators. They have low strength to allow for easy trimming and to facilitate an easy removal of casts from the mounting plates **(Fig. 4.20)**.

## Time Savers

These types of dental stones marketed in 1991 are extremely fast setting dental stone which are ready to use in 5 minutes. They have short working time.

## Resin-added Stones

These types of dental stones are added with small quantity of plastic or resin to reduce its brittleness and improve its resistance to abrasion during carving of wax patterns.

## Balanced Stone

This type of stone contains equal amount of accelerators and retarders.

## Chromatic Stone

This type of dental stone changes its color indicating readiness for use.

## Die Stone—Investment Combination (Divestment)

It is a type of material in which the composition of die stone and investment material is comparable. The divestment is a commercially available gypsum-bonded material which is mixed with colloidal silica liquid to get a die. Wax pattern is made on this die and the entire assembly of pattern and die is invested with divestment material. The material minimizes the distortion of the wax pattern. Since, it is gypsum-bonded, it is only useful for low-fusing gold alloys.

---

## TEST YOURSELF

---

### Essay Questions

1. Classify gypsum products. Describe each gypsum products along with their uses.
2. Differentiate between normal setting expansion and hygroscopic setting expansion of gypsum products.
3. Define setting time? Describe various methods of measuring the setting time in gypsum products.
4. Differentiate the properties of alpha and beta hemihydrates.?

### Short Notes

1. Die stone.
2. Divestment stone.
3. Green strength.
4. Vicat needle.
5. Setting reaction of gypsum products.
6. Crystallization theory.

## Multiple Choice Questions

1. The most common reason for teeth breaking when a stone or plaster model is removed from the impression is due to:
   A. Use of incorrect mixing technique
   B. Removal of cast early from the impression
   C. Incorrect w/p ratio
   D. Waiting too long to remove the cast from the impression

2. The area of the diagnostic cast that records the hard and soft tissues is called as:
   A. Art portion
   B. Base
   C. Anatomical portion
   D. Impression

3. The manufacturing process of gypsum products includes all of the following, *except*:
   A. Use of heat
   B. Use of pressure
   C. Addition of water
   D. Grinding of particles

4. All of the following are differences between plaster and stone, *except*:
   A. Different setting time
   B. Different color
   C. Different mixing technique
   D. Different particle size

5. Teralba is:
   A. Pieces of set gypsum added to plaster of Paris
   B. Metal containing titanium and aluminum
   C. A constituent modelling wax
   D. Allergic reaction to orthodontic wires

6. Dental stone and plaster differ mainly in:
   A. Solubility
   B. Shelf-life
   C. Chemical formula
   D. Particle size and porosity

7. Impression plaster is:
   A. Manufactured by heating calcium dihydrate under steam pressure
   B. More mucostatic than alginate
   C. Borax is used to control setting expansion
   D. All of the above

8. When water/power ratio of dental plaster increases?
   A. Strength and setting time increases
   B. Strength increases but setting time decreases
   C. Strength decreases but setting time increases
   D. Both strength and setting time decreases

9. High dry strength and hardness of type IV compared to type II stone is due to:
   A. Less amount of eater required in solution for wetting the mixture

B. Difference in chemical composition
   C. Difference in mixing times
   D. All of the above

10. Setting of plaster of Paris is due to:
    A. Difference in solubility between hemihydrate and dihydrate
    B. Interaction between hemihydrate and water
    C. Loss of water from hemihydrate
    D. Indirect interaction between hemihydrate and dihydrate

11. If a stone cast is kept under tap water the:
    A. Linear dimension may increase
    B. Linear dimension may decrease
    C. Linear dimension is constant
    D. Change in linear dimension is variable

12. Numerous air bubble on die stone cast when retrieved from polysulfide impression is due to:
    A. Surfactant used on impression before pouring the cast
    B. Did not use wiping motion during mixing of the stone
    C. Mix was vibrated for 15 seconds before pouring
    D. Used stone contaminated with moisture

13. All of the following is considered as positive reproduction of the dental structures, *except*:
    A. A die
    B. An impression
    C. A working cast
    D. A diagnostic cast

14. Diagnostic casts can be used for all of the following, *except*:
    A. Patient education
    B. Checking progress of treatment
    C. Fabrication of orthodontic appliances
    D. As legal document

15. The most appropriate type gypsum product used for orthodontic casts are:
    A. Type I
    B. Type II
    C. Type III
    D. Type IV

16. Initial setting time is measured by:
    A. Loss of gloss
    B. At the end of exothermic reaction
    C. Change in color
    D. None of the above

---

## ANSWERS

| | | | |
|---|---|---|---|
| 1. B | 2. C | 3. C | 4. C |
| 5. A | 6. D | 7. B | 8. C |
| 9. A | 10. A | 11. B | 12. B |
| 13. B | 14. C | 15. C | 16. A |

# BIBLIOGRAPHY

1. Abdelaziz K, Attia A, Coomb E. Evaluation of disinfected casts poured in gypsum with gum Arabic and calcium hydroxide additives. J Prosthet Dent. 2004;92:27-34.

2. Anusavice KJ. Phillip's science of dental materials, 11th edition. Philadelphia Saunders, 2003.

3. Berg E, Neilson O, Skaug N. High-level microwave disinfection of dental gypsum casts. Int J Prosthodont. 2005;18:520-5.

4. Buchanan AS, Worner HK. Changes in the composition and setting characteristics of plaster of Paris on the exposure to high humidity atmospheres. J Dent Res. 1945;24:65-75.

5. Chan TK, Darvell BW. Effect of storage conditions on calcium sulphate hemihydrate-containing products. Dent Mater. 2001;17:134-41.

6. Chong JA, Chong MP, Docking AR. The surface of gypsum cast in alginate impression. Dent Pract. 1965;16:107.

7. Coomb EC, Smith DC. Some properties of gypsum plasters. Br Dent J. 1964;15:237.

8. Earnshaw R, Smith DC. The tensile and compressive strength of plaster and stone. Aus Dent J. 1966;11:415-22.

9. Fairhurst CW. Compressive properties of dental gypsum. J Dent Res. 1960;39:812-24.

10. Fan PL, Powers JM, Reid BC. Surface mechanical properties of stone, resin and metal dies. J Am Dent Assoc. 1981;103(3):408-11.

11. Jorgensen KD. Studies on the setting of plaster of Paris. Odontol Tidskr. 1953;61(5):304-46.

12. Lindquist JT, Brennan RE, Phillips RW. Influence of mixing techniques on some physical properties of plaster. J Prosthet Dent. 1953;3:274.

13. Lindquist TJ, Stanford CM, Knox E. Influence of surface hardener on gypsum abrasion resistance and water sorption. J Prosthet Dent. 2003;90(5):441-6.

14. Lindquist TJ, Stanford CM, Mostafavi H, Xie XJ. Abrasion resistance of a resin impregnated type IV gypsum in comparison to conventional products. J Prosthet Dent. 2002;87:319-22.

15. Lucas MG, Arioli-Filho JN, Nogueira SS, Batista AU, Pereira Rde P. Effect of incorporation of disinfectant solutions on setting time, linear dimensional stability and detailed reproduction in dental stone casts. J Prosthodont. 2009;18:521-6.

16. Mahler DB, Ady AB. Explanation for the hygroscopic setting expansion of dental gypsum products. J Dent Res. 1960;39:578-89.

17. Mahler DB, Asgarzadeh K. The volumetric contraction of dental gypsum materials on setting. J Dent Res. 1953;32(3):354-61.

18. Mahler DB. Hardness and flow properties of gypsum materials. J Prosthet Dent. 1951;1:188-95.

19. Mahler DB. Plaster of Paris and stone materials. Int Dent J. 1955;5:241.

20. O' Brien WJ. Dental materials and their selection, 4th edition. Chicago: Quintessence Publishing, 1997.

21. Peyton FA, Leibold JP, Ridgley GV. Surface hardness, compressive strength, and abrasion resistance of indirect die stones. J Prosthet Dent. 1952;2:381.

22. Phillips RW, Ito BY. Factors affecting the surface of stone dies poured in hydrocolloid impressions. J Prosthet Dent. 1952;2:390.

23. Sanad ME, Combe EC, Grant AA. The use of additives to improve the mechanical properties of gypsum products. J Dent Res. 1982;61:808-10.

24. Smith DC. The setting of plaster. Dent Pract. 1963;13:473.

25. Stern MA, Johnson GH, Toolson LB. An evaluation of dental stones after repeated exposure to spray disinfectants. Part I: Abrasion and compressive strength. J Prosthet Dent. 1991;65:713-8.

26. Sweeney WT, Taylor DF. Dimensional changes in dental stone and plaster. J Dent Res. 1950;29:749-55.

27. Torrance A, Darvell BW. Effect of humidity on calcium sulfate hemihydrate. Aus Dent J. 1990;35:230-5.

28. Von Fraunhofer JA, Spiers RR. Strength testing of dental stone: a comparison of compressive, tensile, transverse and shear strength tests. J Biomed Mater Res. 1983;17:293-9.

29. Wiegman-Ho L, Katelaar JA. The kinetics of the hydration of calcium sulfate hemihydrates investigated by an electric conductance method. J Dent Res. 1982;61:36-40.

30. Winkler MM, Monaghan P, Gilbert JL, Lautenschlager EP. Comparison of four techniques for monitoring the setting kinetics of gypsum. J Prosthet Dent. 1998;79:532-6.

31. Worner HK. Dental Plaster II. The setting phenomenon, properties after mixing with water, methods of testing. Aus Dent J. 1942;46:35.

32. Worner HK. Dental Plasters I. General, manufacture and characteristics before mixing with water. Aus Dent J. 1942:46:1.

33. Yap AU, Yap SH, Teo JC, Tay CM, Ng KL, Thean HP. Microwave drying of high strength dental stone: effects on dimensional accuracy. Oper Dent 2003;28(2):193-9.

# Dental Waxes

*'Your attitude determines your altitude.'*

**—Unknown**

## INTRODUCTION

Dental waxes have wide application in restorative dentistry. Different types of waxes available are inlay pattern wax, bite registration wax, boxing wax, baseplate wax, sticky wax, casting wax, etc. Each type of wax is specially formulated to be used in specific situation.

Dental waxes may be composed of natural and synthetic waxes, fats, fatty acids, natural or synthetic resins and pigments of various types. The working characteristic of each wax is defined by mixing proper proportions of natural and synthetic waxes and resins. The chemical composition and proportion of natural and synthetic waxes impart particular physical properties to the wax, which is to be used for specific purpose.

## DEFINITION

*Dental wax is defined as a low molecular weight ester of fatty acids derived from natural and synthetic components such as petroleum derivatives that soften to a plastic state at a relatively low temperature.*

## HISTORICAL BACKGROUND

Waxes were regarded as valuable natural substance for more than 2000 years. Beeswax is one of the oldest wax known by human beings. Roman and Greek literature has described waxes used in various forms. Waxes were used for softening skin, binding flutes, coatings on arts, making sculptures, candles, etc. In 3000 B.C. beeswax was used by Egyptians in Mummification process. About 1700 A.D. Gottfried Purmann used waxes for prosthetic work. The use of waxes were scientifically investigated in the nineteenth century. In 1935, synthetic liquid paraffin wax was produced by Fischer –Tropsch. Synthetic waxes were found to be more uniform and homogenous in composition than the natural waxes.

## USES

- Used for bite registration
- Used for direct wax patterns for casting
- Used as impression material for edentulous areas
- Used to make indirect wax patterns for casting
- Used for beading and boxing
- Used as base plates for complete dentures
- Used for blocking out undercuts
- Used for mock up in treatment planning.

## COMPOSITION

Dental waxes are composed of natural waxes, synthetic waxes, natural resins, oil, fats, gums and coloring agents. They are organic polymers consisting of hydrocarbon and their derivatives (e.g. alcohols and esters). The average molecular weight of waxes can vary between 400 and 4000. Natural waxes are those waxes which are found in nature whereas synthetic waxes are those that are artificially produced in the laboratory **(Table 5.1).**

**Table 5.1:** Components of dental waxes.

| Natural waxes | Synthetic waxes | Additives |
|---|---|---|
| **Minerals**<br>• Paraffin<br>• Microcrystalline<br>• Barnsdall<br>• Ozokerite<br>• Ceresin<br>• Montan | Acrawax C | **Stearic acid**<br>• Glyceryl tristearate |
| **Plants**<br>• Carnauba<br>• Ouricury<br>• Candelilla<br>• Japan wax<br>• Cocoa butter | Aerosol OT | **Oil**<br>• Turpentine |
| **Insect**<br>• Beeswax | Castor wax | Color |
| **Animal**<br>• Spermaceti | Flexowax C | Natural resins |
|  | Epolene N-10 | **Resin**<br>• Copal<br>• Dammar<br>• Sandarac<br>• Mastic<br>• Shellac<br>• Kauri |
|  | Albacer | **Synthetic resins**<br>• Elvax<br>• Polyethylene<br>• Polystyrene |
|  | Aldo 33, Durawax 1032 |  |

## GENERAL PROPERTIES

Waxes have certain important properties which are required for specific use in dentistry. Some of the important properties are:
• Melting range
• Mechanical properties
• Thermal expansion
• Flow
• Residual stresses
• Ductility.

## Melting Range

• Waxes have melting range rather melting point. The lower range of melting temperature usually controls the applicability of a given wax formulation
• Addition of different waxes can alter their melting range
• The flow of waxes is dependent on temperature besides the forces applied on it. Waxes contract on cooling and expands on heating

• Waxes have highest coefficient of thermal expansion when compared to the other materials in dentistry. They posses high coefficient of thermal expansion and high residual stress
• High coefficient of thermal expansion causes distortion of the fabricated wax patterns. For this reason the wax patterns should be invested as soon as possible. If investing is to be delayed then the patterns should be stored at lower temperature to minimize distortion. If the wax pattern is stored in a refrigerator then first the patterns should be allowed to come to room temperature before investing otherwise the patterns will distort or fracture on removal
• As the wax patterns used in lost wax technique are burnout, wax should not leave any residue behind as this can affect the quality of the restoration
• Crystalline waxes develop greater internal stresses if they are manipulated below the transition temperature.

## Mechanical Properties

• Mechanical properties of waxes are highly dependent on the temperature
• Properties of waxes such as elastic modulus, proportional limit and compressive strength are relatively low as compared to other materials
• As the temperature is reduced, the mechanical properties are improved
• The elastic modulus of carnauba wax is reduced from 1790 to 760 MPa when temperature is raised from 23 to 37°C
• Likewise elastic modulus of paraffin is reduced from 310 to 28 MPa when temperature rises between 23 and 30°C.

**CLINICAL SIGNIFICANCE**
• Inlay wax should be brittle because it should fracture rather than distort on removal from the undercut area
• Dental waxes should show adequate flow at molding temperature but should not or minimally flow at mouth temperature
• In pattern fabrication of cast partial dentures, waxes of different elastic moduli should be used to reduce non-uniform deformation of the wax pattern.

## Thermal Expansion

• Waxes expand with rise in temperature and contract with decrease in temperature
• Dental waxes and their components have largest coefficient of thermal expansion as compared to other materials used in restorative dentistry
• Different waxes have different rates of thermal expansion in different temperature ranges.

## Flow

- Defined as *relative ability of wax to plastically deform when it is heated slightly above mouth temperature*
- Flow is a measure of ability of wax to deform under light forces
- Flow of waxes is dependent on the temperature of wax, amount of force applied and the duration of force application
- It increases with increase in temperature and force. As the temperature approaches its softening range, wax may flow under its own weight
- Type I direct inlay wax should have good flow to reproduce the details of the cavity preparation
- But when it is cooled to mouth temperature, it should not flow so as to minimize the possibility of distortion during removal of the pattern from the prepared cavity
- Likewise, yellow beeswax does not extensively flow until it reaches 38°C and flows about 7% at 40°C. Beeswax is one of the primary constituent of impression wax.

## Residual Stress

- It is the internal stress which is independent of applied force
- Residual stress exists in wax pattern regardless of the method by which it is fabricated
- When the wax specimen is held under compressive force during cooling, atoms and molecules are forced closer to each other. As the specimen cools to room temperature and the force is removed, the movements of the molecules are restricted resulting in residual stresses
- When the wax specimen is heated, residual stresses are released and add to the normal thermal expansion resulting in greater expansion than normal.

*Prevention of residual stresses in a wax pattern:*
- Waxes should not be carved or burnished at temperatures well below their melting range
- Wax patterns are carved with warm (37°C) instruments, and melted wax is added in small increments to prevent rapid or uneven cooling, which promotes residual stresses
- To prevent the release of stress already created, wax patterns should not be subjected to temperature changes or should not be stored at high temperatures
- The time between finishing and investing the pattern should be minimized (<30 minutes) because longer storage times allow residual stresses to be released
- If conditions of time or temperature of the storage of the pattern are suspect, details of the pattern such as proximal contacts and margins should be refinished.

## Ductility

- Ductility of wax increases with the increase in temperature
- Waxes with lower melting temperature have greater ductility than those with higher melting temperatures
- Blended waxes with components having wider melting ranges have greater ductility than those blended waxes with narrow melting range.

## Classification of Dental Waxes

- *According to the origin*
  - Natural waxes
    - Mineral
    - Plant
    - Animal
    - Insect
  - Synthetic waxes
- *According to the application*
  - Pattern wax
    - Inlay wax—Type I and Type II
    - Casting wax
    - Resin wax
    - Baseplate wax—Type I, Type II and Type III
  - Processing wax
    - Boxing wax
    - Carding wax
    - Sticky wax
    - Block out wax
    - Utility wax
    - White wax
  - Impression wax
    - Corrective wax
    - Bite registration wax.

# NATURAL WAXES

## Paraffin Wax (Fig. 5.1)

These waxes form major component of most of the waxes used in dentistry. They are Obtained from high boiling point fractions of petroleum

### Composition

They are straight chain hydrocarbon with 26–30 carbon atoms of the methane series. They also contains small amount of microcrystalline or amorphous phase.

### Properties

- Melting range varies between 40 and 71°C
- Melting temperature usually increases with increasing molecular weight. But presence of oil lowers the melting temperature

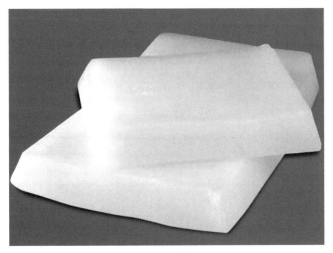

**Fig. 5.1:** Paraffin wax.

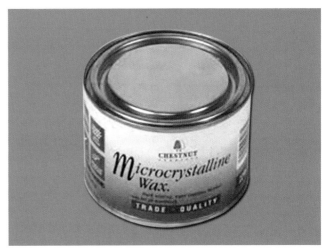

**Fig. 5.2:** Microcrystalline wax.

- Waxes used in dentistry are refined waxes which have less than 0.5% oil
- Has low molecular weight but is sufficient enough to be solid at room temperature

*Drawbacks*

- Not pure because it is difficult to isolate a single molecular weight hydrocarbon.
- Flakes easily on carving and do not give a smooth or shiny surface.
- On solidification there is volumetric contraction ranging between 11% and 15%.

## Microcrystalline Waxes (Fig. 5.2)

These waxes are amorphous waxes which are derived from heavier oils used in the petroleum industry or from the bottom of crude oil tankers.

*Composition*

Consists of Branched chain hydrocarbon with 41–50 carbon atoms, saturated monocyclic and polycyclic compounds and normal alkanes.

*Properties*

- Melting range varies between 60° and 91°C
- These waxes are more tougher and flexible than the paraffin wax
- Have affinity for oil and their hardness and tackiness can change by adding oil
- They are darker in color with high viscosity

*Advantages*

They show less volumetric shrinkage during solidification than the paraffin wax.

## Barnsdall Wax

It is a microcrystalline wax which is used to increase the melting range and hardness and limit the flow of paraffin wax. Their melting point ranges between 70°C and 74°C.

## Ceresin Wax

- These are straight and branched chain paraffin which have higher molecular weight and greater hardness than hydrocarbon waxes
- They are used to increase the melting range of paraffin waxes.

## Montan Wax

- These waxes are mixtures of long chain esters with high molecular weight of alcohols, acids and resins extracted from lignite
- These waxes are mineral waxes which are hard, brittle and lustrous
- They are similar to the plant waxes
- They help in improving the hardness and melting range of paraffin waxes.

## Carnauba Wax

These waxes are derived from leaves of selected variety of tropical palms.

### Composition

Composed of straight chain esters, alcohol, acids and hydrocarbons.

### Properties

- Characterized by high hardness, brittleness and high melting temperatures
- Help in increasing the melting range and hardness of paraffin wax
- It helps in reducing the flow of paraffin wax at mouth temperatures

## Candelilla Wax

- Contains 40–50% of hydrocarbons containing 29–33 carbon atoms with free alcohols, acids, esters and lactones
- They help in hardening of paraffin wax but are not effective in increasing its melting range.

## Japan Wax and Cocoa Butter

- In true sense they are not waxes but are fats
- Japan wax consists of glycerides of palmitic and stearic acids and have high molecular weight acids
- Cocoa butter consists of glycerides of stearic, palmitic, oleic, lauric and lower fatty acids
- Japan wax is tough, malleable and sticky material which melts at 51°C whereas cocoa butter is a brittle material at room temperature
- Japan wax when mixed with paraffin wax improves its tackiness and emulsifying ability
- Cocoa butter is used to protect glass ionomer cements from moisture during its setting and to protect the soft tissues against desiccation.

## Beeswax

It is primary insect wax used in dentistry which is obtained from the honey combs.

### Composition

It is a complex mixture of esters having saturated and unsaturated hydrocarbons and high molecular weight organic acids.

### Properties

- It is brittle at room temperature but is plastic at mouth temperature
- It has intermediate melting range of 60–70°C
- Used to modify the properties of paraffin wax. The flow of paraffin wax is significantly reduced by adding beeswax
- It is major constituent of sticky wax.

## Animal Wax

- Not commonly used in dentistry
- Animal wax like the spermaceti wax is obtained from the sperm whale
- This wax is used to coat the dental floss during its manufacturing.

## Synthetic Wax

- Synthetic waxes are complex organic compounds of varied chemical compositions
- They possess similar physical properties to natural wax but differ in chemical composition
- These are highly refined waxes which have limited use in dentistry in contrast to natural waxes which are usually contaminated and are widely used
- Types of synthetic waxes include:
    - Polyethylene waxes
    - Polyoxyethylene glycol waxes
    - Hydrogenated waxes
    - Wax esters formed after reaction of fatty alcohols and acids.

## Gums

- These are viscous, amorphous exudates that are obtained from plants which hardens when exposed to air
- Mostly formulations contain carbohydrates which when mixed with water either dissolves or form sticky viscous liquid
- Gum Arabic and Tragacanth are natural occurring gums which do not resemble waxes.
- Gum dammer is a copal like resin which is derived from dipterocarpaceous trees found mainly in Southast Asia. It is added to inlay pattern waxes to provide smoothness and gloss and reduce flakiness.

## Fats

- Composed of esters of various fatty acids with glycerol and are called as glycerides
- They are tasteless, colorless and odourless in pure form
- They are softer and have lower melting temperature than waxes
- They can be used to increase the melting range and hardness of compounded wax.

## Resins

- Resins can be of two types—(1) natural resins and (2) synthetic resins
- Natural resins are complex amorphous mixture of organic substances that are obtained from trees and plants
- Types of natural resins—dammer, rosin, sandarac, shellac
- Shellac is obtained from insects

- Natural resins are mixed with waxes to be used in dentistry
- They are relatively insoluble in water
- Synthetic resins are added to paraffin waxes to improve their toughness, film forming characteristics and melting range
- For example, polyethylene and vinyl resins
- Natural and synthetic resins can be dissolved in organic solvents to be used as cavity liners
- Copal resin can be used as cavity liner.

## PATTERN WAX

- An artificial restoration is first made of pattern wax and then this pattern is casted with permanent and durable material such as cobalt chromium, nickel chromium alloy or acrylic resin using lost wax technique
- Pattern waxes include inlay, resin, casting and base plate wax
- Inlay waxes are used to make inlay, onlay, crown and pontics by lost wax technique
- Pattern resin is used to make direct or indirect pattern of crowns, custom post, inlay, etc. These patterns are casted by lost wax technique
- Casting waxes are used for thin sections of certain removable and fixed partial denture pattern
- Base plate wax is used in fabrication of occlusal rims and in construction of full denture patterns
- Two major qualities of pattern waxes are thermal change in dimension and tendency to warp or distort on standing.

## INLAY PATTERN WAX

*It is a specialized dental wax that can be applied to dies to form direct or indirect patterns for the lost wax technique used for casting metals or hot pressing of ceramics* **(Fig. 5.3)**.

### Ideal Requirements

- Wax should be uniform when softened
- Color of the wax should contrast with that of the die or prepared tooth. This aids in better finishing of the margins
- When softened wax is molded, it should not flake or have rough surface
- Wax should be carved in very thin layer without chipping
- During burnout, the wax should be completely eliminated without leaving residue behind
- Wax pattern should be dimensionally stable and rigid at all times until it is eliminated

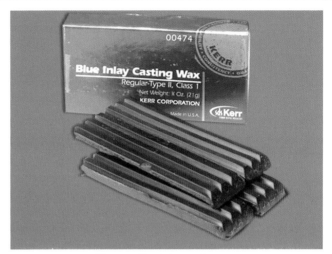

**Fig. 5.3:** Blue inlay casting wax.

- Should have low coefficient of thermal expansion
- Should not adhere to the cavity walls
- Should harden at mouth temperature and remain plastic at temperatures slightly above the mouth temperatures.

### Composition

#### Paraffin Wax (40–60%)

- Main ingredient of inlay wax. It has concentration of 40–60%
- Wax is obtained in wide melting or softening range depending on the molecular weight and distribution of various constituents
- When trimmed it is likely to flake and give a rough surface. Therefore, other modifying agents are added to give smoothness to the wax.

#### Gum Dammar (1%)

- Added in small amounts 1%
- They are natural resins which are added to paraffin to improve its smoothness in molding and to make it more resistant to flaking and carving
- It improves toughness and increases the smoothness and shine of the surface.

#### Carnauba Wax (25%)

- Natural wax obtained from plants
- This type of wax is quite hard and has relatively high melting point
- It is combined with paraffin to decrease the flow at mouth temperature
- It aids in enhancing the glossiness of the wax surface.

### Candelilla Wax

- Added to paraffin to partially or completely replace carnauba wax
- It is less hard and has lower melting point than carnauba wax.

### Ceresin (10%)

- Added to replace part of paraffin
- Improve the toughness and carving of the inlay wax.

### Synthetic Resin

- Currently, carnauba wax is replaced by synthetic wax because they have better uniformity
- Synthetic wax compatible with paraffin are complex nitrogen derivatives of higher fatty acids and other esters of acids derived from montan wax
- As these waxes have higher melting point, more paraffin wax can be incorporated which improves the general qualities of the wax.

## Classification of Dental Inlay Casting Wax

According to American Dental Association (ADA) specification no. 4, dental inlay casting wax is classified as:

*Type I*: Medium wax—used in direct technique
*Type II*: Soft wax—used in indirect technique.

## Supplied As

Sticks of deep blue, green or purple colors which are 7.5 cm long and 0.64 cm in diameter. Are also, available in the form of pellets, cones or small metal ointment jars **(Fig. 5.4)**.

## Properties

### Flow

- It is the relative ability of wax to plastically deform when it is heated slightly above mouth temperature
- Inlay wax should ideally show plasticity or flow slightly above the mouth temperature

- According to ADA specification no.4 requirements for flow of inlay wax is given below:
  - Type I and Type II inlay wax should exhibit flow between 70% and 90% at 45°C
  - Type I should show maximum flow of 20% at 40°C and Type II should show minimum flow 50% at 40°C
  - At 37°C, Type I wax should not flow more than 1%
  - At 30°C Type II wax should not flow more than 1%
  - Each type of wax exhibits sharp transition temperature at which it loses its plasticity. Soft wax has lower transition temperature than hard wax
  - Unlike the metal structure, inlay wax consists of crystalline and amorphous structural regions displaying limited ordering of the molecules
  - Wax lacks rigidity and can flow even at room temperature under stress
  - At lower temperature, 37°C wax permits carving and removal of the pattern from the prepared cavity
  - At higher temperature, 45°C wax should be inserted into the prepared cavity so that it can easily flow and reproduce accurate details.

## Thermal Properties

- Inlay waxes are softened with heat and is inserted either directly into the prepared cavity in tooth or indirectly into the die
- Thermal conductivity of wax is low. Time is needed to uniformly heat the wax and to cool the wax to room temperature
- Inlay wax exhibit high coefficient of thermal expansion. Wax shown expansion of 0.7% with increase of 20°C temperature and shows contraction of 0.35% when it is cooled from 37°C to 25°C
- Inlay wax shows thermal expansion or contraction per degree temperature more than any other material used in dentistry
- This is one of the inherent disadvantages of the wax especially if it is used directly in the mouth.

### Factors Affecting Thermal Expansion

- Wax cooled under pressure
- Wax reheated after cooling under pressure
- Temperature of the die
- Method of pressure application for cooling the wax.

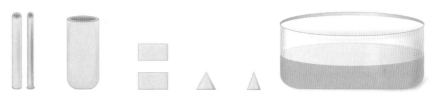

**Fig. 5.4:** Inlay wax is supplied in form of stick, pellets, cones and jars.

## Wax Distortion

- Wax distortion or warping is one of the most critical problems which can occur during wax pattern formation or removal
- This distortion or warping is due to thermal changes and relaxation of residual stresses developed during formation of pattern

### Factors Causing Release of Stresses

- Contraction on cooling
- Occluded air
- Changes occurring during molding, carving and removal of pattern
- Time and temperature of pattern storage
- Wax distortion is present in all dental waxes but is more critical for inlay waxes
- Waxes possess the property of *Elastic Memory*, i.e. tendency of the wax to partially return to their original shape after manipulation.

**CLINICAL SIGNIFICANCE**
- A stick of inlay wax is softened and bent into a horseshoe shape and then chilled in this position. If this wax is placed in water at room temperature for several hours, it has tendency to straighten up **(Figs. 5.5A and B)**
- Patterns made with soft waxes are slightly larger and rougher and also are more sensitive to temperature change than hard waxes.

*Methods to minimize wax distortion are:*
- To invest the pattern immediately after completely shaped
- Pattern should be stored in refrigerator
- Refrigerated pattern should be warmed to room temperature before investing
- Margins of stored pattern should be readapted
- By uniformly heating wax at 50°C for 15 minutes and then applying wax on warm die in increments
- By using warm instruments for carving.

### Manipulation of Inlay Wax

It can be accomplished using either direct technique or indirect technique. For manipulating inlay wax dry heat is usually preferred over the use of water bath. If water bath is used, there are chances of incorporation of water droplets which may lead to splatter on flaming and may distort the pattern.

### Direct Technique

- The inlay stick is softened uniformly over the flame by rotating it until the surface appears shiny **(Fig. 5.6)**
- Softened wax is then shaped according to the prepared cavity
- Soft wax is held in the cavity with finger pressure. It is allowed to cool gradually to mouth temperature
- Sudden rapid cooling with cold water should be avoided as it may result in differential contraction and development of internal stresses
- After the wax has hardened, the pattern is carefully removed with minimum distortion
- Avoid touching the removed pattern with fingers as much as possible to prevent temperature changes.

### Indirect Technique

- Wax patterns are made indirectly over the lubricated die
- Lubricated die can be dipped in melted wax or can be applied using instrument **(Fig. 5.7)**
- Prepared cavity is overfilled with wax and once it is hardened it is carved to proper contour using appropriate carving instrument **(Figs. 5.8A and B)**
- During carving care is taken so that the surface of the die is not abraded
- The completed wax patterns are polished with the help of silk cloth.

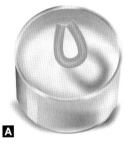 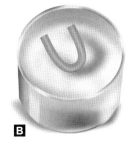

**Figs. 5.5A and B:** Effects of temperature change on wax: (A) Inlay wax stick bent into horse-shoe shape at room temperature; (B) Wax tends to relax after 24 hours.

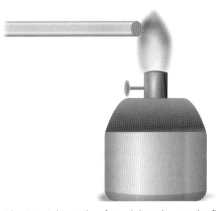

**Fig. 5.6:** Inlay stick softened directly over the flame.

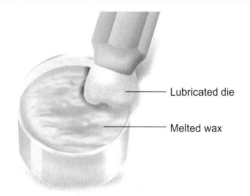

**Fig. 5.7:** Lubricated die dipped in melted wax.

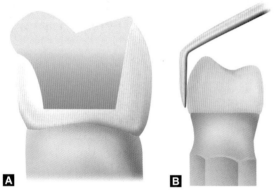

**Fig. 5.8A:** (A). Prepared cavity overfilled with wax; (B). Carving of completed wax pattern.

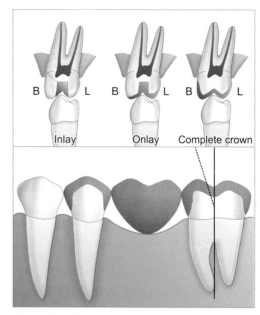

**Fig. 5.9:** Wax pattern fabrication for inlays, onlays and partial dentures.

## Uses

- To fabricate wax patterns for inlays, onlays, fixed partial dentures and single crowns **(Fig. 5.9)**
- Can be used to fabricate pattern by both direct and indirect wax techniques
- Can be used in casting complex restorations.

### Removable Partial Denture Casting Wax

Casting waxes are used to fabricate patterns for metallic framework of removable partial dentures (RPD). These waxes differ from inlay pattern waxes in their physical properties **(Fig. 5.10)**.

### *Supplied As (Fig. 5.11)*

- Wax sheets of 0.40, 0.32 mm thickness
- These waxes are available in the form of round, half round, half pear shaped and wires of 10 cm length
- Preformed meshwork, clasps, grid, etc.

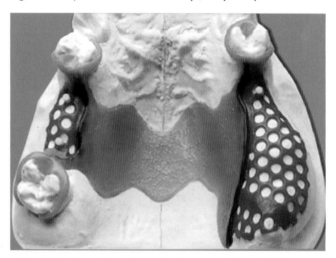

**Fig. 5.10:** Wax pattern fabrication for removable partial denture.

### *Uses*

- To make patterns for metallic framework of removable partial dentures
- Used for postdamming of maxillary denture impressions
- To check high points of articulation
- To produce wax bites of cusp tips for articulation of stone casts.

### *Properties*

- Casting waxes possess certain degree of tackiness which helps in adaptation on the refractory cast

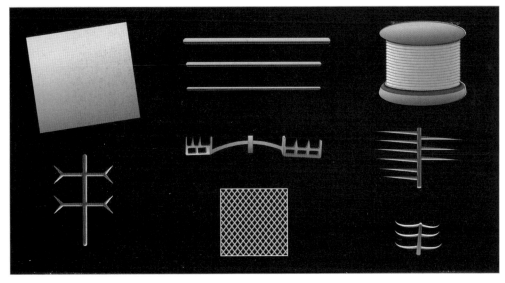

**Fig. 5.11:** RPD casting wax available in different sizes and shapes.

- They show maximum of 10% flow at 35°C and minimum of 60% flow at 38°C
- They have high ductility, i.e. they can be bent double on itself without fracture at 23°C
- Like inlay wax, these waxes vaporize completely without leaving any residue except carbon at 500°C.

## Baseplate Wax

Also called as modelling wax. These waxes are widely used in the fabrication of complete dentures.

### Uses

- To fabricate occlusal rims **(Fig. 5.12)**
- To produce desired contour of denture after teeth are arranged in place
- To check and transfer bite on the articulator
- To make patterns for orthodontic appliances and other prosthesis.

### Composition

- Paraffin-based wax or Ceresin—80%
- Beeswax—12%
- Carnauba wax—2.5%
- Natural or synthetic resins—3%
- Microcrystalline or synthetic waxes—2.5%.

### Supplied As

Pink or red sheets of dimensions—7.6 × 15 × 0.13 cm.

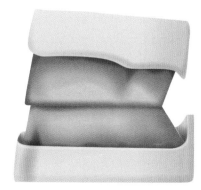

**Fig. 5.12:** Occlusal rim fabricated with modeling wax.

### Classification of Baseplate Wax

According to ADA Specification No. 24, baseplate wax is of following types:
*Class I:* Soft—used for building contours and veneers
*Class II:* Hard—used to fabricate patterns directly in mouth in normal climate
*Class III:* Extra hard—used to fabricate patterns directly in mouth in hot climate.

### Requirements

- Should produce smooth surface after gentle flaming
- Should be easily trimmed with sharp instrument
- Should not irritate the oral tissues
- Sheets should not adhere with each other
- Should not leave residue on porcelain or acrylic teeth
- Color of wax should not impregnate plaster.

## Boxing Wax

Also called as carding wax. It is used to build vertical wall around the impression to produce the desired size and form of the base of the cast. This procedure is called as boxing. It helps in preserving certain landmarks of the impression.

Boxing procedure consists of adapting a long strip of wax around the impression below its peripheral height and then adapting wide strip of wax producing the form around the impression **(Fig. 5.13)**.

### Properties

They have slight tackiness and have sufficient strength and toughness for better manipulation. These waxes are readily adaptable to the impression made with zinc oxide eugenol at room temperature.

### Procedure

* Beading wax of 4 mm width is adapted 3–4 mm below the border of the impression
* Tongue space is adapted in case of the mandibular impression
* Beading wax is sealed to the impression with a wax spatula
* Then a strip of boxing wax is adapted around the beading wax. The height is adapted such that wax strip extends approximately 13 mm above the highest point on the impression.
* Vacuum mixed stone is poured into the boxed impression.

### Advantages

* Preserves border extension
* Preserves border thickness and landmarks
* Controls form and thickness of the base of the cast
* Preserves stone.

## Utility Wax

Also called as Periphery wax or Rope wax. These waxes are soft, pliable and adhesive. They are often used to adjust contour of standard perforated tray to make impression with alginate. They can be used to build up post dam areas on impressions and to make beading on preliminary and final impressions. Sometimes also given to cover sharp brackets and wires in orthodontic treatment **(Fig. 5.14)**.

### Supplied As

They are supplied in form of dark red or orange sheet or stick.

### Composition

Utility wax is composed of beeswax, petrolatum and other soft waxes in varying proportions.

### Properties

They are workable at 21–24°C and are easily adaptable at room temperature. They should have minimum flow of 65% and maximum flow of 80% at normal mouth temperature.

## Sticky Wax

Sticky wax when melted has a property of adhering to surfaces of various materials.

### Composition

Sticky wax is composed of rosin, yellow beeswax, natural resins such as gum dammer and coloring agents **(Fig. 5.15)**.

### Properties

* They are sticky when melted and adheres closely to the surfaces when applied
* Shows shrinkage of not more than 0.5% between 43°C and 23°C
* They are usually dark colored in order to distinguish from plater or stone

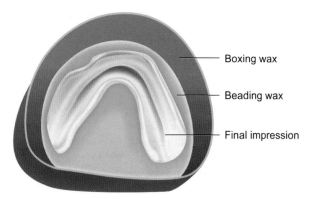

**Fig. 5.13:** Impression beaded and boxed and is ready for pouring with stone.

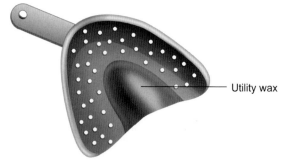

**Fig. 5.14:** Utility wax used to adjust contour of perforated tray.

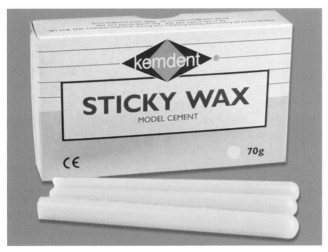

**Fig. 5.15:** Sticky wax.

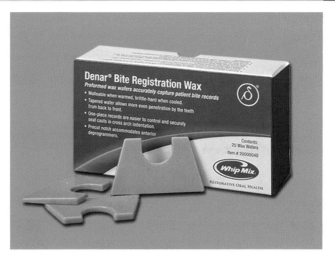

**Fig. 5.16:** Bite registration wax.

- At room temperature they are firm, brittle and free from tackiness.

*Uses*

- Used to join metal parts of denture before soldering
- To join broken pieces of denture.

## IMPRESSION WAXES

### Corrective Impression Waxes

Korecta wax, Iowa wax.

#### Composition

They are composed of Paraffin wax, ceresin, beeswax and metal particles.

#### Uses

These waxes are used to record tissues in functional state. They are veneered over the original impression to contact and record details of the soft tissues. They are useful in recoding posterior palatal seal area, as functional impression material for obturators and to make functional impression for distal extension cases.

#### Properties

These waxes distort when removed from undercut areas. They should be poured immediately. They are very soft at mouth temperature but do not have sufficient body to register details of soft tissues on its own. They are rigid at room temperature. Their use is indicated for edentulous patients because if used in undercut areas (teeth) then they distort on removal.

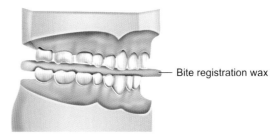

**Fig. 5.17:** Recorded wax bite placed between the models.

### Bite Registration Wax

#### Composition

These waxes are composed of paraffin wax or ceresin. Some waxes may have aluminum or copper particles **(Fig. 5.16)**.

#### Uses

They are used to record relationship of upper and lower teeth and accurately mount the models on articulator **(Fig. 5.17)**.

#### Properties

The flow at 37°C ranges between 2.5% and 22%. They are susceptible to distortion on removal from the mouth.

#### Procedure

These waxes are softened in warm water and placed between upper and lower teeth. Patient is instructed to bite slowly into position. The wax is then allowed to harden and removed from the mouth. The recorded wax bite is chilled and models are placed into the indentations formed by teeth. The assembly is then mounted on the articulator.

# TEST YOURSELF

## Essay Questions

1. Classify Dental waxes. Describe various properties of dental waxes.
2. Describe composition, properties, manipulation and uses of Inlay casting wax.

## Short Notes

1. Processing wax.
2. Sticky wax.
3. Bite registration wax.
4. Utility wax.
5. Wax distortion.

## Multiple Choice Questions

1. Which wax is used to form a base to pour a gypsum model?
   A. Boxing wax
   B. Pattern wax
   C. Sticky wax
   D. Baseplate wax
2. If it is necessary to store a wax pattern or bite registration, it should be stored:
   A. At room temperature
   B. In cool and dry place
   C. Refrigerated
   D. Wrapped in cotton
3. In fabricating a direct wax pattern in the patient mouth with inlay wax. Which is the most critical property:
   A. Melting range
   B. Excess residue
   C. Residual stress
   D. Flow
4. Melting range in case of inlay wax is best described as
   A. Point at which the wax softens
   B. Point at which the wax flows
   C. Temperature at which the heat source is required
   D. A combination of melting points
5. Utility wax are used to:
   A. Hold components together for repair

B. Adapt the periphery of impression trays
   C. For bite registrations
   D. Make corrections in undercut areas of impressions
6. Component of inlay wax which makes it flake resistant
   A. Paraffin
   B. Carnauba
   C. Gum dammer
   D. Candelila
7. Incremental wax buildup is for complete crowns is to compensate for which property of wax:
   A. High thermal expansion
   B. Low modulus of elasticity
   C. Low compressive strength
   D. Low hardness value

## ANSWERS

| 1. A | 2. B | 3. D | 4. A |
|------|------|------|------|
| 5. B | 6. C | 7. A | |

## BIBLIOGRAPHY

1. Anusavice KJ. Phillips' Science of Dental Materials, 11th edition. Saunders St. Louis, Missouri; 2003.
2. Craig RG, Eick JD, Peyton FA. Properties of natural waxes used in dentistry. J Dent Res. 1965;44:1308.
3. Craig RG, Eick JD, Peyton FA. Strength properties of waxes at various temperatures and their practical application. J Dent Res. 1967;46:300.
4. Craig RG, Powers JM. Restorative Dental Materials, 11th edn. Mosby St. Louis, Missouri; 2002.
5. Jorgensen KD, Ono T. Distortion of wax crowns. Scan J Dent Res. 1984;92:253-6.
6. Kotsiomite E, McCabe JF. Improvements in dental wax. J Oral Rehabil. 1997;24:517.
7. Kotsiomite E, McCabe JF. Waxes for functional impressions. J Oral Rehabil. 1996;23:114.
8. McCrorie JW. Some physical properties of dental modelling waxes and of tehrir main constituents. J Oral Rehabil. 1974;1:2.
9. McMillan LC, Darwell BW. Rheology of dental waxes. Dent Mater. 2000;16:337-50.
10. O'Brien WJ. Dental Materials: Properties and Selection. Chicago: Quintessence Publishing; 1989.

# Dental Casting Investment

## CHAPTER OUTLINE

- Requirement of Dental Casting Investment Material
- Composition
- Casting Shrinkage and its Compensation
- Setting Expansion of Investment Materials
- Uses of Investment Materials

- Gypsum-Bonded Investment Material
- Investment for Casting High-Melting Alloys
- Soldering Investment
- Investment of Titanium Alloys

*The best and most beautiful things in the world cannot be seen or even touched.*
*They must be felt with the heart.*

*—Helen Keller*

## INTRODUCTION

The Lost-Wax technique was first described by *William H. Taggart* in 1907 as a means to fabricate dental casting. In this technique, wax pattern is surrounded with a mold made of heat-resistant investment material. This wax is eliminated during the burnout process and empty mold thus created, is filled with a molten metal to complete casting. Slight variation in investing or casting can significantly affect the quality of the final restoration. It is important to understand the commonly used investment materials, which can greatly influence the outcome of the final casting.

## DEFINITION

Dental casting investment: *A material consisting principally of an allotrope of silica and a bonding agent. The bonding substance may be gypsum (for use in lower casting temperatures) or phosphates and silica (for use in higher casting temperatures).* —*GPT 8th Edition*

*According to Craig*—an investment is a ceramic material that is used to form a mold into which a metal or alloy is casted. The process of forming the mold is called as investing.

Investing refers to a process of forming a mold into which the molten metal is forced to obtain a metallic casting. The materials, which can withstand high temperatures

of burnout and casting, are selected for this purpose. Such materials are called as investment materials. These materials include gypsum, phosphate and silicate and they are available as two component system of powder and liquid.

## REQUIREMENT OF DENTAL CASTING INVESTMENT MATERIAL

- Should accurately reproduce the details of the wax patterns
- Should have adequate strength to withstand heat of burnout and casting of molten metal
- Should expand adequately to compensate for solidification shrinkage of alloy
- Should be easily manipulated
- Should be stable at higher temperature
- Should have sufficient porosity to allow escape of air or other gases
- Should be easily divested
- Should produce a smooth surface
- Should not be expensive.

There is no one material, which possesses all these properties. However, most of the required qualities can be fulfilled in an investment material by blending different ingredients.

## Classification of Dental Casting Investment Material

*Based on the type of binder material:*
- *Gypsum-bonded investment*—used for casting gold alloys for fabricating inlays, onlays, crowns and fixed partial dentures
- *Phosphate-bonded investment*—used for casting high-temperature alloys such as those used for metal ceramic frameworks. It can also be used for pressable ceramics and base metal alloys
- *Silica-bonded investment*—used for casting base metal alloys used in removable partial denture castings

*Based on the type of silica used, investments are classified as:*
- Quartz investment
- Cristobalite investment

*Based on the uses (ISO 15912:2006):*
- *Type 1*: Fabrication of inlays, crowns and fixed restorations
- *Type 2*: Fabrication of complete or partial dentures
- *Type 3*: Fabrication of cast used for soldering or brazing
- *Type 4*: Fabrication of refractory dies.

## COMPOSITION

*Basic ingredients of dental casting investment are:*
- Binder material
- Refractory material
- Other chemicals.

### Binder Material

Binder is a material, which helps to bind the particles of refractory substances. The common binding material used for casting gold alloy is α-hemihydrate. For high-temperature castings, investments are phosphate and ethyl silicate, whereas for low-temperature castings gypsum-bonded investments are used.

### Refractory Material

Refractory is a material that is capable of withstanding high temperature without significant degradation. Silica is added as a refractory. It exists in four allotropic forms namely, (1) quartz, (2) tridymite, (3) cristobalite and (4) fused quartz.

Quartz, cristobalite or mixtures of both are usually used as refractory filler in dental investment. When these allotropic forms are heated, there is a change in crystalline form at transition temperature, e.g. quartz inverts from α form to β form at 575°C. The density reduces and volume increases as α form changes to β form resulting in rapid increase of linear expansion. This expansion compensates for the shrinkage of the binding material.

### Functions

- To regulate thermal expansion
- To withstand high temperature without degrading itself.

### Chemical Modifiers

Mixture of refractory materials and a binder is not sufficient to produce all the desirable properties required of an investment; modifiers are added in small amounts to alter various physical properties of the investment. Modifiers can be chemical-modifying agents, coloring agents and reducing agents. Reducing agents are added to provide nonoxidizing atmosphere in the mold during casting.

*Some chemical modifiers are:*
- Sodium chloride
- Boric acid
- Potassium sulfate
- Graphite
- Copper powder
- Magnesium oxide.

## CASTING SHRINKAGE AND ITS COMPENSATION

It is important to understand the concept of casting shrinkage and how investment material helps in its compensation before discussing individual investment materials. In Lost-Wax casting procedure, an accurately fitting wax pattern is prepared on the die and is invested in refractory mold material. On setting, it is kept in a burnout furnace to eliminate the wax without leaving a residue. The empty mold is placed in the casting machine in which the molten metal is forced into the empty mold. The resulting casting is divested and after finishing and polishing the casting is fitted onto the prepared tooth. During this procedure, casting shrinkage occurs and it should be suitably compensated, so that the resulting casting fits accurately on the prepared tooth.

Casting shrinkage occurs due to two reasons:
1. *Wax shrinkage*—due to shrinkage of wax patterns
2. *Alloy shrinkage*—due to shrinkage of metal alloy on solidification.

### Wax Shrinkage

Wax patterns are prepared either by direct method or by indirect method.
- *Direct method*: Type I inlay pattern wax is used to form direct pattern of the prepared tooth and is invested immediately. Type I inlay wax shows large coefficient of thermal expansion, which is about 300–400 ppm/°C and can undergo large thermal contraction when cooled from mouth temperature to room temperature.

- *Indirect method*: In this method, the wax patterns are prepared on the die using softer Type II inlay pattern wax. This wax is applied incrementally on the die material. In this case also, wax shrinkage occurs and shows thermal contraction of 0.3–0.4%.

## Alloy Shrinkage

During the casting procedure, the molten metal is forced into the empty mold and is allowed to solidify before removing the casting. The molten metal first cools down to the liquids temperature and then it solidifies in the mold. A large amount of alloy shrinkage occurs when the alloy cools from the solidus temperature to the room temperature.

Casting shrinkage is combination of both wax shrinkage and the alloy shrinkage.

Casting shrinkage = Wax shrinkage + Alloy shrinkage

Casting shrinkage of commonly used alloys in dentistry is given in **Table 6.1**.

**Table 6.1:** Casting shrinkage of commonly used alloys.

| Types of alloy | Casting shrinkage (%) |
| --- | --- |
| Gold alloy—Type II | 1.56 |
| Gold alloy—Type III | 1.37 |
| Gold alloy—Type IV | 1.42 |
| Cobalt-chromium alloy | 2.3 |
| Nickel-chromium alloy | 2.0 |

## Compensation of Casting Shrinkage

Casting shrinkage is compensated by controlling the mold expansion, large setting expansion and adjusting the thermal expansion of the investment materials. Investment materials are primarily composed of refractory material (silica) and binder, which are mixed with water or colloidal silica. The wax patterns are invested in a metal ring or silicone ring. The casting shrinkage is compensated by the net expansion of the investment material.
Therefore,

Wax shrinkage + alloy shrinkage
= normal setting expansion + hygroscopic setting expansion + thermal expansion

## SETTING EXPANSION OF INVESTMENT MATERIALS

### Normal Setting Expansion

It is the linear expansion, which occurs on setting of the investment material in presence of air. The normal setting expansion can be increased by reducing water-powder ratio, increasing the mixing time or reducing the chemical impurities.

### Hygroscopic Setting Expansion (Low-heat Technique)

This type of expansion occurs when the investment material is allowed to set in the presence of water. It along with normal setting expansion has an additive effect. It occurs by placing the invested casting ring in water before it sets or during setting, by placing wet casting liner inside the casting ring before pouring of investment material or by adding water to the exposed area of investment during setting.

### Thermal Expansion (High-heat Technique)

The refractory material in the investment undergoes changes resulting in expansion. The refractory part in investment material is usually quartz, tridymite, cristobalite or amorphous quartz. When the temperature is raised during the burnout low-alpha form to high-beta form resulting in expansion. This expansion is called as thermal expansion.

#### Ringless Casting System

Greater expansion occurs in flexible ringless casting as compared to metal casting ring especially in case of phosphate-bonded investment material because these materials can withstand high temperature, greater casting force and have high strength. The plastic ring is removed after the investment material sets to allow for expansion. This system is beneficial for casting of those alloys, which require greater mold expansion than the traditional gold-based alloys.

## USES OF INVESTMENT MATERIALS (TABLE 6.2)

**Table 6.2:** Uses of various investment materials.

| Investment material | Use |
| --- | --- |
| Gypsum-bonded investment | Casting of gold-based alloys |
| Phosphate-bonded investment | Casting of base metal alloys, metal ceramic alloys, refractory dies for ceramic buildup |
| Silica-bonded investment | Casting of base metal alloys for removable partial dentures |
| Dental plaster or dental stone | Acrylic dentures |

# GYPSUM-BONDED INVESTMENT MATERIAL

According to American Dental Association (ADA), (specification No. 2) for casting investments for dental gold alloys, there are three types of gypsum-bonded investment materials based on method of obtaining expansion and on the type of appliance to be fabricated. The newer ADA specification number for dental investment is 126 and the ISO is 7490-2000 **(Fig. 6.1)**.

## Classification of Gypsum Bonded Investment

The classification based on the method of compensating casting shrinkage through different types of expansions.
- *Type I*—used for inlays and crowns utilizing mainly *thermal* expansion of the mold to compensate casting shrinkage
- *Type II*—used for inlays and crowns utilizing mainly *hygroscopic* setting expansion of the mold
- *Type III*—used for fabrication of *removable partial dentures* made with gold alloys. Not currently used.

## Composition

### Binder

- About 25–35% of α-calcium sulfate hemihydrate is used
- This type of gypsum is used to cast gold-containing alloys
- Castings made with α-hemihydrate require less water, shrinks less and are more accurate
- Gypsum investments should not be heated above 700°C, as it decomposes above 700°C and contaminates the casting with release of sulfur gases such as sulfur

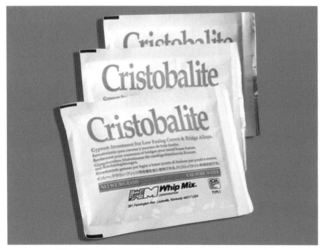

**Fig. 6.1:** Gypsum-bonded investment material.

dioxide and sulfur trioxides. These gases can cause contamination of the metal surface resulting in formation of sulfides, which tends to make the casting more brittle
- The calcium sulfate hemihydrate when mixed water forms calcium sulfate dehydrate, which binds the refractory material together
- It imparts sufficient strength to the mold and contributes to the mold expansion by its setting expansion.

### Refractory Materials

- About 65–75% quartz or cristobalite, or a blend of the two (form of silica)
- Primary function of refractory material is to withstand high temperatures and provide mold expansion by thermal expansion. It also provides high strength to withstand casting forces and provides thermal resistance to disintegration
- Silica when added to gypsum eliminates contraction and change to expansion on heating. It increases setting expansion of stone
- Silica is found in polymorphic forms. Its allotropic forms are quartz, tridymite, cristobalite and fused quartz. These forms are chemically same but have different crystalline structure. The crystalline structure exists in two types: (1) alpha form—(α) and (2) beta form—(β). When the alpha form is heated to high temperature (i.e. above 573°C), it can partially or completely change to beta form. This process is called as *Inversion*. The change from alpha form to beta form results in increase in volume and decrease in density. This increase in volume shows as linear expansion of the investment, which helps in compensating casting shrinkage. The expansion in silica occurs due to crystalline inversion of its alpha form to beta form and by simple thermal expansion. Due to this change, the chemical bonds straighten to form less-dense crystalline structure. The reduction in density results in expansion, which aids in compensating casting shrinkage
- Out of all the four allotropic forms of silica only quartz and cristobalite are used as refractory in dental investments because they provide large thermal expansion.

### Modifying Chemicals

- About 2–3%
- They control setting expansion and setting time of gypsum
- They prevent shrinkage of gypsum when it is heated above 300°C, e.g. boric acid or sodium chloride. These

materials help in retaining the water of crystallization of binder particles and hence prevent shrinkage
- A reducing agent is used to provide nonoxidizing atmosphere in the mold when the gold alloy is casted, e.g. carbon and powdered copper
- Coloring agents are added to differentiate between different investment materials.

## Manipulation

- Powder and water are mixed in a recommended ratio
- Water is dispensed into flexible bowl and powder is added to water **(Fig. 6.2)**. Stiff blade spatula is used initially to mix powder into water. This technique reduces the amount of air incorporated during hand spatulation
- The powder is mixed with water using hand spatulation until all the powder particles are wet **(Fig. 6.3)**
- Then the contents are vacuum mixed. Overspatulation should be avoided, as it increases the thermal expansion **(Figs. 6.4A and B)**
- Properly mixed contents are poured into the casting ring, which is kept on the vibrator **(Fig. 6.5)**.

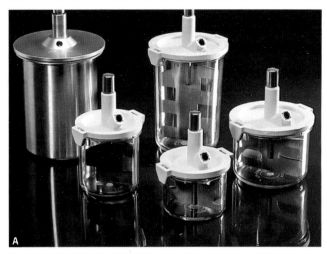

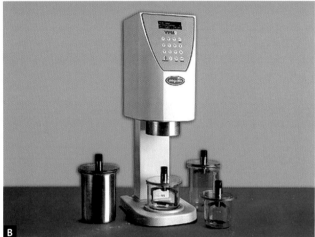

**Figs. 6.4A and B:** Vacuum mixer.

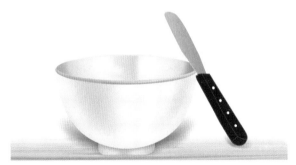

**Fig. 6.2:** Flexible rubber bowl and stiff blade spatula are used for manipulation.

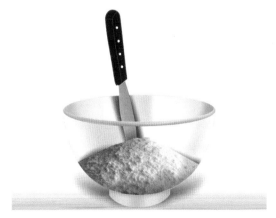

**Fig. 6.3:** Powder particles are hand spatulated.

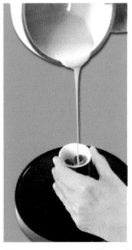

**Fig. 6.5:** Mixed contents are poured into the casting ring.

## Setting Time

- According to ADA specification No. 2, setting time of dental casting investment should be between 5 minutes and 25 minutes.
- Currently available investment material sets between 9 minutes and 18 minutes. This time is sufficient for mixing and investing the pattern before the investment material sets.

*Factors influencing setting time are*:
- Water-powder ratio
- Rate and length of spatulation
- Chemical modifiers—accelerators and retarders
- Temperature.

## Properties of Gypsum-bonded Investment

*Setting expansion:* The objective of setting expansion is to enlarge the mold and partially compensate for casting shrinkage of gold.

Setting expansion is of three types:
1. Thermal expansion
2. Normal setting expansion
3. Hygroscopic setting expansion.

### Normal Setting Expansion

- Setting expansion in the investment takes place due to the normal crystal growth
- Combination of silica and calcined gypsum shows greater setting expansion in comparison to gypsum used alone
- Silica particles most likely interfere with intermeshing and interlocking of the crystals during their formation
- As the crystals grow, they form outward thrust and increases expansion
- According to ADA specification, the normal setting expansion should be less than 0.6%
- Modern investment shows setting expansion of 0.4%
- Setting expansion can be controlled by adding accelerators or retarders.

### Hygroscopic Setting Expansion

- Also called as low-heat technique. This type of expansion is about six or more times greater than the normal setting expansion
- It takes place when gypsum is placed in contact with water during setting
- It is used to augment the normal expansion
- Hygroscopic expansion takes place when the water in which the investment is immersed replaces the water used by the hydration process. It maintains the space

between the growing crystals allowing them to expand outwards
- According to ADA specification No. 2, Type II investments require minimum 1.2% and maximum 2.2% setting expansion in water **(Fig. 6.6)**
- The degree of hygroscopic expansion can be controlled by the quantity of water added to investment during setting. The expansion observed is directly proportional to the quantity of water added during setting and beyond that no expansion occurs. The water added is drawn between the crystals through capillary action resulting in separation and expansion. As the water evaporates the expansion is maintained by the binder.

*Factors influencing hygroscopic expansion are:*
- *Composition:* The amount of silica in the investment material influences the amount of hygroscopic expansion in the investment. Finer the size of the silica particles greater the hygroscopic expansion. Alpha hemihydrate produces greater hygroscopic expansion than the beta hemihydrates in presence of silica
- *Water-powder ratio:* Greater the water-powder ratio of the original investment water mixture, lesser the hygroscopic setting expansion because lesser will be binder crystals per unit volume
- *Spatulation:* If the mixing time is reduced, the hygroscopic time is decreased. More the spatulation time greater will be expansion because the interlocking between the crystals will be delayed
- *Shelf-life of the investment:* Older the investment, lesser the hygroscopic expansion
- *Time of immersion:* Immersion before the initial set produces greater hygroscopic expansion. If the immersion is delayed after the initial set, it results in reduced hygroscopic expansion

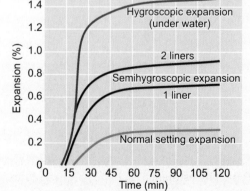

**Fig. 6.6:** Various methods of setting expansion in gypsum-bonded investment material.

- *Confinement:* Investments are confined by the walls of the container resulting in reduced hygroscopic expansion. Confining effect is more pronounced for hygroscopic expansion than normal setting expansion
- *Added water*: The hygroscopic expansion of the investment material is directly proportional to the amount of water added before the initial set of investment. However, if water is added after the initial set, the hygroscopic expansion is less in proportion
- *Flow of wax*: If flow of wax is greater, then greater will be the expansion. The expansion of the investment away from the wax pattern can be increased by:
  - Placing wet casting liner
  - By placing wax pattern toward the outer end of the casting ring
  - By performing ringless casting.

### Thermal Expansion

- Also called as high-heat technique. This type of expansion takes place when the investment is heated in a burnout furnace.
- The invested material is allowed to completely set before placing into the burnout furnace. The temperature is raised to 650°C in the furnace.
- At this temperature, the investment and the metal ring sufficiently expand to compensate for shrinkage of the gold alloy.
- Heated mold aids in eliminating wax pattern and prevents alloy from solidifying before it completely fills the mold.
- Thermal expansion of gypsum-bonded investment is also proportional to the type and quantity of silica present in the composition.
- In order to counterbalance the thermal contraction of gypsum, adequate amount of quartz is needed. If the quartz content is increased to 75%, the thermal contraction of gypsum is completely counterbalanced.
- Thermal expansion of investment containing quartz is influenced by size of quartz particle, type of binder and the resultant water-powder ratio needed to provide workable mix.
- Thermal expansion in investment containing cristobalite occurs at lower temperature than those containing quartz.
- Modern investments usually contain mixture of quartz and cristobalite
- According to ADA specification No. 2, thermal expansion for Type II investment should be between 0% and 0.6% at 500°C and for Type I investment it should be between 1% and 1.6% at 700°C.

*Factors influencing thermal expansion are:*
- *Amount and type of silica used*: Quartz when heated inverts from α quartz (low form) to β quartz (high form) at the transition temperature of 575°C. Likewise, cristobalite changes from α to β form between the transition temperatures of 200°C and 270°C. Despite of lower inversion temperature with cristobalite, it gives much greater expansion than quartz. However, cristobalite-containing investments should be gradually heated to the required temperature because low-inversion temperature and rapid rate of thermal expansion make it prone for greater disintegration **(Figs. 6.7A and B)**.
- *Water-powder ratio*: Greater the water-powder ratio, lesser the thermal expansion achieved during heating.
- *Effect of chemical modifiers*: Addition of sodium, potassium or lithium chlorides in small quantity eliminates contraction caused by gypsum and increases

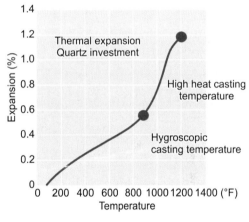

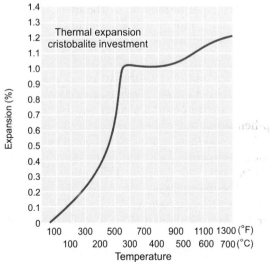

**Figs. 6.7A and B:** Influence of different forms of silica on the thermal expansion of investment material.

thermal expansion. Addition of boric acid has similar effect as it hardens the set material. But drawback of boric acid is that it rapidly disintegrates on heating of the investment resulting in roughened casting

- *Temperature*: Greater the temperature greater will be the expansion. Although, the expansion will not be uniform and will gradually increase with the rise of temperature. But temperature increase should be done with caution because rapid, prolonged or overheating during burnout process can result in fracture of the investment and can produce fins in casting (defects)
- *Confinement*: The coefficient of thermal expansion of metal casting ring should coincide with that of the investment material for effective expansion.

### Thermal Contraction

When investment is cooled from 700°C, it contracts to less than its original dimension. This contraction occurs because of shrinkage of gypsum. If this investment is again reheated, it will expand thermally to the same peak as the first time. However, the investment should not be reheated as it may develop internal cracks.

### Strength

- Compressive strength of the investment material is one of the primary factors considered to evaluate dimensional accuracy of the casting
- According to ADA specification No. 2, the compressive strength for inlay investment should be at least 2.4 MPa when tested 2 hours after setting. The compressive strength increases depending on type and quantity of gypsum binder
- The strength of the mold should be adequate to bear the impact of the molten metal forced in the mold. Also, it should be adequate to resist fracture or chipping of the mold during heating and casting of the gold alloys.

Factors affecting strength of the investment are:
- *Quantity and type of gypsum binder* added, e.g. $\alpha$-hemihydrates increase strength more than the $\beta$-hemihydrates
- *Addition of chemical modifiers* can increase strength of the investment
- *Water-powder ratio*—greater the water content, lesser would be the strength
- *Heating the investment* greater than 700°C may increase or decrease the strength by as much as 65% depending upon the composition. Strength is greatly reduced, if the investment contains sodium chloride
- When *investment cools* to room temperature, its strength is considerably reduced because of fine cracks that form during cooling.

### Porosity

- Lesser the hemihydrates content and more the amount of gauging water used to mix the investment, greater the porosity
- Certain amount of porosity is required to allow gases to escape from the mold cavity during filling of the mold with molten alloy
- Greater the uniformity of the particle size, greater is the porosity. Mixtures of course and fine particles have lesser porosity than investment containing uniform particle size.

### Fineness

Finer-sized particles of the investment result in lesser surface irregularities on the surface of the casting as compared to coarser-sized particles.

### Storage

- Investment material should always be stored in airtight and moisture-free containers. During use, the containers should be opened for shortest time possible to prevent moisture contamination
- They should be purchased in package of small quantities. Preweighed packets of investment powders are available. 2% of less of weight variation between packets suggests excellent quality control, whereas if the variation in weight is 5% or more, it can compromise the properties of the investment material.

### Hygroscopic: Thermal Gold Casting Investment

- This type of investment can be used with either hygroscopic or thermal type of casting techniques
- If hygroscopic expansion technique is used, the investment should be heated to 482°C and if thermal expansion technique is used, investment should be heated to 649°C.

### Limitations of Gypsum-bonded Investment

Above 700°C, a reaction occurs between calcium sulfate and silica:

$$CaSO_4 + SiO_2 \rightarrow CaSiO_3 + SO_3.$$

This sulfur trioxide gas evolved causes:
- Porosity in the casting
- Contributes to the corrosion of the casting.
  For this reason, gypsum-bonded investments are not used for higher fusing alloys like cobalt-chromium. In such cases, phosphate- or silica-bonded materials are chosen.

# INVESTMENT FOR CASTING HIGH-MELTING ALLOYS

- The alloys used for metal ceramic restorations and fabrication of cast partial dentures have high-melting temperatures
- These alloys are cast at mold temperature more than 700°C. Since gypsum investment disintegrates at temperature more than 700°C with the resultant release of contaminating sulfur into the mold, they are not used for these alloys
- Therefore, investment materials which can withstand higher temperatures are selected
- Phosphate-bonded investment and silica-bonded investment material are most suitable for this purpose.

## Phosphate-bonded Investment

Phosphate-bonded investments (ADA Specification No. 42) can withstand much higher temperatures and are much stronger than the gypsum-bonded investment materials **(Figs. 6.8A and B)**. Most of the base metals, palladium-based alloys and titanium-based alloys are cast at temperatures in the range of 850–1,500°C.

### Uses

It is used for investing and casting alloys with higher melting temperatures, for example, nickel-chromium, silver-palladium and gold-platinum.

The use of phosphate-bonded investment material has increased rapidly in modern dentistry due to:
- Increase in the use of metal ceramic and all ceramic restorations
- Increase in use of more economical base metal alloys instead of gold or gold-based alloys
- Greater use of commercially pure titanium and titanium alloys, which need especially formulated investments to reduce interaction of the molten metal with the investment material.

### Supplied As

- Preweighed powder sachets and special liquid bottles **(Fig. 6.9)**.

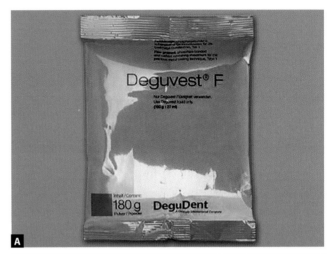

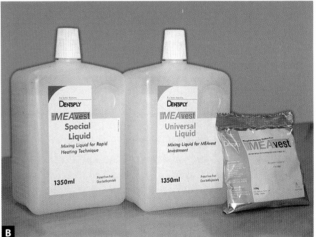

**Figs. 6.8A and B:** Phosphate-bonded investment material.

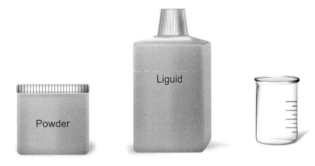

**Fig. 6.9:** Powder and liquid of phosphate bonded investment.

### Composition

*Powder*
- *Refractory fillers*: Silica—in the form of quartz and cristobalite or mixture of both is present in concentration of 80%. These fillers provide high-thermal expansion and high-thermal shock resistance
- *Binder*: Magnesium ammonium phosphate—20%. It provides strength at room temperature. At higher temperatures react with silica to form silicophosphate to

## Classification of Gypsum-Bonded Investment

According to ADA specification No. 42, phosphate-bonded investments are of two types:
1. *Type I:* Used for casting inlays, onlays, crowns and fixed partial dentures. Should have minimum compressive strength of 2.5 MPa
2. *Type II:* Used for casting partial dentures and other cast, removable restorations. Should have minimum strength of 3.0 MPa.

further increase its strength. Originally, phosphoric acid was used, but at present monoammonium phosphate is used as it can be incorporated into the powdered investment. This binder system undergoes acid-base reaction between acidic monoammonium phosphate and basic magnesium oxide

- *Carbon (graphite)*: Carbon added to produce clean castings and facilitate in divesting of gold castings. But, it should not be used for casting base metal alloys, silver palladium or palladium silver alloys, as they make the casting more brittle.

*Liquid*
- Colloidal silica liquid suspensions, which should be stored frost-free environment
- It is three parts of silica liquid in one part of distilled water
- For use in base metal alloys, liquid is diluted by 33%
- Colloidal silica helps in increasing strength of investment as well as increases hygroscopic expansion.

*Setting Reaction*

- The chemical reaction that occurs between the ammonium phosphate and magnesium oxide with water to form hydrated magnesium ammonium phosphate and water. This chemical reaction is exothermic

The setting reaction in phosphate-bonded investment is:

$$NH_4H_2PO_4 + MgO + 5H_2O \xrightarrow{room\ temperature} NH_4MgPO_4.6H_2O$$

- Some of the magnesia present never fully react and the setting reaction continues to occur during increase in temperature during the burnout process
- The water produced during the reaction lowers the viscosity of the mix during spatulation. The magnesium ammonium phosphate formed acts as binder in which the filler particles are embedded in the matrix
- The set matrix consists of multimolecular hydrated magnesium ammonium phosphate, which aggregates around excess magnesium oxide and fillers
- The mix can undergo hygroscopic expansion, if placed in contact with the moisture during setting.

*Setting reaction at high temperature*:
- The setting reaction continues to occur when the set investment is placed in the burnout furnace (high temperature)
- With the rise in temperature sequence of chemical and thermal reactions take place
- At room temperature, magnesium phosphate reacts with primary ammonium phosphate to produce magnesium ammonium phosphate, which provides strength *(Green strength)* to the investment.

- At higher temperature, silicophosphates are formed, which further increase strength of the investment
- This increase in strength enables the investment to withstand the impact of the molten alloys
- The MgO never fully reacts. Thus, a predominantly colloidal multimolecular $(NH_4MgPO_4\ 6H)_{2n}$ is formed, coagulating around excess MgO and fillers
- On heating complex series of reaction occurs which are summarized as follows:

*Room temperature:*
$$NH_4H_2PO_4 + MgO + 5H_2O \rightarrow NH_4MgPO_4.6H_2O + MgO + NH_4H_2PO_4 + H_2O—(1)$$
*Prolonged setting at 25°C/dehydration at 50°C:*
$$NH_4MgPO_4.6H_2O + MgO + NH_4H_2PO_4 + H_2O \rightarrow (NH_4MgPO_4.6H_2O)_n—(2)$$
*Dehydrated at 160°C:*
$$(NH_4MgPO_4.6H_2O)_n \rightarrow (NH_4MgPO_4 + H_2O)_n—(3)$$
*Heated from 300–650°C:*
$$(NH_4MgPO_4 + H_2O)_n \rightarrow (MgP_2O_7)_n—(4)$$
*Amorphous polymeric phase:*
$$(MgP_2O_7)_n \rightarrow MgP_2O_7—(5)$$
*Heated above 1,040°C:*
$$MgP_2O_7 \rightarrow Mg_3 (P_2O_4)_2—(6)$$

*Manipulation*

- Measured quantity of powder is mixed with special liquid using bowl and spatula
- Mix is mechanically spatulated in vacuum for 15 seconds **(Fig. 6.10)**
- This material has poor surface wetting characteristics and has greater chance of air bubble entrapment

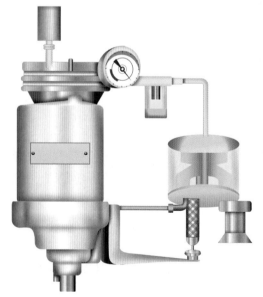

**Fig. 6.10:** Investment mixed in vacuum mixing machine.

- To reduce the amount of air bubbles, the investment should be allowed to set in a pressure pot
- It is important to paint investment material into the wax pattern using a small brush **(Fig. 6.11)**
- After covering the wax pattern, the casting ring is then filled with remaining material with minimum vibration.

## Properties

### Setting and Thermal Expansion
- When the investment powder is mixed with liquid in a ratio as recommended by the manufacturer
- The mix initially expands rather than contract
- Since the mix contains colloidal silica, it is capable of expanding hygroscopically
- This expansion is varied by the proportion of colloidal silica and water
- More colloidal silica and less water results in greater expansion and less colloidal silica and more water results in lesser expansion
- The early thermal shrinkage of phosphate investment shows decomposition of magnesium ammonium phosphate and release of ammonia.

### Strength
- Usually, investment materials are low in strength. Strength is of two types—wet and dry
- Dry strength is that strength of investment under high temperatures whereas wet strength is useful for handling the set material
- High-temperature strength enables the material to withstand the impact of high-melting alloys
- The silica used as liquid helps in increasing the strength of the mixture.

### Setting Time
- The working and setting time of phosphate-bonded investment material is influenced by temperature
- Since the setting reaction is exothermic, it accelerates the rate of setting

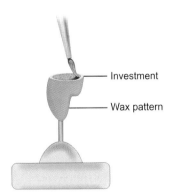

**Fig. 6.11:** Investment material painted with wet brush into the wax pattern.

- Increased mixing time and mixing efficiency result in faster set
- Mechanical mixing under vacuum is better than hand mixing
- Increase in the liquid-powder ratio increases the working time
- Increasing the liquid powder ratio can improve casting surface smoothness and accuracy.

## Advantages

- Possess high strength to bear the impact of high-melting molten alloy
- Provide adequate thermal and setting expansion to compensate for thermal contraction of metal ceramic or cast partial prosthesis
- Do not disintegrate at high temperature of about 1,300°C.

## Disadvantages

- Result in mold breakdown and rougher casting, if heated above 1,375°C
- Divesting is difficult because of its high strength
- For higher expansion, liquid powder ratio is increased, which makes the mold less porous which can result in casting failure because of trapped gases in the mold
- Temperature at the time of mixing is critical.

## Ethyl Silicate-bonded Investment

The use of ethyl silicate-bonded investment material (ADA Specification No. 91) is limited because of its complex and time consuming investment procedure. Also, flammable ethyl alcohol vapor is liberated during hydrolysis reaction making the procedure highly risky.

## Uses

This type of investment material is commonly used for fabricating high-fusing base metal partial dentures with cobalt-chromium alloys. Although it can occasionally be used for casting nickel-based alloys **(Fig. 6.12)**.

## Composition

- *Powder*: Consists of refractory particles of silica and small amounts of calcined magnesium oxide. The magnesium oxide is added to give strength to the gel and to reduce pH of silica gel during mixing
- *Liquid*: Silica gel stabilized in alcohol. Silica gel is produced by adding an acid or salt to sodium silicate or by mixing ethyl silicate with diluted hydrochloric acid

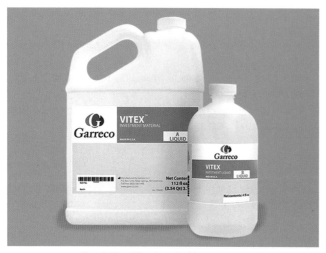

**Fig. 6.12:** Silica-bonded investment.

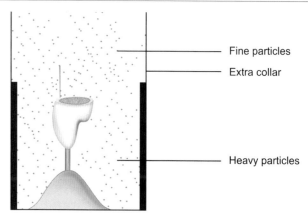

**Fig. 6.13:** Heavy particles of silicate investment settle down and finer particles come on the top.

## Setting Reaction

- Mixing of ethyl silicate investment is more time consuming and complicated than phosphate-bonded investment material
- The binder for this investment is silica. It is formed from an aqueous dispersion of colloidal silica or from sodium silicate
- *Stage I—hydrolysis:*
  - It consists of silica refractory, which is hydrolyzed in presence of hydrochloric acid. The reaction forms colloidal solution of silicic acid and ethyl alcohol.

$$Si(OC_2H_5)_4 + 4H_2O \rightarrow Si(OH)_4 + 4C_2H_5OH$$

### CLINICAL SIGNIFICANCE
This reaction has a disadvantage of producing flammable alcohol and therefore, care should be taken during its handling and burnout process.

Because of this drawback, sodium silicate and colloidal silica are commonly used binders.

- *Stage II—gelation*: Colloidal solution of polysilicic acid is mixed with quartz or cristobalite and small quantity of powdered magnesium oxide is added to the make the mix more alkaline
- *Stage III—drying*: This coherent gel is dried at the temperature below 168°C to give off alcohol and water forming a concentrated hard gel. There is volumetric contraction on drying, which reduces the size of the mold. This contraction is called as *Green shrinkage*
- A faster method to obtain silica gel is by the addition of amines such as piperidine ($C_5H_{11}N$) to the solution of ethyl silicate. Here, hydrolysis and gelation occur simultaneously.

- Mold enlargement is recommended to compensate not only for casting shrinkage of alloy but also green shrinkage and setting shrinkage of investment.

## Setting Expansion

Considerable expansion occurs when this type of investment is heated at high temperature of 1,090–1,180°C. Continuous heating causes considerable expansion, which is capable of compensating both wax shrinkage and alloy shrinkage. The linear thermal expansion of 1.6% occurs at a temperature of 600°C. The quantity of powder incorporated into the mix influences the strength and expansion of the investment material.

## Manipulation

- Powder is mixed with liquid in the ratio as recommended by the manufacturer. The mix is quickly poured into the mold
- The mold is placed on a specialized vibrator, which gives *Tamping action*
- This action allows denser particles to settle at the bottom and the excess liquid with finer particles comes to the top **(Fig. 6.13)**
- After 30 minutes, heavier portion sets and the excess on the top is poured off. This reduces the setting shrinkage to 0.1% as the liquid powder ratio of the set part is greatly reduced.

## Properties

- Compressive strength at room temperature should not be less than 1.5 MPa
- Linear thermal expansion should not be more than 15% from the time as mentioned by the manufacturer
- Setting time should not be more than 30% more than the time mentioned by the manufacturer

- On heating to high temperature, some silica particles converts to quartz, providing added expansion. This type of investment can be heated between 1,090°C and 1,180°C and is compatible with high-fusing alloys.

### Advantages

- Used for high-melting alloys such as cobalt-chromium and nickel-chromium alloys
- Excellent dimensional stability
- Good surface finish
- Can be divested easily than phosphate-bonded investment because of lesser density.

### Disadvantages

- Technique sensitive and complex manipulation
- Has less strength
- Technique sensitive.

## SOLDERING INVESTMENT

- The parts of the restoration to be soldered are temporarily held together by sticky wax
- This assembly is surrounded by investment material before starting the soldering process **(Fig. 6.14)**
- Once the investment material is set, sticky wax is softened and removed and the portion to be soldered is exposed.
- This gap is heated and joined with a solder.

### Classification of Soldering Investment

According to ADA specification No. 93, soldering investment is of two types:
1. *Type I*: Gypsum-bonded soldering investment—used for low-fusing alloys
2. *Type II*: Phosphate-bonded soldering investment—used for high-fusing alloys.

### Requirements

- Should have lower setting and thermal expansion than casting investment parts, so that the joined parts do not shift from its position during setting and heating of the investment

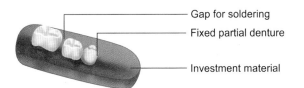

Gap for soldering
Fixed partial denture
Investment material

**Fig. 6.14:** Assembly surrounded by investment material ready for soldering.

- Should have uniform particle size, which need not be very fine
- Should have good fluidity
- Should have compressive strength in range of 2–10 MPa
- Should have linear setting expansion and linear thermal expansion, which should not vary more than 15% of the expansion specified by the manufacturer.

## INVESTMENT OF TITANIUM ALLOYS

- Titanium and its alloys cannot be casted with conventional phosphate or silica-bonded investment material because molten titanium readily reacts with oxygen and is capable of reducing the oxides commonly present in these investments
- Apart from this, titanium is capable of reacting with residual oxygen, nitrogen and carbon resulting in brittle alloy on solidifying
- Therefore, modification of the conventional investment is required.

### Composition

- Refractory used is similar to phosphate and silica-bonded investment material such as silica, magnesia, zirconia or alumina
- Recent formulation consists of magnesia-bonded by aluminous cement having mass fraction of 5% zirconium powder
- The binder for magnesia is in the form of aluminous cement, which forms by mixing with water
- Zirconia used is highly stable and does not contaminate the titanium castings **(Fig. 6.15)**.

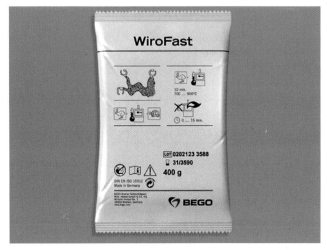

**Fig. 6.15:** Titanium investment material.

## Properties

- Titanium and its alloy have high-melting point of 1,727°C
- As mentioned earlier, the molten alloy can react with the components of the investment material to form a zone of contaminated layer called as α-*case*. This layer makes the alloy more porous and brittle and has poor-corrosion resistance and reduced strength

- To avoid contamination of titanium casting with oxygen, refractory material, which is less readily reduced by titanium, should be used
- To achieve large expansion, spinel reaction of alumina and magnesia takes place when it is burned out at 1,150–1,200°C
- Recently, spodumene ($Li_2O$-$Al_2O_3$-$SiO_2$) (Okuda et al. 1991) has been reduced to achieve increased expansion. This material is capable of expanding irreversibly by heating through temperature of 900–1,100°C.

---

# TEST YOURSELF

## Essay Questions

1. Define investment materials. Classify various investment materials and write their ideal requirements. Write briefly about phosphate investment material.
2. Describe in detail about gypsum-bonded investment material including their composition, setting reaction, setting expansion, uses and properties.

## Short Notes

1. Refractory materials.
2. Thermal expansion of phosphate-bonded investment.
3. Silica-bonded investment material.
4. Composition of gypsum-bonded investment material.
5. Soldering investments.

## Multiple Choice Questions

1. The extent of bubble incorporation in the investment can be minimized by:
   A. Vacuum mixing the investment material
   B. Investing the wax pattern in water
   C. Lowering the water-powder ratio
   D. Using higher water powder ratio
2. High-heat investment in comparison to low-heat investment:
   A. Are used for metal ceramic alloys
   B. Should not be heated above 750°C
   C. Are composed of gypsum
   D. Has greater expansion
3. Dimensional changes that affect the accuracy of metal crown is due to:
   A. Setting expansion of the investment material
   B. Shrinkage of wax pattern during cooling
   C. Shrinkage of metal during burnout
   D. Expansion of the impression material during setting

4. Binder in the investment materials is:
   A. Gypsum
   B. Quartz
   C. Silica
   D. Water
5. Heating of gypsum-bonded investment above 1300°F in the presence of carbon results in:
   A. Increase the strength of gypsum
   B. Greater thermal expansion
   C. Drives excess water present in the investment
   D. Releases sulfur dioxide and blackening of cast
6. Silica-bonded investment material have limited use because of:
   A. Release of methanol vapor
   B. Release of ethanol vapor
   C. Release of sulfur dioxide gas
   D. Less thermal expansion
7. Primary use of asbestos in casting liner is:
   A. Absorb moisture from investment
   B. Aids in expansion of investment
   C. Allow escape of gases
   D. To prevent fracture of investment
8. Hygroscopic expansion in investment material is not:
   A. A physical change
   B. Is 5–6 times the normal setting expansion
   C. Depends on the amount of water added before the final setting
   D. Is directly proportional to the amount of silica
9. Increasing water-powder ratio of gypsum results in investment will result in:
   A. Less setting expansion and reduced strength
   B. More setting expansion and less strength
   C. More setting expansion and more strength
   D. Less setting expansion and more strength

10. High-heat technique requires temperature for thermal expansion at:
    A. 900°F
    B. 1,200°F
    C. 1,500°F
    D. 1,800°F

11. Minimum percentage of gypsum in gypsum-bonded investment should be:
    A. 10%
    B. 15%
    C. 20%
    D. 25%

## ANSWERS

| | | | |
|---|---|---|---|
| 1. A & C | 2. A & D | 3. A & B | 4. A |
| 5. D | 6. B | 7. B | 8. D |
| 9. A | 10. B | 11. B | |

## BIBLIOGRAPHY

1. Allen FC, Asgar K. Reaction of cobalt chromium casting alloy with investments. J Dent Res. 1966;45:1516.
2. Anusavice KJ. Phillip's science of dental materials, 11th edition. St Louis, Missouri: Saunders; 2003.
3. Cooney JP, Caputo AA. Type III gold alloy complete crowns cast in a phosphate bonded investment. J Prosthet Dent. 1981;46:414-9.
4. Craig RG, Powers JM. Restorative dental materials, 11th edition. St Louis: Mosby; 2002.
5. Eliopoulos D, Zinelis S, Papadopoulos T. The effect of investment material type on the contamination zone and mechanical properties of commercially pure titanium castings. J Prosthet Dent. 2005;94:539-48.
6. Jorgensen KD, Okamoto A. Restraining factors affecting setting expansion of phosphate bonded investments. Scan J Dent Res. 1986;94:178-81.
7. Lodovici E, Meira J BC, Filho LER, et al. Expansion of high flow mixtures of gypsum-bonded investments in contact with absorbent liners. Dental Mater. 2005;21:573-9.
8. Mahler DB, Ady AB. An explanation for the hygroscopic setting expansion of dental gypsum products. J Dent Res. 1960;39:578.
9. Matsuya S, Yamane M. Decomposition of gypsum bonded investments. J Dent Res. 1981;60:1418-23.
10. Muller HJ, Reyes W, McGill S. Surfactant containing phosphate investment. Dent Mater 1986;2:42-4.
11. Nieman R, Sarma AC. Setting and thermal reactions of phosphate investments. J Dent Res 1980;59:1478-85.
12. Santos JF, Ballester RY. Delayed hygroscopic expansion of phsopahte bonded investments. Dent Mater. 1987;3:165-7.
13. Shillingburg HT, Hobo S, Whitsett LD, et al. Fundamentals of fixed prosthodontics, 3rd edition. Chicago: Quintessence; 1997.
14. Stevens L. The effect of early heating on the expansion of a phosphate bonded investments. Aus Dent J. 1983;28:366-9.
15. Teteruck WR, Mumford G. The fit of certain dental casting alloys using different investing materials and techniques. J Prosthet Dent. 1966;16:910.

# Die and Die Materials

*'To succeed in your mission, you must have single minded devotion to your goal.'*

*—APJ Abdul Kalam*

## INTRODUCTION

The wax pattern fabrication directly in the mouth is inconvenient, difficult and time consuming. Therefore, most of the wax patterns are fabricated in the laboratory using indirect technique. This technique demands an accurate reproduction of the prepared tooth/teeth, surrounding soft tissues and the adjacent teeth. The accuracy of the master cast and die depends on the accuracy and completeness of the impression.

## DEFINITION

*It is defined as a reproduction of a prepared tooth made from a gypsum product, epoxy resin, a metal or a refractory material.*

## IDEAL REQUIREMENTS OF THE DIE MATERIALS

- Should be dimensionally accurate
- Should be strong and resistant to abrasion
- Should be compatible with separating agent
- Should be able to reproduce surface details accurately
- Should have a contrasting color with wax, alloys and porcelain
- Should have smooth surface
- Should be compatible with all impression materials
- Should be easy to manipulate
- Should be economical.

## Classification of Die Systems

According to the type of material:
- *Gypsum products*
  - Type IV dental stone
  - Type V dental stone
  - Type V dental stone with sulfonates.
- *Metals*
  - Electroformed
  - Sprayed metal
  - Amalgam.
- *Polymers*
  - Epoxy resins
  - Polyurethanes.
- *Divestment*
  - For direct baking of porcelain crowns
  - Refractory dies for wax patterns.
- *Cements*
  - Silicophosphates.

## GYPSUM

Type IV (dental stone, high strength) and Type V (dental stone, high strength and high expansion) are the most commonly used die materials **(Figs. 7.1A and B).**

This type of gypsum has good dimensional accuracy and resistance to abrasion while the wax pattern is formed. The surface detail reproduction is acceptable with these gypsum products. They are capable of reproducing 50 micrometer wide line according to American Dental Association (ADA) specification No. 25. The setting expansion for Type IV stone is 0.1% or less and for stronger Type V stone, it is 0.3%. This increased expansion is useful in compensating large solidification shrinkage of base metal alloys. The use of Type V stone is indicated when inadequate expansion is achieved in fabrication of cast crowns. Type V stone should be avoided in the fabricating dies for inlays as higher expansion produces tight fit, which is unacceptable.

Resin strengthened gypsum products possess high strength and low expansion and are suitable for implant casts. The surface of the die can also be impregnated with low-viscosity resin such as cyanoacrylate to improve the resistance to abrasion. To provide relief space for the cement, die spacer is usually applied over the stone die. The most commonly used die spacer is resins. Also, prior to the fabrication of the wax pattern on the stone die, some separating medium or die lubricant is applied, so as to facilitate wax pattern removal.

### Advantages

- Dimensional accuracy
- Easy to manipulate
- Economical
- Good strength
- Adequate working time
- Can be easily trimmed
- Has good color contrast
- Compatible with all impression material
- Has smooth, hard surface.

### Disadvantages

- Poor resistance to abrasion
- Brittle.

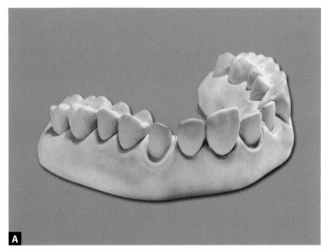

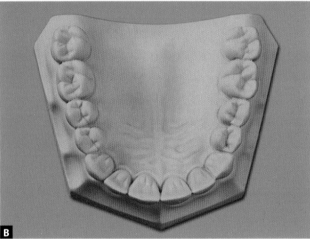

**Figs. 7.1A and B:** Gypsum material commonly used as die material.

## DIE SPACER

Bonding or luting of indirect restoration on the tooth surface requires space for the luting agent. This space is provided by applying die spacer on the die (**Fig. 7.2**). Use of die spacer is one of the most acceptable and common methods used to provide this space. Other methods are inaccurate and do not provide uniform space. Such methods are grinding the inside of the casting, electrochemical milling, etching of the internal surface with aqua regia or carving the wax pattern on the internal surface.

Die spacer is a resin-based solution, which is applied on the axial walls and occlusal surfaces of the prepared tooth on the die before the fabrication of the wax pattern. Two layers of die spacer are applied before fabrication of wax pattern to get desired space for the cementing material. Commonly used die spacers consist of metal oxide powders

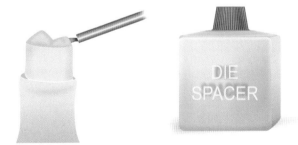

**Fig. 7.2:** Die spacer applied over preparation portion of die.

and adhesives, which are dispersed in ketone-based organic solvent.

**CLINICAL SIGNIFICANCE**

The coat of die spacer should not be applied on the finish line and the application should stop 0.5 mm short of the finish line. This is done to provide better marginal adaptation of the casting on the tooth surface.

# DIVESTMENT (DIE STONE-INVESTMENT COMBINATION)

- This is a combination of die material and investment medium
- In this, gypsum-bonded material called *divestment* is mixed with colloidal silica liquid
- A die is prepared from the mix and wax pattern is fabricated over the die
- The assembly of die and wax pattern is invested in a mixture of divestment and water **(Fig. 7.3)**
- By doing this, possibility of wax pattern distortion on removal from die or during setting is eliminated
- When this material is heated to 677°C, the setting expansion of the material is 0.9% and thermal expansion is 0.6%
- Since, it is gypsum-bonded material, it should not be used for high-fusing alloys
- *Phosphate-bonded die investment* material is similar to divestment and is used for high-fusing alloys.

## Advantage

Highly accurate for conventional gold alloys especially for extracoronal preparations.

# ELECTROFORMED/ELECTROPLATED DIES (FIG. 7.4)

Electroformed dies possess moderately high strength, adequate hardness and excellent abrasion resistance. It is used to overcome the poor abrasion resistance of stone dies. Silver-plated or copper-plated dies are used. This technique involves the deposition of a coat of pure silver or copper on the impression. Individual prepared tooth or full arch impression can be electroplated.

## Procedure

- The surface of the impression material is first coated with finely powdered silver or graphite to make them conduct electricity. This process is called as *Metallizing* **(Fig. 7.5)**

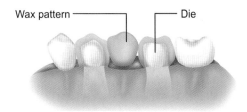

**Fig. 7.3:** Assembly of die and wax pattern invested together.

- This impression is then placed in electroplating bath either copper-forming bath or silver-forming bath. The composition of the electrolytic bath is given in **Table 7.1**
  - The electrolytic bath consists of solution of silver cyanide. It should be handled with caution as any addition of acid solution can result in liberation of cyanide vapor, which is called as "death chamber gas"
- Layer of pure metal is deposited on the impression and is supported with Type IV stone or resin

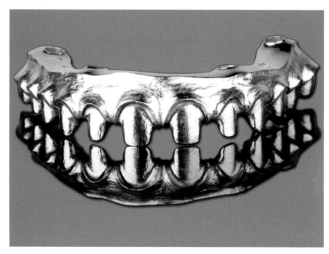

**Fig. 7.4:** Electroplated dies.

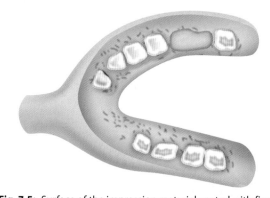

**Fig. 7.5:** Surface of the impression material coated with finely powdered silver or graphite.

| Table 7.1: Composition of copper-forming and silver-forming electrolytic bath. | |
|---|---|
| *Copper-forming electrolytic bath* | *Silver-forming electrolytic bath* |
| Copper sulfate—200 g | Silver cyanide—36 g |
| Concentrated sulfuric acid—30 mL | Potassium cyanide—60 g |
| Phenolsulfonic acid—2 mL | Potassium carbonate—45 g |
| Distilled water—1,000 mL | Distilled water—1,000 mL |

- In silver-plating or copper-plating procedure, greater the concentration of silver or copper in the bath, faster is the deposition of pure silver or copper
- Time required to deposit layer of pure metal on the impression is 10 hours using current of 5–10 mA/cm$^2$ on the cathode surface
- As the stone sets, it is mechanically locked into rough electroformed metal shell **(Fig. 7.6)**
- Impression material is later removed to get die with greater surface hardness and resistance to abrasion.

### CLINICAL SIGNIFICANCE

- Silicone impression materials are difficult to electroplate evenly because of their low-surface energies
- Polysulfide impression material can be silver-plated but difficult to copper plate. These dies are found to be slightly less accurate than the stone die
- Polyether impression material is difficult to electroplate as they are hydrophilic in nature and thus, imbibe water
- Hydrocolloid impression material is very difficult to electroplate and is not done.

### Troubleshooting in Electroforming

- Friable and granular metal deposit on impression
- If the metal anode is too small, it will lead to irregular plating
- Use of overconcentrated solution leads to softening of the rubber base impression and discoloration of the some areas of the cast
- Old electrolytic solution should be discarded and replaced with fresh solution to give best results
- If there is short-circuiting through the electrolyte, it will show faulty conduction on the ammeter.

### Advantages

- Excellent abrasion resistance
- High strength.

### Disadvantages

- Time consuming
- Required special equipment
- Cyanide solution used in silver plating is extremely toxic
- Not compatible with all impression material
- Color contrast and adaptation of wax not as good as the stone die.

## EPOXY RESIN DIE MATERIAL

- Supplied in the form of paste to which a liquid activator is added to initiate hardening **(Fig. 7.7)**
- Hardened resin is more resistant to abrasion and has higher strength than the high-strength stone die
- Recently, fast setting epoxy material is supplied in the form of automixing systems
- The material is injected through the automixing tip directly into the rubber base impression
- Fast setting epoxy hardens quickly and the die can be used to fabricate wax pattern after 30 minutes
- As water retards polymerization of resin, it should not be used with water-containing agar or alginate impression material
- It is most effective with rubber impression material but not compatible with polysulfide impression
- Prosthesis fabricated over the resin dies fits more tightly than those made with gypsum.

### Advantages

- High strength
- Has good abrasion resistance.

### Disadvantages

- Complex technique
- Time consuming
- Polymerization shrinkage
- More expensive than gypsum.

## FLEXIBLE DIE MATERIALS

- Flexible die materials are similar to heavy-bodied elastomer or polyether impression materials

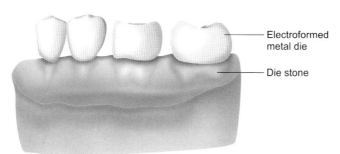

**Fig. 7.6:** Electroformed die supported by stone base.

Electroformed metal die

Die stone

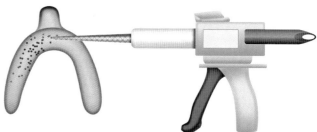

**Fig. 7.7:** Epoxy resins injected into rubber-based impression.

- They are used to fabricate provisional restorations, indirect composite resin inlays or onlays
- When selecting flexible die, it is important to ensure that it is compatible with impression material and provides good surface details.

## Advantages

- Sets more rapid than die stone
- Easier to remove provisional or inlay than from die stone cast.

## Disadvantage

Not compatible with all impression material.

## SILICOPHOSPHATE CEMENT

### Composition

Similar to the filling and cementing materials.

### Advantage

Harder than die stone.

### Disadvantages

- Shrinkage on setting
- Loss of water on standing.

## AMALGAM

Can be condensed.

## Composition

Similar to the restorative material.

## Advantages

- Produces a hard die
- Reproduces fine details and sharp margins.

## Disadvantages

- Can be poured only in a rigid impression material such as impression compound
- Takes a long time to reach maximum hardness
- High-thermal conductivity
- Separating agent is required.

## METAL-SPRAYED DIES

*A bismuth*—tin alloy, which melts at 138°C, can be sprayed directly on to an impression to form a metal shell, which can then be filled with dental stone.

## Advantage

A metal-coated die can be obtained rapidly from elastomeric impression material.

## Disadvantages

- The alloy is rather soft
- Care is needed to prevent its abrasion.

---

## TEST YOURSELF

### Essay Questions

1. Classify die materials. Write ideal requirements of die materials and describe in detail various die material used in dentistry.
2. Critically analyze various die materials used in dentistry.
3. Write in detail about gypsum-based dies. Compare them with electroplated dies.

### Short Notes

1. Die spacers.
2. Epoxy dies.
3. Electroplated dies.
4. Type V die stone.
5. Divestment.

### Multiple Choice Questions

1. Epoxy resins polymerize by:
   A. Condensation
   B. Copolymerization
   C. Cross-linked polymerization
   D. Branched polymerization
2. Gypsum-based die materials are:
   A. Type II and Type III
   B. Type I and Type IV
   C. Type IV and Type V
   D. Type V and Type II
3. Electroplated dies have:
   A. Excellent abrasion resistance
   B. Low strength
   C. Compatible with all impression material
   D. Can be done rapidly

4. Epoxy resin dies have:
   A. Good strength
   B. Cheaper than gypsum
   C. Good abrasion resistance
   D. Show polymerization shrinkage

## ANSWERS

1. C     2. C     3. A     4. A, C & D

## BIBLIOGRAPHY

1. Anusavice KJ. Phillip's Science of Dental Materials, 11th edition. St Louis, Missouri: Saunders; 2003.
2. Craig RG, Powers JM. Restorative Dental Materials, 11th edition. St Louis: Mosby; 2002.
3. Nomura GT, Reisbick MH, Preston JD. An investigation of epoxy resin dies. J Prosthet Dent. 1980;44:45-50.
4. Rosenstiel SF, Land MF, Fujimoto J. Contemporary Fixed Prosthodontics, 3rd edition. Missouri: Mosby; 2001.

# Finishing and Polishing Agents

*'The only limit to our realization of tomorrow will be our doubts of today.'*

*—Franklin D. Roosevelt*

## INTRODUCTION

Finishing and polishing of the restorations are one of the most important aspects of restorative dentistry. Properly finished and polished restorations aids in providing better esthetics, better function and minimize retention of dental plaque thereby improving the oral health. Highly polished restoration significantly reduces tarnish and corrosion of the restorative material. On the contrary, rough-surfaced restorations develop high-contact stresses, are more prone to tarnish and corrosion and give a unesthetic appearance. Rough surfaces on the ceramic cause stress concentration areas leading to loss of functional and stabilizing contacts between the teeth.

## DEFINITIONS

*Abrasion*: Defined as *the wearing away of a substance or structure through some unusual or abnormal mechanical process.*

*—GPT 8th Edition*

*Abrasive*: Defined as *a hard substance used for grinding, finishing, or polishing a less hard surface.*

*Finishing*: Defined as *the process to put final coat or surface on; the refinement of form before polishing.*

*—GPT 8th Edition*

*Polishing*: Defined as *to make smooth and glossy, usually by friction; to give luster to.*

*—GPT 8th Edition*

*Grinding*: Defined as *process of removing material from a substrate by abrasion with relatively coarse particles.*

## GOALS OF FINISHING AND POLISHING PROCEDURE

- To obtain natural contours
- To reduce roughness, scratches and gouges
- To obtain proper occlusion
- To obtain surfaces, which resist plaque accumulation
- To obtain surfaces compatible with oral tissues.

## RATIONALE OF FINISHING AND POLISHING PROCEDURE

The rationale behind finishing and polishing procedure is to use diminishing series of abrasives on the surface of the restoration to first contour, then smoothen and finally polish it to luster. A smooth and polished surface helps in achieving esthetics, minimizes gingival irritation and promotes oral health and function.

## INSTRUMENTS USED FOR FINISHING AND POLISHING PROCEDURE (FIGS 8.1A AND B)

- Diamond
- Carbides
- Bonded stones
- Abrasive disks and strips

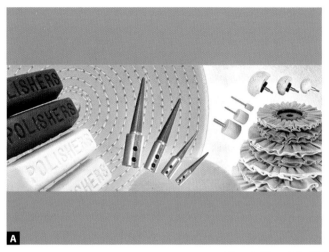 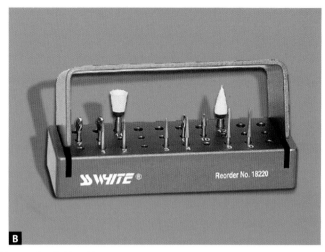

**Figs. 8.1A and B:** Finishing and polishing kits.

- Polymeric cups
- Wheels impregnated with different size of abrasive particles
- Polishing pastes.

## ABRASION

*It is a process of wearing a surface of a material with another through a mechanical process of grinding, rubbing or scrapping.*

The material, which is abraded, is called as *substrate* and the material that causes wear is called as an *abrasive* **(Fig. 8.2)**.

### Types of Abrasion

- *Two body system*—in this type, the abrasive particles are tightly bonded to the abrasive instrument and are used to polish the surface of contact **(Fig. 8.3A)**.
  For example, diamond bur abrading a tooth structure **(Fig. 8.3B)**

- *Three body system*—in this type, the abrasive particles have freedom of movement between two surfaces **(Fig. 8.4A)**.
  For example, prophylaxis paste used with rubber cup against the tooth surface or substrate material **(Fig. 8.4B)**.

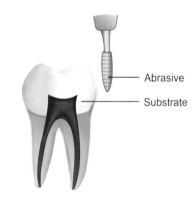

**Fig. 8.2:** Diagram showing abrasive and substrate.

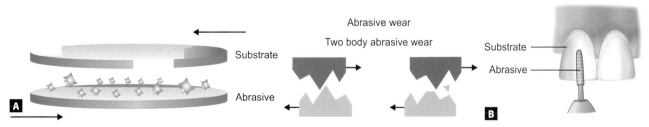

**Figs. 8.3A and B:** Two body abrasion system.

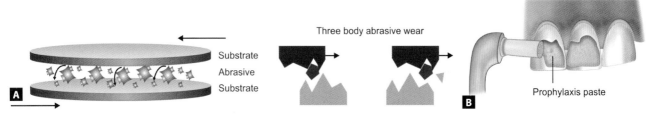

**Figs. 8.4A and B:** Three body abrasion system.

## Types of Abrasion Procedures

- *Cutting procedure* is a process of removing material from the substrate by use of a bladed bur or an abrasive embedded in a binding matrix on a bur or disk. When the blade is pressed into the surface of the substrate, it produces stress, which is more than the elastic limit of the substrate to cut it. The cutting blades of the instrument should have higher elastic limit, greater strength and abrasion resistance to serve for longer duration. This is a unidirectional procedure.

  For example, high-speed tungsten carbide burs are used for cutting procedure. They have several regularly arranged blades, which remove small shavings of the substrate on rotation of the bur

- *Grinding procedure* is a process of removing material from a substrate by abrasion with relatively coarse particles. These instruments contain randomly arranged abrasive particles, which are bonded or glued to paper, plastic, cloth or rotating instrument. When the grinding instrument comes in contact with the substrate, it breaks and removes the fragments. Like the cutting procedure, the grinding procedure is also unidirectional.

  For example, diamond-coated abrasive have randomly coated sharp diamond particles, which produce unidirectional scratches

- *Polishing procedure* is a process of providing luster or gloss on a material surface. Each of its type acts on extremely thin area of the substrate surface. Scratches from previous grinding procedure are removed by progressively using finer abrasives to finally achieve high-luster substrate material. Polishing procedure is a multidirectional procedure and minimal substrate material is removed from the surface **(Fig. 8.5)**.

  For example, rubber abrasive points, fine particle disks and strips, fine particle polishing pastes.

## Factors Influencing Rate of Abrasion

- *Particle size*: Abrasive particles can be fine (0–10 μm), medium (10–100 μm) and course (100–500 μm). Larger the size of the abrasive particles, more rapidly the substrate material is abraded. This is because larger particles plough deeper grooves or cuts into the surface. The procedure of finishing and polishing involves the sequential reduction in size of the abrasive particles. This way the scratches left on the surface by the previous abrasive is removed and replaced by smaller and shallower scratches from the current abrasive. Eventually, the scratches are so small that they are no more visible

- *Particle shape*: Sharp irregularly shaped particles abrade the surface more rapidly than rounded particles. Sharper abrasive has greater cutting efficiency than the blunt one. The abrasive used over a period of time gets dull and clogged with cutting debris and is discarded

- *Difference in hardness*: The difference between the hardness of abrasives and hardness of the substrate is an important consideration in grinding ability of an abrasive. Greater the difference between the hardness of the abrasive and the substrate more efficient is the grinding

- *Speed*: Greater the speed of abrasive tool greater will be the rate of abrasion. Greater speed also increases greater chance of heat generation and risk of overcutting of the substrate

- *Pressure*: Greater pressure produces deeper and wider scratches. But increased pressure also increases greater heat generation and increases the temperature of the substrate. Increase of temperature of the substrate can lead to distortion or physical change of the substrate

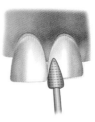

**Fig. 8.5:** Polishing by finer abrasives.

(e.g. crown or restoration). Moreover, if pressure is applied to enhance cutting efficiency it risks of fracturing the restoration especially at the margins

- *Lubrication*: Water is one of the most common lubricant used in dentistry to reduce heat buildup generated during grinding or cutting tooth structure. Lubricant such as water also facilitates the movement of the cutting edge into the substrate surface and helps in removing the debris, which otherwise would have clogged the cutting edge. Removal of debris and reduction of heat generation increase the cutting efficiency of the abrasive and its longevity. However, too much lubrication reduces the rate of abrasion as it prevents some of the abrasive to come in contact with the substrate
- *Physical properties* of the bonding or backing material or substance such as rigidity, elasticity or flexibility
- *Type of substrate* such as metal, composite or ceramics.

## ABRASIVE

Abrasive is a hard substance, which is used for grinding, finishing or polishing a less hard surface.

### Uses of Abrasives in Dentistry

*Abrasives are used for:*
- Grinding ceramics, metal and resin-based composites
- Finishing and polishing of metal, ceramics and resin-based composites
- Cutting metal, ceramics and composites
- Used for dental prophylaxis (teeth cleaning)
- For occlusal adjustment on tooth enamel, metal, ceramics, composites or acrylic
- Finishing and polishing of acrylic dentures
- For preparing cavity or cleaning tooth surface using air abrasion technology
- Used as dentifrices.

### Hardness of Abrasives

- The cutting blades or abrasive particles on the dental instruments should be strong enough to remove particles of substrate material without itself getting dull or fracturing
- Hardness is the surface measurement of the resistance of one material to be plastically deformed by indenting or scratching another material
- Friedrich Mohs ranked hardness of commonly used abrasive from scale of 1–10. Least scratch-resistant material got score of 1 and highly scratch-resistant material got a score of 10 **(Tables 8.1 and 8.2)**.

## Steps in Finishing and Polishing (Table 8.3)

### Step 1—Bulk Reduction and Contouring

Bulk reduction of the substrate material such as metal, resin-based composites or ceramics is done by cutting or grinding procedure.

### Step 2—Finishing Procedure

After bulk reduction and contouring the surface of the substrate is rough with many scratches and imperfections. In this step, the deep imperfections and scratches are

**Table 8.1:** Hardness value of commonly used abrasives.

| Abrasive material | Mohs scale | Knoop hardness number |
|---|---|---|
| Talc | 1 | |
| Gypsum | 2 | |
| Pumice | 6 | 560 |
| Sand | 7 | 800 |
| Tungsten carbide | 9 | 2,100 |
| Aluminum oxide | 9 | 1,900 |
| Silicon carbide | 9–10 | 2,500 |
| Diamond | 10 | 7,000 |

**Table 8.2:** Hardness value of different substrate material.

| Substrate material | Mohs scale | Brinell hardness number |
|---|---|---|
| Acrylic | 2–3 | |
| Glass | 5–6 | 30 |
| Hard gold alloys | 3–4 | |
| Amalgam | 4–5 | 90 |
| Dentin | 3–4 | |
| Enamel | 5–6 | 270 |
| Resin composite | 5–7 | |
| Porcelain | 6–7 | 400 |

**Table 8.3:** Steps of finishing and polishing and the materials used.

| Steps of preparation | Diamond points | Tungsten carbide burs |
|---|---|---|
| Bulk reduction | Particle size of abrasive 100 μm | 8–12 fluted |
| Contouring | Particle size of abrasive 30–100 μm | 12–16 fluted |
| Finishing | Particle size of abrasive 10–20 μm | 18–30 fluted |
| Polishing | Particle size of abrasive 8–20 μm | — |

removed stepwise progressively using finer abrasives. The finished surface looks relatively smooth.

### Step 3—Polishing Procedure

This step involves the final smoothening the surface of the substrate to make it reflective and with high luster. Polishing procedure aims to provide an enamel-like luster to the substrate. After completion of the procedure there should not be any visible scratches. Although, if the surface is seen under high magnification, scratches are detected. Polishing is a multidirectional procedure, which requires minimal removal of the surface material.

### Beilby Layer

*It is a molecular disorganized surface layer of highly polished metal. A relatively scratch-free microcrystalline surface produced by a series of abrasive of decreasing coarseness.*
*—GPT 8th Edition*

This is a microcrystalline layer, which is formed on the metal surface after polishing. During the polishing procedure, heat is generated and the crystalline surface is broken down to form a harder and denser surface layer. This layer is called the Beilby layer, which was first proposed by *Sir George Thomas Beilby* (1850-1924).

### Range of Speed Used in Finishing and Polishing Procedures

The rotational speed of an instrument is measured in revolutions per minute (rpm).

According to Marzouk, the speed of the rotary tool can be classified as:
- Ultra low speed—300-3,000 rpm—provides better tactile sensation and less heat is generated. Useful for excavation of caries and cleaning teeth
- Low speed—3,000-6,000 rpm—provides better tactile sensation. Used during finishing and polishing procedures
- Medium high speed—20,000-45,000 rpm—used during contouring procedures
- High speed—45,000-100,000 rpm—used during cutting teeth and removal of old restorations
- Ultra high speed—100,000 rpm and above—used for gross finishing and contouring. Its advantages are:
  - Greater patient comfort
  - Efficient cutting with smaller and versatile instrument
  - It is faster, producing lesser vibration, pressure and heat generation
  - It offers good control and improves operator efficiency.

## Abrasive Instrument Design

### Abrasive Grits

These are those materials, which are crushed and separated into different particle sizes **(Fig. 8.6)**. The range of different particle sizes are determined by passing the crushed particles through series of mesh sieves. If too coarse abrasive is used, it will result in deep scratches on the substrate, which will be difficult to remove during subsequent finishing procedure.

### Classification of Abrasive Grits

According to the range of particle size:
- *Super coarse*: Abrasive particle size for aluminum oxide, silicon carbide and garnet is 142 μm and for coated diamond, it is 142 μm
- *Coarse*: Abrasive particle size for aluminum oxide, silicon carbide and garnet is 122 μm and for coated diamond, it is 122 μm
- *Medium coarse*: Abrasive particle size for aluminum oxide, silicon carbide and garnet is 70-86 μm and for coated diamond, it is 86 μm
- *Medium*: Abrasive particle size for aluminum oxide, silicon carbide and garnet is 29-32 μm and for coated diamond, it is 52 μm
- *Fine*: Abrasive particle size for aluminum oxide, silicon carbide and garnet is 12-17 μm and for coated diamond, it is 14 μm
- *Superfine*: Abrasive particle size for aluminum oxide, silicon carbide and garnet is 2-5 μm and for coated diamond, it is 6 μm
- *Ultrafine*: Abrasive particle size for aluminum oxide, silicon carbide and garnet is 1 μm and for coated diamond, it is 2 μm.

### Classification of Abrasives

Abrasives are broadly classified as two types:
1. *Bonded abrasives:*
   - Sintered abrasives
   - Resinous-bonded abrasives
   - Vitreous-bonded abrasives
   - Rubber-bonded abrasives.
2. *Nonbonded abrasive:*
   - Polishing pastes.

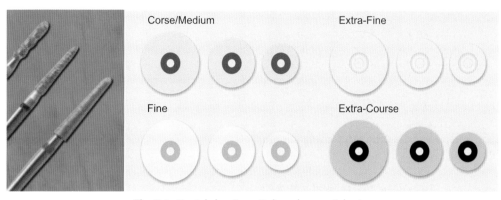

**Fig. 8.6:** Dental abrasive grits based on particle size.

## Bonded Abrasives

In this type, the abrasive particles are bonded with the help of binder to form grinding tools such as wheels, separating disks, points, etc. **(Fig. 8.7)**.

### Mechanism of Bonding

- *Sintering*: Sintered abrasives are strongest type as abrasive particles are fused to each other.
- *Vitreous bonding*: Vitreous-bonded abrasives are combined with glass or ceramic matrix material, which is cold-pressed to the instrument shape **(Fig. 8.8)**.
- *Resinoid bonding*: In phenolic resin. Resin-bonded abrasives are either heat-pressed or cold-pressed and are then heated to polymerize the resin. Heat pressing produces abrasives with very low porosity.
- *Rubber bonding:* In silicone- or latex-based rubber. Rubber-bonded abrasives are made in similar way as the resin-bonded abrasives. The abrasives are bonded with rubber and are used for final polishing **(Fig. 8.9)**.

### Features

- Ideal bonded abrasives are those that hold the abrasive particles for long enough to cut, grind, finish and polish the substrate without heat buildup or loss of cutting efficiency
- Bonded abrasives, which degrade very slowly or rapidly, are undesirable

**CLINICAL SIGNIFICANCE**
- Slow degradation results in clogging of the abrasive particles with grinding debris resulting in reduced cutting efficiency, increased heat generation and increased finishing time
- Whereas rapid degradation results in reduced instrument life and increased cost.

- Prior to using bonded abrasive instrument, it should be trued and dressed:

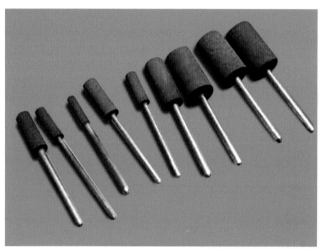

**Fig. 8.7:** Bonded abrasives.

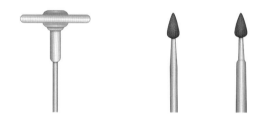

**Fig. 8.8:** Vitreous bonded abrasive wheel and points.

- *Truing* is a process in which the abrasive instrument is run against a harder abrasive block. It helps the abrasive instrument to rotate without eccentricity or run out when placed in contact with the substrate
- *Dressing procedure*: It is used to shape the instrument to its correct size and is used to clean the instrument from clogged debris
  - *Abrasive blinding*: It is clogging of the abrasive instrument with debris. It occurs when the grinding debris occludes the small spaces between the abrasive particles. This causes greater heat generation and reduced abrasive

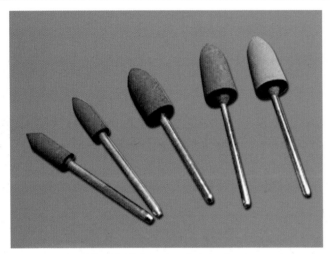

**Fig. 8.9:** Rubber-bonded abrasives.

efficiency. Therefore, frequent dressing of the abrasive instrument is needed to maintain the efficiency of the abrasive.

*Diamond Abrasives*

- Diamond abrasive particles are bonded to metal wheels or bur blank by heat-resistant resin such as *polyimides*
- The grades from super course through fine are plated with a refractory metal film such as nickel
- Nickel plating helps in increasing particle retention and acts as heat sink during grinding procedure
- To further improve their longevity, titanium nitride coating is done on diamond abrasives
- Diamond abrasives should always be used with copious water spray and rotational speed less than 50,000 rpm to reduce heat buildup and clogging
- Disposable diamond burs are popular nowadays because of reduced heat buildup, better instrument efficiency and concern for autoclaving or disinfection
- Diamond cleaning stones are used to remove clogged debris between abrasive particles thereby maintaining grinding efficiency. The diamond bur is run against the moistened cleaning stone for 2–4 seconds **(Figs. 8.10A and B)**
  - Diamond abrasive used for finishing composite restoration are made of diamond of particle size of 40 µm of less and should be used with light pressure and copious water irrigation to avoid heat buildup.

*Abrasive disks and strips:*

- The abrasive disks are coated with different abrasive particles and used primarily for finishing and polishing of restorations **(Fig. 8.11)**
- They are available in different sizes with paper and moisture-resistant backings

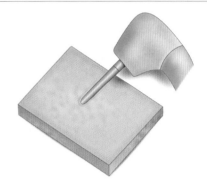

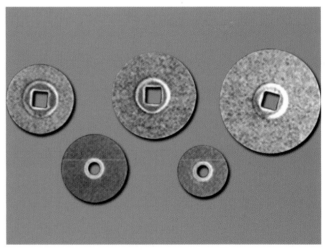

**Fig. 8.10A and B:** (A) Diamond bur cleaned by running against diamond cleaning stone; (B) Diamond cleaning stone.

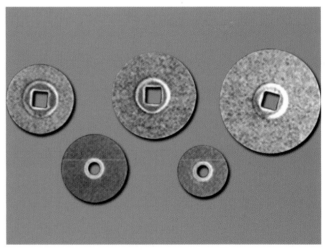

**Fig. 8.11:** Abrasive disk.

- These abrasives are fabricated by securing abrasive particles to flexible backing such as metal, Mylar strip or heavyweight paper.

## Abrasive Disks

- Coated abrasive disks should be used with moisture-resistant backings as moisture acts as lubricant and improves cutting efficiency **(Fig. 8.12)**
  - They are used for contouring, finishing and polishing of the restorations
  - The abrasive particles commonly used are aluminum oxide, garnet, silicon carbide, emery and quartz
  - These disks are supplied as different grits, i.e. coarse to fine. They are used sequentially from coarse grit to fine or ultrafine to get desired result
  - Abrasive disks are mostly used in anterior region and are usually not used in the posterior region
  - Diamond-coated metal disks are used for contouring ceramic crowns in the laboratory.

## Abrasive Strips

- These strips are used to contour and polish proximal and interproximal areas
- Abrasive strips have central part, which does not contain any abrasive in order to facilitate insertion without abrading the contact area
- Like other abrasives, they should be sued sequentially from coarse to fine grit to get desired finish.

*Abrasive brushes and felt devices:*
Abrasive-impregnated brushes and felt are made of polymer bristles, which are used to polish areas which are difficult to reach with burs such as grooves, interproximal areas of ceramic or composite restorations.

### Nonbonded Abrasives

- Polishing pastes are known as nonbonded abrasives, which are used for final polishing
- They are applied to the substrate using nonabrasive device such as rubber cup, felt, synthetic foam or chamois cloth
- Abrasive particles are usually dispersed in water-based or glycerin-based medium for dental use
- Fine or ultrafine aluminum oxide and diamond particles are most commonly used nonbonded abrasives.

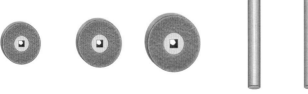

**Fig. 8.12:** Abrasive disks are available in different shape and sizes.

*Factors affecting loose abrasive wear are as follows:*
- Technique of application of abrasive paste
- Field of application of abrasive paste. If used dry, they behave more aggressive and are suitable for finishing and polishing. When used in wet field they produce greater visual surface gloss during polishing procedure
- Type of applicator device used such as felt, rubber cups, soft foam, etc. It is observed that soft foam or felt application gives a smoother finish than the rubber cups.

## Abrasive Motion

The abrasive motion with abrasive instruments can be classified as:
- Rotary
- Planar
- Reciprocal.

### Rotary Motion

The burs in the high-speed instrument make rotary motion and rotate in a clockwise direction. If cutting of the substrate is done in the same direction as the rotation of the bur then the rotating bur tends to slip away from the substrate and produce rough surface. The cutting should be done in the opposite direction to the rotation of the bur to prevent slippage and produce smoother surface.

### Planar Motion

Abrasive disks cut the substrate in the planar motion. This type of motion should be done in one direction to obtain a smooth surface.

### Reciprocal Motion

It is capable of producing two type of motion at one time. It shows cyclic and up and down motions at the same time. Reciprocating handpieces are used to produce such motion. It is used to access interproximal areas to remove overhangs, to create embrasures and to finish subgingival margins.

## Types of Abrasives

Abrasives are broadly classified as natural abrasives and manufactures or synthetic abrasives.

### Natural Abrasives

Naturally occurring abrasive includes abrasives like chalk, Arkansas stone, diamond, pumice, etc.

- *Arkansas stone* **(Fig. 8.13)**:
  - This naturally occurring abrasive stone is found mostly in Arkansas, USA
  - These stones are light gray in color, semitranslucent-containing quartz and silica
  - They are hard, dense and uniformly textured
  - They are helpful in grinding tooth enamel and metal alloys.
- *Chalk* **(Fig. 8.14)**:
  - It is one of the derivatives of calcite, which contains calcium carbonate
  - It has a very low Mohs value of 3 and therefore used as mild-abrasive paste
  - It is used to polish restorative material such as amalgam, gold or tooth enamel
  - It was once used in number of dentifrices but now is replaced with other materials.
- *Corundum* **(Fig. 8.15)**:
  - It is mineral form of aluminum oxide, which is white in color
  - Available as bonded abrasive in different shape and called as white stone
  - Used to grind metal alloys.
- *Natural diamond* **(Fig. 8.16)**:
  - It is the hardest known substance (10 on Mohs scale)
  - It is transparent, colorless mineral-containing carbon
  - Also called as superabrasive, as it can abrade any known substance
  - Supplied in different form including bonded abrasive rotary instruments, flexible metal-backed abrasive strips and diamond-polishing pastes
  - Used to grind hard, brittle substances such tooth enamel, ceramic and resin-based composite.

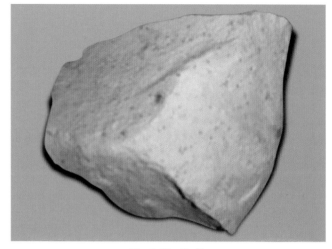

**Fig. 8.14:** Chalk.

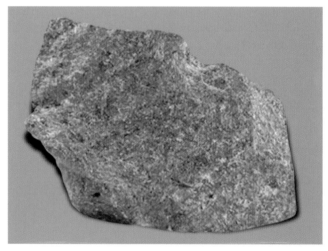

**Fig. 8.15:** Corundum.

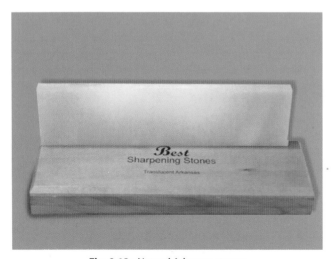

**Fig. 8.13:** Natural Arkansas stones.

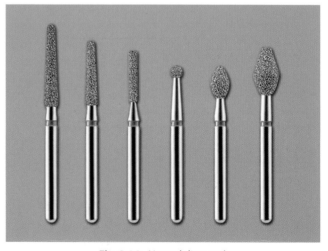

**Fig. 8.16:** Natural diamond.

- *Emery*:
  - Grayish black corundum, which is prepared in fine grain form
  - Used in form of coated abrasive disks and is supplied in various grit sizes
  - It has Mohs value greater than 9
  - Used in finishing metal alloys and acrylic resin materials
  - It is commonly used to make arbor bands, which are attached to the dental lathe and is commonly used to finish acrylic prosthesis.
- *Garnet* **(Fig. 8.17)**:
  - These are composed of several different minerals, which possess similar physical properties
  - Available in different grit sizes and particle sizes bound to paper disks with glue
  - Type of red abrasive, which contains mainly silicates of aluminum and iron and with some silicates of magnesium, cobalt and manganese
  - It can cut both metal and porcelain.
- *Pumice* **(Fig. 8.18)**:
  - It is highly siliceous light gray material
  - It is mostly found near volcanic sites
  - Available mainly in grit form and in some rubber-bonded abrasives
  - It has Mohs value of 6
  - Used to polish acrylic made prosthesis
  - Flour of pumice is used to polish tooth enamel, gold foil, amalgam and acrylic resins.
- *Quartz* **(Fig. 8.19)**:
  - It is a hard, colorless and transparent mineral
  - These particles are usually used to make coated abrasive disks, which are used to grind and finish metal alloy

  - They sometimes can be used to strip tooth enamel as in proximal stripping.
- *Sand* **(Fig. 8.20)**:
  - These are small-sized mineral particles, which predominantly contain silica
  - They can be round- or angular-shaped
  - Used in sand blasting for removing refractory investment material under air pressure
  - They are coated on paper disks and are used for finishing metal alloys and acrylic prosthesis
  - They are also used to finish cast gold restorations.
- *Tripoli* **(Fig. 8.21)**:
  - Fine siliceous powder combined with wax binder to form light-brown cakes
  - It is less abrasive than quartz

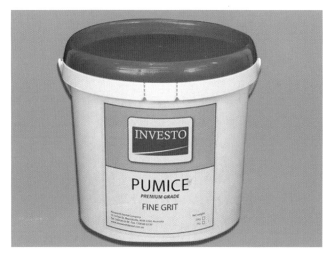

**Fig. 8.18:** Pumice.

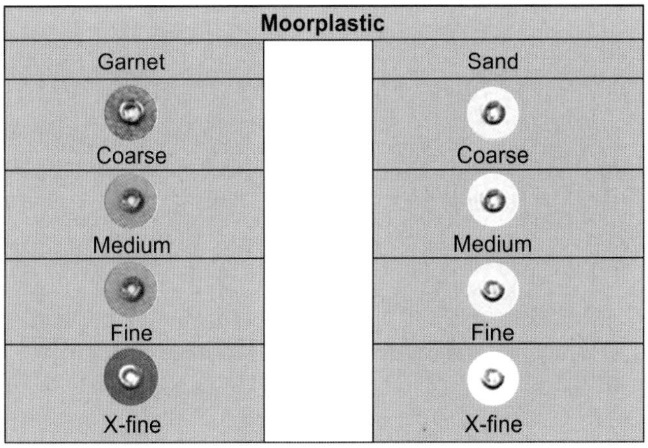

| Moorplastic | | |
|---|---|---|
| Garnet | | Sand |
| Coarse | | Coarse |
| Medium | | Medium |
| Fine | | Fine |
| X-fine | | X-fine |

**Fig. 8.17:** Garnet.

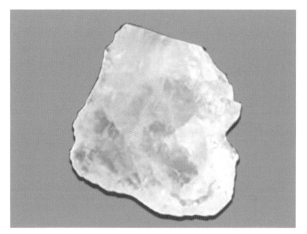

**Fig. 8.19:** Quartz.

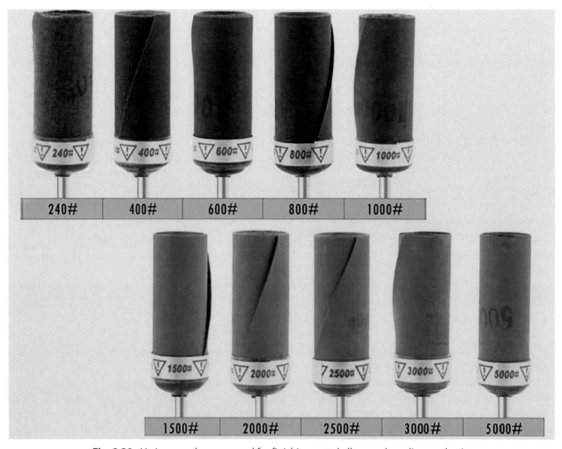

**Fig. 8.20:** Various sand papers used for finishing metal alloys and acrylic prosthesis.

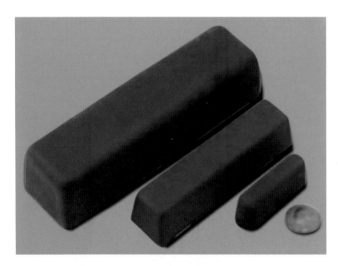

**Fig. 8.21:** Tripoli.

- Can be white, gray, pink, red and yellow types
- It has Mohs value of 6–7
- Gray and red types are commonly used for polishing gold alloys and some acrylic resin materials.
- *Zirconium silicate* (**Fig. 8.22**):
  - These naturally occurring abrasives are off white-colored minerals, which are crushed to various particle sizes
  - Widely used to coat abrasive disks and strips
  - They are also used as prophylaxis paste to polish tooth enamel.
- *Cuttle* (**Fig. 8.23**):
  - Referred to as cuttlefish, cuttle bone or cuttle
  - Fine relatively soft-polishing agent, which is derived from calcified internal shell of the cuttlefish
  - These beige-colored disks are used to finish gold alloys, composites and acrylic resins

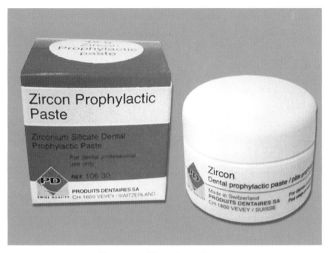

**Fig. 8.22:** Zirconium silicate.

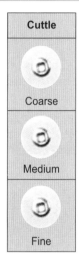

**Fig. 8.23:** Cuttle.

- Used for polishing metal margins and dental amalgam restorations.
- *Kieselguhr*:
  - Material derived from siliceous remains of minute aquatic plants known as diatoms
  - Its coarser form is called as diatomaceous earth
  - Used as filler material in hydrocolloid impression material
  - It is mild abrasive but should be used with caution as it risks respiratory silicosis.

### Synthetic Abrasives

- *Synthetic diamond abrasive (**Fig. 8.24**)*:
  - They have consistent shape and size and have lower cost compared to the natural diamonds
  - Shape of the diamond abrasive determines the type of binder to be used
  - Binder can be either resin or metal
  - Resin-bonded diamonds have sharp edges, which break down and expose new sharp edges
  - Metal-bonded diamonds are more regular and consistent in size
  - Larger synthetic diamond appears greenish because of the chemical reaction with nickel during the manufacturing process
  - This type of abrasive is used in manufacture of diamond burs, saw and wheels
  - Diamond-polishing pastes are manufactured from particles smaller than 5 μm in diameter
  - They are primarily used to cut tooth structure, ceramic and resin-based composite material.
- *Silicon carbide (**Fig. 8.25**)*:
  - This type of abrasive material is the first synthetic abrasive material to be manufactured

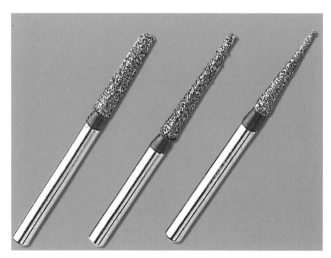

**Fig. 8.24:** Synthetic diamond abrasive.

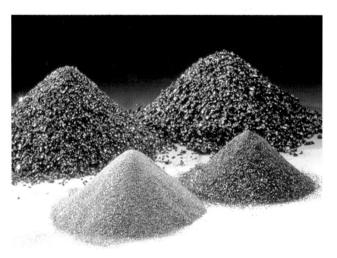

**Fig. 8.25:** Silicon carbide powders.

– They are extremely hard and brittle material, which is pressed into many shapes to form separating disks and many points and wheels called as green stones
– Available as abrasive-coated disks, vitreous-bonded and rubber-bonded instruments
– They are highly efficient in cutting metal alloys, ceramics and acrylic resin materials.

- *Aluminum oxide (Fig. 8.26)*:
  – Synthetic aluminum oxide is much harder than corundum (natural alumina)
  – It has Mohs value of 9
  – It is widely used to produce bonded abrasives, coated abrasives and air-propelled grit abrasive
  – Sintered aluminum oxide is used to make white stones, which are used to adjust dental enamel, for finishing metal alloys, resin-based composites and ceramic materials
  – *White stones* consist of fine-grained aluminum oxide, which is used for smoothing the rough surfaces created by green stones and for adapting gold margins to the tooth enamel
  – *Pink stones* are made of porcelain-bonded aluminum oxide by adding chromium compounds, which are primarily used to finish the areas of metal copings to which porcelain is to be fired.

- *Rouge (Fig. 8.27)*:
  – Consists of iron oxide, which is supplied in cake form
  – It is used for polishing gold alloys
  – Applied with a soft-bristle brush or small muslin buff wheel
  – Also used to produce crocus disks.

- *Tin oxide (Fig. 8.28)*:
  – It is extremely fine abrasive, which is primarily used to polish teeth and metallic restorations intraorally

– It is mixed with alcohol, water or glycerin to form an abrasive paste.

## POLISHING

*It is defined as a procedure that produces a shiny, smooth surface by eliminating scratches, minor surface imperfections and surface stains using mild abrasives.*

- It is a process of providing luster or gloss on a material surface
- Larger particle size abrasive removes larger portion of the substrate material and creates roughness
- Whereas smaller size particles smoothen the roughness created by larger particles
- Very fine abrasives are finally used to produce a smooth shiny surface

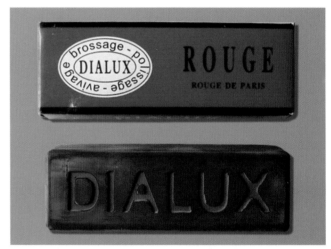

**Fig. 8.27:** Rouge.

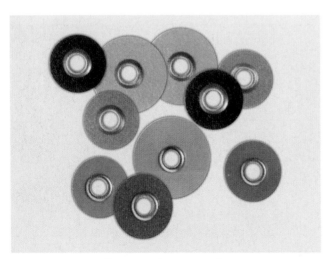

**Fig. 8.26:** Aluminum oxide.

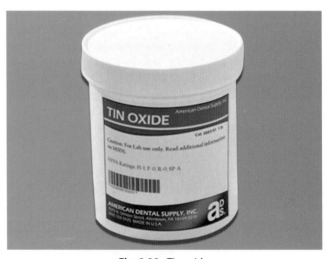

**Fig. 8.28:** Tin oxide.

- Diminishing mild abrasive is used to remove irregularities on the surface of the restoration to produce a smooth, shiny and mirror-like surface
- In order to produce a shiny surface, the scratches should not be more than 0.5 μm.

## Finishing and Polishing Procedure for Different Restorative Materials

### Dental Amalgam *(Figs 8.29A and B)*

- Polished surface of the amalgam restoration is desired as it minimizes plaque accumulation and tarnish of the surface
- Only burnishing the surface does not create the smooth surface

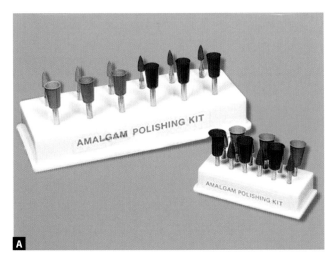

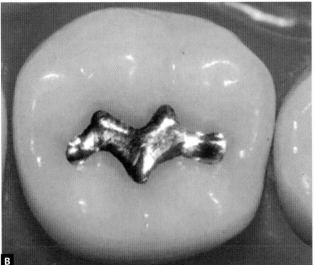

**Figs. 8.29A and B:** Polishing of amalgam restorations using polishing kit.

- Polishing of amalgam restoration is advised 24 hours after the insertion. As these restorations have potential for chipping
- Finishing and polishing of restoration depends on carving and burnishing of amalgam at the time of insertion
- Finishing and polishing is accomplished with rotary instruments using fine-abrasive paste with rubber cup, felt or brush **(Fig. 8.30)**
- Sufficient water should be used during polishing to avoid excess heat buildup
- Fast setting high-copper amalgam can be polished after 15 minutes of placement.

### Gold Alloys

- Gold is highly malleable and ductile material
- Gold restorations can be finished and polished to high luster or gloss **(Fig. 8.31)**
- It is finished and polished by sequentially using coarse, medium and fine abrasives
- Gold restorations are first contoured with carbide burs, green stones
- Then pink stones are used or medium-grade abrasive impregnated with rubber wheels and points

**Fig. 8.30:** Polishing of amalgam restoration using fine grit abrasive point.

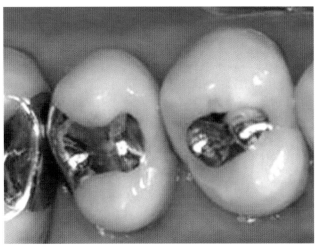

**Fig. 8.31:** Polished gold restoration.

- This step is followed by using fine abrasive impregnated with rubber wheels, cup and points
- Finally, Tripoli or rouge with rag or leather wheels is used to get high luster **(Fig. 8.32)**
- When gold restorations are polished, some minute amounts of abraded surface material are filled into the surface irregularities. This microcrystalline surface is called the *Beilby layer*.

### Resin Composite Restorations

- Resin composite restorations are difficult to finish and polish because they consist of relatively soft polymeric resin and hard filler particles
- This leads to unequal wearing of soft resin and hard filler particles creating peaks and valleys between the filler particles especially in hybrid composites and conventional composites
- However, microfilled composites have greater shiny and smooth surface as compared to conventional or hybrid composites
- Factors, which influence the final finish of the composite restorations, are composition, preparation design, cutting efficiency and postcuring time needed by the material to achieve finished surface
- It has been recommended to delay finishing procedure by 10 minutes after curing in most of the composite to allow complete polymerization of the resin
- Finishing and polishing procedure should always be done in one direction only and the next sequence is done in direction perpendicular to the first one
- Sequence of finishing and polishing of composite restorations **(Fig. 8.33)** is as:
  - Coarse grinding is done using green stone
  - Then 16–30 fluted carbide burs, fine and extra-fine diamond burs are used sequentially
  - White stones or medium and fine abrasive-coated disks are used
  - Final polishing is done using fine and extra-fine polishing paste or silicon-impregnated brushes or diamond-impregnated rubber polishing disks cups or points **(Fig. 8.34)**

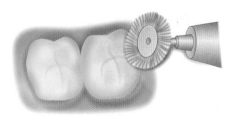

**Fig. 8.32:** Gold restoration polished by using rogue with rag wheel.

### Ceramic Restorations **(Fig. 8.35)**

- Smooth glossy surface on the ceramic restorations can be best achieved by glazing in a porcelain furnace provided the surface is smoothened with abrasives
- Polishing improves the strength of the ceramic surface by eliminating surface pores and microcracks
- Intraoral polishing is done using rotary instruments with copious quantity of water to avoid heat buildup

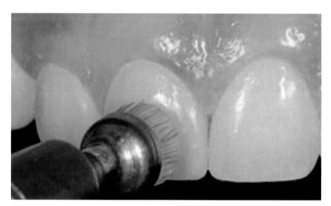

**Fig. 8.33:** Polishing of composite restoration.

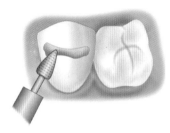

**Fig. 8.34:** Composite restoration polished using rubber abrasive point.

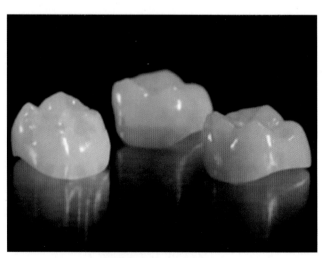

**Fig. 8.35:** Glazed ceramics.

- Sequence of finishing and polishing ceramic restorations are as follows:
  - Restoration is contoured using diamond burs, flexible diamond disks, heatless (silicon carbide) burs or green stones
  - Next finishing is done using white stones or abrasive-impregnated rubber disks, cups or points
  - Polishing is then done with fine abrasive-impregnated rubber disks, cups using diamond abrasive paste
  - Finally, a layer of overglaze or natural glaze is applied and sintered in the porcelain furnace **(Fig. 8.36)**.

## Acrylic Resins *(Fig. 8.37)*

- Denture acrylic resins are relatively soft materials, which are polished using a rag wheel and fine pumice slurry followed by Tripoli or tin oxide
- Overheating during finishing and polishing procedure should be avoided
- Sequence of finishing and polishing is as follows:
  - Denture is contoured using tungsten carbide burs
  - Rubber point and sand paper are used to remove roughness
  - Pumice paste is applied using a rag wheel, felt wheel or bristle brush **(Fig. 8.38)**
  - Finally, Tripoli or tin oxide is applied and polished on rag wheel.

## Air Abrasion Technology (Fig. 8.39)

- It is an alternative method to rotary instrumentation for finishing and polishing procedure
- This type of system can deliver a fine and accurately controlled high-pressure stream of 25–30 µm aluminum oxide particles to remove tooth enamel, dentin and restorative materials
- Air abrasion polishing is done by controlled delivery of air, water and sodium bicarbonate slurry to eliminate surface stains and plaque **(Fig. 8.40)**
- It relies mainly on the transfer of kinetic energy from stream of powder particles on the tooth surface to produce a fractured surface layer resulting in roughness.

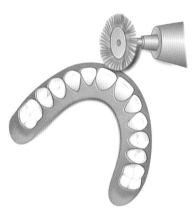

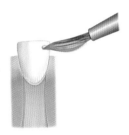

**Fig. 8.36:** Final glaze applied using a brush.

**Fig. 8.38:** Denture base polished using pumic paste on a rag wheel.

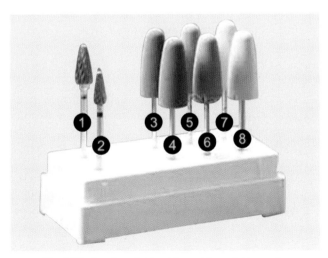

**Fig. 8.37:** Acrylic polishing kit used for polishing resin.

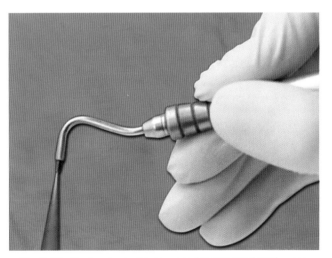

**Fig. 8.39:** Air abrasive technology used to remove dental caries.

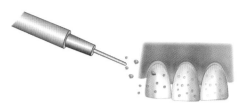

**Fig. 8.40:** Diagram showing air abrasion polishing.

## Uses

- To prepare cavity
- To remove defective composite restorations
- For endodontic access through porcelain crowns
- For repairing crown margins
- During tunnel preparation
- For removal of superficial stains
- For cleaning tooth surface prior to adhesive bonding
- To roughen internal surfaces of indirect restorations before bonding.

## Advantages

- Generates minimal heat or vibration
- Reduces the chances of tooth chipping and microfractures.

## Disadvantages

- Difficult to produce well-defined cavity margins
- Cannot be a substitute for acid-etching procedure
- No tactile sensation
- Abrasive dust interferes with visibility of the cutting site
- Abrasive dust can be inhaled by patient or office personnel.

## Dentifrices

They are usually available as toothpastes, gels and tooth powder.

### Functions

- Has abrasive and detergent action for effectively removing plaque, debris and minor stains
- They aid in polishing the teeth, which helps in increasing light reflectance and enhanced esthetics. Also, polished surface resists plaque accumulation and stains
- Acts as vehicle for delivery of therapeutic agents such as fluorides, tartar-controlling agents, desensitizing agents and remineralizing agents.

### Composition (Table 8.4)

Toothpaste and gel dentifrices contain 50–75% less-abrasive content than tooth powders. Tooth powders should be used with caution as they result in greater dental abrasion and pulpal sensitivity.

*Note*: Composition of dental powders is different than tooth pastes and gels:
- *Abrasive content*: 90–98%
- *Detergent*: 1–6%
- *Humectants*: 0%
- *Flavoring agents*: 1–2%
- *Coloring agents*: 1–2%.

### Factors Influencing Abrasiveness of Dentifrice

*Extraoral factors*:
- Type of toothbrush
- Method of tooth brushing and amount of force applied during brushing
- Frequency and duration of tooth brushing
- Content of abrasive its type, size and quantity in the dentifrice
- Patient's coordination and mental condition.

*Intraoral factors:*
- Quality and quantity of saliva
- Quality and quantity of the existing dental deposits
- Root surface exposure
- Xerostomia induced by salivary gland pathology, drugs or radiation therapy
- Type of dental prosthesis, restorative material or orthodontic appliances.

### Factors Influencing Selection of the Dentifrice

- Tooth brushing habit (frequency, duration, force applied and method of brushing)
- Presence of the type of restorative materials
- Amount of exposed cementum and dentin
- Degree of staining.

### Dental Prophylaxis Paste (Fig. 8.41)

- Prophylaxis paste is used to remove surface stains without roughening or removing the surface of the tooth or restoration
- They usually contain mild-abrasive agents such as pumice
- Usually supplied in paste form
- Mild abrasives commonly used are pumice, silicon dioxide or zirconium silicate

**Table 8.4:** Composition of toothpaste and gels.

| Component | Composition by weight | Material | Function |
|---|---|---|---|
| Abrasive | 20–55 | • Calcium carbonate<br>• Dibasic calcium phosphate dehydrate<br>• Hydrated alumina<br>• Hydrated silica<br>• Sodium bicarbonate<br>• Mixture of above abrasives | Aids in removing plaque and minor stains<br>Aids in polishing tooth surface |
| Detergent | 1–2% | Sodium lauryl sulfate | Aids in debris removal |
| Water | 15–25% | Deionized water | Suspension agent |
| Humectants | 20–35% | Sorbitol, glycerin | Aid in maintaining moisture content |
| Binder | 3% | Carrageenan | Thickener, prevents liquid solid separation |
| Fluoride | 0–1% | • Sodium monofluorophosphate<br>• Sodium fluoride<br>• Stannous fluoride | Aids in prevention of dental caries and increases remineralization of incipient noncavitated enamel lesions |
| Tartar-controlling agents | 0–1% | • Disodium pyrophosphate<br>• Tetrasodium pyrophosphate<br>• Tetrapotassium pyrophosphate | Inhibit supragingival calculus formation |
| Desensitizing agents | 0–5% | • Potassium nitrate<br>• Strontium chloride | Enhance occlusion of dentinal tubules |
| Flavoring agents | 1–2% | • Peppermint<br>• Wintergreen<br>• Oils of spearmint<br>• Cinnamon | For flavor |
| Colorants | 1–2% | Food colorants | For color of paste or gel |

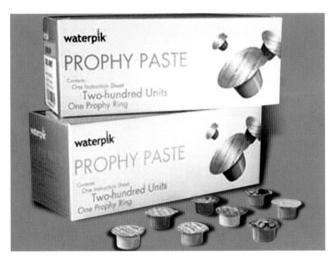

**Fig. 8.41:** Prophylaxis paste.

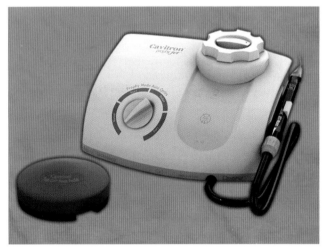

**Fig. 8.42:** Prophy jet system used to remove surface stains and soft deposits.

- Materials like silicon dioxide or zirconium silicate are aggressive abrasive and should be only used in fine powder form
- The abrasive selected as prophylaxis paste should be softer than the tooth but harder than the stain
- Aggressive abrasive should be used with caution on restorations such as composites or acrylics
- Certain prophylaxis paste may contain sodium fluoride or stannous fluoride to aid in preventing caries.

## Prophy Jet (Fig. 8.42)

- This type of prophylaxis system is used to remove surface stains and soft deposits
- It was introduced in 1980's with a specially designed handpiece that could deliver air powdered slurry of warm water and sodium bicarbonate
- Consist of sodium bicarbonate, modified silica and some flavoring agents

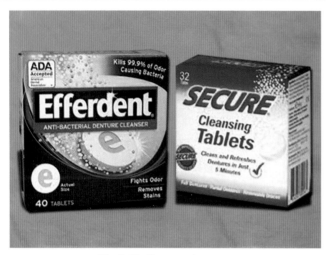

**Fig. 8.43:** Denture cleansers.

- Slurry effectively removes the stains rapidly and provides warm water for rinsing and lavage
- An abrasive powder is loaded in a cleaning device, which is directed on to the tooth surface with steady stream of air and water
- This action helps in removing extrinsic stains and supragingival plaque and calculus
- The flow rate of abrasive powder can be controlled to remove heavy stains.

### Contraindications

- Patient with respiratory disease
- Patient on restricted sodium diet
- Patient with infectious disease
- Patient on medication affecting the electrolytic balance.

### Disadvantages

- Can result in tooth abrasion
- Composite restorations are roughened
- Damage to gingival tissue is transient and is clinically insignificant.

### Denture Cleansers (Fig. 8.43)

- Dentures can accumulate plaque, debris, calculus and stains in a similar manner as natural teeth
- Daily soaking of dentures in denture cleansers is recommended chemical cleansers are:
  - Sodium hypochlorite
  - Alkaline perborates
  - Alkaline hypochlorite
  - Alkaline peroxides
- Usually dentures are soaked in dilute solution of sodium hypochlorite solutions
- The hypochlorite solution provides bleaching action to remove any stains and is an effective germicidal agent
- Dentures should not be soaked in hot water because of chances of distortion
- Patient should be encouraged to clean dentures with soft brush, soap or cleansing paste
- Hard brush should be avoided as it can abrade the denture surface
- Gentle brushing with soft brush and nonabrasive detergent is an effective cleaning method
- Use of organic solvents to clean dentures should be avoided as it may lead to crazing and eventual fracturing of the denture base.

## TEST YOURSELF

### Essay Questions

1. Classify abrasives and discuss in detail different abrasives used in dentistry.
2. Write ideal requirement of abrasive materials and write about different action of abrasives.
3. Describe various natural and synthetic abrasives used in dentistry.
4. Describe various abrasives and polishing agents.

### Short Notes

1. Bonded abrasives.
2. Dentifrices.
3. Diamond abrasives.
4. Beilby layer.
5. Pumice.
6. Finishing and polishing of acrylic dentures.

### Multiple Choice Questions

1. The goal of finishing and polishing of restorations includes:
   A. Removal of excess material
   B. Smoothening of roughened surfaces
   C. Better esthetics
   D. All of the above

2. Moh scale measures:
   A. Hardness of material
   B. Abrasiveness of material
   C. Materials by their relative abrasion resistance
   D. Both A and B

3. Rate of abrasion is influenced by all of the following *except*:
   A. Pressure applied
   B. Size of the particles
   C. Speed used
   D. Manufacturer

4. Which of the following produces smoothest surface on dental ceramic prosthesis?
   A. Aluminum oxide
   B. Tin oxide
   C. Rubber wheel
   D. Glazing

5. Patients should be instructed to clean cast partial dentures with:
   A. Rouge
   B. Household bleaches
   C. Detergent solutions
   D. Fine emery paper

6. Which of the following will not increase rate of abrasion?
   A. Use of lubricant
   B. Increased pressure
   C. Increased speed
   D. Smaller particles

7. Final polish on amalgam restoration is done by:
   A. Green points
   B. Tin oxide
   C. Brown stones
   D. Pumice

8. Prophylaxis paste should not contain diamond particles because:
   A. Abrade enamel
   B. Expensive
   C. Will not remove calculus
   D. Will not remove plaque

9. Which of the hardness scale uses diamond as maximum reference of 10?
   A. Brinell hardness number
   B. Knop hardness number
   C. Vicker hardness number
   D. Moh scale

10. Polishing abrasive for stainless steel crown is:
    A. Aluminum oxide
    B. Chromium oxide
    C. Zirconium oxide
    D. Rouge

11. Hardness of tooth enamel of Moh scale is:
    A. 5
    B. 8
    C. 4
    D. 7

## ANSWERS

| 1. D | 2. D | 3. D | 4. D |
|------|------|------|------|
| 5. C | 6. D | 7. B | 8. A |
| 9. D | 10. B | 11. A | |

## BIBLIOGRAPHY

1. Anusavice KJ, Antonson SA. Finishing and polishing materials. Phillips science of Dental Materials, 11th edition. St. Louis: Saunders Publications; 2003. pp. 351-77.
2. Carr MP, Mitchell JC, Seghi RR, Vermilyea SG. The effect of air polishing on contemporary esthetic restorative material. Gen Dent. 2002;50:238-41.
3. Eide R, Tveit AB. Finishing and polishing glass ionomer cements. Acta Odontologica Scandanavica. 1990;19:861-70.
4. Fairhust CW, Lockwood PE, Ringle RD, Thompson WO. The effects of glaze on porcelain strength. Dent Mater. 1992;8:203-7.
5. Ferracane JL. Materials in dentistry. Principles and applications, 1st edition. Philadelphia: Lippincott Williams; 1995.
6. Fruits TJ, Miranda FJ, Coury TL. Effects of equivalent grit sizes utilizing different polishing motions on selected restorative materials. Quintessence Int. 1996;27:279-85.
7. Goldstein RE. Finishing of composites and laminates. Dent Clin N Am. 1989;33:305-18.
8. Jefferies SR. Abrasive finishing and polishing in restorative dentistry. A state of the art review. Dent Clin N Am. 2007;51:379-97.
9. Jones CS, Billington RW, Pearson GJ. The in vivo perception of roughness of restorations. Brit Dent. 2004;196:42-5.
10. Powers JM, Bayne SC. Friction and wear of dental materials. In: Henry SD (Ed). Friction lubrication and wear technology, ASM Handbook, Vol 18. Material Park, OH: American Society of Metals International; 1992. pp. 665-81.
11. Pratten DH, Johnson GH. An evaluation of finishing instruments for an anterior and posterior composite. J Prosthet Dent. 1988;60:154-8.
12. Rosenblum M. Abrasion, grinding and polishing. In: O'Brien WJ (Ed). Dental Materials: Properties and selection. Chicago: Quintessence Publishing Co; 1989. pp. 437-48.
13. Stookey GK, Burkhard TA, Schemehirn BR. In vitro removal of stain with dentrifices. J Dent Res. 1982;61:1236.
14. Williamson RT, Kovarik RE, Mitchell RJ. Effects of grinding, polishing and over glazing on the flexural strength of a high leucite feldspathic porcelain. Int J Prosthodont. 1996;9:30-7.
15. Yazici AR, Antonson D. Effect of prophylactic pastes on composites surface gloss. J Dent Res. 2011;90:3046.

# Section  3

# Impression Materials

# Introduction to Impression Materials

*'Do No Harm.'*

—*Latin Phrase*

## INTRODUCTION

Impression materials are most important auxiliary materials which are widely used in dentistry to record intraoral structures for the fabrication of restorations. An accurately fitting restoration greatly depends on the accuracy of the impression. Materials used for making impressions should be thoroughly understood for a successful outcome. Usually, the choice of the material for impression making largely depends on the operator's choice, experience and treatment need. This section highlights the commonly used impression materials in dentistry.

## HISTORICAL BACKGROUND

*1728: Pierre Fauchard* known as "father of dentistry" published treatise describing many dental restorations and procedures

*1730:* Sealing wax was introduced

*1756: Phillip Pfaff* first described method to make impression with wax

*1760s: Pfaff* first used plaster of Paris for making models

*1789:* Full dentures made by *John Greenwood* for George Washington, then President of the United States of America

*1820:* Impression trays were first introduced.

*1839: Charles Goodyear* first used low-cost vulcanized rubber to fabricate dentures.

*1857:* Impression compound was first used.

1883: *Stanford,* a British Pharmacist first discovered algin which was precursor for alginate.

*1925: Alphous Poller* of Vienna first introduced reversible hydrocolloid.

*1928:* Hydrocolloid was marketed as Dentacol.

*1935:* Sears promoted the use of agar for impression making in fixed partial dentures.

*1953:* Polysulfide impression material introduced.

*1960s:* Polyether impression material was developed in Germany.

*1970s:* Condensation silicones used as an alternative impression material to polysulfide.

*1980s:* Addition polysilicones introduced as improvement to condensation silicones.

## IMPRESSION TRAYS

*It is defined as a device that is used to carry, confine and control impression material while making an impression.*

Impression tray is a receptacle into which a suitable impression material is placed to make a negative likeness. The impression is poured with plaster or dental stone to obtain a cast or a model which is a positive replica of the teeth and adjacent structures.

*Requirements of the impression tray:*

- Impression tray should be rigid
- It should be dimensionally stable
- It should be smooth and should avoid injury to the mucosa
- It should provide uniform space for the impression material
- It should not distort the vestibular area.

### Types

Impression trays are of four types:

1. Stock trays
2. Custom trays
3. Triple trays

4. Bite registration trays.
* *Stock trays* are further classified as **(Figs. 9.1A to C):**
  Type I—disposable or nondisposable
  Type II—metallic or nonmetallic

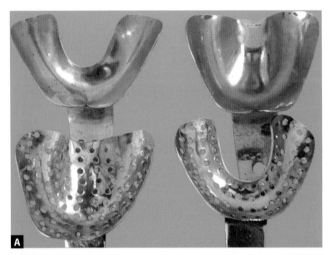

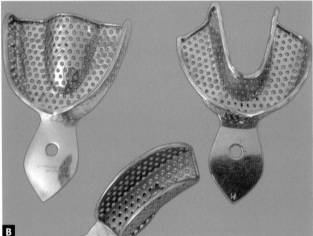

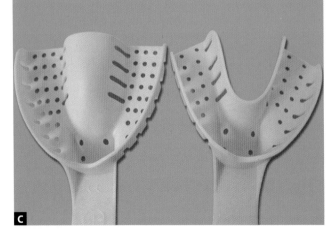

**Figs. 9.1A to C:** Types of stock trays.

Type III—perforated or nonperforated: These trays may or may not be rim locked. *Rim locked trays* have thickened flange edges which aid in mechanical retention of the impression material.

* *Custom trays*: These are special trays which are made to custom fit the mouth of the patient. They are usually made of chemically cured, light cured or thermoplastic resins on the primary cast. Also called as *final impression trays* or *individualized trays*
* *Triple trays*: Also called as *double bite* or *check bite trays*. It is a stock sectional impression tray that is used to make an impression of the treated teeth and the opposing teeth at the same time. With proper use, it can accurately record the centric occlusion of the patient
* *Bite registration trays*: These are U-shaped plastic frames with a thin fiber mesh stretched between the sides of the frame. Bite registration material is loaded on the frame and the patient is instructed to bite in maximum intercuspation. The recording material is thin enough so that it does not interfere with the closure of the upper and the lower teeth **(Fig. 9.2)**.

## IMPRESSION

### Definition

*Impression is defined as a negative likeness or copy in reverse of the surface of an object; an imprint of the teeth and adjacent structures for use in dentistry.*

*—GPT, 8th Edition*

According to *Heartwell*, impression is defined as *the negative form of the teeth and/or other tissues of the oral cavity recorded at the moment of crystallization of the impression material.*

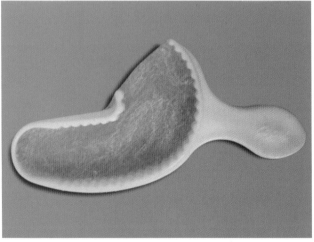

**Fig. 9.2:** Bite registration tray.

# IDEAL REQUIREMENTS OF IMPRESSION MATERIALS

The requirements of impression materials are discussed in the following section. There is no impression material which fulfills all the requirements.

- It should have good dimensional accuracy
- It should be biocompatible
- It should be easy to manipulate and have reasonable cost
- It should have adequate flow properties
- It should have adequate mechanical strength
- It should not tear or permanently deform during removal
- It should be nontoxic, nonirritating
- It should allow disinfection without deterioration in its properties
- It should be compatible to die and cast materials
- It should be sufficiently flexible to allow removal of the impression from the undercuts without tearing
- It should have appropriate setting time and characteristics
- It should have adequate shelf life
- It should be easy to use with the minimum of equipment.
- It should have satisfactory consistency and texture.
- It should readily wet oral tissues.
- It should not release any gas during the setting of impression or cast.

## Classification of Impression Materials

- *Based on the elasticity of the materials (Table 9.1)*:
- *Based on the type of reaction (Table 9.2)*:
- *Based on their use*:
  - *Materials used for obtaining impressions in dentulous mouth*:
    - Alginate
    - Agar
    - Nonaqueous elastomeric impressions.
  - *Materials used for obtaining impressions of edentulous mouth*:
    - Impression compound
    - Impression plaster
    - Zinc oxide(ZnO)-eugenol
    - Impression wax
    - Agar.
- *Based on the viscosity or type of tissue displacement (Table 9.3)*.

**Table 9.1:** Classification of impression materials based on the elasticity.

| Elastic | Inelastic or rigid |
|---|---|
| • Hydrocolloid<br>  – Agar<br>  – Alginate<br>• Nonaqueous elastomer<br>  – Polysulfide<br>  – Polyether<br>  – Silicones<br>    - Condensation<br>    - Addition | • Impression compound<br>• Impression waxes<br>• Impression plasters<br>• Zinc oxide-eugenol impression pastes |

**Table 9.2:** Classification of impression materials based on the type of reaction.

| Chemical reaction (irreversible) | Thermally induced physical reaction (reversible) | |
|---|---|---|
| • Plaster of Paris<br>• Zinc oxide-eugenol<br>• Alginate<br>• Nonaqueous elastomers | Thermoplastic<br>• Impression compound<br>• Waxes | Nonthermo-plastic<br>• Agar |

**Table 9.3:** Classification of impression materials based on the viscosity or type of tissue displacement.

| Mucostatic | Mucocompressive |
|---|---|
| Impression plaster, agar, alginate | Impression compound |

## TEST YOURSELF

### Essay Questions

1. What is an impression tray? Classify and write about various impression trays.
2. Define impression? What are ideal requirements for impression materials? Write briefly about historical background of impression materials.

### Short Notes

1. Ideal requirements of impression materials.
2. Impression trays.
3. Triple trays.
4. Bite registration trays.

## Multiple Choice Questions

1. Which of the following impression material can be changed from sol to gel state when set?
   A. Agar and alginate
   B. Zinc oxide-eugenol impression paste
   C. Addition silicones
   D. Polyether

2. Requirements of impression tray do not include:
   A. Should be flexible
   B. Should be dimensionally stable
   C. Should provide uniform space for impression materials
   D. Should not injure soft tissues

3. All are elastic impression materials, *except:*
   A. Alginate
   B. Addition polysilicone
   C. Polyether
   D. Impression paste

## ANSWERS

1. A     2. A     3. D

## BIBLIOGRAPHY

1. Anusavice KJ. Phillip's Science of Dental Materials, 11th Edn. Elsevier, St. Louis, 2003.
2. Anusavice KJ, Shen C, Rawls HR. Phillip's Science of Dental materials, 12th edition, Elsevier Inc, St. Louis; 2013.
3. Craig RG, Powers JM. Restorative Dental Materials, 11th Edn. Elsevier, St. Louis; 2002.
4. Craig RG. Review of dental impression materials. Adv Dent Res. 1988;2:51.
5. Donavan JF, Chee WW. A review of contemporary impression materials and techniques. Dent Clin N Am. 2004;48:445-70.
6. Giordano R. Impression materials: basic properties. Gen Dent. 2000;48:510-6.
7. Gladwin MA, Bagby MD. Impression materials. Clinical Aspects of Dental Materials. Lippincott Williams and Wilkins. Philadelphia; 2000.
8. Leinfelder KF, Lemons JE. Impression materials. Clinical Restorative Materials and Techniques. Lea and Febiger. Philadelphia; 1988.
9. Lloyd CH, Scrimgeour SN (Eds). Dental materials: Literature review. J Dent. 1997;25:193.
10. Rubel BS. Impression materials: A comparative review of impression materials most commonly used in restorative dentistry. Dent Clin N Am. 2007;51:629-42.

# Elastic Impression Materials

*'Coming together is a beginning, staying together is progress and working together is success.'*

*—Henry Ford*

## INTRODUCTION

Elastic impression materials were introduced to overcome the inability of rigid inelastic material to be used in undercut area. These materials have adequate flexibility to be removed from the undercut area without getting distorted. Materials which are flexible are polymeric in nature and are cross-linked.

*Elastic impression materials are of two types:*
1. Hydrocolloids
2. Elastomers (Discussed in detail in Chapter 11)

## HYDROCOLLOIDS

A *colloid* is a glue-like material which is composed of two or more substances in which one substance does not go into solution but is suspended within another substance.

*Hydrocolloids* are water based colloids that function as elastic impression materials. These are polysaccharide materials which form cross-linked network through hydrogen bonding, e.g. agar and alginate.

*Some terms which are essential to understand before discussing individual materials are:*
- Sol—small solid particles are suspended in colloidal liquid solutions
- Gel—network of fibrils that form a weak, elastic brush heap structures
- Liquefaction temperature—the temperature at which the gel converts into sol
- Gelation—conversion of sol into gel

- Imbibition—water absorbed by the gel
- Syneresis—loss of water from the surface of gel due to evaporation.

*Types of hydrocolloids are:*
- Reversible hydrocolloids
- Irreversible hydrocolloids.

## REVERSIBLE HYDROCOLLOID—AGAR

Agar hydrocolloid (ADA Specification No. 82) was the first elastic impression material used successfully in dentistry. It was introduced by *Alphous Poller* of Vienna in 1925. He initially named it as "Nogacoll". Although it was marketed as Dentacol in 1928.

Agar hydrocolloid impression materials are compounded form of reversible agar gels. It is an organic hydrophilic colloid extracted from certain *seaweed*. It is a sulfuric ester of a linear polymer of galactose. Though highly accurate, it has been largely replaced by alginates and elastomers due to its cumbersome manipulation.

### Applications

- For making impression of edentulous and dentulous arches without deep undercuts
- For duplication of master casts
- Impression of operative and crown and bridge procedures before the advent of elastomers
- As tissue conditioners
- Used for bite registration in triple tray technique.

**Table 10.1:** Composition of hydrocolloid—agar.

| Ingredient | Percentage | Function |
|---|---|---|
| Agar | 12–15% | Colloidal particles as basis of the gel, i.e. brush heap structure |
| Potassium sulfate | 1% | Ensures set of gypsum material; acts as accelerator |
| Borax | 0.2% | Strengthens gel |
| Alkyl benzoate | 0.1% | Antifungal agent |
| Water | 85% | Dispersing medium for the colloidal suspension; controls flow properties of sol |
| Colors and flavors | Traces | For appearance and taste |
| Wax, silica, rubber | 0.5–1.0% | As filler material to control strength, viscosity and rigidity |
| Thymol | Traces | Bactericidal agent |
| Glycerin | Traces | Plasticizer |

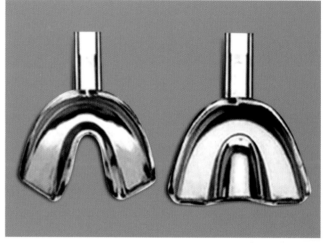

**Fig. 10.2:** Special metal stock tray to make impressions.

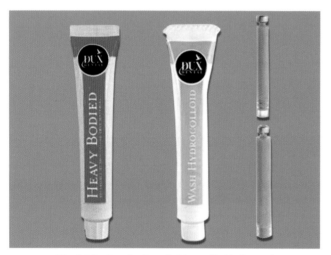

**Fig. 10.1:** Agar hydrocolloid supplied in form of collapsible tubes.

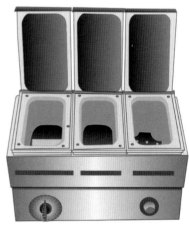

**Fig. 10.3:** Hydrocolloid conditioner with three compartments.

## Composition

The composition of hydrocolloid—agar has been shown in **Table 10.1**.

## Supplied As (Figs 10.1)

- Gel in collapsible tubes for impression
- As syringe material, they have similar composition but with lower concentration of agar (6–8%)
- In bulk containers for duplication.

## Manipulation

The manipulation of agar hydrocolloid requires a special equipment specific for its use. Special metal stock trays

called as *water cooled trays* are used to carry liquefied sol into the patient mouth **(Fig. 10.2)**. These trays have tubing running through them that connects the water lines by rubber hoses to circulate tap water through the tray. The running water cools the impression material so that it gels within a reasonable time (setting time—5 minutes). These trays also allow adequate thickness of the material to minimize the dimensional changes.

### Preparation and Conditioning of the Material

For preparation of the material to be used for impression, a special heating unit called as hydrocolloid conditioner is required **(Fig. 10.3)**. This conditioner has three water bath chambers, each of which are set a different temperature. These three chambers are **(Figs. 10.4A to C)**:

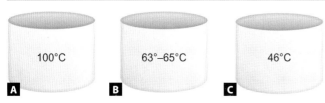

**Figs. 10.4A to C:** Three chambers of hydrocolloid conditioner (A) Liqueifaction; (B) Storage; (C) Tempering.

1. *Boiling or liquefaction section*: 10–12 minutes in boiling water (100°C). In case the material needs liquefaction, additional 3 minutes are required. In higher altitudes, the boiling point of water lowers and it may not be enough to liquefy the gel. In such a situation, propylene glycol is added to water to obtain liquefaction temperature of 100°C
2. *Storage section*: 65–68°C is ideal it can be stored till needed even for several hours. The syringe material does not require storage as it flows when it is forced out from the syringe
3. *Tempering section*: 46°C for about 2 minutes. Tempering prevents burn to the oral tissues or potential pulp damage of the prepared tooth. The syringe material is never tempered because it should be maintained in the fluid state to increase adaptation to the tissues.

In case the hydrocolloid sol is required urgently. Portion of sol is taken from the storage section and the tray is filled with it. A gauze pad is covered on the top of the tray material and it is placed in the tempering section for 3–10 minutes. Once the temperature is lowered sufficiently so that it does not harm the oral tissues it is ready for use. The gauze is removed and the tempered sol is placed in the mouth to make impression. The purpose of the gauze piece is to prevent absorption of water.

*Impression making:* The syringe material is taken from the storage compartment and is applied to the base of the preparation and injected around the prepared teeth. The tempered hydrocolloid sol is loaded into the water cooled rim locked trays and placed into position in the patient mouth with light pressure. Gelation of the sol is accelerated by circulating cool water at around 18–21°C for 3–5 minutes. The tray is positioned in the mouth until complete gelation has occurred and it has attained sufficient strength to resist deformation. Adequate time is needed for gelation as the material sets from periphery to the center and premature removal of the tray from the mouth should be avoided **(Fig. 10.5).**

*Removal of tray:* The impression should be removed rapidly with a snap rather than slowly. This is because if the material is removed slowly it has greater chance of tearing.

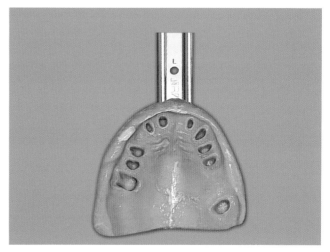

**Fig. 10.5:** Impression made with reversible hydrocolloid.

## Advantages

- It is a hydrophilic impression material and can be used in a moist field
- It has good elastic properties, good recovery from distortion. It has 98.8% of elastic recovery, i.e. the material regains 98.8% of its shape after elastic strain during removal from the undercuts
- It can be reused as a duplicating material
- Long working time and low material cost
- No mixing technique
- High accuracy and fine detail recording
- Long shelf life.

## Disadvantages

- Only one model can be used
- Extensive and expensive equipment required
- It cannot be electroplated
- Impossible to sterilize for reuse
- Low dimensional stability and tear strength
- Impressions to be poured immediately
- Thermal discomfort
- Difficult to see margins and details.

## Properties

- *Sol-gel transformation*: When agar powder is mixed in water, it forms a glue-like suspension that entraps water. This is called as *sol*. Heating this will disperse agar in the water faster. When this sol is chilled, it converts into *gel* which is semisolid or jellylike. In a gel state, the dispersed phase form chains or fibrils which branch and intermesh to form *brush heap structure*. When the agar gel is again heated, it changes into a liquid suspension, i.e. sol. This process is reversible and, therefore, called as reversible hydrocolloid.

- *Thixotropic gel*: Agar is a thixotropic material because of its ability to flow under pressure or force. This property helps the material to stay in the confines of impression tray until carried into the mouth. Once pressure is applied during impression making the material flows to record details
- *Strength*: The agar gel can sustain considerable shear stress without flow, provided the applied stress is rapid. The strength and stiffness of the gel is dependent on the concentration of the hydrocolloid. Its strength can increase with the addition of modifiers such as fillers and chemicals. The tear strength of agar hydrocolloid is comparable to alginate but is much less than that of elastomer. Since it has poor tear strength, it should not be used in areas with undercuts. The compressive strength of agar hydrocolloid is 8,000 g/cm$^2$ and its tear strength is 800–900 g/cm$^2$. The impressions made with hydrocolloid should be removed with a snap because this minimizes the chances of rupture or tearing of the impression
- *Dimensional stability*: The agar gels if left in open lose water and contracts. This process of loss of water by evaporation from its surface is called as *syneresis*. Likewise if the agar gel is placed in water it absorbs water and swells by a process called as *imbibition*. Contraction or swelling of the gel leads to dimensional changes in the poured cast and ultimately the final prosthesis. The effects of dimensional changes can be minimized by pouring the impression immediately. If the impression cannot be poured immediately then it is best stored in 100% relative humidity (humidor) or wrapped in a damp towel and sealed in a zippered plastic bag
- *Gelation, liquefaction and hysteresis*: Most of the materials melts and solidifies at the same temperature but in case of agar hydrocolloid it does not coincide. The gel converts into sol when it is heated between 70°C and 100°C called as *liquefaction temperature*. When cooled from this temperature range, the sol converts into a gel. This temperature is called the *gelation temperature* (37°C). This temperature difference between the gelation and liquefaction temperature is called as *hysteresis*
- *Flexibility*: The American Dental Association (ADA) specification requirements for flexibility allow a range of 4–15%. Most of the agar hydrocolloids meet this requirement. Since it has poor tear strength it should be avoided in areas of undercuts
- *Working and setting time*: Working time for agar hydrocolloid is 1.25–4.5 minutes and setting time is 1.5–5.0 minutes
- *Elastic recovery*: Recovery from deformation at 10% compression for 30 seconds is 98.2%
- *Reproduction of details*: A reproduction of up to 25 μm is achievable with agar hydrocolloids.

# LAMINATE TECHNIQUE OR AGAR-ALGINATE COMBINATION TECHNIQUE

It is a syringe tray combination impression technique which minimizes the equipment requirement of agar hydrocolloid. Here a syringe type of agar hydrocolloid is heated in boiling water for 6 minutes and stored at 65°C water bath for 10 minutes of use. The tray is loaded with freshly mixed chilled alginate. The prepared tooth is injected with syringe agar hydrocolloid material. Immediately the loaded alginate tray is placed over the agar hydrocolloid. The alginate material sets in about 3 minutes whereas the agar material sets in 4 minutes. The alginate material helps in setting of the agar hydrocolloid material. During the setting of alginate and gelling of agar hydrocolloid, a bond is created which holds both the impression materials together. To obtain an effective bond both the impression materials should be used when they are in a flowable state. The tensile bond strength varies between 600 g/cm$^2$ and 1,100 g/cm$^2$.

## Advantages

- Elimination of water cooled impression trays
- Simplification of heating equipment
- Easy to manipulate
- Good accuracy and low cost
- Compatibility with die materials.

## Disadvantages

- Bonding between agar and alginate is not usually adequate
- Greater viscosity of alginate displaces agar hydrocolloid.

## Wet Field Technique

In this technique, the tooth surfaces which are to be recorded are flooded with warm water. Then a syringe agar is injected over and around the prepared surface. Immediately tray loaded with agar hydrocolloid is seated over the syringe material. The hydraulic pressure of the viscous tray material forces the syringe material to flow evenly over the surface to be recorded. Theoretically, there is less chance that these materials will tear when the impression is removed from the mouth.

**CLINICAL SIGNIFICANCE**

- It should be ensured that viscosity of the sol should be sufficient to record teeth and adjacent tissues accurately
- It is advisable to wait longer after gelation of agar before removal of impression because this will increase the tear strength of the material
- The impression made with this material should be poured as soon as possible
- Gelation occurs from the periphery toward the center of the mass which is accompanied by shrinkage stress. Therefore, rapid cooling of the tray is not advised as it will lead to build up of stress near the tray area.

## IRREVERSIBLE HYDROCOLLOID OR ALGINATE

Alginate (ADA Specification No. 18) is one of the most widely used impression material today. It is an irreversible hydrocolloid as it sets by chemical reaction. The alginate hydrocolloid was developed as a substitute for the agar impression material when it became scarce during the World War II. This material is derived from *"Algin"* which is a peculiar mucous extract yielded by Algae (brown seaweed). Chemically, it is a linear polymer of anhydrous β-D-mannuronic acid of high molecular weight **(Fig. 10.6)**.

This material is widely used because of the following reasons:

- Ease of manipulation and use
- Minimum equipment requirement
- Flexibility of the set materials
- Accuracy if handled properly
- Relatively inexpensive
- Comfortable for the patient.

### Composition

The composition of alginate has been shown in **Table 10.2**.

### Clinical Uses **(Fig. 10.7)**

- Used for making impressions for diagnostic casts (study models)
- Used for preliminary impression for complete dentures
- Used for making impression for fabrication of provisional restorations
- Used for making impression for fabricating custom trays for fluoride or bleaching
- Used in repairs of partial and complete dentures
- Used for making impressions for making opposing cast for crown and bridge treatments
- For duplicating models
- For fabricating sports protector and night guard appliance
- Used for making impression in presence of undercuts and in mouth with excessive saliva
- Used for impression for partial denture frameworks
- For fabricating maxillofacial prosthesis.

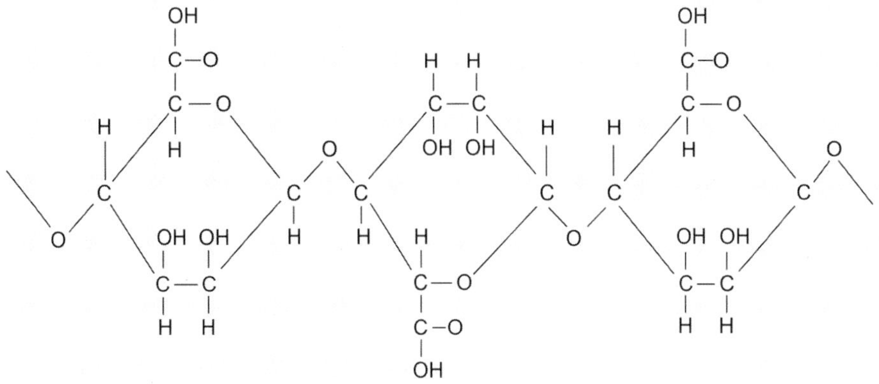

**Fig. 10.6:** Chemical formula of alginic acid.

**Table 10.2:** Composition of alginate.

| Ingredient | Percentage | Function |
|---|---|---|
| Sodium or potassium alginate | 15–20% | Primary reactive ingredient; colloidal particles as basis of the gel |
| Calcium sulfate dihydrate | 14–20% | Forms irreversible gel with alginate and controls the rate at which cross-linking cations are released |
| Potassium sulfate or potassium zinc fluoride | 10% | Ensures set of gypsum material |
| Trisodium phosphate | 2% | Acts as retarder to control setting time |
| Diatomaceous earth | 55–60% | Fillers to increase thickness and strength |
| Organic glycol | Small quantity | Reduce dust when handling powder |
| Flavoring agents | Small quantity | Improve taste of material |
| Coloring agents | Small quantity | Give a pleasant color |
| Disinfectants such as quaternary ammonium compound or chlorhexidine | Small quantity | Provides self-disinfection |

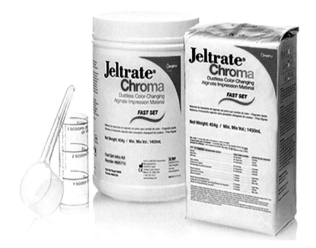

**Fig. 10.7:** Alginate impression material.

## Advantages

- Easy to manipulate and mix
- Minimum requirement of equipment
- Accurate if handled properly
- Flexibility of the set impression
- Relatively inexpensive
- Comfortable to the patient
- It is hygienic as it is not reusable
- Can be used in undercut areas
- Provides good surface detail even in presence of saliva.

## Disadvantages

- Has low tear strength
- Dimensionally unstable
- Cannot be electroplated
- Cannot be corrected
- No proper storage medium
- Cannot capture fine details of the preparation needed for precise fit of the restoration.

## Types

Based on the setting time alginate is of two types:
1. *Type I:* Fast set.
2. *Type II:* Normal or regular set.

## Supplied As

Alginate can be supplied as:
- *Single component*: In this supplied as powder to which water is mixed to initiate chemical reaction
- *Two component*: In this system one component is supplied in the form of alginate sol and the other contains calcium reactor. They are available both in syringe viscosity and tray viscosity.

## Setting Reaction

When alginate powder is mixed with water it forms a sol which converts into gel after a chemical reaction. The calcium ions in the calcium sulfate dihydrate react preferentially with phosphate ions from the trisodium phosphate and pyrophosphate to form insoluble calcium phosphate. First calcium phosphate is formed rather calcium alginate as it has lower solubility. Because of this reason, trisodium phosphate is added as retarder to delay the setting reaction. The amount of retarder added determines the time of set and differentiate between the fast set and regular set alginate.

$$2Na_3PO_4 + 3CaSO_4 \longrightarrow Ca_3(PO_4)_2 + 3Na_2SO_4$$
$$\text{(Retarder)} \qquad\qquad \text{(Reactor)}$$

Once the phosphate ions are depleted, the calcium ions react with soluble sodium alginate to form insoluble calcium alginate which along with water form an insoluble gel. This reaction is irreversible as the material sets by chemical reaction. Unlike the agar hydrocolloid, it cannot be converted to sol state.

$$Na_{2n}Alg + n\,CaSO_4 \longrightarrow nNa_2SO_4 + Ca_nAlg$$
$$\text{(Reactor)} \qquad\quad \text{(Gel)}$$

The *final gel structure* consists of fibrous network of calcium alginate with water occupying the intervening capillary spaces. At least one of the dimensions of the network is colloidal and this *brush heap structure is called as alginate hydrocolloid* **(Fig. 10.8)**.

Manufacturers control the setting time by the amount of sodium phosphate. They also adjust the concentration of filler to control the flexibility of the set impression material. Also, sometimes certain compounds are used as retarders instead of phosphates. These compounds are called as *sink compounds*, e.g. $Na_2CO_3$, $Pb_2SiO_4$, and $BaSO_4$.

## Properties

- *Working time and setting time*: According to the ADA Specification No. 18, regular or normal set alginate has a working time (from start of mix to seating in the mouth) of 2–3 minutes whereas the fast set alginate has working time of 1.25–2 minutes. The setting time for regular set alginate is 2–5 minutes and for fast set alginate is 1–2 minutes.

  *Factors influencing the setting time of alginate are:*
  - *Temperature of water*: Cold water increases the setting time whereas warm water reduces the setting time
  - *Altering the water powder ratio*: Not recommended as it can adversely affect the physical properties of the mix
  - *Addition of retarder*: Increases the setting time and is controlled by the manufacturer.

- *Permanent deformation*: The ANSI-ADA Specification No. 18 requires 95% recovery (5% permanent deformation) when alginate is compressed 20% for 5 seconds. There are many commercially available alginate which have 96–98% recovery (2–4% permanent deformation). The alginate impression material is flexible but not exactly elastic. A thickness of 2–4 mm is needed between the impression tray and the teeth in order to resist tearing and deformation. Like the agar hydrocolloid, the alginate impression should be removed by rapid snap to prevent deformation of the critical areas

- *Dimensional stability*: Alginate impressions are dimensionally unstable because of imbibition and syneresis. Therefore, the impressions should be poured immediately after disinfecting it. If it cannot be poured immediately then it should be wrapped in a damp towel and sealed in a zipped bag or kept in a humidor

- *Strength*: The tear strength of alginate impression material is less than the compressive strength. Thin sections of alginate are more prone for tearing of the impression. If the material is handled properly, it has adequate tear strength. The ADA Specification No. 18 requires minimum compressive strength of 3,570 $g/cm^2$. Although most of the commercially available alginate have strength varying between 5,000 $g/cm^2$ and 9,000 $g/cm^2$.

  *Factors influencing gel strength are*:
  - *Water-powder ratio*: Any alteration than recommended ratio will reduce the gel strength
  - *Mixing time*: Over or under mixing will reduce the gel strength
  - *Time of removal of impression*: If the impression is removed from the mouth after 1–2 minutes beyond the setting time, it will increase the tear strength
  - *Thickness of alginate*: Thin sections of alginate are more prone of tearing.

- *Flexibility*: According to the ADA Specification No. 18, the flexibility of alginate should be between 5% and 20% in compression. The compression is measured between stress of 100 $g/cm^2$ and 1,000 $g/cm^2$. Most of the commercially available alginate have flexibility between 12% and 18% but some hard set alginates have flexibility between 5% and 8%. Alteration in water-powder ratio influences the flexibility of the set alginate. Thicker mix results in lower flexibility

- *Reproduction of detail*: The impression material should record the details of the oral tissues and this detail should be transferred to the gypsum die. The ADA specification requires a minimum capability of transferring a line of 0.075 mm wide to a gypsum model or die material. There are many products available which exceed this minimum limit

- *Shelf life*: Alginate impression materials have shorter shelf-life. They deteriorate rapidly at higher temperatures. The alginate should be stored in cool dry place

- *Adhesion*: Since alginate does not adhere well to metal tray. The stock tray should be perforated to provide mechanical interlocking for retention of the material or an adhesive should be applied on the tray

- *Electroplating*: The alginate impression material cannot be electroplated

- *Biological properties*: Silica particles present in the alginate powder can cause health hazard during dispensing. The dust particles can be airborne. Some manufacturers have coated alginate powder with organic glycols in order to make it *dust free*.

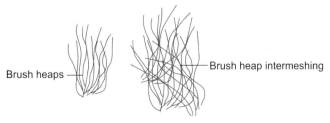

**Fig. 10.8:** Brush heap structure.

## Manipulation

### Objectives for Making Alginate Impression

- Recording of all teeth in upper and lower arches
- Recording of entire alveolar process
- Recording of the retromolar area of the lower arch
- Recording of the hamular notch in the upper arch
- A detailed, undistorted and bubble free reproduction of the oral tissues.

### Selection Criteria for Maxillary Impression Tray (**Fig. 10.9**)

- Tray should cover the anterior teeth with incisors contacting the flat arch portion of the tray about 4 mm from the raised palatal part of the tray
- Tray should be 4 mm wider than the most apical portion of the alveolar process at the molar region
- Tray should cover the tuberosity.

### Selection Criteria for Mandibular Impression Tray (**Fig. 10.10**)

- Lower tray should cover all teeth and retromolar pad
- Tray should be 4 mm wider that the buccal and lingual positions of the posterior and the labial and lingual positions of the anterior teeth
- Tray should be placed such that the teeth are in the center.

### Dispensing of Alginate

- The recommended amount of the water for either upper or lower impression is measured using liquid dispensing vial
- The measured quantity of water is poured into the rubber bowl
- The temperature of water should be between 22°C and 23°C

- The alginate powder is usually available in bulk. The powder is fluffed by tumbling the container several times before opening
- Powder scoop is filled with alginate powder and tapped lightly with the spatula in order to endure full measure free from large voids
- Excess powder is dropped back into the container
- The recommended *water-powder ratio* is 2:1.

### Mixing of Alginate (**Figs. 10.11A to D**)

- Powder is sifted in water contained in a rubber bowl. If water is poured over the powder, then water is prevented from flowing to the bottom of the bowl thereby increasing the mixing time
- A stiff, wide bladed curved metal or plastic spatula is used to mix powder with water
- The spatula which is flexible enough to adapt to the walls of the bowl is selected
- Initially proper wetting of powder particles with water should be ensured
- Then the mix is spatulated vigorously against the side of the rubber bowl until a smooth, homogeneous creamy mix is formed which is free from voids
- The spatula is moved in vigorous figure of 8 motion with the mix being swiped or stropped against the sides of the rubber bowl to press out the air bubbles
- Mechanical mixing devices can also be used for mixing alginate. The advantages are rapid mixing, ease of use and consistent mix
- The final mix should be smooth, creamy which does not drip off the spatula when it is raised from the bowl
- The mixing time, working time and setting time of alginate are given in **Table 10.3**.

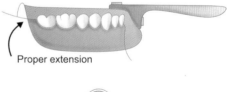

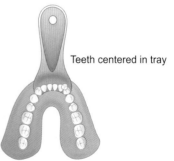

**Fig. 10.10:** Selection of mandibular impression tray.

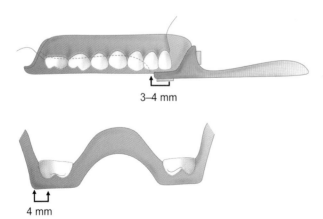

**Fig. 10.9:** Selection of maxillary impression tray.

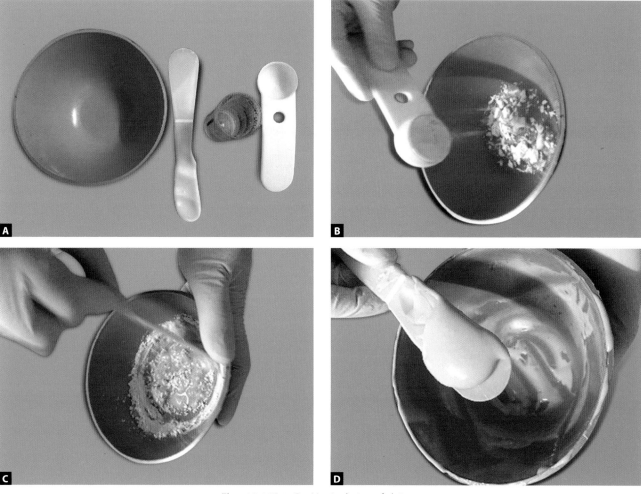

**Figs. 10.11A to D:** Manipulation of alginate.

**Table 10.3:** Mixing time, working time and setting time of alginate.

| Types | Mixing time | Working time | Setting time |
|---|---|---|---|
| I-Fast set | 45 sec | 1.25 min | 1–2 min |
| II-Normal set | 60 sec | 2 min | 2–4.5 min |

### Control of Gelation Time

- By manufacturers: by adding retarders
- By dentist
  - *Cold water*: Longer is the gelation time
  - *Warm water*: Shorter is the gelation time.

### Loading of the Tray

- The tray is evenly filled with mixed alginate with the help of the spatula
- It should be ensured that air bubbles are not entrapped during loading

- The tray is loaded till the mix is even with the top sides of the tray
- Perforated tray is usually preferred for alginate impression because it provides mechanical retention
- If a plastic tray or metal rim locked tray is used, then alginate tray adhesive should be used.

### Seating of the Tray and Impression Making

- For the *mandibular impression*, the operator position is in the 7 o'clock position. The loaded tray is rotated into the mouth and aligned over the teeth with the tray handle in the midline
- The tray is first seated posteriorly and then anteriorly
- The lower lip is pulled out to allow the alginate to flow into the vestibule and the patient is instructed to touch the palate with the tongue and relax
- The borders are molded outward, upward and inward
- The tray is stabilized with the index and middle finger over the right and left sides of the arches

- For the *maxillary impression*, operator stands at the 11 o'clock position
- The tray is rotated into position, aligned over the teeth and centered in the midline
- The tray is first seated posteriorly and then anteriorly
- Patient should be seated in an upright position when the tray is placed to minimize the collection of saliva
- Excess alginate is quickly swiped away to avoid gagging or breathing problems.

*Handling of the Impression*

- Once set the alginate impression should be removed with a snap
- The impressions are rinsed with cold water
- Impressions are inspected under light and any unsupported alginate is removed
- Impressions are disinfected appropriately
- After disinfection, the impressions are poured with stone of choice.

**CLINICAL SIGNIFICANCE**

Pressure should not be applied when the loaded tray is placed in position in the mouth because the material first set inward therefore any pressure at this stage will result in stress incorporation. When the impression is removed from the mouth, the stresses tend to relieve and distortion can occur in the impression.

## MODIFIED ALGINATES

- *Chromatic or color indicator alginates*: In this type of alginate, chemical indicators are added to aid the operator in depicting various stages during manipulation. The indicator reflects various stages of reaction which has been reached
- *Dust free alginates*: Some manufacturers coat the powder particles with glycol to make it dust free
- *Siliconized alginates*: For better properties of alginates, the powder particles are incorporated with silicon polymers. Such materials are supplied in two consistencies—tray and syringe viscosities. These materials have better tear strength as compared to unmodified alginates
- *Hard and soft set alginates*: These alginates are differentiated by adjusting the percentage of fillers to control the flexibility of the set impression material
- *Alginates containing disinfectants*: Some manufacturers are adding disinfectants to the alginate powder to provide antimicrobial properties. Quaternary ammonium salts or chlorhexidine are commonly added

- *Sol form alginates*: Some alginates are supplied in the form of sol containing water but without $Ca^{++}$ ions. A reactor of plaster of Paris is added to the sol to complete reaction.

## COMPARISON BETWEEN HYDROCOLLOIDS

Comparison between hydrocolloids has been shown in **Table 10.4.**

**Table 10.4:** Comparison between hydrocolloids.

| Properties | Agar | Alginate |
|---|---|---|
| Flexibility | 20% | 14% |
| Elasticity and elastic recovery | 98.8% | 97.3% |
| Reproduction of details | 25 μm | < agar |
| Tear strength | 715 g/cm² | 350–700 g/cm² |
| Compressive strength | 8,000 g/cm² | 500–8,000 g/cm² |
| Dimensional stability | Better | Poor |
| Reuse | Possible | Not possible |
| Manipulation | Conditioner and rim lock trays | Perforated or nonperforated stock trays |

## DISINFECTION OF ALGINATE IMPRESSION

The disinfection procedure for hydrocolloid impression should be rapid as the impression should be poured immediately. Disinfectants commonly used are sodium hypochlorite, iodophor, glutaraldehyde and phenylphenol solution. The current protocol for disinfecting hydrocolloid impression is to use household bleach in 1:10 dilution, iodophors or synthetic phenol. Once the impression is rinsed, it is sprayed liberally over the exposed surface. The impression is then wrapped immediately in a disinfectant soaked paper towel and placed in a sealed plastic pouch for 10 minutes. After that the impression is quickly unwrapped and poured with stone of choice **(Table 10.5)**.

## DUPLICATING MATERIALS

Duplicating materials (ADA Specification No. 20) are those materials which are used to make an accurate replica of master cast or model. Hydrocolloids both reversible and irreversible are used to duplicate dental casts used in the construction of prosthetic and orthodontic appliances. Duplicating of models is required because:
- Original master cast is required to check the accuracy of the metal framework and for processing acrylic portion of cast partial denture

**Table 10.5:** Troubleshooting in alginate impression.

| Problem | Cause | Remedy |
|---|---|---|
| Set prematurely | • More powder in mix<br>• Prolonged mixing warm water or high room temperature | • Use correct water/powder ratio<br>• Use timer to gauge working time<br>• Use cool water to slow the set |
| Set slowly | • Water used is cold<br>• More water in mix | • Use warmer water<br>• Use correct water/powder ratio |
| Grainy surface | • In homogeneous mix of powder and water | • All powder particles should wet and mix to creamy consistency |
| Incomplete coverage of teeth or tissues | • Selected tray is small<br>• Tray not seated completely | • Proper tray selection<br>• Use mouth mirror to check complete seating of tray |
| Voids on occlusal surface | • Air entrapment during tray seating | • Alginate wiped on occlusal surface before placing loaded tray |
| Large voids at vestibule or midpalate region | • Trapped air<br>• Insufficient alginate in the tray<br>• Improper seating of the tray<br>• Lip interference | • Place alginate in the vestibule before placing the tray<br>• Use adequate amount of alginate<br>• Seat the tray posteriorly first before seating anteriorly<br>• Lips are pulled out to create space for alginate |
| Distortion | • Movement of tray during gelation<br>• Removal before complete gelation<br>• Improper removal from mouth<br>• Delay in pouring of cast | • Tray movement should be avoided during gelation<br>• Tray should be removed after complete gelation<br>• Tray should be removed with a jerk<br>• Impression should be poured immediately |
| Rough and chalky cast surface | • Inadequate cleaning of the impression<br>• Excess water on the surface of impression<br>• Premature removal before gelation<br>• Improper mixing of powder and water<br>• High water/powder ratio | • Impression should be cleaned properly<br>• Excess water should be removed before pouring<br>• Impression should be removed after complete set<br>• Proper mixing should be done<br>• Powder and water should be mixed in proper ratio |
| Torn alginate | • Impression is removed too slowly<br>• Mix is thin | • Impression should be removed with a snap<br>• Mix should be done in proper proportion |
| Excess alginate at the back of the tray | • Tray seated anterior first and then posteriorly, forcing the material on back side<br>• Tray overfilled with alginate | • Tray should be placed first posteriorly then anteriorly<br>• Tray should be filled excessively |

• Cast on which wax pattern is formed should be made with refractory investment so that it can withstand high casting temperature.

## Classification of Duplicating Materials

According to the ADA Specification No. 20, duplicating materials are of two types:
1. *Type I:* Thermoreversible
   i. *Class I:* Aqueous—hydrocolloid—agar
   ii. *Class II:* Nonaqueous—PVC gel
2. *Type II:* Nonreversible
   i. *Class I:* Aqueous—alginates
   ii. *Class II:* Nonaqueous—elastomers.

Requirements for duplicating materials according to the ADA Specification No. 20 are:
• Maximum permanent deformation for both type I and type II Duplicating materials are 3%, i.e. minimum elastic recovery should be 97%

• Strain in compression for both type I and type II materials are 4–25%
• Minimum compressive strength for type I materials should be $2200 \text{ g/cm}^2$ and for type II materials are 4–25%
• Minimum tear resistance for both types of materials is 900 g/cm.

### Duplicating Procedure

Agar hydrocolloid duplicating materials are most commonly used and most preferred material for duplication. The composition of agar duplication material is similar to the agar impression material except it has higher water content. For the duplicating process, the sol form of agar is poured into the duplicating flask containing master cast positioned in the center. The liquid sol is poured in the hole through the flask until it overflows from the other vent. After the gelation of the agar, the master cast is removed with a jerk to minimize permanent deformation. The mold is poured immediately with refractory material to obtain a refractory or duplicating cast.

*The benefits of using agar material are:*
- Reversibility
- Acceptable reproduction of details
- Can be stored in sol form for a long period of time

- Have adequate strength and elastic properties.

*Drawbacks of using agar:*
- Subject to dimensional changes
- Chances of tearing.

---

# TEST YOURSELF

## Essay Questions

1. Classify various impression materials. Write in detail about alginate impression material.
2. What are hydrocolloids? Discuss in detail composition, types, setting reaction, properties and uses of Alginate impression material.
3. Classify hydrocolloid impression materials. Discuss Agar – agar materials in detail.
4. Discuss trouble shooting in alginate impression materials.

## Short Notes

1. Duplicating materials.
2. Laminate technique.
3. Siliconized alginate.
4. Wet field technique.
5. Brush heap structure.
6. Syneresis and imbibition.

## Multiple Choice Questions

1. Which of the following impression material can be changed from sol to gel state when set?
   A. Agar and alginate
   B. Zinc oxide-eugenol impression paste
   C. Addition silicones
   D. Polyether
2. Which is the least accurate impression material?
   A. Agar hydrocolloid
   B. Polyether
   C. Condensation silicone
   D. Alginate
3. Elastic irreversible impression material is:
   A. Impression compound
   B. Agar hydrocolloids
   C. Impression paste
   D. Alginate
4. Retarder used in irreversible hydrocolloid is:
   A. Borax
   B. Trisodium phosphate

C. Calcium sulfate dihydrate
D. Calcium alginic acid

5. Sol to gel and gel to sol transformation in reversible hydrocolloid is:
   A. Independent of temperature and is a chemical change
   B. Independent of temperature and is a physical change
   C. Dependent on temperature and is a physical change
   D. Dependent on temperature and is a chemical change
6. Setting reaction of alginate involves:
   A. Insoluble alginate and calcium ions
   B. Insoluble alginate and phosphate ions
   C. Soluble alginate and calcium ions
   D. Soluble alginate and trisodium phosphate
7. Disinfection in impressions:
   A. Should be done for all impressions
   B. Should be done only in those patients with infectious disease
   C. Is done to protect patient from surface bacteria
   D. Is not required
8. Irreversible hydrocolloid is:
   A. Hydrophobic
   B. Can be converted to sol by heating the gel
   C. Cannot be converted back to sol from gel state
   D. Does not tear easily
9. Reversible hydrocolloid is:
   A. Has excellent tear strength and can be removed from deep undercuts without tearing
   B. Hydrophobic
   C. Pouring can be delayed for several days
   D. can record accurately in wet field
10. Setting time of alginate can be controlled by:
    A. Mixing time
    B. Temperature of water used
    C. Accelerators and retarders
    D. Altering water-powder ratio

---

## ANSWERS

| | | | |
|---|---|---|---|
| 1. A | 2. D | 3. D | 4. B |
| 5. C | 6. C | 7. A | 8. C |
| 9. D | 10. B | | |

# BIBLIOGRAPHY

1. Anusavice KJ, Shen C, Rawls HR. Phillip's science of dental materials, 12th edition Elsevier Inc, St. Louis; 2013.
2. Anusavice KJ. Phillip's science of dental materials, 11th Edn. Elsevier, St. Louis, 2003.
3. Cottone JA, Molinari JA. State of art infection control in dentistry. J Am Dent Assoc 1991;122:33-41.
4. Craig RG, Powers JM. Restorative dental materials, 11th edn. Elsevier, St. Louis; 2002.
5. Craig RG. Review of dental impression materials. Adv Dent Res. 1988;2:51.
6. Davis BA, Powers JM. Effect of immersion disinfection on properties of impression materials. J Prosthodont. 1994;3:31.
7. Donavan JF, Chee WW. A review of contem-porary impression materials and techniques. Dent Clin N Am. 2004;48:445-70.
8. Finger W. Accuracy of dental duplicating materials. Quint Dent Tech. 1986;10:89.
9. Giordano R. Impression materials: basic properties. Gen Dent. 2000;48:510-6.
10. Gladwin MA, Bagby MD. Impression materials. Clinical Aspects of Dental Materials. Lippincott Williams and Wilkins. Philadelphia; 2000.
11. Johnson GH, Craig RG. Accuracy and bond strength of combinations of agar/alginate hydrocolloid impression materials. J Prosthet Dent. 1986;55:1.
12. Miller MW. Syneresis in alginate impression materials. Br Dent J. 1975;139:425-430.
13. Rubel BS. Impression materials: A comparative review of impression materials most commonly used in restorative dentistry. Dent Clin N Am. 2007;51:629-42.
14. Rudd KD, Morrow RM, Rhodes JE. Dental laboratory procedures. Vol 2. Removable Partial Dentures. St Louis: Mosby; 1986.
15. Takahashi H, Finger WJ. Dentin surface reproduction with hydrophilic and hydrophobic impression materials. Dent Mater. 1991;7:197-201.

# Elastomeric Impression Materials

ADA Specification No. 19; ISO Specification No. 4823:2015

## CHAPTER OUTLINE

- Polysulfides
- Silicone Rubber Impression Material
- Polyether Rubber Impression Material
- Disinfection of Elastomeric Impression
- Recent Advances in Elastomers
- Impression Techniques

*'Any fact facing us is not as important as our attitude towards it, for that determines our success or failure.'*
— ***Norman Vincent Peale***

## INTRODUCTION

Elastomers are highly accurate impression materials which have properties similar to rubber, and therefore are called as rubber base impression materials. These materials are group of rubbery polymers which are either chemically or physically cross-linked. As rubbers they can be stretched and quickly recover the original shape once the stress is released. Owing to their accuracy, they are extensively used in restorative dentistry for constructing indirect esthetic restorations, fixed partial dentures, inlays, onlays, veneers, partial denture frameworks and complete dentures.

Elastomers are defined as three-dimensional polymer network which has good elasticity and has a wide elastic range within an intended working temperature range. In dentistry, four types of elastomers are commonly used namely—polysulfides, polyethers, condensation silicones and addition silicones. All these elastomeric impression materials are capable of recording intraoral and extraoral structures with adequate accuracy.

According to the ADA Specification No. 19, these impression materials are referred to as nonaqueous elastomeric impression materials.

### Classification of Elastomeric Impression Materials

- *According to chemistry:*
  - Polysulfides
  - Polysilicones—condensation and addition
  - Polyether.
- *According to viscosity:*
  - Light body or syringe consistency
  - Medium or regular body
  - Heavy body or tray consistency
  - Very heavy body or putty consistency.

- *According to the ADA classification:* Based on selected elastic properties and dimensional changes
  - Type I
  - Type II
  - Type III.

### General Properties

- Excellent reproduction of surface details
- Elastomers are generally hydrophobic in nature as they do not wet well by water because it forms a high contact angle with them. Among the elastomers the most hydrophilic materials are the polyethers. Some manufacturers add surfactant to the addition silicones to make them more wettable and hydrophilic. Also before pouring the elastomeric impression, surfactant should be sprayed into the impression before it is poured with gypsum to replicate fine details **(Fig. 11.1)**
- *Elasticity and viscoelasticity*: Elastomers show good elastic properties (repeated pouring is possible). All elastomeric impression materials are viscoelastic in nature. The polyvinyl siloxane (PVS) shows the highest elastic recovery among the available materials. These materials exhibit least amount of permanent deformation when removed from the undercut area. Although, the heavy body putty material shows elastic property while it is in the working stage. Such a material if compressed excessively during seating of impression can show distortion on removal because of rebound phenomenon **(Fig. 11.2)**
- *Dimensional accuracy and dimensional stability*: Dimensional inaccuracies are lower but exist due to various reasons. They may be due to polymerization

shrinkage, thermal contraction from mouth temperature to room temperature, loss of byproduct, absorption of disinfectant or water, incomplete recovery after removal due to viscoelastic behavior and incomplete recovery due to plastic deformation. Dimensional change occurs more in polysulfides and condensation silicone material in comparison to polyether and addition polysilicone because of loss of byproducts. For this reason impression of condensation silicone and polysulfides should be poured within 30 minutes whereas impressions with addition silicone and polyether can be poured within a week showing least amount of distortion. The polyether impression should be stored in cool, dry place to maintain its accuracy otherwise it has tendency to absorb water or fluids. The dimensional accuracy of elastomers is time dependent with greatest accuracy reported immediately after complete polymerization. The accuracy reduces if the impression is stored for extended period of time

- Elastomers have excellent tear strength
- Elastomers are electroplatable
- It exhibits extended shelf life
- Generally it has higher cost

- *Requires tray adhesive or mechanical interlocking*: Since elastomers are rubbery in nature they do not adhere well to the metal or acrylic surface. Therefore, a tray adhesive is needed to prevent the material from separating from the tray and causing distortion **(Fig. 11.3)**
- *Rebound phenomenon*: Since elastomers are rubbery in consistency, they have certain amount of recovery or rebound from deformation. Rebound phenomenon reduces distortion in the cast that is poured from the impression. The addition silicones and polyether have the highest amount of rebound, condensation silicones have moderate and polysulfides have least amount of rebound
- *Tear strength*: It is measured by the amount of force required to tear a specific test specimen divided by the thickness of the specimen. A tear strength test measures the resistance of an elastomeric impression material

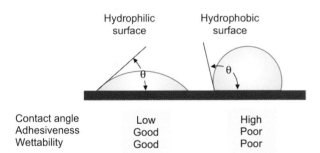

**Fig. 11.1:** Diagram to explain contact angle, wettability and adhesiveness in hydrophilic and hydrophobic surfaces.

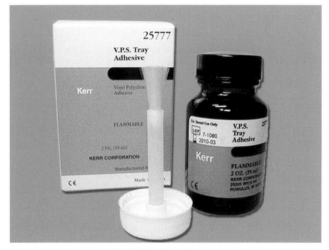

**Fig. 11.3:** Tray adhesive.

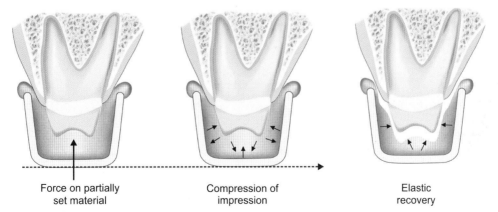

**Fig. 11.2:** If heavy body putty is compressed excessively during impression, it shows distortion on removal due to rebound phenomenon.

to tear when subjected to tensile load perpendicular to the surface flaw. The tear strength of elastomers from low to high is in the order—silicones, polyether and polysulfides. Although studies show that some polyethers and addition silicones have high tear strength than some of the polysulfides. However, despite polysulfides having greater tear strength, they have high susceptibility to permanent deformation

- *Elastic recovery*: A set impression should be sufficiently elastic so that it returns to its original dimension without distortion on removing from the mouth. PVS has best elastic recovery followed by polyether and polysulfides.

## Supplied As

- All elastomers—two paste systems (base and catalyst)
- Putty consistency supplied in jars.

Elastomeric impression materials are two-component setting materials (chemically) that are delivered as two tubes of pastes.

The pastes can be mixed together with:

- *Mixing pads (manually)*: Both base and catalyst pastes are taken on pad in equal quantity and then mixing is done manually to obtain uniform mix. Mixing is done in circular motion for 45 seconds till the mix is free from streaks
- *Automixing guns (by manually expressing the two pastes through a mixing tip)*: This mixing system is also referred as static automixing system. In this system, the base and catalyst are stored in separate cylinders of a plastic cartridge. The plastic cartridge is fitted into the extruder gun which has two plungers. As the gun is pressed, these plungers force the base and catalyst through the stationary plastic internal spiral in correct volume and dispenses as premixed. The uniform mix is directly flowed over the prepared tooth and the impression tray. Condensation, addition polysilicones and polyether are available in these systems

- *Mixing equipment (electrically driven pumps for proportioning of materials from larger tubes through a Kenics mixing tip)*: This system is called as automated mixing system or dynamic mechanical system. It consists of paste mixing machine for base and catalyst cartridges and a plastic mixing tip. It uses a motor to force materials through the syringe onto the impression tray with the help of parallel plungers. The amount of material left in the mixing tip is greater than that left in static system. Through this method even high viscosity materials can be mixed with less effort. Addition polysilicone and polyether impression materials are available in this system **(Figs. 11.4A and B)**.

## Rheological Behavior of Elastomers **(Fig. 11.5)**

- The type of mixing technique depends on the rheological behavior of the mixture, the viscosity of a fluid is proportional to the shear rate
- The viscosity of Newtonian liquid is constant and independent of the shear rate
- The viscosity of pseudoplastic liquid decreases with increasing the shear stress (the viscosity decreases by tenfolds)
- The viscosity of a dilatant liquid increases with increasing the shear rate
- Materials that are *Newtonian or dilatant* are hard to mix through a mixing tip. *Silicone* and *polysulfide* elastomers are examples of those situations, respectively. Therefore, they must be mixed manually on a mixing pad
- *Polyether* and PVS are examples of materials that undergo shear-thinning. This property of addition

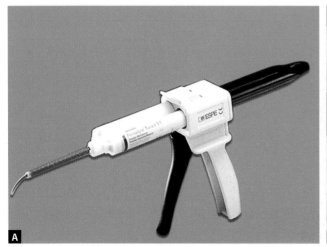 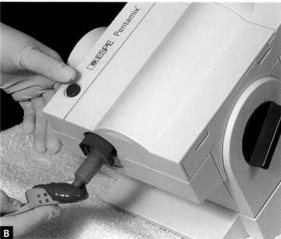

**Figs. 11.4A and B:** (A) Automixing gun; (B) Automated mixing equipment .

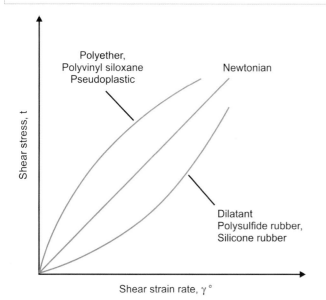

**Fig. 11.5:** Rheological properties of elastomers.

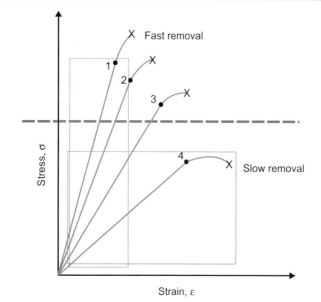

**Fig. 11.6:** Effects on slow or fast removal of elastomeric impression.

polysilicone and polyether impression material allows the dentist to use a monophasic impression making technique

- Pseudoplastic materials when subjected to low shear rates during spatulation or while an impression is made in a tray. These materials when used in a syringe, the viscosity decreases as the material passes through the syringe tip (the viscosity decreases by tenfolds)
- Rapid removal of an elastomeric impression material leads to the least chance for plastic deformation if the procedure involves rapid elastic deformation
- All polymers are *strain rate sensitive*. We should remove the impression with a snap. This creates a rapid loading rate. If the stress is applied quickly, then all the energy is stored elastically and the material does not undergo plastic deformation **(Fig. 11.6)**
- This is important in the region of the greatest deformations (e.g. the margins)
- Fast removal rates, generate elastic deformations
- Slow removal rates cause plastic deformation and distort the impression in critical areas.

## Uses

- Impression material for all applications including:
  - Fixed partial dentures
  - Dentures and edentulous impressions.
- Border molding of special trays (polyether)
- Bite registration
- As duplicating material for refractory casts.

## POLYSULFIDES

They are also called as rubber base. Polysulfides are the oldest elastomers introduced as mercaptan/Thiokol. They have greater dimensional stability and better tear strength than agar or alginate hydrocolloids. They have greater accuracy than hydrocolloids but least among other elastomers. They are supplied as two pastes in tubes.

### Composition

#### Base Paste

- Liquid polysulfide polymer (80–85%)—contains reactive mercaptan group
- Inert fillers (titanium dioxide, zinc sulfide—16–18%)—reinforcing agent (copper carbonate or silica)
- Plasticizer (dibutyl phthalate) (1–2%)—provides viscosity to the paste
- Accelerator (sulfur or zinc sulfate) (0.5%)—to accelerate the reaction
- It is supplied as white color paste.

#### Catalyst or Reactor Paste

- Lead dioxide (60–68%)—most common catalyst—causes the mercaptan groups to form polymer of polysulfide rubber. T-butyl hydroperoxide can be used as an alternative to lead dioxide
- Dibutyl phthalate (30–35%)—as plasticizer

- Sulfur (3%)—as accelerator
- Other substances like magnesium
- Oleic or stearic acid (2%)—acts as retarder
- It is supplied as dark brown or dark gray color paste. When the catalyst paste is mixed with the base paste, it gives the blue-green color.

### Tray Adhesive

Butyl rubber or styrene/acrylonitrile dissolved in a volatile solvent such as chloroform or a ketone.

## Availability

Available as two paste systems:
1. Base and accelerator
2. Three viscosities—light, medium and heavy bodies **(Fig. 11.7)**.

## Chemistry and Setting Reactions

The reaction occurs when molecules of the long chain polysulfide polymer with its functional mercaptan groups react with oxygen from the lead dioxide. This results in lengthening of the polymer chains and a cross-linking of adjacent chains. Cross-linking is important for forming elastic rubber-like material. The byproduct released during the setting reaction is water. The setting reaction begins as soon as the mixing is started and continues till spatulation is completed. Soon resilient network begins to form and once the material is completely set it can be removed from the undercuts easily. The setting reaction is slightly exothermic recording a slight increase in temperature from 3°C to 5°C.

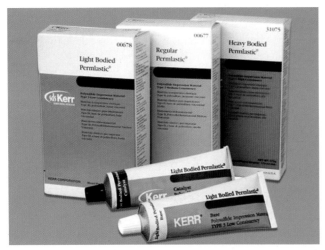

**Fig. 11.7:** Polysulfide impression material.

$$\text{HS-R-SH HS} \xrightarrow{\text{PbO}_2 + \text{S}} \text{R-S-S-R-SH} + \text{H}_2\text{O}$$
$$\text{Mercaptan} + \text{Lead dioxide} \longrightarrow \text{Polysulfide} + \text{Water}$$

The setting reaction in polysulfides is sensitive to moisture and temperature. In hot and humid conditions, it sets faster whereas in cold conditions it sets slowly. Water formed as a byproduct is lost from the set material and has a significant effect on the dimensional stability of the impression.

## Manipulation

An equal lengths of base and catalyst paste are dispensed on a mixing pad. A stiff blade spatula is used to first mix the base and catalyst paste together with its tip in a circular motion for 5–10 seconds. Then the side of the blade is used to mix the materials using wide sweeping strokes until a homogeneous mix is achieved. Properly mixed material should have uniform color and consistency. The process of mixing should be complete in 45 seconds. Since polysulfides are hydrophobic in nature, they will not flow into areas of moisture. The operating field should be well isolated. As mentioned setting reaction is sensitive to moisture and temperature. Increase in either one will accelerate the setting reaction.

The heavy or regular viscosity material is loaded into the custom tray which is having a uniform space of 2 mm for the impression material. Inside surface of custom trays are painted with a tray adhesive for better mechanical interlocking of the material. On the other hand, the low viscosity material is syringed on the prepared tooth surface. The loaded tray is then seated over the low viscosity material until it sets. Light body or low viscosity material takes longer to set than higher viscosity material. The impression is removed with a steady force on setting. The working time is 5–7 minutes whereas the final setting time varies between 8 minutes and 12 minutes. The impression should be poured within 30 minutes otherwise polymerization shrinkage will occur. Dies can be poured with gypsum or epoxy materials. The impression can be electroplated resulting in greater abrasion resistant dies.

## Uses

- Used for impression making in fixed partial denture and removable partial dentures
- Used for complete denture impressions
- They have limited use now as they have number of drawbacks.

## Properties

- *Setting time*: It ranges between 8 minutes and 14 minutes. Light body material requires longer time to set than regular or heavy body. Setting time can alter by temperature change and moisture contamination
- *Permanent deformation during compression*: Polysulfides have slightly higher permanent deformation than the hydrocolloids which are less than 3%. The permanent deformation values of 2–3% is obtained when the material is held under 12% compression for 30 seconds. During removal, the compression of impression should be avoided
- *Tear strength*: They have about eight times higher tear strength than hydrocolloids. The strength and permanent deformation of polysulfides continue to improve after they are set
- *Loss of water*: Polysulfides lose water but to a less extent than the hydrocolloids which are produced as byproduct resulting in certain degree of distortion
- *Compatibility with die and model materials*: Polysulfides as other elastomeric materials are compatible with gypsum and epoxy or metal dies which can be electroplated. The metal or epoxy dies have greater resistance to abrasion than gypsum dies
- *Taste and odour*: Polysulfide elastomers have very unpleasant taste and odour which resemble rotten eggs because of the presence of sulfur. They are very messy to work with and are difficult to clean. If the material drops on the patient's or operators clothing, then it is very difficult to remove. Orange solvent is usually used to remove the stains
- *Shrinkage on setting*: Polysulfide impressions shrink 0.3–0.4% during the first 24 hours. The models and dies should be prepared immediately
- *Flexibility*: During removal polysulfide impressions have high flexibility. High viscosity materials have lower flexibility
- *Reproduction of surface details*: Polysulfide provides excellent reproduction of surface details and is capable of reproducing a fine line of width 0.025 mm
- *Shelf-life*: Polysulfide materials have excellent shelf life but should not be stored in warm conditions. The caps should be tightly replaced after use. Storing in a refrigerator extends its shelf life
- *Radiopacity*: It is radiopaque because of the presence of lead dioxide.

## Advantages

- Capable of reproducing surface details accurately
- Polysulfides are compatible with gypsum materials and epoxy resins
- Can be electroplated
- Have excellent shelf life when stored at lower temperature
- Tear resistance is about eight times more than the hydrocolloids.

## Disadvantages

- Has unpleasant odor
- Staining is due to lead dioxide.

## SILICONE RUBBER IMPRESSION MATERIAL

Developed to overcome some of the disadvantages of polysulfide. There are two types of silicone impression materials which have been developed and are named based on the type of polymerization reaction.

| Classification of Silicone Rubber Impression Material |
| --- |
| Based on the type of polymerization reaction, it is classified as:<br>• Condensation silicones<br>• Addition silicones. |

### Condensation Silicones

Condensation silicone materials were first developed as an alternative to polysulfide materials. These materials are also known as conventional silicone. It has superior properties than the polysulfide elastomers such as ease of manipulation, odourless, pleasant taste, reduced working and setting times.

#### Supplied As

Base paste and accelerator or catalyst paste. It is available in light, medium, heavy and putty consistency **(Fig. 11.8)**.

#### Composition

High molecular weights are used with more viscous materials. The reinforcing agent increases from 35% for low viscosity to 75% for the putty consistency.

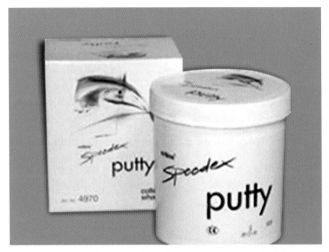

**Fig. 11.8:** Condensation silicone impression material.

- *Base paste:*
  - *Moderately low weight polydimethyl siloxane:* Contains reactive—OH groups
  - *Silica or microsized metal oxide:* Provides proper consistency to the paste and stiffness to the set rubber
  - *Color pigment:* To provide color to the paste.
- *Accelerator or catalyst paste:*
  - Orthoethyl silicate: Cross-linking agent
  - Stannous octoate: Catalyst.

### Setting Reaction

When base paste is mixed with a catalyst paste, a condensation reaction takes place between dimethyl siloxane and orthoethyl silicate to form silicone rubber and ethyl alcohol. The ethyl alcohol which is produced as a byproduct is rapidly lost by evaporation thereby leading to relatively high dimensional instability from shrinkage. The dimensional changes in condensation silicones are higher in first 24 hours as compared to polysulfides. In condensation silicones with putty consistency have higher amount of fillers which helps in reducing dimensional changes. The setting time for condensation silicones is 5–7 minutes. Any increase in temperature and moisture reduces the setting and working time of this type of silicones. After setting the impression should be poured within few minutes to reproduce an accurate detail.

Hydroxy terminated + Tetraethyl  Tin octoate  Silicone + $C_2H_5OH\uparrow$
Polydimethyl siloxane  orthosilicate ———→ rubber

Tray adhesive – Polydimethyl siloxane and Ethyl silicate

### Properties

- Pleasant odor and color as compared to polysulfides
- They are nontoxic but direct skin contact of the catalyst paste should be avoided because of its allergic potential
- They have short mixing time of 45 seconds and short setting time of 6–7 minutes as compared to polysulfides
- They are prone for greater dimensional changes in first 24 hours as compared to polysulfides
- They have lesser dimensional stability because of:
  - High curing shrinkage (0.4–0.6%)
  - Permanent deformation due to shrinkage caused by the evaporation of ethyl alcohol is also high (1–3%).
- Permanent deformation of condensation silicones is lower than that of polysulfides because they have higher cross-linking in silicones
- Excellent reproduction of surface details and is highly elastic
- Hydrophobic—needs a dry field
- Flexibility of silicones is lower
- Tear strength of condensation silicones is 3,000 g/cm which is lesser than that of polysulfides

- Electroplatable (silver/copper)
- Has adequate shelf life but is shorter than that of polysulfides
- Biologically inert
- Compatible with all gypsum products
- They have poor wetting characteristics and surfactant should be used before pouring the casts.

## Uses

Used primarily for impression for fixed partial dentures but have largely been replaced by addition silicones.

## Manipulation

Condensation silicones are usually encouraged to be used as *putty wash impression* material. Desired quantity of putty is taken with a scoop and the appropriate amount of catalyst paste or liquid is dispensed. Both are mixed using a stiff blade spatula until it is free from streaks for 30 seconds. Direct contact with skin should be avoided during mixing. Mixed putty is loaded in a perforated or nonperforated tray which is coated with an adhesive. The loaded impression tray is placed over the teeth before the preparation of the teeth. The putty material is allowed to set. After cavity preparation, the wash impression material is syringed over the prepared surface and into the putty impression. The loaded putty tray is seated over the wash material until it sets. The putty wash impression is removed and is inspected for details. This system increases the accuracy of the impressions as putty has a lower dimensional change than the wash material. Since the wash material is used in thin layer the dimensional change is insignificant.

## Advantages

- Unlike polysulfides, it has pleasant odour and taste
- Has less permanent deformation than the polysulfides.

## Disadvantages

- Has limited shelf life
- Impression cannot be stored for long before pouring
- Dimensional stability is affected because of release of ethyl alcohol as byproduct.

## Addition Silicones

Addition silicones are also called as *PVS* or *vinyl polysiloxane* impression materials. Addition silicones were developed as an improvement over the condensation silicones. These materials are more dimensionally stable and accurate than the condensation silicones.

## Supplied As

Two paste systems. One is the base paste and other is the catalyst paste. PVS materials are supplied as low, medium, high or very high viscosity (putty) material. They are available in the form of base and catalyst tubes or automixing cartridges **(Fig. 11.9)**.

*Automixing or dual cartridge system:* In this system, the base paste is supplied in one cartridge and catalyst paste in another cartridge with a mixing gun. The cartridge is placed in a mixing gun and with the help of ratchet device plungers it forces the pastes through a *static mixing tip*. During extrusion the two pastes are folded over one another and the mixed material flows out of the tip. For every use, a new mixing tip is used. A very high viscosity addition silicone (putty material) is supplied in boxes and is dispensed with scoops. The putty material is mixed by hand.

Addition silicones can also be mixed using a mechanical mixer using a *dynamic mixing tip*. The base and catalyst paste are supplied in form of cartridges and are placed in the allotted slots in the mixer. The mixer is switched on and the mix is dispensed directly into the tray. The mix with automatic mixing systems result in very few bubbles as compared with hand mixing.

*Monophasic materials:* Addition silicones are also available as monophase materials, i.e. as a single consistency material which can be used both as a low and high viscosity material. When they are under high shear force such as been extruded from the syringe, they have low viscosity and when they are under low shear force such as loaded into impression tray using spatula they have high viscosity *(shear thinning)*.

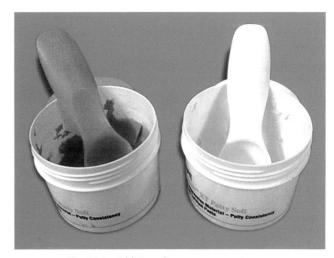

**Fig. 11.9:** Addition silicone putty consistency.

## Composition

- *Base paste:*
  - Polymethyl hydrogen siloxane
  - Other siloxane prepolymers
  - Hybrid silicones
  - Fillers.
- *Accelerator paste:*
  - Divinyl polysiloxane
  - Other siloxane prepolymers
  - *Platinum salt*: Catalyst (chloroplatinic acid)—acts as activator
  - Palladium (hydrogen absorber)
  - Retarders
  - Fillers.

## Setting Reaction

Addition silicones undergo polymerization reaction of chain lengthening and cross-linking with reactive vinyl groups that produce a stable silicone rubber.

Hydrogen containing siloxane + Vinyl terminal siloxane + Chloroplatinic acid → Silicone rubber

$$CH_3 \qquad CH_3 \qquad\qquad CH_3 \qquad CH_3$$
$$Si\text{-}H + CH_2\text{=}CH\text{-}Si \xrightarrow[\text{activator}]{\text{Pt salt}} Si\text{--}CH_2\text{--}CH_2\text{--}Si$$
$$CH_3 \qquad CH_3 \qquad\qquad CH_3 \qquad CH_3$$

Hydrogen containing siloxane + Vinyl terminal siloxane
+ Chloroplatinic acid ⟶ Silicone rubber

Hydrogen containing siloxane is multifunctional and the vinyl terminal siloxane is difunctional. In this reaction, no byproduct is formed and therefore minimal dimensional change occurs during polymerization. PVS amongst all the elastomers and hydrocolloid impression materials have the smallest dimensional change (0.05%) on setting.

### CLINICAL SIGNIFICANCE

Some addition silicones can produce hydrogen gas through secondary reaction. For this palladium, powder is added to absorb the hydrogen gas released during the reaction. PVS material which produces hydrogen, the impression should be poured immediately before the formation of the gas or pouring is delayed for 1–2 hours so that most of the gas formed is released.
- Setting time varies between 3 minutes and 7 minutes
- Increase in temperature reduces the setting time.

## Properties

- Excellent reproduction of surface detail. It can easily reproduce lines smaller than 0.025 mm
- Relatively shorter mixing time (45 seconds) and setting time (5–7 minutes)
- Have pleasant odour and color
- *Dimensional stability*: Best dimensional stability
  - Low curing shrinkage (0.17%)
  - Lowest permanent deformation (0.05–0.3%)
- *Dimensional change*: After 24 hours dimensional change is least among elastomers, i.e. 0.1% which is very low
- *Permanent deformation*: At the time of removal from mouth is 0.2% (99.8% elastic recovery) is lowest among all impression materials
- *Tear strength*: It is good. It varies between 2,000 g/cm and 4,300 g/cm depending on the consistency
- *Hardness*: The shore A hardness increases from low to high consistency
- Multiple pouring of PVS impressions are possible. The impressions remain dimensionally stable for at least a week without distortion
- Impressions should be either poured immediately with gypsum or should be delayed for 1–2 hours. Epoxy dies should be poured after storing the impression overnight.

### CLINICAL SIGNIFICANCE

Latex gloves adversely affect the setting of addition silicone impressions. Sulfur compound contained in latex retard the setting of silicones. For this, vinyl gloves should be used.

- Extremely hydrophobic, some manufacturers add a surfactant (detergent) to make it more hydrophilic. They require a dry field before impression making
- Can be electroplated with silver and copper
- Good shelf life of 1–2 years
- Good tear strength (3,000 g/cm)
- *Flow*: PVS impression materials show less flow than the condensation silicones.

## Uses

- They are the most popular impression materials for crown and bridge procedures
- They can be used as a bite registration material
- Especially formulated addition silicone material can be used to make dies for indirect composite inlays
- They can be used to make final impressions of the edentulous arches.

## Manipulation

Addition silicones are supplied in light, medium, heavy and putty consistencies. The most popular dispensing system for light body, medium body and heavy body materials is in the form of cartridges having two chambers one for base and other for catalyst. A mixing tip fits at the end of the cartridge which is either fitted into hand operated gun type dispenser or in motor driven dispenser. On pressing both the base and catalyst paste flow through the interwined spiral that mixes the material thoroughly till the time it exits from the end of the tip. One advantage of this mixing system is that it ensures proper ratio of the two materials without incorporation of bubbles or voids. The extruded material is directly syringed around the prepared tooth and some of it is syringed into the space in the stock tray.

## Advantages

- Has excellent dimensional stability
- Impression made with PVS can be kept up to a week without pouring
- PVS material available in various consistencies such as extra low, low, medium, heavy and extra heavy.

## Disadvantages

- Cannot be mixed with latex gloves as it inhibits the setting reaction of PVS
- Although byproducts are not there but residual hydrides are present which react with moisture in the atmosphere and form hydrogen gas. Therefore, the impression should not be poured immediately. Gypsum should be poured after at least 30 minutes and epoxy resins after 24 hours
- Due to its inherent hydrophobic nature, moisture control should be done before making impression. To make it hydrophilic, manufacturers are adding nonionic surfactant.

# POLYETHER RUBBER IMPRESSION MATERIAL

Polyether impression materials were introduced in Germany in 1960s. They are polymer based elastomers which have excellent mechanical properties and dimensional stability. They are hydrophilic and have excellent wetting properties but have short working time and have high stiffness.

## Composition

Base paste:
- Polyether polymer (moderately low molecular weight): Undergoes cross-linking to form rubber
- Colloidal silica: Acts as fillers
- Glycol ether or phthalate: Acts as plasticizer.

Accelerator paste:
- Aromatic sulfonate ester: Acts as cross-linking agent
- Colloidal silica: Acts as fillers
- Phthalate or glycol ether: Plasticizer
- Octyl phthalate (thinner): It reduces the viscosity of the unset material and increases working time (retarder).

## Supplied As

Polyether impression material is supplied as base and catalyst tubes or automixing cartridges. They are available in three viscosities: low, medium and heavy bodied **(Fig. 11.10)**.

## Setting Reaction

$$CH_3-C-CH_2-C-O-R-O-C-CH_2-C-CH+ \longrightarrow \text{Cross-linked rubber}$$

Equal lengths of base paste and the catalyst paste when mixed together addition polymerization occurs. The ionized form of sulfonic acid provides the initial source of cation and in each stage of the reaction it involves the opening of

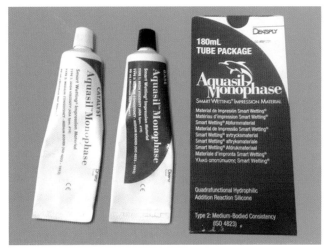

**Fig. 11.10:** Polyether elastomeric impression material.

the aziridine ring producing new cations. There is simple chain lengthening with formation of cross-linked rubber without any byproducts. As the reaction progresses, the viscosity of the mix increases eventually forming a rigid cross-linked rubber.

Polyether + Sulfonic ester → Cross-linked rubber
Exothermic reaction

Imine terminated polyether + Sulphonic acid ⟶ Polyether rubber

## Properties

- *Odor and taste*: It is pleasant **(Table 11.1)**
- *Working and setting time*: Polyethers have relatively short working and setting times as compared to other elastomeric materials. Mixing time is 30 seconds and setting time is 3–5 minutes. Increase in moisture and temperature further reduces the setting time
- *Dimensional stability*: It is very good. This is because of:
  - Addition polymerization reaction where no byproducts are formed
  - Curing shrinkage is low (0.24%)
  - Permanent deformation is low (1–2%).
- *Stiffness*: Very stiff (flexibility of 3%), needs extra space, around 4 mm is required. Undercuts should be blocked before making polyether impression.

**CLINICAL SIGNIFICANCE**

Higher stiffness and hardness of polyether impression materials demands greater force to remove the impression from the mouth.

- *Hydrophilic*: Amongst all the elastomers, polyethers are hydrophilic; therefore, impression should not be stored in water or disinfecting solution
- Electroplatable with silver and copper
- Polyether impressions can be poured multiple time within a week and can be sent to the laboratory without pouring. The impression remains dimensionally stable for several days
- Shelf-life extends up to 2 years
- *Tear strength*: The tear strength of polyethers is least for low viscosity, i.e. 1,800 g/cm, for medium viscosity it varies between 2,800 g/cm and 4,800 g/cm and for high viscosity it is 3,000 g/cm.
- *Strain in compression*: It varies between 2% and 3%.

## Manipulation

The polyether materials are supplied in three forms of mixing systems.
- Manual mixing—two tubes one base and other catalyst
- Automatic cartridge and mixing gun
- Mechanical mixer with dynamic mixing tip.

*Manual mixing:* Equal lengths of base and catalyst paste are extruded on a paper mixing pad. Mixing is done using stiff blade spatula. A uniform mix which is free of streaks is obtained in 30–45 seconds. The working time and setting time can be increased or decreased by increasing or decreasing the amount of catalyst paste up to 25%. Sometimes a thinner can be added as equal length of the base paste to increase the working time and flexibility of the mix.

| Table 11.1: Properties of different elastomeric materials. | | | | |
|---|---|---|---|---|
| Property | Polysulfide | Condensation silicone | Additional silicone | Polyether |
| Working time (min) | 4–7 | 2.5–4 | 2–4 | 3 |
| Setting time (min) | 7–10 | 6–8 | 4–6.5 | 6 |
| Tear strength (N/m) | 2,500–7,000 | 2,300–2,600 | 1,500–4,300 | 1,800–4,800 |
| Byproduct | $H_2O$ | Ethanol | – | – |
| Custom tray | Yes | No | No | No |
| Unpleasant odour | Yes | No | No | No |
| Multiple casts | No | No | Yes | Yes |
| % contraction (24 h) | 0.40–0.45 | 0.38–0.60 | 0.14–0.17 | 0.19–0.24 |
| Stiffness (1 ≥ Stiff) | 3 | 2 | 2 | 1 |
| Distortion (1 ≥ Dist) | 1 | 2 | 4 | 3 |

*Automatic cartridge and mixing gun:* Automatic cartridge is inserted into the gun and the static mixing tip is placed on the end of the cartridge. Procedure same as explained in addition silicone manipulation.

Mechanical mixer with dynamic mixing tip: Procedure same as explained in addition silicone manipulation.

The uniform mix is loaded into the tray which is coated with tray adhesive on the inner surface for better retention. The tray should be selected such as that it provides at least 4 mm of thickness of the impression material. The loaded tray is placed in the mouth and the material is allowed to set. Once completely set the impression is slowly pulled to break the seal and then removed with a single stroke. After removal, the impression is rinsed with water and blown dry to inspect for details. It is then disinfected.

## Advantages

- Have excellent dimensional stability
- Has *pseudoplastic* properties, i.e. same mix can be used both for a tray and a syringe material
- Permits multiple pouring and produces accurate casts
- Has shorter setting time
- Long shelf life
- Since hydrophilic have better wetting
- Cast pouring can be delayed for few hours to even a week.

## Disadvantages

- Expensive
- Very high stiffness removal difficult especially from undercuts
- Low tear strength
- Electroplating difficult.

## Clinical Applications

- For making final impression in fixed prosthodontics
- Can be used as bite registration material
- For impression making in partial edentulous and completely edentulous arches.

## DISINFECTION OF ELASTOMERIC IMPRESSION

All dental impressions should be adequately disinfected in order to prevent transmission of infection to gypsum casts and to the laboratory personnel. The most commonly used disinfectant for elastomeric impressions are: (1) neutral glutaraldehyde, (2) acidified glutaraldehyde, (3) neutral-phenolated glutaraldehyde, (4) phenol, (5) iodophor, and (6) chlorine dioxide. The elastomeric impressions are immersed in disinfectant solutions for 10 minutes except for chlorine dioxide where they are immersed for 3 minutes only. Disinfection of polyether impression by immersion is not recommended except for very short duration of 2–3 minutes. Some of the recommended disinfection solutions for impression materials are given further in **Table 11.2**.

## RECENT ADVANCES IN ELASTOMERS

### Visible Light Cured Impression Material

- Polyether urethane dimethacrylate
- Introduced in early 1988 by *Genesis* and *LD Caulk*
- *Two viscosities*: Light and heavy.

### Composition

- Polyether urethane dimethacrylate
- Photoinitiators
- Photoaccelerators
- Silicon dioxide (filler).

*Chemistry:* Similar to light cured composites.

### Properties

- Long working time and short setting time
- Blue light is used for curing with transparent impression trays
- Tear strength: 6,000–7,500 g/cm$^2$ (highest among elastomers)
- Other properties are similar to addition silicone.

**Table 11.2:** Recommended disinfectants for impression materials.

| Material | Disinfectants | Method of disinfection |
| --- | --- | --- |
| Polysulfide | Glutaraldehyde, chlorides, iodophors, phenolics | Immersion |
| Silicones | Glutaraldehyde, chlorides, iodophors, phenolics | Immersion |
| Polyether | Chlorides or iodophors | Immerse with caution; use disinfectant with short exposure |
| Alginate | Chloride compounds or iodophors | Immersion with caution; use disinfectant with short exposure |
| Zinc oxide-eugenol | Glutaraldehyde or iodophors | Immersion preferred; for bite registration use spray disinfectant |
| Impression compound | Chlorides or iodophors | Immersion or phenolic spray |

*Manipulation*

- Both light body and heavy body are cured with visible light having larger diameter probe
- Curing time approximately 3 minutes.

*Advantages*

- Controlled working time
- Excellent properties.

*Disadvantages*

- Special transparent trays
- Difficult to cure in remote area.

## IMPRESSION TECHNIQUES

### Single Mix Impression Technique

This technique is also called as monophasic impression technique or single viscosity technique. Usually medium viscosity of addition polysiloxane or polyether is used to make impression. The equal lengths of base and catalyst paste are taken and mixed with spatula. One part of the mix is loaded into the tray and the other part is loaded into the syringe. Here custom tray is fabricated to make impression. The mix is extruded onto the prepared tooth and the loaded tray is placed in position. The impression is allowed to set before removal. The success of this technique is dependent on the shear thinning (pseudoplastic) property of the material.

### Multiple Mix Impression Technique

In this impression technique, two different viscosities of impression materials are used. One is light body which is a syringe material and other is heavy body which is a tray material. Both the materials are mixed simultaneously and the syringe material is directly extruded onto the prepared tooth surface and the tray material is then inserted into the mouth and seated over the syringed material. The tray material forces the syringe material to adapt to the prepared tooth surface. It should be ensured that both the materials are loaded within the working time to get proper bond between them.

### Putty Wash Impression Technique

This impression technique was originally developed for condensation silicones to reduce dimensional accuracy. In this technique, putty consistency material is loaded in the stock tray and a preliminary impression is made. This impression is essentially made to make a custom tray. There are two ways to create space for light body material either cutting away tray material or by placing a wet polyethylene sheet on teeth before making preliminary impression. Once the space is created, the light body material is injected on the prepared tooth and the tray is placed in position over the syringed material.

Another variation in this technique is to inject the wash material on the prepared tooth and simultaneously placing the putty loaded stock tray over it. Problem with this technique is that there is high risk of displacement of the wash material with the putty material in the critical area.

### Triple Tray Technique

In this technique, a sectional tray is required where both the maxillary, mandibular and intercuspal positions can be recorded. A high viscosity elastomeric impression material is loaded on the sectional triple tray and preliminary impression is made. This tray is removed and cleaned and dried. The prepared tooth is syringed with light body material and the tray is placed back in the exact position of occlusion. The final impression made displays the maxillary and mandibular interocclusal position.

## TEST YOURSELF

### Essay Questions

1. Classify various impression materials. Write in detail about various elastomeric impression material.
2. Classify elastomeric impression materials. Discuss in detail additional polysilicones impression materials.
3. What are different disinfectants used for elastomeric impression materials. Critically evaluate each of them.
4. Discuss in detail polyether impression materials including setting reaction, properties and its manipulation.

### Short Notes

1. Polysulfides.
2. Polyether.
3. Monophase materials.
4. Rebound phenomenon.
5. Putty wash impression technique.
6. Visible light cure impression material.

## Multiple Choice Questions

1. Which of the following impression material can be changed from sol to gel state when set?
   A. Agar and alginate
   B. Zinc oxide eugenol paste
   C. Addition silicones
   D. Polyether

2. Which impression material produces alcohol as byproduct?
   A. Condensation silicone
   B. Polysulfides
   C. Polyether
   D. Addition silicone

3. Disadvantage of polyether impression material is:
   A. High modulus of elasticity and rigidity
   B. High linear coefficient of thermal expansion
   C. Hydrophobic
   D. Requires greater setting time

4. Which impression material is called as room temperature vulcanization?
   A. Silicones
   B. Polysulfides
   C. Polyether
   D. Methyl methacrylate

5. The accelerator used in silicone elastomer is:
   A. Stannous octoate
   B. Lead peroxide
   C. Ethyl siloxane
   D. Palladium

6. Impression with which type of impression material if poured immediately then cast shows crater like depressions is:
   A. Polyether
   B. Polysulfides
   C. Condensation silicone
   D. Addition silicone

7. Contraction permissible in type I and type II elastomer is:
   A. 0.5%
   B. 1.0%
   C. 1.5%
   D. 2.0%

8. Multipouring of casts is possible with which impression material:
   A. Polysulfides
   B. Addition silicones
   C. Condensation silicones
   D. Alginate

9. Rubber base impression should be poured within one hour because:
   A. They become more elastic with time
   B. Polymerization continues leading to dimensional inaccuracy
   C. Undergo syneresis and imbibition
   D. Cannot be poured immediately

10. Most common cause of distortion of rubber base impression material is:
    A. Improper base accelerator ratio
    B. Prolonged mixing
    C. Premature removal of impression
    D. Failure to retract gingiva

11. Automixing system can be used for:
    A. Addition silicones
    B. Agar hydrocolloids
    C. Polysulfides
    D. Impression paste

12. Elastomer with longest curing time:
    A. Addition silicones
    B. Condensation silicones
    C. Polyether
    D. Polysulfides

13. Elastomer which records most accurate reproduction of details is:
    A. Polysulfide
    B. Condensation silicone
    C. Addition silicone
    D. Polyether

## ANSWERS

| | | | |
|---|---|---|---|
| 1. A | 2. A | 3. A | 4. A |
| 5. A | 6. D | 7. A | 8. B |
| 9. B | 10. C | 11. A | 12. D |
| 13. C | | | |

## BIBLIOGRAPHY

1. Anusavice KJ. Phillip's Science of Dental Materials, 11th edn. Elsevier, St. Louis; 2003.
2. Anusavice KJ, Shen C, Rawls HR. Phillip's Science of Dental materials, 12th edn. Elsevier Inc, St. Louis, 2013.
3. Adabo GL, Zanarotti E, Fonseca RG, et al. Effect of disinfectant agents on dimensional stability of elastomeric impression materials. J Prosthet Dent. 1999;81:621-4.
4. Braden M, Causton B, Clarke RL. A polyether impression rubber. J Dent Res. 1972;51:889.
5. Baumann MA. The influence of dental gloves on the setting of impression materials. Br Dent J. 1995;179:130.
6. Chee WW, Donavan TE. Polyvinylsiloxane impression materials: a review of properties and techniques. J Prosthet Dent. 1992;68:728-32.
7. Ciesco JN, Malone WF, Sandrik JL, et al. Comparison of elastomeric impression materials used in fixed prosthodontics. J Prosthet Dent. 1981;45:89-94.
8. Craig RG, Powers JM. Restorative Dental Materials, 11th edn. Elsevier, St. Louis; 2002.
9. Craig RG. Review of dental impression materials. Adv Dent Res. 1988;2:51.

10. Chen SY, Liang WM, Chen FN. Factors affecting the accuracy of elastomeric impression materials. J Dent. 2004;32:603-9.

11. Craig RG, Urquiola NJ, Liu CC. Comparison of commercial elastomeric impression materials. Oper Dent. 1990;15:94-104.

12. Davis BA, Powers JM. Effect of immersion disinfection on properties of impression materials. J Prosthodont. 1994;3:31.

13. Donavan JF, Chee WW. A review of contemporary impression materials and techniques. Dent Clin N Am. 2004;48:445-70.

14. Finger W. Accuracy of dental duplicating materials. Quint Dent Tech. 1986;10:89.

15. Herfort TW, Gerberich WW, Macosko CW, et al. Tear strength of elastomeric impression materials. J Prosthet Dent. 1978;39:59.

16. Johnson GH, Craig RG. Accuracy of addition silicone as a function of technique. J Prosthet Dent. 1986;55:197.

17. Johnson GH, Craig RG. Accuracy of four types of rubber impression materials compared with time of pour and a repeat pour of models. J Prosthet Dent. 1985;53:484.

18. Mandikos MN. Polyvinylsiloxane impression materials : an update on clinical use. Aust Dent J. 1998;43:428-34.

19. Mc Cabe JF, Carrick TE. Recording surface detail on moist surfaces with elastomeric impression materials. Eur J Prosthodont Rest Dent. 2006;14:42-46.

20. Petri CS, Walker MP, O'Mahony AM, et al. Dimensional accuracy and surface detail reproduction of two hydrophilic vinyl polysiloxane impression materials tested under dry moist and wet conditions. J Prosthet Dent. 2003;90:365-72.

21. Pratten DH, Covey DA, Sheats RD. Effect of disinfectant solutions on the wettability of elastomeric impression materials. J Prosthet Dent. 1990;63:223-7.

22. Pratten DH, Craig RG. Wettability of a hydrophilic addition silicone impression material. J Prosthet Dent. 1989;61:197-202.

23. Rubel BS. Impression materials: A comparative review of impression materials most commonly used in restorative dentistry. Dent Clin N Am. 2007;51:629-42.

24. Rupp FD, Axmann D, Jacobi A et al. Hydrophilicity of elastomeric non aqueous impression materials during setting. Dent Mater. 2005;21:94-102.

25. Salem NS, Combe EC, Waats DC, et al. Mechanical properties of elastomeric impression materials. J Oral Rehab. 1988;15:125.

26. Shillingburg HT, Herbert T. Fundamentals of Fixed Prosthodontics. 3rd Edition. Quintessence, 1997.

27. Stackhouse JA Jr. The accuracy of stone dies made from rubber impression materials. J Prosthet Dent. 1970;24:377.

28. Wassell RW, Ibbetson RJ. The accuracy of polyvinyl siloxane impression materials made with standard and reinforced stock trays. J Prosthet Dent. 1992;64:748-57.

29. Williams JR, Craig RG. Physical properties of addition silicones as a function of composition. J Oral Rehabil. 1988;15:639.

# Rigid Impression Materials

*'Never leave till tomorrow, which you can do today.'*

—*Benjamin Franklin*

## INTRODUCTION

Inelastic impression materials are those materials which exhibit insignificant amount of elastic deformation when subjected to bending or tensile stresses. If the applied stress exceeds their tensile, shear or compressive stress, then they fracture without exhibiting any plastic deformation, e.g. impression plaster, impression compound, ZnO-eugenol impression paste.

## IMPRESSION PLASTER

Chapter 4 Page no. 55 to study in detail.

## IMPRESSION WAX

Refer to Chapter 5 page no. 83 to study in detail.

## IMPRESSION COMPOUND

It is also called as *modeling plastic* (ADA Specification No. 3). It is one of the oldest dental impression materials. They are rigid thermoplastic mucocompressive impression materials. These are softened by placing in hot water or by warming over the flame. Depending on the temperature at which they are softened, they are divided into high fusing and low fusing compounds **(Fig. 12.1)**.

- *Supplied as*—sheets, sticks, cylinders and cones.
- *Uses:*
  - For making primary impressions of the edentulous arches
  - To secure rubber dam retainers
  - To modify the fit of stock trays
  - As a base in wash impression techniques
  - To obtain peripheral seal.

### Classifications of Impression Compound

- *Type I*: Low fusing compound—fusion temperature approximately above 45°C, e.g. impression compound, green stick compound
- *Type II*: High fusing compound—fusion temperature approximately above 75°C, e.g. tray compound.

### Properties

- *Fusion temperature*: It is that temperature at which amorphous material begins to soften. The fusion temperature of impression compound is 43.5°C
  - The "plateau" or horizontal straight-line portion of the curve, characteristic of a pure crystalline material is ill-defined

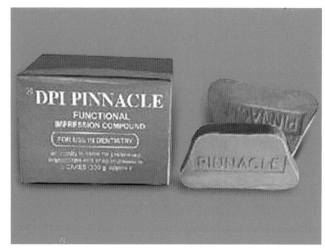

**Fig. 12.1:** Impression compound.

- The fusion temperature of approximately 43.5°C is not a solidification temperature since the glass transition temperature for this particular compound is approximately 39°C
- The practical significance of fusion temperature is that it indicates a definite reduction in plasticity during cooling
- The fusion temperature of impression compound should be such that at the time of insertion it should flow enough to register the details of the oral mucosa and not cause discomfort or tissue irritation.

- *Thermal conductivity*:
  - Thermal conductivity is low
  - During softening of the material, the outside always soften first and the inside at the last.
- *Thermal contraction*:
  - The average linear contraction of impression compound from mouth temperature to room temperature of 25°C may vary between 0.3% and 0.4%
  - The volume expansion over the same temperature range may be as great as 1.38–2.29%.
- *Flow*:
  - According to the ADA Specification No. 3, flow of impression compound at 37°C should not be more than 6% and flow at 45°C should not be less than 85%
  - Impression compound should have adequate flow to adapt to tissues to accurately record the surface detail. The compound should soften at a point just above mouth temperature to register surface details
  - Once the compound has solidified, any deformation should be completely elastic, so that the impression can be withdrawn without distortion of flow
  - Impression compound is the most viscous of the impression materials. Viscosity is about 70 times greater than that for impression plaster and more than 100 times greater than values for some of the light-bodied elastomers
  - The very high viscosity of impression compound is significant in two ways:
    1. It limits the degree of fine details which can be recorded in an impression
    2. It characterizes compound as a mucocompressive material.
- *Dimensional stability*:
  - Softening the compound by a method that will not affect its physical properties adversely by overheating or prolonged heating is important
  - In the mouth, adequate cooling of the compound is essential to avoid distortion when the impression is removed

- If the surface of the compound is hard, but the inside is soft, warpage (distortion) will occur immediately after the impression is withdrawn
- Storage in a warm environment or for extended periods of time promote dimensional changes
- So, a cast or die should be constructed as soon as possible after the impression has been obtained—at least within the first hour.
  ***Factors producing significant internal stresses within the compound impression are*:**
  - The high value of coefficient of thermal expansion
  - The poor thermal conductivity
  - The relative large temperature drop from softening temperature to room temperature.
- *Reproduction of details*:
  - Impression compound has a high viscosity, so reproduction of surface detail is not very good.
- *Rigidity*:
  - Impression compound is fairly rigid after setting and has poor elastic properties.
- *Biological properties*:
  - It is nontoxic and nonirritant to the oral tissues.

## Composition

The composition of impression compound has been shown in **Table 12.1.**

**Table 12.1:** Composition of impression compound.

| Ingredients | Percentage | Functions |
| --- | --- | --- |
| Natural or synthetic resins, e.g. copal resin or rosin | 20% | Provides thermoplasticity and increases flow and cohesiveness |
| Waxes (bees wax, carnauba wax or paraffin wax) | 7% | Produces smooth surface |
| Stearic acid, shellac, gutta-percha | 3% | Acts as plasticizers. They enhance the flow, plasticity, workability of the compound. They help in hardening of compound |
| French chalk, talc, diatomaceous earth | 50% | Acts as fillers. They help in improving strength and reduce thermal expansion and contraction |
| Rouge (ferric oxide) | Traces | Added as coloring agents. Provides reddish brown color to the compound |

## Clinical Applications

- For recording prosthetic impressions, such as preliminary impressions of edentulous arches, the material is supplied in rectangular/circular sheets of about 5–7.5 cm and 0.65 mm thick
- Peripheral seal materials, supplied as stick forms of 10 cm long and 1 cm in diameter, are used for border extensions on impression trays
- For copper band impressions of inlays and crowns, the material is supplied in stick form. Working temperature of green stick is 122–129°F and black stick is 133–135°F.

## Manipulation

Temperature controlled water bath or open flame is required to soften the impression compound. Open flame heating of compound is not recommended as it can lead to burning of important constituent of the impression compound.

## Techniques for Kneading Impression Compound

- Wet kneading
- Dry kneading.

The impression compound is softened by immersing in hot water bath (at temperature of about 60°C). Since the material has low thermal conductivity, the softening procedure takes several minutes. A napkin or cotton cloth is placed in the bowl to avoid sticking of the heated material to the walls of the bowl. Once the material is softened uniformly, it is kneaded with fingers to uniformly achieve a state of plasticity. Uniformly softened compound is placed in the nonperforated tray and is molded to the shape of the tray. The ridges are preformed with fingers and are then inserted in the patient's mouth. The impression is allowed to cool below the fusion temperature. Because of low thermal conductivity of the impression compound, the surface of the impression hardens before the inner portion. Therefore, sufficient time is allowed before removing the impression from the mouth to avoid warpage or distortion. Once the impression compound is completely hardened, it is removed from the mouth. The impression is washed and dried and inspected for accuracy. The impression then is disinfected and thereafter poured with gypsum material **(Fig. 12.2)**.

---

**CLINICAL SIGNIFICANCE**

- Direct flame for heating should be avoided as important constituents are volatized
- Prolonged heating in the water bath is avoided as it can lead to leaching out of ingredients making the compound more grainy and sticky
- Unnecessary kneading of compound should be avoided as it can lead to incorporation of water in it. This will increase flow after hardening.

---

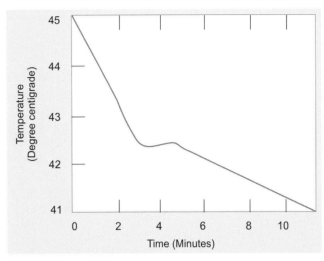

**Fig. 12.2:** Time-temperature cooling curve for impression compound.

- Sufficient time for hardening is allowed in order to avoid warpage or distortion of the compound
- Impression should be poured with gypsum as soon as possible as any delay can lead to distortion because of relaxation of the internal stresses.

## Disinfection of the Impression

- The impression should first be rinsed to remove blood, debris and saliva
- Disinfection is done by immersion for a minimum of 10 minutes and maximum of 30 minutes in a glutaraldehyde (e.g. Cidex) or an iodophor (e.g. Biocide)
- A 20-minute immersion in 2% ID210 solution has no adverse effects on the dimensional stability or surface detail reproduction
- ID210 is a virucidal, synergistic combination of aldehydes, quaternary ammonium compound and a nontoxic surfactant.

## Advantages

- It is reversible and reusable
- Has long shelf life
- Economical
- Nontoxic and nonirritant which is well-tolerated by oral tissues
- Can be added and remolded.

## Disadvantages

- It is rigid and nonelastic which cannot be used in undercut areas
- It is mucocompressive and can lead to displacement of soft tissues on recording
- Not capable of recording fine surface details

- Has low thermal conductivity
- Should not be reused as it cannot be sufficiently sterilized.

## Green Stick Compound (**Fig. 12.3**)

It is also called as tracing compound or border molding compound.

It is a low fusing impression compound which is supplied as cylindrical rods of dimensions 8–10 cm in length and 6 mm in diameter. It is commonly used for border molding of custom trays. It can also be used for copper tube impression for making impression of a single tooth. Its fusion temperature varies between 43°C and 45°C.

## Tray Compound (Type II Impression Compound)

Type II impression compound is viscous when it is softened and is stiff when hardened. It has less flow than impression compound is more rigid. It has high fusion temperature of more than 70°C. It is composed of thermoplastic resins, waxes, fillers and color pigments. They are used to prepare special trays which are used to make final impressions. Its major drawback is that they have poor strength and is dimensionally unstable and is, therefore, not preferred for fabricating custom trays.

## ZINC OXIDE-EUGENOL IMPRESSION PASTE

Zinc oxide-eugenol impression pastes produces a rigid impression with a high degree of accuracy and good reproduction of surface detail. It is also called as metallic oxide paste (**Fig. 12.4**).

Types of material—rigid, inelastic and mucostatic impression material.

## Uses

- For recording secondary or corrective wash impressions of edentulous arches in the fabrication of complete dentures
- As bite registration material
- As surgical paste
- For stabilization of base plates in bite registration
- Noneugenol pastes are used to record secondary impressions in patients who are sensitive to eugenol
- As temporary filling material
- As root canal filling material
- As temporary relining material for dentures.

### Classification of Zinc Oxide-Eugenol Impression Paste

- Based on hardness after setting, it is of two types:
  - *Type I*: Hard set—it has shorter setting time and has higher resistance to penetration when set
  - *Type II*: Soft set—they are tougher but not as brittle on setting.
- Based on the eugenol content:
  - *Type I*: Eugenol containing impression paste
  - *Type II*: Noneugenol paste.

## Composition

This impression material is dispensed as two separate pastes namely base paste and the reactor or catalyst paste.

*Base paste:* The ingredients, percentage and functions of base paste have been shown in **Table 12.2**.

*Catalyst or reactor paste:* The ingredients, percentage and functions of catalyst or reactor paste have been shown in **Table 12.3**.

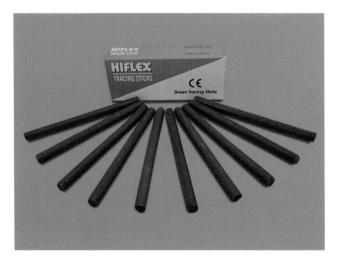

**Fig. 12.3:** Green stick compound.

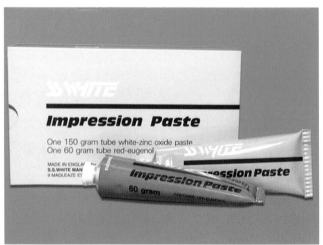

**Fig. 12.4:** Zinc oxide-eugenol impression paste.

**Table 12.2:** Ingredients, percentage and functions of base paste.

| Ingredients | Percentage (%) | Functions |
|---|---|---|
| Zinc oxide | 87 | Reactive ingredient |
| Fixed vegetable or mineral oil | 13 | Acts as plasticizers and helps in masking the action of eugenol |

**Table 12.3:** Ingredients, percentage and functions of catalyst or reactor paste.

| Ingredients | Percentage (%) | Functions |
|---|---|---|
| Oil of cloves or eugenol | 12 | • Reactive ingredient<br>• Oil of cloves contains 70–80% of eugenol and produces less burning sensation than eugenol |
| Gum or polymerized rosin | 50 | • Facilitates speed or reaction<br>• Aids in producing smoother and homogeneous mix<br>• Provides body and coherence to the mix |
| Fillers (silica type) | 20 | Improves strength of the paste |
| Lanolin | 3 | Acts as plasticizers |
| Resinous balsam | 10 | Increases flow and improves mixing qualities |
| Calcium chloride | 5 | Accelerates the setting reaction |
| Color pigments | Traces | Provides color to the paste |

## Setting Reaction

- The reaction between ZnO and eugenol is very complex and has never been completely defined
- When a base paste is mixed with catalyst paste, an acid-base reaction takes place when ZnO reacts with moisture (water) to yield zinc hydroxide. The zinc hydroxide produced further reacts with eugenol to form zinc eugenolate salt (chelate product) and water as a byproduct

- The water which is produced as byproduct is utilized for further reaction and therefore the reaction is called as *autocatalytic reaction*
- The setting reaction is *ionic* in nature and ionic medium is increased by the presence of certain ionizable salts which acts as accelerator whereas water provides the ionic medium
- The setting reaction in ZnO-eugenol paste is called as acid-base reaction, chelation reaction, autocatalytic reaction and ionic reaction.

Structural formula for eugenol

(Eugenol)   (Excess)   (Zinc eugenolate)

$$ZnO + H_2O \text{ (moisture)} \longrightarrow Zn(OH)_2$$

$$Zn(OH)_2 + 2HE \longrightarrow ZnE_2 + 2H_2O$$

(Base)     (Acid)

Zinc Eugenolate
(chelate product)

Zinc oxide eugenolate
(Chelate compound)

## Properties

- *Setting time*: Initial setting time is defined as the time elapsed from the time of mixing until the material ceases to pull away or string out when its surface is touched with a metal rod of specified dimension.

  According to the ADA specification no.16, the initial setting time for both soft and hard impression pastes is 3–6 minutes.

  Final setting time is defined as the time from beginning of mixing until the material gets maximum hardness so that the impression can be withdrawn from the mouth with a minimum distortion.

  Final setting time for type I material is less than 10 minutes. Final setting time for type II material is less than 15 minutes.

  Factors influencing setting time are:
  - *Temperature*: Higher the temperature shorter the setting time. Similarly setting time can be increased by lowering the temperature. For example, by heating spatula or glass slab, the setting time can be reduced. Likewise, if the glass slab is cooled not below the dew point, the setting time can be increased
  - *Humidity*: If a drop of water is added to the mix, the setting time is reduced
  - *Ratio of base to catalyst paste*: If more base paste (ZnO) is taken, the setting time is increased and if more catalyst paste (eugenol) is taken then the setting time is reduced
  - *Mixing time*: If the mixing time is increased then the setting time reduces as vice versa

  - *Chemical modifiers*: Addition of accelerators reduces the setting time whereas the addition of retarders increases the setting time. Addition of petrolatum jelly or inert oils increases the setting time.
- *Consistency and flow*:
  - The mix which is having good flow and thinner consistency will produce an accurate impression
  - The mix which has thick consistency or high viscosity can compress the tissues
  - The thickness of the mix used normally is about 1 mm.
- *Rigidity*:
  - Zinc oxide impression pastes are rigid and inelastic materials and should not be used to record the undercuts
  - The set material can distort or fracture when removed from the undercuts.
- *Strength*:
  - It is not a critical requirement for this impression material since it is supported by a tray
  - The strength of the hardened impression paste is about 7 MPa after 2 hours from the start of mixing.
- *Hardness*:
  - Hardness of the set material is measured by Krebs penetrometer
  - Penetration hardness for type I material is < 0.5 mm
  - For type II material it varies between 0.8 mm and 1.5 mm.
- *Dimensional stability*:
  - The ZnO impression paste is highly dimensionally stable
  - The dimensional change during setting is about 0.1%.

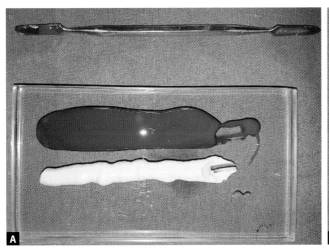
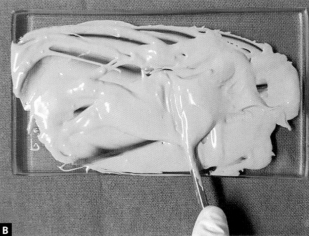
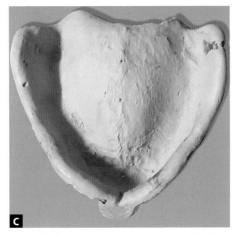

**Figs. 12.5A to C:** Manipulation of Impression paste: (A) Base and catalyst pastes are taken in equal lengths; (B) Spatula is moved in sweeping motion to get uniform mix; (C) Final impression made with Impression paste.

- There is no dimensional change after setting or hardening
- If the tray material is dimensionally stable the impressions can be preserved indefinitely without change in shape resulting from warpage.
- *Reproduction of details*: The low initial viscosity of the mixed paste in addition to its pseudoplastic nature allows recording of fine details accurately.
- *Shelf life*: Shelf life of ZnO paste is good.
- *Biological properties*: These materials are non-toxic but some patients can be allergic or sensitive to eugenol. Such patient should be treated with noneugenol pastes.

## Manipulation (**Figs. 12.5A to C**)

- The two pastes are mixed on a glass slab or oil impervious paper. A flexible stainless steel spatula is used to mix both the base and the catalyst pastes
- Both the base and the catalyst pastes are squeezed of the same lengths and diameter on the glass slab or paper. The ratio being 1:1

- The two strips are mixed with the first stroke of the spatula. Thereafter, the spatula is moved with a broad stroke in a sweeping motion. The mixing is continued for about 1 minute until a uniform color mix is produced
- Once the uniform mix is achieved it is collected and spread on the custom tray and is inserted in the patient's mouth
- Petrolatum jelly is applied around the lips before the impression is placed in the mouth in order to avoid the sticking of the material to the skin
- The loaded impression tray is firmly held in position until the material is hardened
- After the material has completely set it is removed from the mouth
- The impression is rinsed under tap water to remove saliva or debris
- The impression is then disinfected and thereafter poured with gypsum material
- The master cast is separated from the impression by immersing in hot water for 5–10 minutes.

## Disinfection of the Impression

The final impression is disinfected by immersing in 2% alkaline glutaraldehyde solution.

## Advantages

- Dimensionally stable
- Mucostatic in nature and produces accurate details
- Separating medium is not required
- Easy to manipulate
- Economical
- Has adequate shelf life
- Can be added or readapted if required.

## Disadvantages

- Rigid and inelastic cannot be used in undercut areas
- Some patients sensitive to eugenol
- Requires special trays
- Instruments are difficult to clean because of its sticky nature.

## Modifications of Zinc Oxide-Eugenol Impression Pastes

*Noneugenol pastes:* Occasionally, eugenol may produce an allergic response in some patients. There may be a stinging or burning sensation when eugenol contacts the oral tissues. In such patients noneugenol pastes should be used.

Noneugenol materials are based upon the reaction between ZnO and a carboxylic acid such as orthoethoxybenzoic acid (EBA), to form an insoluble soap (saponification reaction). The carboxylic acid may be present as a liquid or as a powder dispersed in a medium such as ethyl alcohol.

$$ZnO + 2RCOOH -> (RCOO)_2 Zn + H_2O$$

The reaction is not greatly affected by temperature or humidity. Bactericidal agents and other medicaments can be incorporated without interfering with the reaction.

*Bite registration paste:* Zinc oxide-eugenol impression paste can be used as bite registration paste by slight modification in its composition. The basic composition of bite registration paste is same as conventional impression paste except more plasticizers are added. This paste is used to record the occlusal relationship of maxillary and mandibular teeth during various prosthodontics procedures.

Benefit of using bite registration paste is that it does not provide any resistance during jaw closure. Therefore, provides more accurate record. The bite record is more dimensionally stable than that made with wax.

*Surgical pastes:* Modification of ZnO-eugenol impression paste can be used as a surgical paste after certain surgical procedures such as gingivectomy. The paste is used as an intraoral bandage to protect the wound and aid in retention of the medicament and promote healing.

The composition of the surgical paste is similar to that of conventional impression paste, except it contains:
- More fillers—to prevent fracture and dislocation of the material during mastication
- More eugenol—it provides more sedative effect and is mild antiseptic
- Greater amount of plasticizer—to improve plasticity and allow easy moldability
- Greater medicaments—may contain antibiotics or other bactericidal agents.

## Properties

- Surgical paste is generally softer and has slower setting reaction
- Has adequate strength to resist displacement during mastication
- Is not brittle otherwise it will readily shear under localized stress
- Can produce irritation or burning sensation in eugenol sensitive patients
- Can cause gastric disturbances in some patients.

## TEST YOURSELF

### Essay Questions

1. Classify various impression materials. Write in detail about impression compound.
2. Classify impression materials. Describe in detail composition, setting reaction, properties, and uses of Zinc oxide-eugenol impression paste.

### Short Notes

1. Inelastic impression materials.
2. Bite registration paste.
3. Impression compound.
4. Impression plaster.
5. Impression wax.
6. Noneugenol pastes.
7. Green stick compound.

## Multiple Choice Questions

1. Which of the following is an inelastic impression material ?
   A. Condensation silicones
   B. Polyether
   C. Alginate
   D. Impression compound
2. Zinc oxide-eugenol impression paste is:
   A. Used alone as a wash material in custom acrylic tray
   B. Used as wash with compound in preliminary complete arch impression
   C. Used for making impression of the prepared crown with inflamed gingiva
   D. Mixed to the same consistency as zinc oxide eugenol temporary filling material
3. In Noneugenol impression paste, eugenol is replaced by:
   A. Clove oil
   B. Carboxylic acid
   C. Ethoxybenzoic acid
   D. Alginic acid
4. Rigid reversible impression material is:
   A. Agar agar
   B. Impression plaster
   C. Elastomers
   D. Impression compound

## ANSWERS

1. D    2. A    3. B    4. D

## BIBLIOGRAPHY

1. Anusavice KJ. Phillip's Science of Dental Materials, 11th edition Elsevier, St. Louis; 2003.
2. Anusavice KJ, Shen C, Rawls HR. Phillip's Science of Dental Materials, 12th edition Elsevier Inc, St. Louis; 2013.
3. Braden M. Rheology of dental composition (impression compound). J Dent Res. 1967;46:620.
4. Brauer GM, White EE, Moshonas MG. Reaction of metal oxides with o-ethoxybenzoic acid and other chelating agents. J Dent Res. 1958;37:547.
5. Craig RG, Powers JM. Restorative Dental Materials, 11th edn. Elsevier, St. Louis, 2002.
6. Craig RG. Review of dental impression materials. Adv Dent Res. 1988;2:51.
7. Davis BA, Powers JM. Effect of immersion disinfection on properties of impression materials. J Prosthodont. 1994;3:31.
8. Donavan JF, Chee WW. A review of contemporary impression materials and techniques. Dent Clin N Am. 2004;48:445-70.
9. Leinfelder KF, Lemons JE. Impression materials. Clinical Restorative Materials and Techniques. Lea and Febiger. Philadelphia, 1988.
10. Lloyd CH, Scrimgeour SN (Eds). Dental materials: Literature review. J Dent. 1997;25:193.
11. Myers GE, Peyton FA. Physical properties of the zinc oxide-eugenol impression pastes. J Dent Res. 1961;40:39-48.
12. Rubel BS. Impression materials: A comparative review of impression materials most commonly used in restorative dentistry. Dent Clin N Am. 2007;51:629-42.

# Denture Base Materials

# Denture Polymers and Polymerization

*'Destiny is not a matter of chance, it is a matter of choice; it is not a thing to be waited for, it is a thing to be achieved.'*
**—William J. Bryan**

## INTRODUCTION

Synthetic polymers often termed as plastics are used extensively in prosthetic dentistry. Before the introduction of acrylic polymers to dentistry in 1937, the principal polymer used was vulcanized rubber for denture bases. Polymers introduced since then are vinyl acrylics, polystyrene, epoxies, polycarbonates, polyvinyl acetate polyethylene, cis- and trans-polyisoprene, polysulfides, silicones, polyethers and polyacrylic acids.

Resins find a special place in dentistry because of their wide applications. They have earned this place on the basis of performance, plus the apparently unlimited ability of dental researchers, educators and clinicians to develop new techniques and materials to meet specific needs.

## HISTORY

Before 1770 AD, dentures were fabricated from hardwood; ivory and bone with natural teeth held by screws or other means.

- *1774*: *Duchateau de Chemant* designed first porcelain dentures
- *1795*: *John Greenwood* made dentures for George Washington with ivory and wood held by springs
- *1840*: *Vulcanite rubber* discovered by *Charles Goodyear*
- *1855*: Vulcanite rubber was introduced as denture-based material with porcelain mounted on them. The vulcanite-based material ruled the field of prosthetics for denture-based material for nearly 75 years
- *1868*: *John Hyatt* introduced nitrocellulose

- *1909*: *Dr Leo Baekeland* found phenol formaldehyde resins. This material was known as Bakelite
- *1922*: *Staudinger H* proposed that polymers consist of long chain of atoms held together by covalent bonds
- *1930's*: *Dr Walter Wright* and *Vernon* Brothers developed methyl methacrylate
- *1940's*: Around 90% of all dentures were made of acrylic dentures.

## VULCANITE

It contains rubber with 32% sulfur and metallic oxides for color pigment **(Fig. 13.1)**.

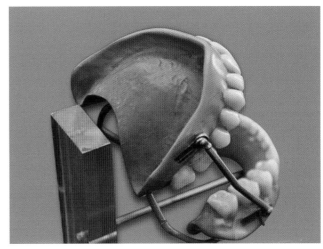

**Fig. 13.1:** Vulcanite denture.

## Advantages

- Nontoxic and nonirritant
- Excellent mechanical properties.

## Disadvantages

- Poor esthetics
- Poor color stability
- Taste and odor were not acceptable.

## PHENOL FORMALDEHYDE

In 1909, Dr Leo Baekeland found phenol formaldehyde resin, which was known as "Bakelite" **(Fig. 13.2)**.

Disadvantages of phenol formaldehyde are:
- Dimensionally unstable
- Lack of strength
- Lack of color stability.

## NITROCELLULOSE

In 1868, *John Hyatt* introduced first plastic moldable material by dissolving nitrocellulose under pressure. He called this material as celluloid. This material had better esthetics than vulcanized rubber but its major drawback was bad taste and foul smell.

## Disadvantages

- Dimensionally unstable
- Excessive warpage
- High-water absorption
- Poor-color stability
- Contains unpleasant tasting plasticizers.

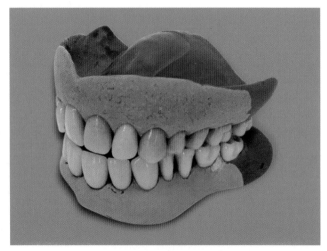

**Fig. 13.2:** Bakelite dentures.

## POLYMETHYL METHACRYLATE RESINS

In 1937, *Walter Wright* introduced more satisfactory plastic denture-based materials called methyl methacrylate resins. By 1945, most of the dentures were constructed of methyl methacrylate polymers.

Pure polymethyl methacrylate (PMMA) is stable and transparent resin. This material does not discolor in ultraviolet (UV) light and has excellent aging property. It is stable to heat although softens at 125°C. It can be thermoplastically molded and its optical and color properties remain stable intraorally. It is found to be soluble in various organic solvents such as chloroform and acetone.

Its tensile strength is 60 MPa, with density of 1.19 g/cm³. Its modulus of elasticity is 2.4 GPa.

*Methyl methacrylate resins satisfy the needs of:*
- Esthetics
- Dimensional stability
- Simple procedure of processing.

## Classification of Resins

### Based on Thermal Behavior

- *Thermoplastic:* This type of resins can be softened on heating and can be hardened on cooling. Such type of reaction is reversible. For example, polystyrene, PMMA, polyethylene
- *Thermosetting:* This type resins are those that hardened during fabrication but do not softened on reheating. For example, silicones, cis-polyisoprene, bisphenol A diacrylates.

### Based on Spatial Structure

- *Linear polymer*:
  - Linear homopolymer
  - Random copolymer of linear type
  - Linear block copolymer.
- *Branched polymer*:
  - Branched homopolymer
  - Graft or branched copolymer.
- Cross-linked polymers

### Based on the Origin

- *Natural*—For example rubber
- *Synthetic*—For example polyvinyl chloride, nylon, polyethylene
- *Semisynthetic*—For examplecellulose rayon, cellophane

## Based on Use

- Elastomers
- Plastic
- Fiber (nylon)
- Liquid epoxy resins.

## Based on the Composition of Main Chain

- *Inorganic*—main chain does not contain carbon atoms
- *Organic*—main chain contains carbon atoms.

## Requisites for Dental Resins

The ideal requirements of the dental resins are given below, although no single resin meets all these requirements.

### Biocompatibility

- Resins should be tasteless, odorless, nontoxic, nonirritating and compatible to the oral tissues
- Should be completely insoluble in saliva or in other fluids
- Should be impermeable to oral fluids such that resins do not become unhygienic or disagreeable in taste or odor.

### Physical and Mechanical Properties

- Should have adequate strength and resilience to bear the functional forces and excessive wear that can occur in oral cavity
- Should be dimensionally stable
- Should have low-specific gravity especially for the maxillary denture.
- Should have good thermal conductivity for patient to detect temperature changes in the oral cavity.

### Manipulation

- Should be easy to handle and manipulate
- Should have a relatively short-setting time
- Should not generate dust or toxic vapors during handling and manipulation
- Should be insensitive to factors such as saliva or blood contamination, oxygen inhibition, etc.
- It should be easy to polish and repair.

### Esthetic Properties

- Should have adequate translucency or transparency to match the appearance of oral tissues it replaces
- Should be capable of characterizing the resins.

### Economic Considerations

Cost of resin should be relatively low.

### Chemical Stability

Should be chemically stable and inert.

## POLYMER

It refers to a long-chain organic molecule that is made of many mers. A mer (mono) is a chemical structural unit, which joins to form a polymer. The conversion of polymer takes place by a process of polymerization, which is a series of chemical reaction by which macromolecules is formed.

### Definition

*Polymer: Defined as a chemical compound consisting of large organic molecules built by repetition of smaller monomeric units.*

*—GPT 8th Edition*

*Monomer: Defined as any molecule that can be bound to a similar molecule to form a polymer.*

*—GPT 8th Edition*

*Copolymer resin: Defined as polymers formed from more than one type of molecular repeat unit.*

*—GPT 8th Edition*

### Uses

- Used in dentures as denture bases, for relining, rebasing and artificial teeth **(Fig. 13.3)**
- For fabricating customized impression trays

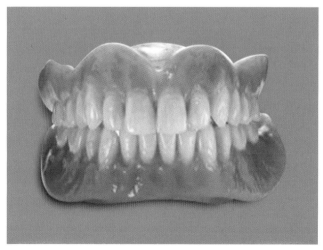

**Fig. 13.3:** Dentures made with acrylic resins.

- As equipment such as mixing bowls
- Used as resin-based cements for luting-fixed restorations
- For manufacturing artificial teeth
- Used in various maxillofacial prosthesis
- Used for fabricating temporary crown and bridge materials
- Used to give esthetic facings (acrylic) on fixed metal bridges
- For fabrication of athletic mouth protectors
- Used as pit and fissure sealants and root canal sealants
- Used as cavity-filling materials in the form of composites
- Used in fabricating removable orthodontic and pedodontic appliances
- Used for making brackets, cements to bond brackets and spacers
- Used as splinting material and veneers.

## Properties

### General Properties

- Longer the chains, i.e. higher the molecular weight ($M_w$), slower the dissolution of the polymers
- $M_w$ represents the molecular weight of the average chain of the polymers and $M_n$ represents the average number of mer repeating units in a chain.
- Polymers have tendency to absorb solvent, swell and soften rather than dissolve
- Cross-linking prevents complete chain separation and retards dissolution
- If the polymers are highly cross-linked, it has very less chances of dissolution
- Small amount of swelling of the polymers can compromise the fit of the prosthesis
- Absorbed molecules spread polymer chains apart and facilitate slippage between the chains. This lubricating effect is called as *plasticization.*

### Deformation and Recovery

When forces are applied on the resins, it can cause elastic strain, plastic strain or combination of both strains.
- Elastic deformation occurs when resins completely recover on removing the stresses. Since the recovery is complete there is no change of shape of the resin
- Plastic deformation occurs when resins are irreversibly or permanently deformed on removing the applied stresses. This leads to change in shape of the resin
- Viscoelastic deformation is due to the combination of both elastic and plastic strain. Here, when the applied stress is removed, recovery only occurs of the elastic strain. Here, since the recovery is only partial, there is

some change or alteration in shape of the resin. This phenomenon is termed as "*Viscoelastic recovery*".

### Rheometric Properties

- Rheometry or flow behavior of solid polymers depends on the elastic/plastic deformation and elastic recovery when stresses are removed
- The term viscoelasticity includes combination of elastic and plastic deformations
- Plastic flow is the irreversible change, which occurs when polymer chains slide over one another leading to a permanent deformation. Branched and cross-linked polymers show plastic flow.

> **CLINICAL SIGNIFICANCE**
>
> Elastic recovery occurs in resins, when randomly coiled chains straighten and recoil to its original dimension on removing the applied force. Polymers usually show both elastic and plastic properties. Therefore, elastomers do not completely recover and exhibit some amount of plastic deformation on removal of stress. Likewise, plastics exhibit greater amount of plastic deformation and very small amount of elastic recovery.

### Thermal Properties

- Properties of polymers can be altered by changes in temperature. Higher the temperature, softer and weaker will be the polymers
- Polymers can be classified as thermoplastic polymers and thermosetting polymers based on the change in temperatures
- Thermoplastic polymers—also called as thermosoftening plastics are made of linear and/or branched chains that soften on heating above glass transition temperature ($T_g$). These materials can be repeatedly softened and reshaped on heating and cooling. This cycle of heating and cooling can be repeated infinitely. These resins are soluble in organic solvents and can be melted. The setting reaction is reversible as they have relatively weaker bonds between the molecular chains. Such materials have good flexural and impact strengths. For example, PMMA, polyethylene, polystyrene
- Thermosetting polymers are those polymeric materials, which become permanently hard when heated above the temperature at which it begins to polymerize and that does not soften again on reheating to the same temperature. Since, they undergo chemical change they cannot be resoftened and the change is irreversible. They have greater abrasion resistance and are dimensionally

stable. On heating, these resins will decompose and char rather melt. They are usually cross-linked and are insoluble in solvents. Longer linear polymers have higher $T_g$ than the shorter linear polymer because they have greater $M_w$ and therefore require greater thermal energy to reach $T_g$, e.g. Silicones, cis-polyisoprene, cross-linked PMMA.

*Behavior of polymers to heat:* When linear polymers are heated above the $T_g$, vibrations and rotations of chains occur. These motions among molecules force the polymer chains to separate and break. This induces chain slippage causing reduction of strength and modulus of elasticity of the resin and increase of thermal expansion. This behavior will be seen less as cross-linking of the resins increases. Greater the cross-linking of the polymers, lesser will be tendency of chain slippage making it progressively more thermal resistant.

## Dissolution Properties

Polymers are not completely soluble in any liquid. They usually absorb a solvent becomes soft and swollen but does not dissolve. The solubility of a polymer depends on the type of polymer whether it is branched, cross-linked or a homopolymer. Cross-linked polymers show least dissolution. Again, longer the length of the chain of the polymer lesser is the dissolution. Elastic polymers absorb and get swollen up more than the plastic polymers. The absorbed solvent molecules spread the polymer chains and permit slippage to occur between chains. This phenomenon is called as "*Plasticization*". Swollen polymers lead to misfit of the prosthesis such as partial or complete dentures.

### CLINICAL SIGNIFICANCE

The cross-linked polymer shows least dissolution because it forms a three-dimensional network between the linear chains that is capable increasing its strength and rigidity but reducing water sorption. Cross-linked polymers are widely used in manufacturing of acrylic teeth to reduce water sorption or dissolution in any solvent and for increased strength.

## Plasticizers

*Plasticizers are those materials, which are added to polymers to soften it and to decrease their fusion temperature.*
- *Function of plasticizers*:
  - Improve solubility of polymers
  - Decrease brittleness of polymers
  - Reduce softening (or) fusion temperature.

### Classification of Plasticizers

- *External plasticizers* are not a part of the polymers and are added. They should have very high-molecular attraction to the polymers otherwise there are chances of leaching out during fabrication procedure. They increase the intermolecular space by penetrating the polymer. Usually, external plasticizers are not used in dentistry
- *Internal plasticizers* are part of the polymer, e.g. butyl methacrylate when added to methyl methacrylate before polymerization, the resin polymerizes internally by butyl methacrylate.

## Structure of Polymers

Polymers consist of large chains of molecular structures, which have infinite configurations and conformations. Lengths of chains, their branches and cross-linking determine the properties of polymers. The molecular chain structures can have both organic and inorganic polymer networks. Longer the chain, greater the chances of entanglements along this chain, and greater the difficulty in breaking these chains. Therefore, polymers with greater chain length have increased rigidity, strength and melting temperatures. The length of polymer chain is expressed as $M_n$ depending on the average number of mer units repeating in the chain, whereas the weight of the polymer chain is expressed as $M_w$ depending on $M_w$ of the average chain. Usually, average $M_w$ of the commonly used denture resins varies from 8,000 to 39,000, although $M_w$ of the cross-linked denture teeth can have much greater value.

As the polymerization of the polymer progresses, there is leaching of low $M_w$ compounds which are capable of causing adverse reactions. Again on polymerization, there is leaching of residual monomer, which reduces the average $M_w$ of the polymer after complete polymerization. For example, denture base resins with $M_w$ 22,400 will reduce to 7,300 after complete polymerization, which has only 0.9% of residual monomer.

Molecular weight of the polymer is usually always more than the $M_n$ length of the polymer chain. There is an exception, if all the molecular chains are of equal lengths then $M_w = M_n$.

*Polydispersity:* It is defined as the measure of the range and distribution of chain sizes. It is denoted by the ratio of $M_w/M_n$. Polymers having different value of polydispersity, but same value of $M_w$ will vary in properties such as rigidity, melting temperature and strength.

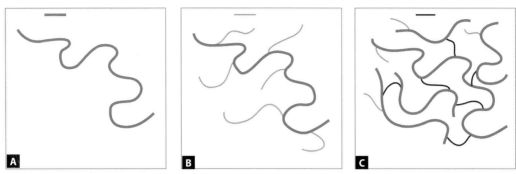

**Figs. 13.4A to C:** Structure of polymers: (A) linear; (B) branched; and (C) cross-linked.

It is important to study structure of polymers as it helps in determining and predicting the nature of each polymer. Broadly polymers are of three types **(Figs. 13.4A to C)**:
1. Linear
2. Branched
3. Cross-linked.

### Linear Polymer

- *Linear homopolymer*: Such resins have all the chemical units or mers of same type **(Fig. 13.5A)**
- *Random copolymer of linear type*: They have two types of chemical units or mers, which are randomly placed along the chain **(Fig. 13.5B)**
- *Linear block copolymer*: They have segments of chain where the chemical units or mers are the same, which are sequentially repeated along the main polymer **(Fig. 13.5C)**.

### Branched Polymer

Branched polymers consist of extra arms growing from the main polymer chain. These entanglements are temporary as they can get disentangled with relatively low energy.
- *Branched homopolymer*: This type of resin contain same type of mer units **(Fig. 13.6A)**
- *Branched random copolymer*: This resin type have two types of mer units distributed randomly **(Fig. 13.6B)**
- *Graft or branched copolymer:* This type of resin contains one type of mer unit on the main chain and has another type of mer units on the other chain **(Fig. 13.6C)**.

### Cross-linked Polymers *(Fig. 13.7)*

- They are those types of polymers, which are made up of homopolymer cross-linked with a single cross-linking agent
- The linear and the branched molecules are separate and discrete whereas the cross-linked molecules are a network structure that may result in the polymer becoming one giant molecule. Cross-linking may involve

interlinking of small $M_w$ polymers, which can have some giant molecules or even a single giant molecule.
- Cross-linking results in three-dimensional network, which increases its rigidity and makes it more resistant to different solvents
- The spatial structure of polymers affects their flow properties and increases their $T_g$

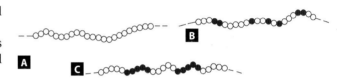

**Figs. 13.5A to C:** Linear polymers; (A) Homopolymer; (B) Random Copolymer; (C) Block polymers.

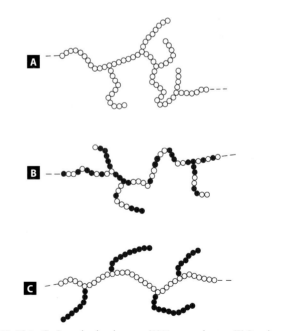

**Figs. 13.6A to C:** Branched polymers; (A) Homopolymer; (B) Random copolymer; (C) Graft copolymer.

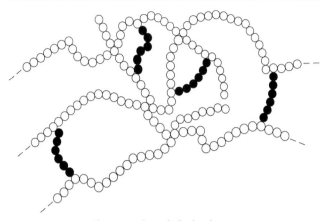

**Fig. 13.7:** Cross-linked polymer.

- In general, cross-linked polymers flow at a higher temperature than linear (or) branched polymers. Another distinguishing feature of some cross-linked polymers is that they do not absorb liquids as readily as linear (or) branched.

**CLINICAL SIGNIFICANCE**

Cross-linked polymers have chains, which are linked to each other with chemical bond and therefore require greater amount of energy to break this bond as compared to branched polymers.

## Molecular Structure

Polymers have different molecular structures, which vary from amorphous, i.e. highly disordered or random pattern to highly ordered chain alignment or combination of both. The amorphous structure of polymers has molecular chains, which are randomly coiled and entangled, whereas the crystalline structure have chains aligned in orderly manner. But usually, polymers have molecular structures, which have combination of both amorphous and crystalline structures in varying ratio. The crystalline nature of polymers improves strength, hardness, modulus of elasticity and melting temperature but reduces ductility, i.e. increases brittleness.

Factors, which reduce crystallinity of the polymers, are:
- Presence of plasticizers
- Copolymerization of chain alignment
- Branching of polymer chain
- Random arrangement of groups, which separate polymer chains.

## Chemistry of Polymers

- Polymers are formed by a process called polymerization, which consists of monomeric units becoming chemically linked together to form high $M_w$ molecules

- Types of polymerization:
  1. Addition
  2. Condensation or step growth polymerization.

### Addition Polymerization

- Most common form of polymerization for number of dental materials
- In this type, the mer units are activated and added one at a time in sequence to form a growing chain
- Here, the monomers add sequentially to the end of the growing chain
- It starts from the active center to form a chain
- Theoretically, the chain can grow indefinitely until the entire monomer is exhausted
- It is capable of producing giant molecules of unlimited size
- There are two types of monomers, which bring about addition polymerization:
  1. *Vinyl groups*: Monomers based on opening of carbon-carbon double bonds, which join to form single bond. Most commonly used in dentistry by methacrylate monomers
  2. *Imine-containing compounds*: Monomers based on ring opening reactions in which three atom rings are opened and join with another broken ring to form a single bond. These imine-containing compounds consist of two carbons and one nitrogen ring. Ring opening monomers are commonly found in the polyether impression material
- It occurs in four stages namely—(1) initiation, (2) propagation, (3) chain transfer, and (4) termination.

### Stages in Addition Polymerization *(Fig. 13.8)*
*Induction or initiation stage:*
- This is the first stage, which is controlled by activation and initiation
- The initiation of polymerization reaction requires a source of free radicals
- These free radicals are released by activating chemical such as benzoyl peroxide or heat or by UV light/visible light
- In dentistry, heat, chemical and visible light are most commonly used
- Addition polymerization takes place in the presence of unsaturated group and free radicals. Free radicals are those atoms, which have an unpaired electron
- The free radical initiates polymerization reaction by bonding its electron with the double bond of the monomer. The broken monomer bond releases another electron for further reaction

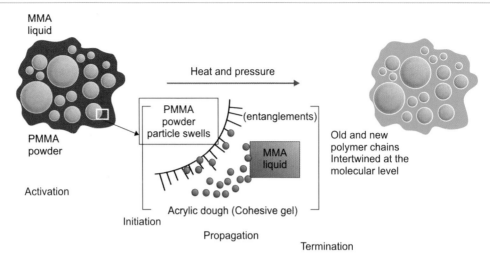

**Fig. 13.8:** Stages of addition polymerization.
*Abbreviations:* PMMA, polymethyl methacrylate; MMA, methyl methacrylate.

- Most commonly used initiator is benzoyl peroxide (for polymerization of Polymethyl methacrylate, which is activated rapidly between 50°C and 100°C
- During the induction period, the initiator molecule becomes energized and breaks down into free radicals. These radicals react with monomer molecule to initiate chain growth
- This initiation period depends on purity of monomer molecule. Any impurity increases the length of the period by consuming the activated initiator molecules higher the temperature, the more rapid the formation of free radicals and consequently shorter the induction period
- The polymerization process for dental resins is activated by one of the three energy sources:
  1. *Heat activation:* The free radicals are released by heating benzoyl peroxide, which initiates and propagates polymerization of monomer by producing two free radicals. Benzoyl peroxide is rapidly activated between 50°C and 100°C and starts releasing free radicals above 50°C. Most of the dental resins are polymerized by this energy source. Higher temperatures bring about rapid formation of free radicals and reduce the induction period
  2. *Chemical activation:* System consists of two reactants, which when mixed together generate free radicals by chemical reaction. These resins are called as self-cure or cold-cure resins or autopolymerizing resins. Tertiary amine activator and benzoyl peroxide initiator, when mixed together initiate polymerization. Tertiary amines release the free radicals by reducing thermal energy needed to break the initiator at room temperature. It actually forms

a complex with the initiator (benzoyl peroxide) to reduce the thermal energy to form free radicals
  3. *Light activated:* This system requires light source to activate the initiator to form free radicals. During inception of this system, UV light was used but was replaced by visible light due to certain drawbacks such as its limited penetration depth, loss of intensity and damage to retina and unpigmented oral tissues. Currently, visible light with a wavelength of about 470 nm is used to generate free radicals by activating camphorquinone and an organic amine, e.g. dimethylaminoethyl methacrylate. Since polymerization cannot take place without exposure to light, they are usually supplied as single paste system. Care should be taken that they are stored in dark without any light exposure. This system is highly technique sensitive because of factors such as the light source, its intensity, angle of exposure and distance of light source from the resins. One distinct advantage is that it provides operator adequate working time to contour the resin.

*Propagation:* The free radical-monomer complex formed in the initiation stage acts as a new free radical center to form a dimer with another monomer. This reaction continues until all the monomer is converted to the polymer. Thus, in reality, polymerization is never complete. However, the growth center stops to grow when one of the reactive centers is eliminated by the termination reaction. This process continues simultaneously as series of chain reaction. This reaction occurs rapidly with release of heat (exothermic reaction).

*Chain transfer:* In this stage, a new free radical is formed by transfer of the active free radical to another monomer molecule. The new free radical helps in further growth of the molecule.

*Termination:* Addition polymerization reactions are most often terminated by direct coupling of two free radical chain ends or by exchange of hydrogen atom from one growing chain to another. Chain termination can also result from chain transfer.

*Inhibition reaction:*

Polymerization reaction can be inhibited by:

- *Impurities*: An impurity can react with the activated initiator, e.g. addition of small amount of common inhibitor such as hydroquinone to monomer inhibits spontaneous polymerization, if no initiator is present, and retards the polymerization in the presence of an initiator
- Addition of inhibitor influences the storage stability and working time of the resin. Usually, for this reason, dental resin contains small amount of inhibitor (0.06%), e.g. hydroquinone
- *Oxygen*: Reacts rapidly with free radicals, and its presence retards the polymerization reaction. It is observed that the rate of reaction and degree of polymerization is reduced, if the polymerization takes place in open environment in comparison to that in oxygen-deficient environment
  *Factors affecting the role of oxygen on polymerization are:*
  - Temperature
  - Intensity of light
  - Concentration of oxygen.
  *Matrix strip* is commonly used in clinical practice to prevent the influence of air directly on the resin. This matrix strip helps to shape the resin and block the contact of oxygen during curing.

### Step Growth Polymerization or Condensation Polymerization

It is step growth type of polymerization or condensation polymerization involves the formation of byproducts.

- This process of polymerization is not commonly used in dentistry. In this reaction, two or more molecules react to form a structure which is a simple non-macro molecular in nature. It is often accompanied by formation of byproducts such as water, hydrogen gas, ammonia or alcohol. These byproducts compromise the properties or manipulation of the materials
- The formation of polymers by step growth is rather slow because the reaction proceeds in a stepwise fashion from monomer to dimer to trimer, and so forth until a large polymer molecule is formed.

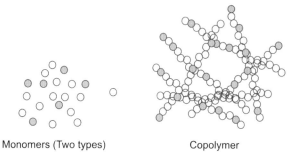

Monomers (Two types)          Copolymer
**Fig. 13.9:** Copolymerization.

## Copolymerization (Fig. 13.9)

It is a process of forming a copolymer by combining two or more chemically different monomers to yield specific physical properties of a polymer. The process of formation of copolymers is called as copolymerization. In a copolymer, the number and position of the different type of repeating units may vary. The composition of the copolymers depends on the relative chemical reactivity of two or more monomers.

### Types

- *Alternating copolymers*: In alternating copolymers, different mers are alternatively distributed along the polymer chain
  A – B – A – B – A – B – A – B
- *Random*: In this type of copolymer, the different mers are randomly distributed along the chain such as:
  A – B – A – A – A – A – B – A – A
- *Block type*: In this type, the mer units occur in relatively long sequences along main polymer chain
  A – A – A – A – A – A – A – B – B – B – B – B
- *Graft type*: Here, sequences of one of the monomer area grafted onto the backbone of second monomer species.

A – A – A – A – A – A – A – A
        |   |
        B   B
        |   |
        B   B
        |   |
        B   B

---

**CLINICAL SIGNIFICANCE**

Copolymerization process improves the physical and mechanical properties of the resulting resin. There are number of resins, which are copolymerized in dentistry. Some examples are methyl methacrylate, methacrylic esters, acrylic esters, etc. If small quantity of ethyl acrylate is copolymerized with methyl methacrylate, it improves the flexibility and fracture resistance of the denture. Polymer segments can be grafted on the linear chain to alter the properties of the resin. Grafting of the polymers also helps in altering the adhesive properties of the resins.

## Cross-linking Polymer

- The formation of chemical bonds or bridges between linear polymers is referred to as *cross-linking*. This forms three-dimensional networks. These cross-linked polymers may be produced by presence of small amount of different monomer units with reactive double bonds on each end of the molecules
- Cross-linking affects the physical properties of a polymer by limiting the movement of the polymer chains relative to each other when the material is stressed. Thus, the deformation is elastic rather than plastic. Extensively, cross-linked polymers are harder, more brittle and more resistant to the action of solvent crazing or surface cracking and surface stresses than noncross-linked materials. The more recent acrylic resins are of cross-linked variety.

## Factors Influencing Properties of Polymers

- Molecular weight and chemical structural units of monomers
- Degree of polymerization or conversion factor and $M_w$ distributions
- Copolymerization and spatial organization
- Crystallinity
- Temperatures.

## TEST YOURSELF

### Essay Questions

1. What are polymers? Differentiate between the addition and condensation polymerization reaction.
2. Discuss in detail various stages of polymerization.
3. Discuss in detail dental polymers.
4. Describe application of resins in dentistry.
5. Discuss properties of polymers.
6. Classify polymers. Write briefly ideal requirements of polymers.

### Short Notes

1. Copolymerization.
2. Condensation polymerization.
3. Cross-linked polymers.
4. Polydispersity.
5. Role of plasticizers in polymers.
6. Thermal properties of polymers.
7. Rheological properties of polymers.
8. Branched-chain polymers.

### Multiple Choice Questions

1. Polymer is formed by:
   A. Joining monomer molecules together in a long chain through carbon bonds
   B. Fusing acrylic powder beads together at high temperature
   C. Breaking down complex high-molecular weight molecules by heating atom
   D. Linking nitrogen atoms together with hydrogen bonds
2. Denture polymers cannot be polymerized in the oral cavity by which mode of activation:
   A. Heat
   B. Chemical
   C. Microwave
   D. Light
3. Cross-linking agents in denture acrylics improve:
   A. Craze resistance
   B. Internal color
   C. Tissue compatibility
   D. Surface hardness
4. Hardness of denture acrylic resin is:
   A. Less than gingival tissues
   B. Less than the cast metal
   C. More than tooth enamel
   D. More than glass
5. In which polymerization reaction water or alcohol byproduct is formed during the reaction:
   A. Addition
   B. Condensation
   C. Cross-linking
   D. Ring-opening
6. Addition polymerization reaction occurs in which stages:
   A. Wet, flexible and stiff
   B. Sandy, stringy and dough
   C. Initiation, propagation and termination
   D. Solution, gel and solid
7. Cross-linking of polymers:
   A. Occurs when long chains are linked end-to-end
   B. Occurs when long-chain polymers are mixed together and chain wrap around each other
   C. Used to improve physical properties of the final resin product
   D. Results in weaker material

8. Addition polymerization:
   A. Is initiated by a free radical that opens the bond between the carbon atoms of the monomer
   B. Is an endothermic reaction
   C. Is not a common method of polymerization
   D. Results in porosity after completion

## ANSWERS

| | | | |
|---|---|---|---|
| 1. A | 2. C | 3. A | 4. B |
| 5. B | 6. C | 7. C | 8. A |

## BIBLIOGRAPHY

1. Asmussen E. NMR-analysis of monomers in restorative resins. Acta Odontol Scand. 1975;33:129.
2. Braden M. Characterization of the setting process in dental polysulfide rubbers. J Dent Res. 1966;45:1016.
3. Cook WD. Rheological studies of the polymerization of the elastic impression materials. Viscocity measurements. J Biomed Mater Res. 1982;16:331.
4. Craig RG, Powers JM. Polymers and polymerization. Restorative Dental Materials, 11th edition. St. Louis: Mosby; 2003.
5. Leinfelder KF, Lemons JE. Dental polymers. Clinical Restorative Materials and Techniques. Philadelphia: Lea and Febiger; 1988.
6. Rueggeberg FA. From vulcanite to vinyl, a history of resins in restorative dentistry. J Prosthet Dent. 2002;87:364-79.
7. Ward IM. Mechanical properties of solid polymers, 2nd edition. New York: Wiley-Interscience; 1983.
8. Williams JR, Craig RG. Physical properties of addition silicones as a function of composition. J Oral Rehabil. 1988;15:639.

CHAPTER 14

# Denture Base Resin

ADA Specification No. 12; ISO Specification No. 1567:1999

## CHAPTER OUTLINE



*'Study as if you were to live forever. Live as if you were to die tomorrow.'*

***—Mahatama Gandhi***

## INTRODUCTION

Acrylic resin was introduced to dentistry in 1936 and it received a great response from the dental professionals such that by 1946, 98% of all dentures were made with methyl methacrylate polymers or copolymers. Denture polymers have wide application in dentistry and various other forms of polymers such as vinyl acrylic, polystyrene, epoxy resins, nylon, vinyl styrene, polycarbonate, silicones, light-activated urethane polyacrylate, rubber reinforced acrylics, etc. are used.

## ACRYLIC RESINS

The most common acrylic resins used in dentistry were polymethyl methacrylates (PMMA). Pure polymethyl methacrylate is a colorless and transparent solid. It can be tinted to provide almost any shade and degree of translucency. Its color and optical properties remain stable under normal intraoral conditions.

### Definition

*Any of a group of thermoplastic resins made by polymerizing esters of acrylic or methyl methacrylate acids.*

*—GPT 8th Edition*

Acrylic resins are synthetic polymers, which are derived from acrylic acid. They are formed when liquid monomer is mixed with polymer beads to undergo polymerization. The resins commonly used in dentistry are esters of acrylic acid and methacrylic acid. Based on the method of polymerization, resins are of following types:

- Heat-cured resins
- Self-cured or chemically cured or autopolymerizing resins
- Light-cured resins.

### Applications

- Used for fabricating complete dentures **(Fig. 14.1)** and removable partial dentures
- For fabrication of denture bases

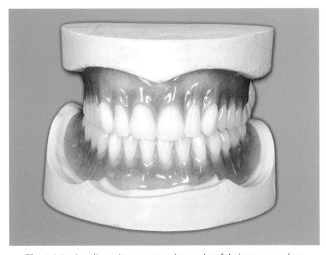

**Fig. 14.1:** Acrylic resins commonly used to fabricate complete dentures.

- Denture tooth material
- For relining and rebasing of dental prosthesis
- For repair of dentures
- As tissue conditioners
- For fabricating custom impression trays
- For fabricating orthodontic retainers and removable tooth movement devices
- For fabricating mouth guards and night guards
- For fabricating fluoride and bleaching trays
- Used as facing in crowns for esthetics
- For fabrication of provisional crowns and partial dentures
- For fabrication of surgical, interim and definitive obturators
- Specialized resins used as esthetic tissue replacement in congenital defects or defects due to trauma or surgery
- In fabrication of maxillofacial prosthesis such as eye, ear or nasal prosthesis.

## IDEAL REQUIREMENTS OF DENTURE BASE MATERIALS

Denture base materials should have the following ideal requirements:

- *Biological requirements*—should be nontoxic, nonirritating, tasteless and odorless. They should be impermeable to oral fluids and should inhibit microbial growth
- *Physical properties*—should be adequate strength to bear masticatory forces. They should be dimensionally stable and resists thermal changes. To reduce the bulk, they should have low-specific gravity
- *Esthetics*—should have adequate translucency and should be color stable. They should allow characterization to enhance esthetic

- *Manipulation*—they should be easy to handle and manipulate
- *Polishability*—should be finished and polished to high luster
- *Repair*—should be easily relined and repaired
- *Economic*—cost of material should be low.

### Classification of Denture Base Materials

- *Based on durability*:
  - *Temporary denture bases*—shellac baseplate, cold-cure resins
  - *Permanent denture bases*—metal denture bases, heat-cure acrylic resin.
- *Based on materials*:
  - *Metallic*—gold alloys, cobalt-chromium (Co-Cr) alloys
  - *Nonmetallic*—acrylic resins, vinyl resins, shellac baseplate.
- *Based on mode of activation (ISO classification)*:
  - *Cold-cure or self-cure resins*—polymerize at room temperature
  - *Heat-cure resins*—polymerize at temperature more than 65°C
  - *Light-cure resins*—polymerize in presence of light
  - *Microwave-activated resins*—polymerizes in microwave
  - *Thermoplastic resins*—moldable polymers.

## HEAT-CURED DENTURE BASE RESINS

These resins are most commonly used acrylic resins in dentistry, which can fabricate all types of denture bases. **(Fig. 14.2)**. Such resins require heat for polymerization, which can be provided using a water bath or a microwave oven.

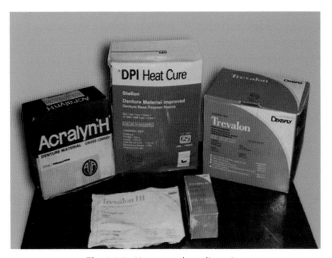

**Fig. 14.2:** Heat-cured acrylic resins.

## Composition

This is supplied in the form of powder, liquid or the gel form.

### Powder

- *Polymethyl methacrylate*: Main constituent to dissolve in monomer and reduce polymerization shrinkage. They are in the form of high-molecular weight prepolymerized spheres or beads, which are mixed with the liquid
- *Benzoyl peroxide initiator*: 0.5–1.5% to provide free radicals
- *Pigments*: Like mercuric sulfide, cadmium sulfide, cadmium selenide, ferric oxide, carbon black, etc. help in characterization of the denture
- *Dyes*: Usually not used as they tend to leach out of plastics due to oral fluids
- *Opacifiers*: Zinc or titanium oxides to improve its radiopacity
- *Dyed synthetic fibers*: Nylon or acrylic added to mimic minute blood vessels of oral mucosa
- *Plasticizers-dibutyl phthalate*: Used to reduce the softening temperature. They partially neutralize secondary bonds or the intermolecular forces.

### Liquid

It usually supplied in dark-brown, amber-colored bottles, so as to prevent evaporation and polymerization by some ionizing agents.

- *Methyl methacrylate*: They are in the form of nonpolymerized methyl methacrylate monomer. It possesses one carbon-carbon double bond per molecule
- *Hydroquinone inhibitor*: 0.003–0.1% prevents undesirable polymerization during storage. It also retards the polymerization process and increases the working time
- *Dibutyl phthalate plasticizers*: Sometimes added to make the polymer softer—disadvantage is they gradually leach out of the plastic into the oral fluids
- *Glycol dimethacrylate cross-linking agents:* 1–2% volume—they provide increased resistance to crazing and deformation. Structurally although similar to methyl methacrylate, it has two carbon-carbon double bonds per molecule, which helps in forming net-like interconnections between the polymer chains enhancing resistance to deformation.

## Properties

- *Tensile strength*: 48.3–62.1 Mpa—they are brittle and typically low in strength in comparison to other dental materials
- *Compressive strength*: 75.9 Mpa—this depends on composition of the resin, technique of processing, degree of polymerization, water sorption, etc.
- *Impact strength*: 0.98–1.27 J/m$^3$—addition of plasticizers can increase the impact strength
- *Elongation:* 1–2%—it is an indication of toughness of plastic. Low elongation is seen in brittle materials
- *Elastic modulus:* 3.8 Gpa
- *Hardness*: 15–17 Knoop hardness number (KHN). Low KHN of the heat-cure resins show that they can be easily scratched and abraded. Fillers may increase resistance to abrasion. Wear resistance of resins is low
- *Water sorption*: 0.69 mg/cm$^2$—the resins absorb water through diffusion and these water molecules occupy spaces between the polymer chains
- *Water solubility*: 0.02 mg/cm$^2$. A small amount of monomer may be leached out
- *Residual monomer*: 0.2–0.3%
- *Dimensional stability*: Good—this depends on the proper processing technique, type of investing medium used, method of resin packing and the temperature during processing
- *Creep*: These resins display viscoelastic behavior, act as rubbery solids. The creep rate depends upon the temperature, residual monomer and plasticizers. Cross-linking agents reduce creep rates
- *Crazing*: They are small linear cracks on the surface of the denture. Give a hazy or foggy appearance to the dentures. They occur due to the mechanical separation of polymer chains under tensile stress. They begin at the surface and are oriented at right angles to the tensile forces. Crazing occurs due to:
  - Mechanical stresses
  - Solvent action like ethyl alcohol
  - Incorporation of water
- *Denture warpage*: Caused due to the release of stresses incorporated during processing like:
  - Uneven or rapid cooling
  - Packing resin in rubbery stage
  - Improper deflasking

These stresses are released during denture polishing, immersion of denture in hot water, etc.

- *Polymerization shrinkage volumetric shrinkage:* Ratio of polymer-monomer = 3:1, then volumetric shrinkage is 7%
  - *Linear shrinkage* = 0.2–0.5%

Affects the denture base adaptation and cuspal interdigitation

- *Porosity*: It is the presence of surface and subsurface voids, and affects the physical, esthetic and hygienic properties of the denture

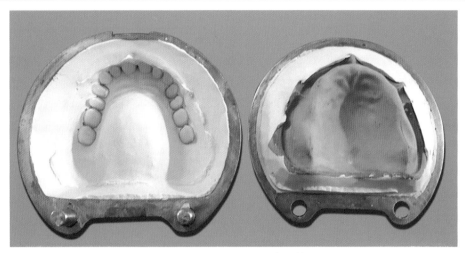

**Fig. 14.3:** Preparation of mold.

*Causes*:
- – Vaporization of unreacted monomer in the thicker sections of denture
- – Inhomogeneity of the mix
- – Rapid temperature elevation
- – Inadequate pressure or material in the mold
- • *Color stability*: Good.

## Storage

The heat-activated polymer and monomer should be stored according to the manufacturer's instructions, which are usually defined with specific temperature and time limit.

**CLINICAL SIGNIFICANCE**

The monomer should be stored in *airtight amber or brown-colored bottles* and in cool environment. This prevents the monomer from undergoing polymerization due to exposure to ultraviolet (UV) radiation and heat.

## Manipulation and Processing

### Compression Molding Technique

The technique can be described in following steps:

*Preparation of mold* **(Fig. 14.3):** After the final wax, contouring and finishing the wax denture is sealed onto the master cast. This assembly is removed from the articulator and thin layer of separator is applied to prevent adherence of dental stone during the flasking process. The lower

portion of the flask is filled with freshly mixed dental stone and the master cast is placed into this mix. The dental stone is then contoured to facilitate wax elimination, packing and deflasking procedures.

Once the mix reaches the initial set, it is coated with separator such as petroleum jelly. The upper portion of the flask is then positioned on the lower portion. Wax denture assembly placed in the flask for investing. A surface tension-reducing agent is applied on the exposed wax surfaces and the second mix of dental stone is poured into the flask until all the surfaces of the denture are embedded into the flask **(Fig. 14.4)**. The occlusal and the incisal surfaces of the teeth

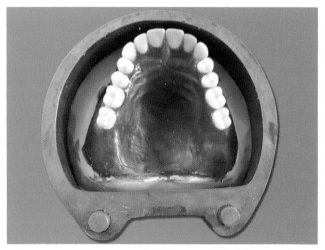

**Fig. 14.4:** Wax denture assembly placed in the flask for second pour.

are minimally exposed to easily deflask subsequently. The mixed stone is allowed to set and then cold mold seal is applied. After this, additional stone is mixed and filled into the remainder of the flask and then the lid is closed.

After the complete setting of the dental stone, the flask and clamp assembly is placed in boiling water for 4 minutes. The flask is removed from the boiling water and both upper and lower member of the flask are carefully separated. The softened wax and the record base are completely removed. On the other hand, it should be ensured that the teeth are firmly secured into the investing stone of the remaining segment. Residual wax, if any is removed from the mold cavity using wax solvent and is later on rinsed with clean boiling water.

*Selection and application of separating media:* Various separating media used are:
- Solution of alginate compounds—commonly used
- Tinfoil—obsolete—no more used now
- Cellulose lacquers
- Evaporated milk
- Soap
- Sodium silicate
- Starches
- *Purpose of separating media*:
  - To prevent diffusion of water from the mold surface into the denture base resins
  - To prevent leaching of free monomer from denture base resins into the mold surface. The most popular separating medium is water-soluble alginate solution. On application of this medium on the mold surface, it forms relatively insoluble film of calcium alginate. The separating medium is applied on the warm mold surface in thin layers by means of fine brush **(Figs. 14.5A and B)**
- *Mechanism of action*:
  - The separating medium is applied in two coats on the warm gypsum cast as well as the invested plaster or stone. The sodium alginate interacts with the calcium in the gypsum to form a thin layer of separating medium, which forms a barrier against the acrylic flowing into the gypsum

**CLINICAL SIGNIFICANCE**

The separating media should not be applied on the exposed portion of the teeth because this will result in compromised bonding between the teeth and the denture base. Also, the mold is positioned such that there is no pooling of the separating medium. The separating medium is allowed to dry before packing procedure.

*Polymer-monomer ratio:* The accepted polymer-monomer ratio is 3:1 by volume and 2.5:1 by weight. This provides

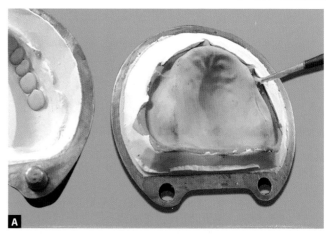
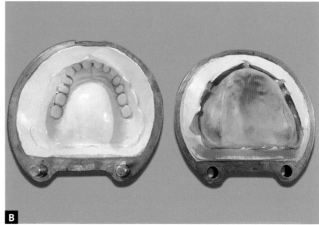

**Figs. 14.5A and B:** Application of cold mold seal.

sufficient monomer to thoroughly wet the polymer particles. Adequate quantity of monomer minimizes the chances of polymerization shrinkage. To reduce dimensional changes, the manufacturer provides powder in the form of prepolymerized PMMA beads and the liquid in form of unpolymerized methyl methacrylate called monomer. When 3:1 powder-liquid ratio is used then the volumetric shrinkage is limited to approximately 6%.

- *Rationale behind polymerization shrinkage:*
  The methyl methacrylate has two carbon-carbon double bonds per molecule as mentioned earlier. Each molecule possesses an electrical field, which repels other molecules. Because of this, the distance between the molecules is greater than the length of the carbon-carbon bond. When these molecules are chemically bonded a new carbon-carbon linkage is formed, which brings both the molecules close to each other. This reduces space occupied by the molecules and hence polymerization shrinkage occurs
- *Compensation mechanism of polymerization shrinkage:*
  The inevitable polymerization shrinkage is compensated initially by the setting expansion of the gypsum mold

and later when polymerized acrylic resin is exposed to water in mold it swells and expands.

A proper polymer-to-monomer ratio is of considerable importance in the fabrication of well-fitting denture bases with desirable physical properties.

- If too much monomer is used, it results in:
  - Greater polymerization shrinkage
  - Additional time will be required to reach packing consistency
  - There will be a tendency for porosity to occur.
- If too little monomer is used:
  - Not all the polymer beads will be wetted by monomer and the cured acrylic will be granular
  - Dough will be difficult to manage.

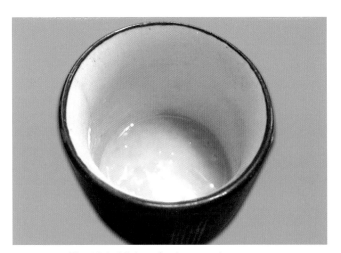

**Fig. 14.6:** Mixing of polymer and monomer.

*Mixing of polymer-monomer* **(Fig. 14.6):** When polymer and monomer are mixed in prescribed ratio, a workable mass is formed. Polymer and monomer are usually mixed in a porcelain jar, as it prevents adherence of mixed resin to its walls. This mass goes through five distinct physical stages:

- *Stage 1—sandy stage*: There is no or minimal interaction between polymer particles and monomer at molecular level. Consistency of the mix—coarse or grainy
- *Stage 2—stringy*: In this stage, the monomer attacks the polymer particles. These polymer chains are dispersed in liquid monomer increasing the viscosity of the mix. Stage characterized by *stringiness or stickiness* when material is touched or drawn apart
- *Stage 3—doughlike*: In this stage, increased numbers of polymer chains enter the monomer. The polymer chains are dissolved to form a mix, which looks like a pliable dough. This consistency of the mix is not sticky or tacky to the mixing jar or spatula. The properties of the mix are ideal for compression molding. The packing should be done in this stage **(Fig. 14.7)**
- *Stage 4—rubbery or elastic*: In this stage, the mix becomes rubbery. This is because the monomer gets either dissipated by evaporation or further penetrates into remaining polymer beads. It results in a mass, which rebounds when compressed or stretched. It is not possible to mold by conventional compression technique
- *Stage 5—stiff*: In this stage, there is further evaporation of the free monomer resulting in a very dry mix, which is resistant to mechanical deformation.

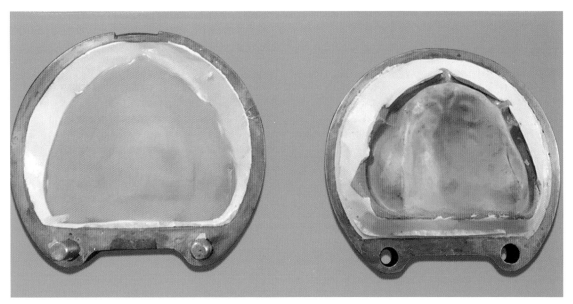

**Fig. 14.7:** Packing is done in dough stage.

*Dough forming time:* American Dental Association (ADA) specification No. 12 (ISO 20795-1:2008: Dentistry—base polymers) requires that dough-like consistency be attained in less than 40 minutes from start of mixing process. Clinically, most resins reach dough-like stage in less than 10 minutes.

*Working time:* It is the time in which the mixed resin remains in the dough stage. ADA specification No. 12 requires the dough to remain moldable for at least 5 minutes. The working time of the resin may be extended by refrigeration. Drawback of refrigeration is that moisture condenses on the resin when removed from refrigerator and this will compromise the physical and esthetic properties of the processed resin. Moisture contamination can be avoided by storing the mix in an airtight container. When the stored container is removed from the refrigerator, it should not be opened until it comes to room temperature.

*Packing:* Packing is the process of placement and adaptation of the denture base resins into the mold cavity. This step is one of the most critical steps, which required that the mold cavity should be properly filled with the mixed resin in dough stage. Excessive resins should be avoided as this may result in excessively thick denture base and it may even displace the prosthetic teeth from the mold. Likewise packing too little material will result in porosity and void formation in the denture base.

The mixed resin in dough stage is removed from the container and is rolled into a rope-like shape. Just before packing, little monomer is painted on the cervical portion of the prosthetic teeth to aid in better bonding to the denture base. The rope-shaped resin is bent like a horseshoe and is placed on the prosthetic teeth and rolled over such that it covers the entire mold. It should be ensured that adequate material is packed into the mold. A thin polyethylene sheet is placed over the master cast and the curing flask is reassembled.

A proper polymer-to-monomer ratio is of considerable importance in the fabrication of well-fitting denture bases with desirable physical properties.
- *Overpacking*: Exhibits excessive thickness and resultant malpositioning of prosthetic teeth
- *Underpacking*: Leads to noticeable denture base porosity.

The flask is subjected to slow pressure under bench press in order to ensure even flow of flash (excess resin) from the mold space. Excessive flash is displaced eccentrically. The pressure is applied on the flask till there is complete closure of the flask. Flask is removed from the press and is carefully opened to remove the excess resins. Carefully, the polyethylene sheet is removed from the surface of the resin with continuous tug **(Fig. 14.8)**. The process of placing

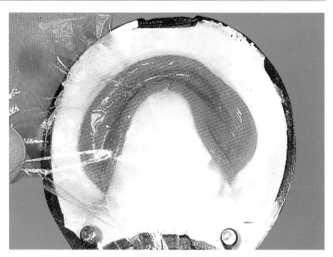

**Fig. 14.8:** After trial closure, sheet is removed.

polyethylene sheet during trial closure is done until all the excess resins are removed **(Fig. 14.9A)**.

Finally definitive closure is done where no polyethylene sheet is placed. The flask halves are properly oriented in position such that there is complete contact of the two metal edges of the flask. The closed flask is placed under pressure for 30 minutes before curing in flask carrier (sometimes called "bench curing"). The flask carrier maintains even pressure on the flask assembly during denture processing **(Fig. 14.9B)**.

*Rationale of bench curing:*
- Allow equalization of pressure through the mold
- Allow uniform distribution of monomer through the dough mass
- Allow better bond between the resin teeth and the base material because the teeth are exposed to monomer for a longer duration.

*Curing (polymerization):* Polymerization of heat-activated resins begins when they are heated above 60°C. Heat in these resins behaves as activator. Benzoyl peroxide present in the resin decomposes to yield-free radicals, which initiate the polymerization reaction. The initiation reaction occurs when the released free radicals react with the available monomer molecule. This reaction occurs very rapidly and terminates in two ways: (1) by directly connecting with two growing chains, or (2) by transferring the single hydrogen ion from one chain to another.

Polymerization of denture base resins is an exothermic reaction, where heat is evolved. The amount of heat-evolved influences the properties of the processed denture. When the temperature of the water bath reaches above 70°C, there is rapid increase of temperature of the resin, which in turn rapidly decomposes benzoyl peroxide. This results

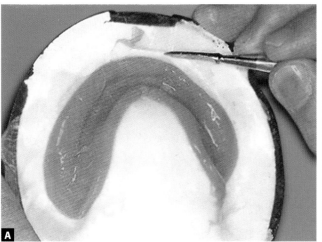
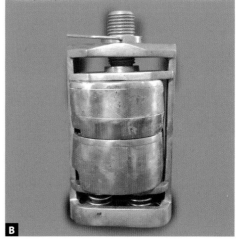

**Figs. 14.9A and B:** Excess flash is removed and two halves of flasks are closely packed.

in increased rate of polymerization and increased rate of exothermic heat.

*Curing cycle:* The heating process used to control polymerization is termed as the polymerization cycle (or) curing cycle. Electrically controlled curing water baths can be used as they enable better control of the curing process. Sudden rapid heating of the resin should be avoided, as it can cause boiling of monomer, which may result in porosity in the polymerized denture base resin.

The recommended curing cycles are:

- *Technique I*—involves processing the heat-cure resins at a constant temperature of 74°C for 8 hours in a water bath or longer without terminal boiling temperature
- *Technique II*—consists of processing the heat-cure resins at 74°C in a water bath for 8 hours and then slowly increasing the temperature to 100°C for 1 hour
- *Technique III*—involves processing the resin at 74°C in a water bath for approximately 2 hours and then slowly increasing temperature of water bath to 100°C and processing for 1 hour.

*Cooling:*

- Following completion of chosen polymerization cycle the denture flask is cooled slowly to the room temperature. Rapid cooling is avoided, as it may lead to warping of denture base because of the difference in thermal contraction of resin and investment material. Slow uniform cooling minimizes this potential problem
- Flask removed from water bath should be bench cooled for 30 minutes. Subsequently, flask should be immersed in cool tap for water for 15 minutes.

*Deflasking, finishing and polishing:*

- Cured acrylic denture is retrieved from the flask and this process is known as deflasking

- The process of deflasking should be done carefully in order to avoid flexion and breakage of acrylic denture
- Retrieved denture is finished and polished using various grades of abrasives stones and sand paper
- Finally, finely ground pumice powder in water is used to finish final dentures for high luster.

### Injection-molding Technique *(Figs. 14.10A and B)*

- Dentures can be fabricated by injection molding technique using specially designed flasks
- The flasking and the dewaxing procedures are similar to that followed in compression-molding technique. In this technique, wax sprues are attached to the waxed denture, which is invested in stone. These sprues are connected to the inlet or pressure port. After this, the remaining half of the flask is precisely positioned and the investment procedure is completed. The flasks are then placed in water bath for wax elimination as described in compression-molding technique
- After dewaxing procedure, a hollow sprue connects the mold cavity to the external opening on the flask
- The flask is placed on the carrier, which maintains pressure on the assembly during resin introduction and processing
- The denture base resin is mixed and placed in the cylinder. As soon as the material reaches the proper consistency, it is injected into the empty mold under high pressure. The pressure is maintained during polymerization cycle
- The flask is placed in the water bath for polymerization
- As this material is polymerizing, added resin is injected into mold to offset polymerization shrinkage
- This technique can be used for microwavable and pour-type resins

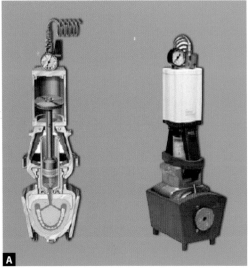
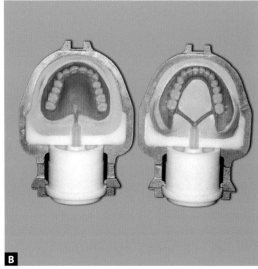

**Figs. 14.10A and B:** Injection molding technique.

- After the polymerization procedure is completed, the dentures are recovered, adjusted, finished and polished
- Studies show that denture bases fabricated by this method produces slightly better clinical accuracy than those fabricated with compression-molding method.

*Advantages:*
- Better dimensional accuracy
- Residual monomer content is less
- Has good impact strength
- Reduced risk of monomer vapor inhalation.

*Disadvantages:*
- High cost of equipment
- Difficult mold design problems
- Special flask is required.

*Materials used in injection-molding technique:*
- Acrylic
- Polycarbonate
- Nylon or polyamides
- Polystyrene.

# MICROWAVE-POLYMERIZED RESINS (FIG. 14.11)

- Heat-cure resins can also be polymerized using microwave energy
- The composition of microwavable-polymerized resins is similar to conventional heat-cure resins. Although, special liquid rather normal liquid is used
- With normal liquid chances of porosities are higher

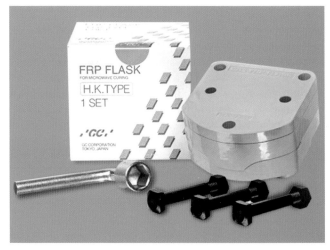

**Fig. 14.11:** Microwave-polymerized resins with special flask.

- In this technique, a especially formulated resin and a nonmetallic flask (usually polycarbonate) is used
- A conventional microwave oven is useful to supply the required thermal energy for polymerization
- Major benefit of this technique is speed with which polymerization is accomplished as the processing time is only 4–5 minutes. Possible drawback of this technique is rapid rate of polymerization can result in overheating of the thick section of denture base resulting in internal porosity
- The physical properties and fit of microwave resins are comparable to conventional resins processed through compression-molding technique.

## Supplied As

Powder and liquid system.

## Microwave Polymerization Techniques

- Compression-molding technique
- Injection-molding technique.

## Technical Considerations

Microwave produces electromagnetic field to generate heat required to break the initiator benzoyl peroxide into two free radicals. Microwaves target the monomer only and as the reaction proceeds lesser monomer particles are left to absorb same amount of energy. This *self-regulatory mechanism* generates sufficient energy to rapidly complete the polymerization of the resins. It is for this reason that polymerization time with microwavable resins is less. Also, this technique eliminates the need to transfer external heat from the flask, investment material and stone cast to the resin. As there is no external heat source, the flask remains cool and is not damaged. As the heat dispersed is more efficient and rapid, the chances of polymerization shrinkage and porosity are less as compared to conventional heat-activated resins.

## Advantages

- Reduced curing time
- Good color stability
- Good denture base adaptation
- Minimal residual monomer
- Reduced dough-forming time.

## Disadvantages

- Increased porosity
- Flasks are expensive
- Added equipment
- Poor bonding to denture teeth.

## HIGH-IMPACT RESISTANT RESINS (FIG. 14.12)

- These denture base resins have similar composition to conventional heat-cure resins, but they have much higher impact strength
- Cost of these resins is higher
- In these resins, the PMMA in the powder is substituted with a copolymer. This copolymer is made of rubbery monomer, which gives an illusion of a shock absorber
- Additionally, the liquid of these resins does not have a cross-linking agent
- These materials not only have high-impact strength but accurate fit and low-creep value.

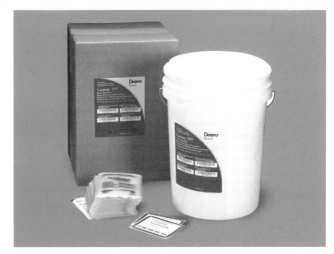

**Fig. 14.12:** High-impact-resistant resins.

## RAPID HEAT-POLYMERIZED RESINS

- These resins also have similar composition as heat-cure acrylic resins except they have altered initiator system
- This initiator system allows the resins to be processed in boiling water in 20 minutes. Curing occurs at much shorter time than compared to conventional heat-cure resins
- Benefit of these resins is faster processing in comparison to conventional resins
- Drawbacks are greater amount of residual monomer and greater porosity in thickness of more than 6 mm. Whereas in conventional heat-activated resins have little porosity up to thickness of 20 mm of denture base.

## CHEMICALLY ACTIVATED OR AUTOPOLYMERIZING OR SELF-CURE OR COLD-CURE RESINS

These resins are activated by the chemical activators present in them and therefore, can be polymerized at room temperature. In cold-cured acrylic resin the chemical initiator benzoyl peroxide is activated by another chemical, dimethyl-para-toluidine (tertiary amine), which is present in the monomer. When powder is mixed with liquid, tertiary amine decomposes benzoyl peroxide to produce free radicals, which initiate polymerization reaction. The hydroquinone presents in the liquid initially inhibits the reaction by destroying free radicals. Thereby increasing the working time for manipulation. Once hydroquinone is used, the reaction then proceeds rapidly and changes from dough stage to rubbery stage. It is an exothermic reaction. When the reaction is complete the mixed resin becomes rigid.

Some cold-cure resins are called as *pour resins* because these resins can be poured into the processing mold of agar hydrocolloid to form a denture base. They are mixed thin, fluid consistency.

## Supplied As

Usually supplied in the powder-liquid form **(Fig. 14.13)**.

## Composition

### Liquid

- Methyl methacrylate—monomer. It helps in dissolving polymer
- Tertiary amine—acts as activator for self-cure resins
- Dibutyl phthalate—plasticizing agent
- Glycol dimethacrylate 1–2%—acts as cross-linking agent
- Hydroquinone 0.006%—acts as inhibitor. It prevents polymerization of monomer during storage.

### Powder

- Polymethyl methacrylate and other copolymers—polymer beads
- Benzoyl peroxide—acts as initiator
- Compounds of mercury sulfate; cadmium sulfate—dyes
- Zinc or titanium oxide—reduces translucency
- Dibutyl phthalate—plasticizing agent
- Dyed organic fillers, inorganic particles like glass fibers or beads—to simulate natural tissues.

## Properties

- Polymerization in cold-cure acrylic resin is not as complete as that of heat-cure resins. This indicates that there is great amount of unreacted monomer in cold-cure resins. The amount of residual monomer is about 3–5%

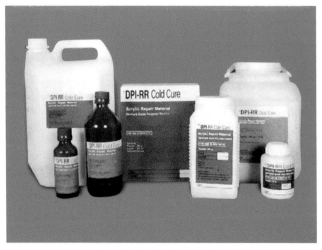

**Fig. 14.13:** Cold-cure resins.

- This unreacted monomer can cause two major problems. Firstly, it behaves as plasticizers that reduce transverse strength of denture resin. Secondly, the residual monomer serves as a potential tissue irritant thereby compromising biocompatibility of denture bases. From physical standpoint, chemically activated resins display slightly less shrinkage than heat-activated counterparts. This imparts greater dimensional accuracy to chemically activated resins. The polymerization shrinkage is less because of less complete polymerization resulting in greater dimensional accuracy
- The color stability of chemically activated resins generally is inferior to that of heat-activated resins. This property is related to presence of tertiary amines within the chemically activated resins. Organic sulfinic acids may be added to improve the color stability
- Porosity in cold-cure resins is greater than heat-cured resins
- Cold-cure resins give greater *creep* values
- They have low *impact strength*—15 J/m
- The *transverse strength*—84 Mpa
- *Water sorption*—0.5–0.7 mg/cm$^2$ (almost same as that of heat-cure resins)
- *Water solubility*—0.05 mg/cm$^2$.

## Technical and Processing Considerations

- Compression-molding technique is often used to mold cold-cure resins. Therefore, the preparation of mold and resin-packing procedure is similar to that of heat-cure resins
- The monomer and polymer are mixed following the manufacturer's instructions to achieve dough-like consistency. The working time of cold-cure resins is less than that of heat-cure resins
- Working time can be increased by refrigerating the monomer bottle before mixing or keeping the mixing jar in refrigerator. This decreases the rate of polymerization and the resin is in the dough stage for a longer period of time (increased working time)
- Since, the working time with chemically activated resins is less than that of heat-activated resins care should be taken that only adequate resin is packed into the mold. So that minimal trail closures of the curing flask is required
- Once the final closure of flask is done, the pressure should be maintained till the completion of the polymerization process. The time needed for polymerization can vary depending on the type of material used
- Chemically activated resin requires 30 minutes for initial hardening but the polymerization reaction occurs for longer duration. To ensure complete polymerization, the flask is held under pressure for minimum of 3 hours

- The residual monomer content after polymerization for cold-cure resins varies between 3% and 5% and for heat-cure resins it varies between 0.2% and 0.5%. It is advisable to achieve high degree of polymerization for chemically activated resins because incomplete polymerization will lead to denture instability and can cause tissue irritation.

Comparison between heat-cure resins and cold cure resins is summarized in **Table 14.1**.

## Fluid Resin Technique

- In this technique **(Figs. 14.14A to F)**, highly flowable chemically cured resins are used for fabricating dentures. These resins are supplied in form of powder and liquid components
- The monomer-polymer ratio is 1:2.5. When powder and liquid are mixed with proper proportions, it results in low-viscosity resins
- The mix is poured into the mold without doing any trial closures. The flowable resin is subjected to atmospheric pressure and allowed to polymerize at ambient temperature.

### Technical Considerations

- The waxed denture is positioned in a specially designed flask. The waxed denture is sealed to the master cast, so that it does not move during investment procedure

- The flask is filled with reversible hydrocolloid investment material (agar) or irreversible hydrocolloid or less commonly soft stone or silicone mold
- After complete gelation of the hydrocolloid, the cast assembly with attached teeth is carefully removed from the mold
- The wax elimination is done using hot water. The teeth are retrieved and carefully positioned into its respective position in the mold
- The sprues and vents are cut from outside of the flask to the mold cavity
- Cast is repositioned over the teeth. There exists a space between teeth and cast, which was previously occupied by wax. The flowable resin is mixed according to the manufacturer's instructions
- Now, the mixed resin is flowed through the sprue into the empty space in the mold
- The flask assembly is placed into a pressure pot at room temperature for complete polymerization
- For polymerization, it is kept for 30–45 minutes in the pressure pot (pressurized chamber). Application of pressure eliminates air bubbles, which are formed during mixing and manipulation of resin resulting in better adaptation of the denture base and also reducing porosity in the dentures
- On completion of polymerization, the denture is retrieved from the flask
- Sprues are cut and the denture is finished and polished in conventional manner. The finished and polished dentures are kept in water to prevent distortion and dehydration.

**Table 14.1:** Comparison between heat-cure and cold-cure resins.

| Property | Heat-cure resins | Cold-cure resins |
|---|---|---|
| Composition | Powder and liquid system | Powder and liquid system |
| Activator | Heat | Dimethyl-para-toluidine |
| Initiator | Benzoyl peroxide | Benzoyl peroxide |
| Residual monomer | Less—0.2–0.5% | More—3–5% |
| Properties | Superior strength, low creep, lesser distortion, less initial deformation | Lesser strength, greater creep, greater distortion, higher initial deformation |
| Porosity | Less | Greater |
| Curing temperature | Greater than 60°C | Room temperature |
| Processing time | More | Less |
| Processing procedure | More technique sensitive | Simple |
| Equipment | Expensive | No heating equipment required |
| Color stability | Good | Poor |
| Molecular weight | Higher | Lower |
| Deflasking | Difficult | Easier |
| Polymerization | Heat and pressure | Room temperature |
| Polymerization shrinkage | Slightly more (0.53%) | Less (0.26%) |

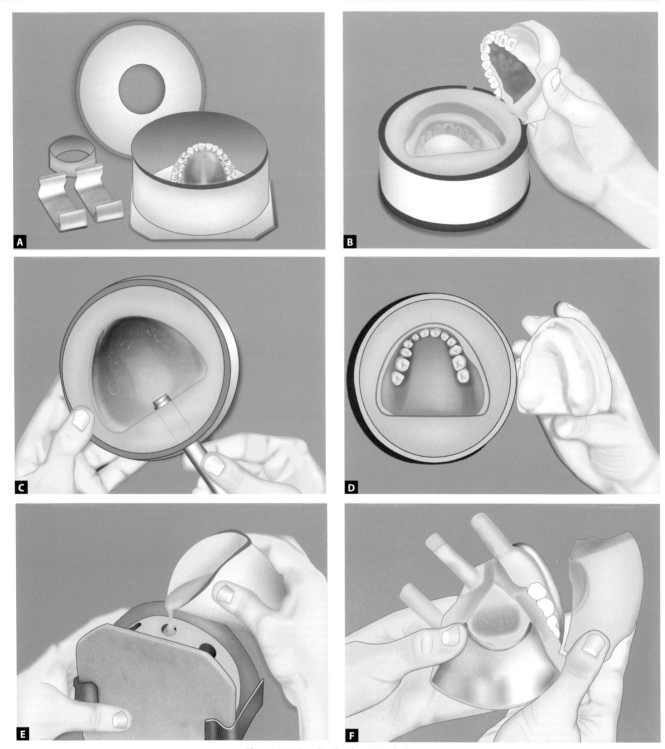

**Figs. 14.14A to F:** Fluid resin technique.

*Advantages:*
- Greater adaptation to underlying soft tissues
- Less chances of damage to the prosthetic teeth
- Reduced cost of material
- Flasking, deflasking and finishing procedures are simplified.

*Disadvantages:*
- Greater chances of displacement of denture teeth during processing
- Air-bubble entrapment
- Bonding between the denture teeth and denture base is poor
- Technique-sensitive procedure.

**CLINICAL SIGNIFICANCE**

When compared with heat-cure resins, pour-type acrylics are characterized by lower impact strength and fatigue strengths, higher creep values, lower transverse bond strength, lower water sorption and higher solubility.

## LIGHT-ACTIVATED DENTURE BASE RESINS

In this type of denture base resins, visible light is used as the activator. These resins are resin-based composites, which are made of urethane dimethacrylate, silica and high-molecular weight resin monomer.

### Supplied As

They are supplied as single component in the form of sheets or ropes, which are packed in lightproof plastic pouches to prevent polymerization **(Fig. 14.15)**.
- *Matrix*: Urethane dimethacrylate (composite)
- *Fillers*: Microfine silica
- High-molecular weight acrylic resin monomers
- Organic fillers—acrylic resin beads
- Initiator for polymerization—camphorquinone 5%
- Activator—visible light.

### Classification of Light-Activated Resins

Based on their uses, light-activated resins can be classified as:
- *Base-forming resin*—this type of resin is adapted to the cast. The cast and denture base assembly is placed into the high-intensity light chamber to induce polymerization
- *Teeth-setting resin*—then teeth setting resin is applied on the base-forming resin to attach teeth. The assembly with teeth is again placed in high-intensity light chamber to polymerize and maintain the teeth in proper position
- *Contouring resin*—lastly contouring resin is applied to get desired contour. The final denture is then placed into the light chamber to complete polymerization. The polymerized denture is retrieved, finished and polished conventionally.

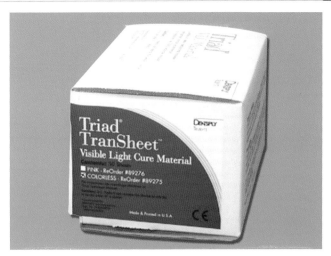

**Fig. 14.15:** Light-polymerized acrylic resins.

### Technical Considerations

For light-activated resins, conventional investing and packing in curing flask are not possible because light cannot penetrate the flask to polymerize.
- After complete wax try-in is done. The trial denture is waxed and carved in the conventional manner
- A roll of light-activated material is taken and is contoured on the occlusal surfaces of the teeth to form a template having three reference areas on the master cast
- The template is cured in the light chamber for 10 minutes
- The waxed denture with master cast and the template are placed in boiling water to eliminate wax completely
- The cleaned master cast is coated with a release agent. A sheet of light-activated resin is adapted on the master cast
- The base is then polymerized in a light chamber
- A strip of light-activated acrylic resin is placed below the teeth after they have been coated with a bonding agent
- Using the template, the teeth are repositioned into original position
- The denture is finally polymerized in the light chamber. The light chamber consists of a rotating table on which the cast assembly (cast with denture) is placed for polymerization. The depth of polymerization depends on the light intensity, angle of illumination and distance of light from the resin
- Polymerized denture is finished and polished in conventional manner.

The light-curing system **(Fig. 14.16)** also comprises of:
- A coating for the denture base material to prevent surface inhibition of polymerization by oxygen
- Arch form teeth in four arch sizes
- A bonding agent to bond the teeth to the base
- The curing unit has four tungsten halogen lamps, which use a wavelength of 400–500 nm.

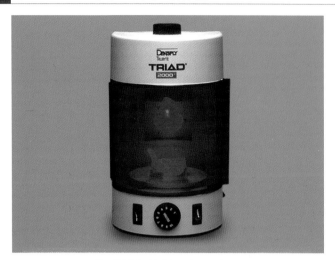

**Fig. 14.16:** Light-curing system.

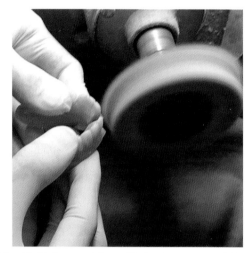

**Fig. 14.17:** Fracture of mandibular denture on polishing.

## Properties

- Transverse strength—80 MPa
- Knoop hardness number—18
- Modulus of elasticity—2.1 GPa
- Impact strength—13 J/m
- Polymerization of light-activated resins takes about 10 minutes
- Rockwell recovery of light-activated resins is about 72% after 10 minutes at 30 kg. The recovery index shows the viscoelasticity of the denture resins. It depends on factors such as effect of plasticizers, free monomers and degree of cross-linking.

## Advantages

- Extended working time
- Reduced porosity
- Light in weight
- Monomer free
- Nontoxic, nonallergenic
- Reduced polymerization shrinkage.

## Disadvantages

- Time consuming
- Technique sensitive
- Curing flask cannot be used.

# GENERAL PROPERTIES OF DENTURE BASE RESINS

## Strength Properties

Conventional heat-cured acrylic resins are commonly used for partial or complete dentures. They are low in strength, brittle on impact and fairly resistant to fatigue failure. The tensile strength varies between 48.3 Mpa and 62.1 Mpa. The compressive strength is 75.9 Mpa. The strength of the resins varies directly in relation to the degree of polymerization of the respective resins. If the degree of polymerization is higher, the strength of the resin will also be higher. Therefore, heat-cured resins have greater strength than the cold-cure resins. Usually, the strength of the heat-processed dentures is adequate unless the thickness of the denture base is thin especially in the midline. If it is thin then there is high chance of midline fracture of the denture. Dentures can also fracture, if too much of force is applied during polishing of the dentures especially the mandibular denture **(Fig. 14.17)**.

## Impact Strength

It is the amount of energy absorbed by a material when it is hit with a sudden blow. The impact strength of polyvinyl acrylic is almost twice than that of polymethacrylate resins. Ideally, a denture bases should have sufficient high-impact strength to prevent breakage on accidental dropping, but not at the expense of other properties. If plasticizers are added, it will increase the impact strength but will reduce the hardness, proportional limit, elastic modulus and compressive strength.

## Hardness and Abrasion Resistance

Resins have low-hardness value, i.e. they can be easily scratched and abraded. Cross-linked PMMA is only slightly harder than regular PMMA. The incorporation of fillers may alter resistance to abrasion but the hardness of plastic matrix remains unchanged.
- *Heat-cure resin*—18–20 KHN
- *Cold-cure resin*—16–8 KHN.

The patient should be advised to clean the dentures using soft-bristle brushes and instructed not to apply too much of force during cleaning.

## Thermal Conductivity

Denture bases have poor thermal conductivity and it is for this reason that patient does not appreciate the hot or cold food as the temperature is not readily transferred to the underlying tissues. This induces artificial feeling in the patient. Another problem is chances of tissue burn when hot food item such as tea or coffee is ingested and the patient does not realize the hotness until it contacts the tissues of the throat.

## Fatigue Strength and Fracture Toughness

During chewing, dentures are subjected to large number of small cyclic stresses. Fatigue strength is the property, which represents number of cycles before failure occurs at a certain stress. There is greater tendency of fracture in the presence of notch, crack or deep scratch on the denture. Therefore, during deflasking, the dentures should not be overstressed.

## Modulus of Elasticity

Acrylic denture bases have adequate rigidity (modulus of elasticity 2,400 Mpa) for use in complete and partial dentures. But, the rigidity of acrylic dentures is low when compared with metal denture bases.

## Polymerization Shrinkage

- There is considerable change in density of the mass from 0.94 g/cm$^3$ to 1.19 g/cm$^3$ when methyl methacrylate monomer is polymerized to PMMA. This difference in density causes volumetric shrinkage of 21%. When prepolymerized PMMA powder particles are mixed with the monomer in ratio of 3:1. The mix after complete polymerization produces volumetric shrinkage of 7%
- Despite of high-volumetric shrinkage still denture base resins produce clinically acceptable dentures. This is because the shrinkage occurs evenly through the surface of the dentures. Therefore, adaptation of the denture bases to the underlying tissues is not affected significantly
- Apart from volumetric shrinkage, linear shrinkage also occur, which effects denture base adaptation and cuspal interdigitation
- Linear shrinkage of cold-cure acrylic is 0.26% as compared to 0.53% for heat-cure acrylic resins. The amount of linear shrinkage is determined by measuring the distance between two predetermined reference points in the second molar regions of the complete tooth arrangement. The distance is measured both before and after compete polymerization. The difference in readings determines the linear shrinkage. The greater value of linear shrinkage suggests greater discrepancy in the initial fit of the denture.

The thermal shrinkage is mainly responsible for linear shrinkage phenomenon in heat-cure resins. The resin is soft during initial stage of cooling and hardens thereafter. As the resin hardens, it contracts at the same rate as the surrounding dental stone.

Change of state from soft rubbery state to hard glassy state occurs during cooling is because the resin approaches the glass transition temperature ($T_g$) to the room temperature. Once the resin is cooled beyond the $T_g$, the resin becomes hard and glassy. During cooling, internal stresses are build up in the denture base because of polymerization. The magnitude of stress buildup depends on the maximum temperature and rate of cooling. Higher temperature will cause greater distortion and internal stress buildup. Therefore, it is important to allow the dentures to cool slowly after curing process. This will allow the residual stresses to relax and will cause less distortion when the denture is removed from the cast. If the residual stresses are not allowed to relax, it will lead to greater amount of distortion leading to poorly fitting denture especially in the palatal area (**Fig. 14.18**).

- Similarly, when custom trays are fabricated, there will be similar type of polymerization shrinkage and contraction stresses. If the custom tray is used immediately after fabrication, it will show greater amount of distortion and will not fit properly in the patient's mouth. Moreover, if impression is made using such tray, it will lead inaccurate replication of the tissues as the tray is dimensionally unstable. It is therefore advised to fabricate the custom trays 1 day before the impression procedure.

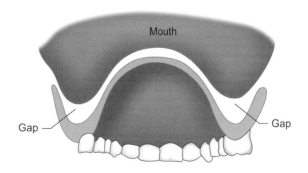

**Fig. 14.18:** Poorly fitting upper denture.

Following the above discussion, complete dentures processed with cold-cure acrylic resins display better adaptation than those processed with heat-cure resins. Since, thermal shrinkage is negligible in cold-cure resins adaptation is better. However, other factors such as type of investment material, temperature and method of resin introduction are responsible for dimensional accuracy of the denture.

- Dentures processed with heat-cure or cold-cure resins using compression-molding techniques display minimal increase in overall vertical dimension of the dentures in comparison to those processed with fluid resin techniques, which result in reduced vertical dimension **(Table 14.2)**.

## Porosity

Porosities in the dentures can give it an unesthetic appearance, can weaken the denture base and can interfere in maintaining proper denture hygiene. It is usually observed that porosity develops in the thicker portion of the denture base. The reason for this is due to evaporation of the unreacted monomer when the temperature of the resin goes beyond the boiling point of the resin. But, it is not necessary that same type of porosity will occurs throughout the denture base. Porosities can be localized or generalized throughout the denture base. Different type of porosity can occurs at different location in the same denture base. Generally, porosities can be avoided by proper manipulation of the monomer and polymer following manufacturer's instructions and proper temperature control during polymerization.

### Classification of Porosity

*Based on the location:*
- Internal porosity
- External porosity.

*Based on the causes:*
- Gaseous
- Granular
- Air inclusion
- Contraction.

**Table 14.2:** Polymerization shrinkage with different denture base resins.

| Material | Linear shrinkage (%) |
|---|---|
| High-impact resins | 0.12 |
| Vinyl resins | 0.33 |
| Conventional heat-cure resins | 0.43 |
| Pour-type resin | 0.48 |
| Rapid heat-cure acrylic resin | 0.97 |

### Internal Porosity

*Gaseous Porosity*

Appearance is in the form of void or bubbles within the mass of polymerized acrylic. It is usually not present on the surface of the denture.
- *Location:* It is confined to thicker portion of the denture
- *Causes:* Vaporization of unreacted monomers and low-molecular weight polymers
- *Remedy:* It can be avoided by using long- and low-temperature curing cycle.

### External Porosity

*Causes*
- Lack of homogeneity
- Lack of adequate pressure
- Air inclusion porosity.

*Lack of homogeneity or granular porosity:* If the dough is not homogeneous at the time of polymerization the portion containing more monomer will shrink more than the adjacent areas. This localized shrinking results in void. The resin appears white. It can be avoided by using proper powder liquid ratio and mixing it well. The mix is more homogeneous in dough stage therefore packing should be done in dough stage only.

*Lack of adequate pressure or contraction porosity:* This type of porosity is caused due to lack of adequate pressure or lack of adequate dough in the mold during the polymerization process. Voids occurring due to this reason are not spherical but are of irregular shapes. The resultant resin appears lighter and more opaque because of these voids.

*Air inclusion porosity:* Another type of porosity is most often associated with fluid resins. Such porosities appear to be caused by air inclusion incorporated during mixing and pouring procedures. If these inclusions are not removed, sizable voids may be produced in the resultant denture base. Careful mixing, spruing and venting are advised to reduce the incidence of air inclusion.

## Water Absorption

Resins and other organic denture base materials vary considerably in the amount of water they take up when immersed in water. The absorption of water affects their mechanical properties and dimension. The process of absorption is aided by diffusion mechanism. Here, the water molecules penetrate the PMMA mass and occupy the positions between the polymer chains. Absorption of water molecules in the polymerized mass behaves as plasticizers, which interfere with the entanglement of polymer chains and secondly causes slight expansion of the polymerized mass. The changes of this are relatively minor and do not exert any significant effect on fit or function of the processed bases. Laboratory reports suggest that for every 1% increase in weight due to water absorption leads to 0.23% of linear expansion in the resin. The linear expansion due to water absorption is almost equal to the thermal shrinkage, which occurs during the polymerization process.

The diffusion coefficient of water in heat-activated denture resins is $0.011 \times 10^{-6}$ cm$^2$/second at 37°C and for chemically activated resin, it is $0.023 \times 10^{-6}$ cm$^2$/second.

## Solubility

The acrylic resins are virtually insoluble in fluids commonly come in contact with the oral tissues. However, they are soluble in ketones, esters and aromatic chlorinated hydrocarbons. Alcohol causes crazing in some resins. A small amount of monomer may be leached out when stored in water. The solubility of resins is low. The degree of solubility did not seem to affect the clinical performance of dentures.

## Processing Stresses

During processing of denture base resins, stresses are incorporated in the resin. The release of these stresses produces dimensional changes, which are cumulative in nature. Although the dimensional changes are very small. The total dimensional changes as a result of processing and water sorption are in the range of 0.1–0.2 mm.

## Crazing

*Crazing* is the phenomenon of forming flaws or microcracks on the surface of the denture because of stress relaxation, which can adversely affect the esthetic and physical properties of the denture.

### Mechanism

Tensile stresses are mainly responsible for crazing in denture base resins. It is produced by mechanical separation of the individual polymer chains that occurs on the application of the tensile stresses. Crazing occurs at the surface of the resins and is oriented at right angles to the tensile forces.

### Appearance

In transparent resins, crazing imparts foggy or hazy appearance; whereas in tinted resin, it gives a whitish appearance **(Figs 14.19A and B)**.

### Causes

- Can occur when dentures are frequently subjected to complete drying and then placing in water for water sorption
- Prolonged exposure to alcohol
- Can occur at the cervical portion of porcelain teeth because of difference in thermal expansion between porcelain and acrylic resins
- Prolonged contact with denture cleansers containing chlorine
- During denture repair when monomer comes in contact with the cured resin.

### Remedy

- Crazing can be reduced by using cross-linked denture base resins and cross-linked teeth
- Avoid using porcelain teeth.

## Creep

Denture base resins show viscoelastic behavior, i.e. these materials behave as rubbery solids, which can recover elastic deformation over time provided the induced stresses are removed. If these stresses are not removed, additional plastic deformation may occur, which is called creep. The

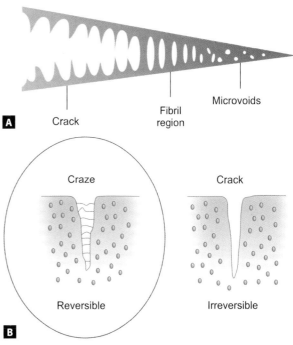

**Figs. 14.19A and B:** Crazing in acrylic resins.

rate at which this deformation takes place is called as creep rate. This rate can be elevated by increasing in temperature, applied load, residual monomer and presence of plasticizer. At low stresses, the creep rate for both heat-cure and cold-cure resins are similar, but as the stresses increase creep rate increases rapidly for cold-cure resins.

## BIOCOMPATIBILITY

- The monomer used in acrylic resins has potential-irritating effect and can cause allergic reaction. The presence of unreacted residual monomer after polymerization can cause allergic reaction in sensitive patients. It can be prevented by storing the dentures in water for a day, so that the residual monomer can leach out
- Dental technicians and other personnel should manipulate monomer in well-ventilated room, so as to minimize inhalation of monomer vapors. Continuous inhalation of vapor can cause mild headache.

### CLINICAL SIGNIFICANCE

Acrylic dentures are also site for growth of microorganisms. It can cause staining, discoloration of dentures as well as irritation of the oral tissues. One of the most common microbial growths is due to *Candida albicans*. These growth can be prevented by maintaining good oral hygiene practice, regularly cleaning the dentures and by soaking dentures in nystatin solution or in chlorhexidine.

## REPAIR OF RESINS

According to ADA specification no. 13, fractured segments of dentures can be repaired by using heat-cure, cold-cure or light-cured resins. The fractured segments are first realigned and joined by means of an adhesive or sticky wax. Petrolatum jelly is applied on the impression surface of denture. Thin mixture of dental stone is poured into the impression surface to get the repair cast. Once the stone sets, the broken denture segments are removed. Cold mold seal is applied onto the repair cast and the broken segments are repositioned on the cast. Fractured segments are roughened and retentive slots are prepared to provide space for the repair resins. Fractured segments are approximated and repositioned on the repair cast. Appropriate resin is selected and used to repair the fractured dentures. Usually, cold-cure resins are preferred as they polymerize as room temperature **(Fig. 14.20)**. Heat-cured resins and light-cured resins require water bath and light chamber for polymerization. Moreover, heat produced by water bath and light chamber causes stress release and can cause distortion of original fracture segments of the denture.

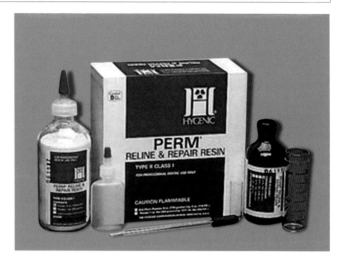
**Fig. 14.20:** Repair resins.

When using cold cure resins to repair denture. Small amount of monomer is painted on the fractured edges on the denture to soften the old resin, which will also help in better bonding with the repair resin. Small quantity of polymer and monomer is added in the space between the fractured segments in increments. After completely filling the space, some extra repair resin is added in order to compensate for the polymerization shrinkage.

Factors influencing selection of repair resins:
- Time needed for repair
- Strength of repair material
- Dimensional accuracy of repair.

## RELINING AND REBASING DENTURE BASES

Relining is the process of replacing the tissue surface of an existing denture whereas rebasing is the process of complete replacement of the denture base.

In both the procedures, the existing denture is used as the impression tray to obtain impression of the soft tissues. A stone cast is poured and then the entire assembly is invested in a denture flask. Subsequently, the denture flask is opened, the impression material is removed. The impression surface is cleaned to improve the bond between the reline material and original denture base. Then separating medium is applied on the gypsum mold. Thereafter, relining resin of choice is mixed following manufacturer's instructions and introduced into the empty mold created after removal of impression material. The flask is closed and polymerized following compression-molding technique. In relining procedure, the reline resin is subjected to low-polymerization temperature in order to minimize distortion of the original denture base. Cold-cure resins can be used as it polymerizes preferred, since it polymerizes at room temperature and minimizes distortion of the remaining denture base. After completion of the polymerization procedure, the relined dentures are retrieved, finished and polished. The finished dentures are finally placed intraorally and checked for fit and accuracy. Drawbacks of these resins are that they have tendency to discolor, can separate from the original denture base or can harbor microorganisms especially fungi.

Certain cold-cure resins are available, which can be used intraorally directly for relining purposes. But, most of these resins evolve enough heat to cause injury to the oral tissues. Apart from cold-cure resins, heat- and light-activated resins or activated through microwave energy can be used. But, these resins generate significant heat, which is capable of distorting the original denture base.

### Rebasing Resin Dentures

The procedure for rebasing of dentures is similar to the relining procedure. Impression is made by using the existing denture as the custom tray. This impression is poured to get a stone cast. The assembly of cast and denture is mounted on an appropriate instrument, which correctly maintains the vertical and horizontal relationship between the stone cast and the denture teeth. The resultant assembly provides indices for the occlusal surfaces of the denture teeth. The denture is removed and the entire base is removed and each tooth is repositioned into these indices. The original cast is waxed and contoured to the desired form. The completed tooth arrangement is sealed to the cast and the assembly is invested in a denture flask. The packing and curing and finishing of the denture are done conventionally.

## SOFT LINING MATERIALS

*A soft (resilient) lining material is defined as a soft-elastic and -resilient material forming all or part of the fitting (impression) surface of a denture.* It usually acts as a cushion between the hard denture base and tissues to reduce the masticatory forces transmitted by prosthesis to underlying tissues. Because of soft tissue contour changes, during service, it is sometimes necessary to alter tissue surface of prostheses to ensure proper fit and function. In some instances, it may be achieved by selective grinding procedure. In other instances, tissue surface may be replaced by relining or rebasing existing dentures.

- The earliest soft lining material recorded (soft rubber) was used by *Twitchell* in 1869. In 1940, a soft natural rubber known as *"velum"* was used with vulcanite. However, this material had high-water absorption, and it became foul and ill-fitting after a period of time.
- Silicone rubber materials based on polydimethylsiloxane (PDM) have been used as soft liners since 1958.

### Classification of Soft Lining Material

*Based on duration of use:*
- Short-term soft denture liner
- Long-term soft denture liner

*Based on techniques:*
- Direct technique (chairside technique)
- Indirect technique (laboratory procedure)

Materials used for direct technique are chemical cure, light-cure and tissue conditioners.

Materials used for indirect technique are heat-cure acrylic and heat-cure silicone.

Soft lining materials **(Fig. 14.21)** can also be classified as:
- Heat-polymerized acrylic resin
- Autopolymerized acrylic resin
- Heat-polymerized silicone
- Autopolymerized silicone
- Treatment liners (tissue conditioners).

### Ideal Properties of Soft Liners

For maximum efficiency, soft lining materials should exhibit the following properties:
- Should be easily processed using conventional laboratory equipment
- Should exhibit minimal dimensional changes during processing and such changes should be same as that of denture base materials
- Water absorption should be minimal. Ideally, water absorption should be close to that of the acrylic resin denture base polymers
- Should have minimal solubility in saliva. Ideally, the plasticizer should not leach out with time; however, if leaching occurs, it should be minimal

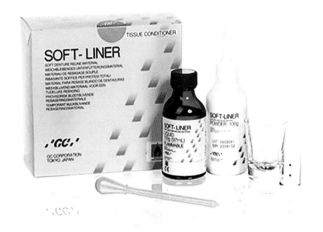

**Fig. 14.21:** Soft relining material.

- Should retain their resiliency
- Should bond sufficiently well to PMMA to avoid separation during use
- Should have adequate tear strength to resist rupture during normal use. This is because the propagation of small crack at the periphery of soft lining could lead to failure and detachment of the material
- Should be easily cleaned and not affected by food, drink or tobacco
- Should be nontoxic odorless and tasteless to encourage long-term wear by the patient
- Should be esthetically acceptable and their color should match that of the denture base material.

*Rationale:* To absorb some of the energy produced by masticatory impact. Hence, a soft liner serves as a "shock absorber" between the occlusal surface of denture and underlying oral tissue.

## Types of Resilient Liners

### Chemically-activated Liners

Supplied as powder form and are subsequently mixed with liquids containing 60–80% of plasticizers. They generally have PMMA or polyethyl methacrylate as principle structural component. The plasticizer used is large molecule such as dibutyl phthalate, which reduces entanglement of polymers and allows the individual chains to "slip" over one another. This slippage movement permits cushioning effect on the underlying tissues. It is important to note that the liquid used here does not contain acrylic monomer. According to their durability and duration of use, these reliners are called as short-term soft liners or tissue conditioners.

### Heat-activated Liners

This type of liners is more durable and lasts for longer period of time. Although, they also degrade over time and cannot be considered permanent.

- Heat-activated soft liners are supplied as powder-liquid systems. The powder contains polymers and copolymers and the liquid contains monomers and plasticizers
- When mixed these materials form pliable resins exhibiting (glass transition temperature) $T_g$ below mouth temperature
- Although plasticizers impart flexibility they also present certain difficulties. Plasticizers have tendency to leach out making the soft liners more rigid
- As PMMA is replaced by higher methacrylates (ethyl, n-propyl, n-butyl) the $T_g$ becomes progressively lower. As

a result, less plasticizer is required and effect of leaching can be minimized.

### Silicone Rubber

These are highly successful soft liner material. They do not possess leachable plasticizers and therefore retain their elastic properties for a longer period of time. But, their drawback is that they lose adhesion to underlying denture bases over period of time.

## Classification of Silicone Rubber

*Types of silicone rubber:*
- *Chemically activated*—supplied as two component system
- *Heat-activated*—supplied as single component system in the form of gel or paste.

### Technique

Using of chemically and heat-activated silicone is similar. First impression surface of the denture base is trimmed. Adhesive is applied on the trimmed surface to facilitate bonding of the resins. The resilient liner is mixed according to the manufacturer's instructions and is applied on the denture base and is compression molded. After polymerization, the dentures are retrieved and is finished and polished.

### Limitations in Use of Soft Liners

- *Reduction in denture base strength*: The replacement of part of the denture base with a soft lining material reduces the overall strength of the denture and inevitably increases its tendency to fracture
- *Loss of softness and resiliency*: Soft liners with plasticizers integrated tend to leach out and cause the lining to harden, limiting its usefulness
- *Colonization of Candida albicans*: Porosity of soft lining material allows water absorption and the diffusion of nutrients, which permit mycotic growth especially *Candida albicans*
- *Difficulty in keeping soft lining clean using normal denture cleaning methods*: The use of conventional denture cleaners may cause bleaching, and surface may become bubbled, if an oxygenating cleaner is used. It has been reported that hypochlorite cleansers should be employed in daily maintenance of these liners to prevent microbial colonization
- *Dimensional instability*: Some soft liners lose their plasticity with time, which may cause dimensional changes

- *Failure of adhesion*: A common problem of soft-lined dentures is the failure of adhesion between the soft lining and denture base
- *Difficulty in finishing and polishing*: Soft lining materials are difficult to trim, finish and polish. If excess force is used, they may over heat or tear, leading to poor surface finish.

## RESIN IMPRESSION TRAYS AND TRAY MATERIALS

Tray made of resin to make impression is called as custom trays. Custom trays are fabricated on the primary cast. An appropriate spacer is adapted on the cast to provide adequate relief. Thereafter, separating media is painted on the cast. A resin dough (most often cold-cure acrylic resin), if formed by mixing polymer and monomer in proper ratio. The dough is adapted onto the cast and allowed to polymerize. The dough is rolled into sheet of thickness 2 mm, which is adapted onto the cast. Tray handle is added to permit removal of tray from the patient's mouth. After completion of polymerization, the custom trays are finished and polished.

Resin impression trays undergo significant dimensional changes in first 24 hours following fabrication and therefore its use should be avoided. At the end of this prescribed period, the fit of the tray is evaluated intraorally and necessary modifications are made. Subsequently, spacer is removed and master impressions are made using appropriate impression material. Both chemically activated resins and light-activated resins are used for fabricating custom trays. Chemically activated resins can cause contact dermatitis to the personnel handling them **(Figs. 14.22A and B)**.

Recently, another material, which has been used for tray fabrication is the *light-activated urethane dimethacrylate.* This type of resin material is supplied in the form of sheet and gel. Sheet form is more preferred for custom tray fabrication. Procedure is similar, which is described above except for polymerization the cast along with the tray is placed in specialized light chamber for a specified time. After polymerization, the trays are finished and polished as required to remove sharp edges, which may injure the oral mucosa. Custom trays fabricated using urethane dimethacrylate resins are more dimensionally stable. However, their drawback is that the tray produced is brittle and produces fine particles during grinding procedure. These resins are also more expensive and require high-intensity light for polymerization.

## DENTURE CLEANSERS

There are various types of agents available to clean artificial dentures. Some of these agents are dentifrices, denture

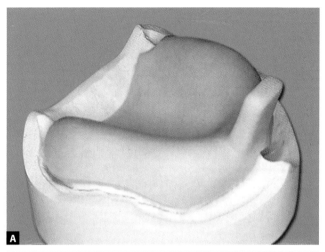

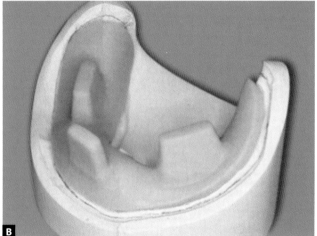

**Figs. 14.22A and B:** Types of impression trays.

cleansers, mild detergents, household cleansers, vinegar and bleaches. These agents can be used by immersing the dentures in them or by brushing. The most commonly used commercial cleansers are based upon or require immersion techniques. These cleansers are marketed in powder and liquid form.

### Immersion Denture Cleansers

#### Composition

- Alkaline compounds
- Detergents
- Sodium perborate
- Flavoring agents.

#### Mode of Action

When these agents are dissolved in water, sodium perborate decomposes to form an alkaline peroxide solution. This peroxide subsequently releases oxygen that loses debris through mechanical means.

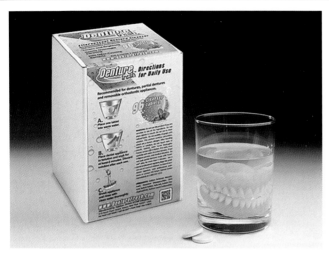

**Fig. 14.23:** Denture cleansers.

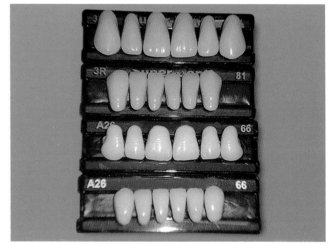

**Fig. 14.24:** Acrylic denture teeth.

## Household Bleaches

Household bleaches (hypochlorites) can also be used in dilution for denture cleaning. Concentrated solutions should be avoided as they may affect denture coloration. The use of bleaches should be avoided as they have tendency to discolor dentures especially those which are relined with silicones. The metal prosthesis in particular should not be cleaned with bleaches as they are capable of producing significant blackening of the metal denture base.

Patient should be educated on the use of denture cleansers at the time of denture insertion. Tooth brushing with dentifrices, mild detergents or soaps can be used for effective cleaning of the dentures **(Fig. 14.23)**. Tooth brushing has mild effect on the resin surface of the denture. Use of mild detergents and soaps with brushes has been found to be nondestructive to the denture surface. Household cleansers such as kitchen abrasives are contraindicated for cleaning dentures. Prolonged use of such hard abrasives will wear out the resin tooth and denture surface and significantly affect the esthetic and function of the denture.

## RESIN TEETH FOR PROSTHETIC APPLICATIONS

According to ADA specification no. 15. Resin teeth are mostly made of PMMA resins. The resins used for teeth production are somewhat similar to that used for denture base except that they have more cross-linking agents. Greater use of the cross-linking agents displays increased stability and improves the clinical properties. To permit greater chemical bonding between teeth and denture base, cross-linking is reduced at the cervical portion of the teeth. Retention can be further enhanced by grinding the ridge lap area of the resin tooth to create roughness. Failures can occur between bonding of teeth and denture base, if the ridge lap area of the teeth is contaminated with wax or separating media.

### CLINICAL SIGNIFICANCE

It should be ensured that during wax elimination process with boiling water, all the residual wax is removed and the exposed cervical portion of teeth is cleaned. For better bonding the cervical portion should be wet with monomer just before the mixed resin dough is placed in contact for packing.

Resin teeth are insoluble in oral fluids but are soluble in certain ketones and aromatic hydrocarbons. The mechanical properties of resin teeth are compressive strength (76 MPa), abrasion resistance, elastic modules (2,700 MPa), elastic limit (55 MPa) and hardness (18–20 kg/mm$^2$) are low when compared with other restorative materials or with human enamel and dentin **(Fig. 14.24)**.

To further improve the wear resistance of the prosthetic teeth, hybrid teeth are introduced. This type of teeth contains both composite resins and PMMA. Composite resins component is mainly concentrated at the occlusal and incisal surfaces of the prosthetic teeth to improve wear resistance. However, the chemical bond between the composite resins and the PMMA is inferior in comparison to the cross-linked teeth. To overcome this issue of bonding, the ridge lap area and the lingual surface of the hybrid teeth are made of PMMA.

## RESINS AS MAXILLOFACIAL MATERIALS

Maxillofacial materials are used to correct facial defects resulting from cancer surgery, accidents or even congenital deformities. Nose, ears, eyes and orbits or any other part of head and neck may be replaced by this prosthesis.

## Historical Background

- *Before 1600 AD:* Egyptians and Chinese used natural waxes, resins and metals to fabricate auricular, nasal and ocular prosthesis
- *1600s AD: Ambroise Pare* first described fabricated obturator consisting of a simple disk attached to sponge
- *1855: Charles Goodyear* first developed vulcanite rubber and used in velar design
- *1894: Tetamore* fabricated a nasal prosthesis using light-weight cellulose nitrate
- *1905: Ottofy, Baird* and *Baker* used black vulcanized rubber to fabricate maxillofacial prosthesis
- *1937:* Acrylic resins were first introduced and replaced vulcanite rubber
- *1942: AH Bulbulian* introduced the use of prevulcanized latex in facial prosthesis
- *1965: Barnhart* first used silicone rubber for constructing and coloring facial prosthesis
- *1975: Koran* and *Craig* investigated the properties of silicone elastomers, PVC and polyurethane
- *1982: Udagama* and *Drane* first introduced the new silicone elastomer (medical adhesive type A or Dow Corning A-891)
- *1990: Gonzalez* described the use of polyurethane elastomers
- *1990s:* Rapid prototyping technique used in maxillofacial prosthodontics
- *2008:* 3D printing used to bioprint maxillofacial prosthesis.

### Classification of Maxillofacial Materials

*Based on usage of maxillofacial materials:*
- *Impression materials:*
  - Irreversible hydrocolloids
  - Impression compounds
  - Impression plaster
  - Condensation and addition silicones
  - Impression waxes
  - Impression pastes.
- *Moldable and sculpting materials:*
  - Plaster
  - Waxes
  - Modeling clay
  - Plastolene.

- *Definitive materials:*
  - Acrylic resins
  - Acrylic copolymers
  - Vinyl polymers and copolymers
  - Polyurethane elastomers
  - Silicone elastomers—heat temperature vulcanizing (HTV) and room temperature vulcanizing (RTV)
  - Metal implants.

## Ideal Requirements

- Should be biocompatible
- Should be easy to fabricate
- Should have good esthetic property, i.e. should simulate the color, texture, form and translucency of the adjacent natural skin
- Should be easily moldable
- Should have adequate working time
- Should be easily duplicated
- Should be soft, flexible, resilient and simulate feeling of real flesh
- Should be dimensionally stable
- Should be light in weight
- Should be easily cleaned without damage or deterioration
- Should have sufficient edge strength even in thin margins
- Should have low-thermal conductivity
- Should be durable and resistant to stains
- Should be stable when exposed to UV light, oxygen or adhesive solvent.

Various materials which are used to fabricate definitive prosthesis are:

## Acrylic Resins

They were used commonly to fabricate maxillofacial prosthesis. They are usually derivatives of ethylene and contain a vinyl group in their structural formula. Heat polymerization is preferred to autopolymerization resins because of color stability and because of the presence of free-toxic tertiary amines.

### Uses

- Used in fabrication of intraoral and extraoral prosthesis
- Used in cases where there is little movement of the tissue bed during the function
- Used as core for silicone facial prosthesis.

### Properties

- Curing of resins can be initiated by UV light or heat or by chemical activation
- It is soluble in organic solvents such as chloroform and acetone
- Water absorption of 0.3% is observed after 24 hours
- It is a hard resin with KHN varying between 18 and 20
- Modulus of elasticity is 350,000 pounds per square inch
- Tensile strength is 8,500 pounds per square inch.

### Advantages

- Can be relined and repaired
- Are color stable
- More durable
- Are compatible with most adhesive system and can be easily cleaned
- Easy to manipulate
- Because of its superior strength, it can be used in thin margins
- Capable of intrinsic and extrinsic coloration
- Compatible with most adhesive system.

### Disadvantages

- Greater rigidity
- Duplication of prosthesis is not possible because of mold destruction during processing
- Due to water sorption the weight increases by 0.5% after 1 week
- Use doubtful at the movable tissue bed
- Relatively high-thermal conductivity
- Crazing is occasionally observed.

### Acrylic Copolymers

These are acrylic copolymers, which are formulated with a foaming agent. These materials are soft and elastic but are not used because of poor-edge strength, poor durability, degradation on sunlight exposure and chances of discoloration. With heat or an initiating chemical the foaming agent releases gas that is incorporated in the material as it polymerizes. The resulting prosthesis is spongy having a solid skin, e.g. Palamed, Polyderm.

### Disadvantages

Tacky surface predisposes to dust collection and staining. The deposited dust particles are especially cleaned with *benzene.*

### Latex

Latex is a soft and inexpensive material, which can be used to create lifelike maxillofacial prosthesis. These materials are weak, which degenerate rapidly and show color instability. Although they are not used to fabricate long-term maxillofacial prosthesis. Recently, synthetic latex is used, which is a terpolymer of butyl acrylate, methyl methacrylate and methyl methacrylamide. Colorant can be applied on the tissue side to provide increased translucency. They also cannot be used for long-term prosthesis and therefore have limited application.

### Vinyl Polymers and Copolymers

Vinyl polymers were introduced as plastisols in 1940s. They are composed of PVC and plasticizers. PVC is a clear hard resin, which is odorless and tasteless. Copolymers of vinyl chloride and vinyl acetate have greater flexibility but are chemically less resistant than polymethyl chloride. They darken when exposed to UV light and heat. Therefore, they require heat and light stabilization to prevent discoloration during fabrication and use. Polyvinyl acetate is stable to light and heat but is having abnormally low-softening point. Likewise, realistic (PVC compound) solidifies into a flexible material when heated, e.g. realistic, mediplast.

### Advantages

- Easy to handle
- Flexible and provides acceptable initial appearance
- Both intrinsic and extrinsic staining can be done
- Available in wide variety of colors to match patient's skin tone.

### Disadvantages

- Leaching of plasticizer results in discoloration and hardening of the prosthesis
- Can be easily stained, if exposed to UV light, peroxides and ozone
- Lack lifelike translucency and tends to absorb sebaceous secretions, cosmetics and solvent
- Thin edges tear easily
- Require metal molds because they polymerize at high temperature.

### Silicone Elastomers (**Figs. 14.25 A to C**)

Silicones are long-chain molecules, which were introduced in 1946 and are one of the most widely used materials for fabricating facial prosthesis. These polymers are translucent,

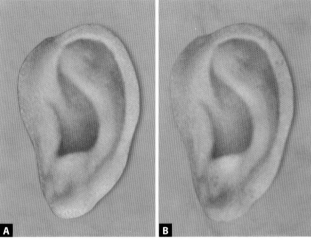

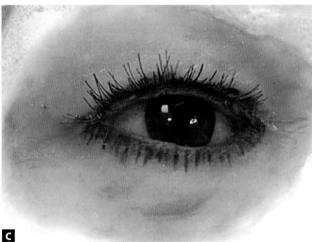

**Figs. 14.25A to C:** Silicone elastomers used in maxillofacial prosthodontics

white-color fluids whose viscosity is dependent on the length of the polymer chain. Additives are added to give color to the prosthesis and filler are added to provide strength. Antioxidants and vulcanizing agent are used to convert the raw mass from plastic to rubbery resin during curing. Cross-linking of the polymers is called as *Vulcanization*. It may or may not require heat to vulcanize and is dependent on the catalyst or the cross-linking agent.

### Classification of Silicone Elastomers

*Based on the method of vulcanization:*
- Room temperature vulcanization silicones (RTV)
- Heat-temperature vulcanizing silicones (HTV).

### Room Temperature Vulcanization Silicones

They are composed of comparatively short-chain silicone polymers, which are partially end blocked with hydroxyl groups. They are supplied as single component system,

which vulcanizes by evaporation of acetic acid at room temperature. They are composed of diatomaceous earth particles (fillers), stannous octoate (catalyst) and ortho-alkyl silicate (cross-linking agent). They give natural flesh like appearance by blending suitable earth pigments with the silicone, e.g. Silastic 382, 399; Silastic 386.

*Advantages*
- These are color stable
- These are biologically inert
- Ease of handling and processing
- Retain physical and chemical properties at wide range of temperatures

*Disadvantages*
- These have poor edge strength
- These are costly
- Poor tear strength
- These are rigid
- Poor wettability.

### Heat-temperature Vulcanizing Silicones

These silicones are composed of dichlorobenzoic acid, platinum salts, finely divided silica (filler) and benzoyl peroxide (vulcanizing agent). The amount of filler particle added can be altered depending on the requirement of strength, hardness and elongation. The solid HTV elastomers can undergo more intense mechanical milling than the soft putty RTV silicone. They are supplied as putty-like consistency materials, which require milling, packing in two or three parts mold at temperature of 180°C for half an hour under pressure, e.g. MDX-4-4210, SE-4524U.

*Advantages*
- Excellent thermal stability
- These are color stable
- Biologically inert
- Superior strength
- Good tear strength.

*Disadvantages*
- Lack elasticity
- Low-edge strength
- Opaque and life less appearance
- Metal molds are required
- Require milling machine and press
- Time-consuming fabrication process.

### Extrinsic and Intrinsic Coloration

Coloration of the maxillofacial prosthesis is important to simulate the natural appearance of the adjacent tissues. Good matching of prosthesis to the natural tissues enhances patient satisfaction and acceptability. The maxillofacial prosthesis can be colored or stained in three ways:

1. Intrinsic coloration
2. Extrinsic coloration
3. Combination of both intrinsic and extrinsic coloration.

*Intrinsic coloration:* Metallic oxide pigments or dry earth pigments are commonly used to provide color to the prosthesis like giving more natural skin tone or simulating blood vessels. These pigments are mixed with silicones during processing to provide the effect.

*Extrinsic coloration:* These pigments are applied externally on the maxillofacial prosthesis to provide the lifelike appearance. The pigments are either sprayed or applied carefully to enhance the effect. Color stabilizers are used to stabilize the color on the prosthesis because there is high chance of discoloration on regular use of the prosthesis.

### Adhesives

These components are applied on the external surface of the maxillofacial prosthesis to bond it with the adjacent natural tissues. Dow Corning 355 is the most commonly used adhesive to provide strong bond with the skin. This adhesive is easy to remove from the skin but difficult from the silicone. Other retentive aids, which are commonly used in maxillofacial prosthesis are double-sided tapes, Velcro, Pros-Aide adhesive, etc.

## TEMPORARY RESINS

These are used to provide temporary coverage following tooth preparation. These are cemented in place with temporary cements. Chemically activated resins have become popular as provisional restorations. They have reduced the use of polycarbonate crowns and aluminum shell because they are easy to fabricate and provide adequate esthetic. They are available in various shades to approximate color of patient's teeth **(Fig. 14.26)**.

### Basic Requirements of Provisional Restorations

- Should protect the pulp
- Should have adequate marginal seal
- Should maintain positional stability
- Should enhance patient comfort, esthetics and phonetics
- Should restore masticatory function
- Should promote periodontal health
- Should distort minimally
- Should have adequate strength
- Should have adequate retention
- Should have radiopacity
- Easy to manipulate

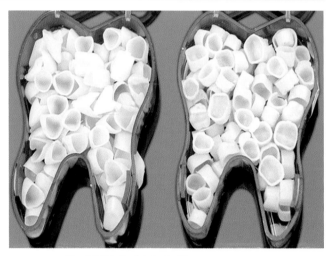

**Fig. 14.26:** Prefabricated temporary crowns.

- Easy to trim and adjust
- Have color stability.

### Disadvantages of Resins Used as Temporary Crown and Bridge Material

- Heat generated during polymerization is harmful to the teeth
- Marginal opening can be caused by polymerization shrinkage
- Allergic reaction seen may be due to monomer component.

## OCCLUSAL SPLINTS

Occlusal splints are used in the treatment of patients with temporomandibular joint pain or excessive bruxism. The splint is waxed on a model of the patient's teeth, usually the maxilla. The model and wax pattern are invested in a denture flask and the wax is boiled out. After cooling, separating media is painted on the mold and allowed to dry. A clear heat-accelerated (activated) acrylic resin is packed into the mold and processed. Chemically activated acrylic resin is also used but less often. The properties of acrylic splints are similar to those of heat-activated acrylic materials **(Fig. 14. 27)**.

## INLAY PATTERNS

Chemically accelerated acrylic is used to fabricate inlay patterns and post and cores by direct method. These materials are brightly pigmented and having good dimensional stability. The pattern is made by painting the

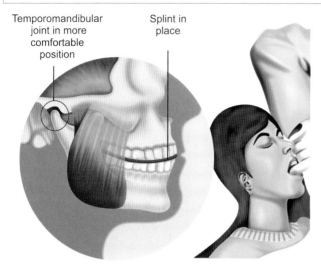

Temporomandibular joint in more comfortable position

Splint in place

**Fig. 14.27:** Occlusal splints placed in mouth.

powder-liquid onto the die or tooth in layers and allowing it to polymerized. After polymerization, the pattern can be modified with stones and burs. If required inlay wax may be added to complete the patterns. For burnout procedure, longer time is needed for complete burnout.

## RESINOUS DIE MATERIAL

Resin materials have been used as die materials for number of years. The commonly used resin die materials are:
- Epoxy resin
- Resin-modified gypsum
- Polyvinyl siloxane die material.

### Epoxy Resin

This type of resin contains epoxy resin and a hardener. Both the components when mixed are poured into the impression to obtain die.

### Advantages

- Good abrasion resistance
- Less brittle.

### Disadvantages

- Polymerization shrinkage is more
- Cannot be poured in hydrocolloid impression.

### Resin-modified Gypsum

This type of die material is a combination of resin and gypsum. They result in more dimensionally accurate dies. They have adequate abrasion resistance.

### Polyvinyl Siloxane Die Material

It is a flexible elastomeric die material having composition similar to polyvinyl siloxane impression material.

### Advantage

Does not break while removing from impression.

### Disadvantages

- Requires a separator when used with polyvinyl siloxane impression material
- Use of separator may result in inaccuracy.

## POLYMERS USED AS IMPLANTS

Polymeric implants in the form of PMMA and polytetrafluoroethylene were first used in 1930s. The low-mechanical strength of the polymers has precluded their use as implant materials because of their susceptibility for mechanical fracture during function. Also, the physical properties of the polymers are greatly influenced by changes in temperature, environment and composition and their sterilization can be accomplished only by gamma irradiation or exposure to ethylene oxide gas. Contamination of these polymers is another disadvantage, because electrostatic charges often attract dust and other impurities from the environment.

The use of polymers for osseointegrated implants is now confined to components. The intramobile zirconia (IMZ) implants are either titanium plasma sprayed or HA-coated (hydroxyapatite) and incorporate a polyoxymethylene (POM) intramobile element (IME). The IME is placed between prosthesis and implant body to initiate mobility, stress relief and shock absorption capability to mimic that of natural tooth. When incorporated into the IMZ implant, the IME initiates the biomechanical function of the natural tooth unit, periodontal ligament and alveolar bone **(Fig. 14.28)**.

The IME is designed to ensure a more uniform stress distribution along the implant interface. Studies have demonstrated that the shock-absorbing element also helps in reducing occlusal load.

## ALLERGIC REACTIONS

Some components of acrylic resins produce allergic reactions in the patient. Residual monomer is the most common irritant, which can cause allergic reaction. Although in a properly processed denture, the amount of residual monomer is less than 1%. It has been validated if the denture is left in water for 17 hours, surface monomer is completely eliminated.

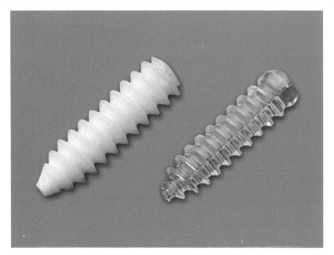

**Fig. 14.28:** Polymers used in implants.

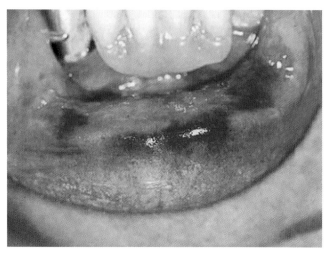

**Fig. 14.29:** Contact dermatitis due to acrylic denture.

Contact dermatitis has been reported in cases with prolonged and repeated contact with monomer. This condition is most commonly found in technicians manipulating acrylic resins. During manipulation, the personnel should use gloves. Monomer polymer should be manipulated in well-ventilated areas to avoid inhalation of monomer vapor **(Fig. 14.29)**.

## TEST YOURSELF

### Essay Questions

1. Classify denture base resins. Discuss in detail about heat-cure resins.
2. Write ideal requirements of denture base resins. Write the composition and polymerization cycle of heat-cure resins.
3. Describe in detail soft resilient liners.
4. Discuss chemically activated resins and light-activated resins.
5. Discuss general properties of denture base resins.
6. Describe compression molding technique in detail.

### Short Notes

1. Injection molding resins.
2. Pour resins.
3. Porosities in denture base resins.
4. Copolymerization.
5. Denture cleansers.
6. Separating medium.
7. Repair resins.
8. HTV (heat-vulcanizing silicone).
9. Tissue conditioners.
10. Resin teeth.
11. Polymerization shrinkage.
12. Comparison between heat-cure and cold-cure acrylic resins.

### Multiple Choice Questions

1. Liquid of monomer of heat-cure resins have all of the following, *except*:
   A. Hydroquinone
   B. Methacrylate
   C. Dimethyl-para-toluidine
   D. Ethylene glycol dimethacrylate
2. Recommended monomer-polymer ratio of heat-cure resins by volume is:
   A. 1:3
   B. 3:1
   C. 2:1
   D. 1:2
3. Monomer in liquid bottle turns milky white due to:
   A. Partial polymerization
   B. Inhibitor getting exhausted
   C. Opening of double bonds in methyl methacrylate
   D. All of the above

4. All of the following describe function of separating medium *except*:
   A. To prevent water from gypsum to contaminate setting of acrylic resins
   B. To facilitate separating of upper and lower halves of the curing flask
   C. To prevent monomer to penetrate the gypsum mold
   D. To reduce the number of trail closure

5. In comparison to heat-cure resins, cold-cure resins have:
   A. Low-molecular weight
   B. High-residual monomer content
   C. Greater porosity
   D. Greater strength

6. Tissue conditioners should be used in presence of:
   A. Sharp ridges
   B. Excessive resorption of residual ridges
   C. Abused and traumatized tissues
   D. Knife-edged ridges

7. Benefits of cold-cure resins in comparison to heat-cure resins are:
   A. Short-processing time
   B. Can be used for chairside reline procedure
   C. Has better color stability
   D. Lesser warpage of denture in repair

8. Initiation in heat-cure resins is due to:
   A. Hydroquinone
   B. Para-Toluidine
   C. Tertiary amines
   D. Benzoyl peroxide

9. Which of the following statements about the monomer of methyl methacrylate is true?
   A. Has boiling point of 83.2°C
   B. Does not react with fully polymerized acrylic resins
   C. Has two carbon-carbon double bonds per molecule
   D. Has one carbon-carbon double bond per molecule

10. All are benefits of acrylic teeth over porcelain teeth, *except*:
    A. Have greater wear resistance
    B. Chemically bonds with the denture base
    C. Can be easily grinded and shaped to fit in the available space
    D. Are kind to the opposing teeth or ridges

11. Pressure pot is used for polymerization of chemically activated resins to:
    A. Increase strength of acrylic
    B. Reduce porosity
    C. Reduce polymerization shrinkage
    D. All of the above

12. Porosity in acrylic denture cannot cause:
    A. Increases staining
    B. Growth of microorganism

C. Reduces strength
D. Reduces thermal conductivity of denture

13. If cast partial denture is soaked in chlorinated denture cleanser:
    A. Stains from cast metal are removed and it becomes shiny
    B. No effect
    C. Cast metal can corrode
    D. Cast metal will dissolve and fracture

14. Heat-cure resins are packed in the denture flask at which stage of polymerization:
    A. Dough stage
    B. Stringy stage
    C. Sandy stage
    D. Rubbery stage

15. Acrylic resins are made soft and pliable by:
    A. Reducing monomer content in mix
    B. Reducing polymer content in mix
    C. Adding aromatic ester
    D. Adding benzoyl peroxide

16. All are true about short-term soft liners, *except*:
    A. Are called as tissue conditioners
    B. Can readapt to the tissues as healing takes place
    C. Can be adversely affected by denture cleansers
    D. Do not require frequent replacement as they absorb water and become soft over time

17. Indications of long-term soft liners are all, *except*:
    A. Chronic soreness caused by hard acrylic resins
    B. Sharp, knife-edged ridges
    C. Severe tissue undercuts
    D. Soft tissues with chronic fungal infections

18. If the acrylic denture is left on the table for few days, it will:
    A. No effect
    B. Crack
    C. Lose water and shrink
    D. Oxidize and get discolored

19. Fabrication of Custom acrylic trays are not:
    A. Fabricated with cold-cure and light-cure acrylic
    B. Require wax spacer inside the tray for even thickness of impression material
    C. Fabricated directly over the cast
    D. During curing becomes hot

20. During repairing of the denture all steps are performed, *except*:
    A. Fractured segments are reassembled and joined with sticky wax
    B. Fracture segments are handheld and repair resin is directly applied to the fracture site and chemically cured
    C. The fracture segments are wet with monomer to increase chemical bond with repair resin

D. Small portion of old resin is removed surrounding the fracture site to create space for better bonding and strength

## ANSWERS

| | | | |
|---|---|---|---|
| 1. C | 2. A | 3. D | 4. D |
| 5. D | 6. C | 7. C | 8. D |
| 9. D | 10. A | 11. D | 12. D |
| 13. C | 14. A | 15. C | 16. D |
| 17. D | 18. C | 19. C | 20. B |

## BIBLIOGRAPHY

1. Andreopoulos AG, Polyzois GL. Repairs with visible light curing denture base materials. Quint Int. 1991;22:703.
2. Anusavice KJ. Phillip's science of dental materials, 11th edn. St. Louis: Saunders. 2003.
3. Arab J, Newton JP, Llyod CH. The effect of elevated level of residual monomer on the whitening of the denture base and its physical properties. J Dent. 1989;17:189.
4. Arima T, Murata H, Hamada T. The effects of cross linking agents on the water sorption and solubility characteristics of denture base resin. J Oral Rehabil. 1996;23:476.
5. Bartoloni JA, Murchison DF, Wofford DT, Sarkar NK. Degree of conversion in denture base materials for varied polymerization techniques. J Oral Rehabil. 2000;27:488.
6. Bates JF, Stanford GD, Huggett R, Handley RW. Current status of pour type denture base resins. J Dent. 1977;5:177.
7. Blagojevic V, Murphy VM. Microwave polymerization of denture base materials: a comparative study. J Oral Rehabil. 1999;26:804.
8. Braden M. Tissue conditioners. I. Composition and structure. J Dent Res. 1970;49:145.
9. Braden M. Tissue conditioners. II. Rheologic properties. J Dent Res. 1970;49:496.
10. Chalian VA, Drane JB, Standish SM. Maxillofacial Prosthetics. Baltimore: Williams and Wilkins; 1971.
11. Chandler HH, Bowen RL, Paffenbarger GC. Physical properties of a radiopaque denture base material. J Biomed Mater Res. 1971;5:335.
12. Clancy JMS, Boyer DB. Comparative bond strengths of light-cured, heat cured and autopolymerizing denture base reins to denture teeth. J Prosthet Dent. 1989;61:457.
13. Compagnoni MA, Barros Barbosa D, de Souza RF, Pero AC. The effect of polymerization cycles on porosity of microwave-processed denture base resin. J Prosthet Dent. 2004;91:281.
14. Craig RG, Powers JM. Restorative dental materials, 11th edn. St. Louis: Mosby Inc. 2003.
15. Craig RG. Denture materials and acrylic base materials. Curr Opin Dent. 1991;1:235.
16. Hadary AE, Drummond JL. Comparative study of water sorption, solubility, and tensile bond strength of two soft lining materials. J Prosthet Dent. 2000;83:356.
17. Jagger DC, Jagger RG, Allen SM, Harrison A. An investigation into the transverse and impact strength of 'high strength' denture base acrylic resins. J Oral Rehabil. 2002;29:263.
18. Jagger RG, Huggett R. The effect of crosslinking on sorption properties of a denture base materials. Dent Mater. 1990;6:276.
19. Jones DW, Sutow EJ, Hall GC, Tobin WM, Graham BS. Dental soft polymers: plasticizers composition and leachability. Dent Mater. 1988;4:1.
20. Kalachandra S, Turner DT. Water sorption of plasticized denture acrylic lining materials. Dent Mater. 1989;5:161.
21. Machado C, Sanchez E, Azer SS, Uribe JM. Comparative study of the transverse strength of three denture base materials. J Dent. 2007;35:930.
22. Martinez LJ, Von Fraunhofer JA. The effects of custom tray materials on the accuracy of master casts. J Prosthodont. 1998;7:106.
23. Nikawa H, Jin C, Hamada T, Murata H. Interactions between thermal cycled resilient denture lining materials, salivary and serum pellicles and Candida albicans in vitro. Part I. Effects on fungal growth. J Oral Rehabil. 2000;27:41.
24. Nogueira SS, Ogle RE, Davis EL. Comparison of accuracy between compression and injection molded complete dentures. J Prosthet Dent. 1999;82:291.
25. Phoenix RD, Mansueto MA, Ackerman NA, Jones RE. Evaluation of mechanical and thermal properties of commonly used denture base resins. J Prosthodont. 2004;13:17-27.
26. Phoenix RD. Introduction of a denture injection system for use with microwaveable acrylic resins. J Prosthodont. 1997;6:286.
27. Polyzois GL. Mechanical properties of 2 new addition vulcanizing silicone prosthetic elastomers. Int J Prosthodont. 1999;12:359.
28. Robinson JG, McCabe JF. Impact strength of acrylic resin denture base materials with surface defects. Dent Mater. 1993;9:355.
29. Sanders JL, Levin B, Reitz PV. Porosity in denture acrylic resins cured by microwave energy. Quintesence Int. 1987;18:453.
30. Shlosberg SR, Goodacre CJ, Munoz CA, Moore BK, Schnell RJ. Microwave energy polymerization of poly(methyl methacrylate) denture base resin. Int J Prosthodont. 1989;2:453.
31. Smith LT, Powers JM, Ladd D. Mechanical properties of new denture resins polymerized by visible light, heat and microwave energy. Int J Prosthodont. 1992;5:315.
32. Takamata T, Setcos JC, Phillips RW, Boone ME. Adaptation of acrylic resin dentures influenced by the activation mode of polymerization. J Am Dent Assoc. 1989;118:271.
33. Takamata T, Setcos JC. Resin denture bases. Review of accuracy and methods of polymerization. Int J Prosthodont. 1989;2:555-62.
34. Vallittu PK. A review of fibre reinforced denture base resins. J Prosthodont. 1996;5:270.
35. Wang X, Powers JM, Connelly ME. Color stability of heat activated and chemically activated fluid resin acrylics. J Prosthodont. 1996;5:266.

# Section 5

## Direct Restorative Materials

# Dental Amalgam

ADA Specification No. 1; ISO Specification No. 24234:2015

*'The price of greatness is responsibility.'*

—*Winston Churchill*

## INTRODUCTION

Dental amalgam has been one of the most common restorative materials used in dentistry for past 150 years. The dental amalgam alloy primarily consists of silver, tin, copper and sometimes indium, zinc, palladium or selenium. These alloy particles are wetted with mercury to initially form into a plastic form that is directly placed into the prepared cavity of the tooth. After hardening, dental amalgam is carved to generate the desired anatomic form.

Today, the popularity of amalgam has reduced because of the recognized advantages and esthetics of composite restorative material. However, dental amalgam is still used as posterior restorative material because of its ease of manipulation, clinical longevity, reduced cost and versatility to restore carious lesions in most positions in the mouth.

The term "amalgam" was derived from Greek word "emollient" which means paste.

## DEFINITION

- *Dental amalgam is defined as a restorative material which is composed of silver-based alloy mixed with mercury*
- *Dental amalgam alloy is defined as an alloy of silver, copper, tin and other elements that is formulated and processed in the form of powder particles or a compressed pellet.*

## HISTORY

- *650 AD*: First reference of silver paste made in China
- *1528:* Amalgam was first introduced in Germany by *Johannes Stockerus*
- *1578: Li Shihchen* formulated amalgam as mixture of Hg (100 part), Sn (900 part) and Ag (45 part)
- *1603: Kreilius TD* advocated amalgam filling with copper sulfides dissolved in strong acids and mixed with mercury
- *1800 D' Arcet* (France): 1st dental amalgam alloy of Bi (eight part), Pb (one part), Sn (three parts) and Hg (one part) which plasticized at 100°C and called it as *mineral cement*
- *1818: Louis Regnart* credited as "Father of Amalgam". He increased amount of Hg and lowered the plasticizing temperature of mineral cement to 68°C
- *1819: Charles Bell* (England) first introduced the room temperature mixed amalgam and called it as "Bell's Putty"
- *1826: M Taveau* (Paris) used combination of Ag and Hg to form silver mercury paste
- *1833: Crawcour brothers* introduced silver mercury paste in the USA and named it as "Royal Mineral Succedaneum" meaning "substitute for gold"
- *1843* beginning of first amalgam war: American Society of Dental Surgeons disapproved all filling materials including amalgam except gold and referred to it as

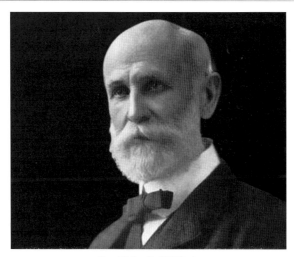

**Fig. 15.1:** Dr GV Black.

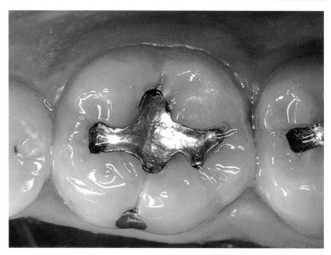

**Fig. 15.2:** Amalgam restoration.

toxic. This started the "First Amalgam War" and the members signed a pledge to stop using amalgam in clinical practice

- *1855:* First amalgam war came to an end by breakup of the society
- *1855: Elisha Townsend* formulated the Ag-Sn-Hg alloy.
- *1860: JF Flagg* originally explored the effect of copper, but copper was not effectively pre-alloyed with silver or tin
- *1895: GV Black* gave standardized cavity preparations and manufacturing processes for dental amalgam products **(Fig. 15.1)**
- *1926: A Stock* became poisoned with Hg through 25 years of exposure "Second Amalgam War"
- *1929: American Dental Association (ADA) specification No 1 for dental amalgam* was adopted and revised in 1934, 1960, 1970 and 1980
- *1930: Gayler* again investigated the effect of copper and found that the copper content above 6% produced excessive expansion, although corrosion reducing effect of high-copper was not known
- *1952:* Minamata bay disaster (Japan)
- *1959: Eames* promoted low mercury to alloy ratio and called it *Eames technique or No-squeeze cloth technique*
- *1963: Innes and Youdelis* added silver-copper spheres to conventional amalgam alloys and highlighted the effect of copper on corrosion resistance
- *1974: Asgar* introduced the single composition high-copper amalgam
- *1980: Huggins* publicly condemned the use of amalgam stating that mercury is responsible for cardiovascular and nervous problems. This started the "Third Amalgam War". Based on his concern the United States and other First World countries demonstrated that there was

no cause and effect relationship between the dental amalgam and medical problems

- *1980: Showell* introduced the amalgapins
- *1991: FDI, National Institute of Health* concluded that there is no basis for claims that amalgam is a health hazard
- *1992* (Sweden): First country in the world to recommend phasing out of amalgam use in practice
- *1998 ADA and US Public Health Service:* Expressed their support on use and safety of dental amalgam
- *1998: Gallium alloys* were introduced which has properties similar to amalgam.

## INDICATIONS

- Moderate to large class I and class II restorations **(Fig. 15.2)**
- Class V restorations which are not esthetically critical
- Caries control restorations done provisionally for those teeth that are badly broken down and which require assessment of pulpal health before final restoration
- Foundations for badly broken down teeth that requires enhanced retention and resistance form
- Post-endodontic restorations
- Tooth with fractured cusp
- When the entire occlusal contact has to be restored.

## CONTRAINDICATIONS

- Avoided in esthetically critical areas such as anterior teeth, premolars and in some cases molars
- Class III and class V restorations in esthetically critical areas
- Small to moderate restorations in posterior teeth.

# ADVANTAGES

- Ease of manipulation
- Greater compressive strength
- Excellent wear resistance
- Increased clinical longevity
- Lower cost
- Less technique sensitive
- Self-sealing
- Maintain anatomic form
- Isolation less critical as compared to composite restorations.

# DISADVANTAGES

- Brittle and non-insulating
- Unesthetic
- Weakens tooth structure
- Greater removal of tooth required, thus less conservative
- Do not bond to the tooth
- Mercury toxicity
- Subject to corrosion and galvanic action
- More technique sensitive if bonded
- Tooth preparation more difficult.

## Classification of Amalgam

- *According to amalgam particle geometry (Figs. 15.3A to C):*
  - Lathe-cut alloys (irregular spindle shaped)
  - Admixed alloys (combination of lathe-cut and spherical alloy)
  - Spherical alloys (sphere shaped particles).
- *According to amalgam alloy particle size:*
  - Regular cut
  - Fine cut
  - Microfine cut.
- *According to copper content:*
  - *Low copper amalgam:* Copper content less than 6%
  - *High copper amalgam:* Copper content more than 6%.
- *According to zinc content:* Zinc acts as scavenger or deoxidizing agent. It helps in producing clean and solid castings. However, it is capable of causing abnormal expansion if zinc-containing amalgam is moisture contaminated during manipulation. This abnormal expansion is called as "delayed expansion".
  - *Zinc containing amalgam:* Zinc content more than 0.01%
  - *Non-zinc containing amalgam:* Zinc content less than 0.01%

- *According to addition of noble metals:*
  - Palladium
  - Gold
  - Platinum
  - Indium.
- *According to chronology of development:*
  - *First generation:* Three parts Ag (silver) + 1 part Sn (tin) (peritectic)
  - *Second generation:* Three parts Ag + 1 part Sn + 4% Cu to reduce plasticity and improve hardness and strength + 1% Zn to reduce brittleness and act as oxygen scavenger
  - *Third generation:* Blending spherical Ag-Cu (eutectic) to original powder
  - *Fourth generation:* Addition of Cu (copper) to original Ag and Sn powder up to 29% to form ternary alloy so that Sn is bonded to Cu
  - *Fifth generation:* Ag + Cu + Sn + In
  - *Sixth generation:* Alloy Pd (10%), Ag (62%) and Cu (25%) to first, second, third generation.
- *According to the composition:*
  - Unicomposition (same chemical composition)
  - Admixed (spherical eutectic high Cu + lathe-cut low Cu).
- *According to number of alloyed materials:*
  - *Binary:* Ag-Sn
  - *Ternary:* Ag-Sn-Cu
  - *Quaternary:* Ag-Sn-Cu-In.

# COMPOSITION

## Low-Cu Alloy

(Lathe-cut or Spherical Alloy Particle Shape)
- Silver: 63–70%
- Tin: 26–28%
- Coper: 2–5% (<6%)
- Zinc: 0–2%.

## High Cu Alloy

Innes and Youdelis in 1963 introduced the high-copper amalgam with the aim of improving the properties of low-copper amalgam. In the low-copper alloy they increased the content of copper between 5% and 12%. High copper amalgam is of two types:
1. *Admixed alloys:* They are also called as *blended alloys* as it is composed of two-thirds of lathe-cut alloy particles and one-third of spherical silver-copper eutectic alloys. The admixed alloys are made by mixing silver-tin with silver-copper particles **(Table 15.1)**.

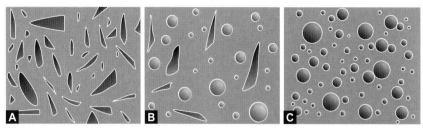

**Figs. 15.3A to C:** Types of amalgam alloy: (A) Lathe-cut alloys; (B) Admixed alloys; and (C) Spherical alloys.

**Table 15.1** Composition of lathe-cut alloy particles and spherical silver-copper eutectic alloys.

| Lathe-cut alloys particle shape 1/3 | | Spherical particle shape 2/3 | |
|---|---|---|---|
| Ag | 40–70% | Ag | 40–65% |
| Sn | 26–30% | Sn | 0–30% |
| Cu | 9–20% | Cu | 20–40% |
| Zn | 0–2% | Zn | 0–1% |

*Eutectic alloys are those alloys which exhibit complete liquid solubility but limited solid solubility. For example, silver-copper eutectic alloys.*

2. Single composition or unicomposition: In this type of alloy, all the particles in the alloy powder have same composition. Unicompositional alloy have copper content in the range of 13–30%.
   - Silver: 60%
   - Tin: 27%
   - Copper: 13–30%
   - Zn: 0–1%
   - Indium: 0–5%
   - Platinum: 0–1%.

Types of single composition alloys:
- *Ternary alloy in spherical form*:
  - Silver: 60%
  - Tin: 25%
  - Copper: 15%.
- *Ternary alloy in spheroidal form*: Composition same as spherical form.
- *Quaternary alloy in spheroidal form*:
  - Silver: 59%
  - Copper: 13%
  - Tin: 24%
  - Indium: 4%.

### Functions of Individual Alloying Metals

- Silver:
  - Major constituent in the alloy
  - Improves strength and corrosion resistance
  - Decreases creep and increases setting expansion
  - Its presence makes the alloy whitish
  - It can also regulate setting time to some extent.
- Tin:
  - Controls rate of reaction between silver and mercury
  - Reduces hardness and strength of set amalgam
  - Reduces resistance to tarnish and corrosion
  - It decreases setting expansion.
- Copper:
  - Reduces brittleness of resulting amalgam
  - Enhances strength and hardness
  - Increases setting expansion.
- Zinc:
  - Acts as scavenger or deoxidizer
  - Improves plasticity of set amalgam
  - Decreases tarnish and corrosion
  - Prevents oxidation of alloys during manufacture
  - Causes *delayed expansion* if amalgam alloy is contaminated with moisture during manipulation.
- Palladium:
  - Increases hardness and resistance to corrosion
  - Whitens the alloy.
- Indium and platinum:
  - It increases plasticity of the alloy
  - It also provides resistance to deformation.
- Mercury:
  - Sometimes present in alloy powder in range of 2–3% and are referred to as *preamalgamated alloys*
  - These alloys enhanced the rate of reaction.

## MANUFACTURING OF ALLOY POWDER

### Lathe-Cut Powder

Lathe-cut powder is manufactured by heating the constituent metals until they are melted to form a molten alloy which is poured into the mold to form an ingot. This process is protected from oxidation. The formed ingot is slowly cooled and annealed. This annealed ingot of alloy is placed into milling machine or lathe to produce the lathe-cut powder. Chip sizes are needle like which can be reduced in size by ball milling. The lathe-cut particles are filtered by passing through fine sieves. The larger particles sieved are again subjected to ball milling to achieve particle sizes ranging between 50 μm and 100 μm length, 10 μm and 60 μm width and 10 μm and 30 μm thickness. The powder particles are then acid washed to improve its reactivity.

### Spherical Alloy Powder

Spherical alloy powders are manufactured by atomization process. The desired elements are melted to form molten alloy. This liquid alloy metal is atomized by spraying into a large chamber through a small hole in a crucible under high inert pressure to form fine spherical droplets. As the chamber is large the liquid globules solidify before reaching the bottom to retain spherical shape. The resulting particles can also be oblong or spherical depending on the atomizing and solidification technique.

### Homogenizing Annealing

An ingot of silver-tin alloy has cored structure containing nonhomogeneous grains of varying composition because of rapid cooling conditions. A homogeneous heat treatment is performed to reestablish the equilibrium phase relationship by placing the ingot into an oven and heating below the solidus temperature. After heating, the ingot is cooled to room temperature. The manner in which the ingot is cooled influences the proportion of phases present in the ingot. If cooled rapidly, phase distribution is almost unchanged. If cooled slowly, β phase is primarily retained.

### Particle Treatments

Lathe-cut particles are subjected to various surface treatments in order to make it more reactive. Acid washed powders are more reactive than unwashed powders. Stresses induced during cutting and ball milling process is relieved by annealing process in order to retain its reactivity and properties. The manufactured lathe-cut alloy powder particles are subjected to *aging process*. This process allows

for relief of stresses incorporated during milling of the ingot. It helps in improving the shelf life of the powder particles. Currently aging is done by controlled heating the particles at the temperature of 60–100°C for 1–6 hours **(Table 15.2).**

## METALLURGICAL PHASES IN DENTAL AMALGAM

Metallurgical phases in dental amalgam are given in Table 15.3.

**Table 15.3:** Phases in dental amalgam.

| Phases | Formula |
| --- | --- |
| $\gamma$ | $Ag_3Sn$ |
| $\gamma_1$ | $Ag_2Hg_3$ |
| $\gamma_2$ | $Sn_{7-8}Hg$ |
| $\varepsilon$ | $Cu_3Sn$ |
| $\eta$ | $Cu_6Sn_5$ |
| Silver copper eutectic | Ag-Cu |

## SETTING REACTION (TABLE 15.4)

**Table 15.4:** Differences between low-copper and high-copper amalgam.

| Low copper | High copper |
| --- | --- |
| More mercury is required for reaction | Less mercury is required |
| $Ag_2Hg_3$ ($\gamma_1$ phase) is dominant phase | $Cu_6Sn_5$ ($\eta$ phase) is dominant phase |
| Tarnish and corrosion due to γ2 phase | Very less corrosion due to copper rich phase |
| Low compressive strength (145–343 Mpa) | High compressive strength (262–510 Mpa) |
| Creep rate is higher (0.8–8%) | Creep rate is less (0.4%) |
| Modulus of elasticity is low | Higher modulus of elasticity |
| Setting reaction is slow | Setting reaction is faster |
| Subject to greater dimensional changes | Subject to lesser dimensional changes |
| Requires less speed and lesser energy for amalgamation | Requires higher speed and greater energy for amalgamation |
| Copper content ≤6% | Copper content varies between 6% and 30% |
| Has irregular lathe-cut shaped alloy particles | Have spherical smooth-shaped alloy particles |
| Produced by milling of annealed ingot of alloy | Produced by atomization of molten alloy |
| Mixture is less plastic, requires greater condensation pressure | Mixture is more plastic and requires lesser condensation pressure |

**Table 15.2:** Comparison between the lathe-cut powder and spherical powder particles.

| Lathe-cut powder particles | Spherical powder particles |
| --- | --- |
| Resists condensation pressure better | More plastic provides less resistance to condensation pressure |
| Require more mercury for trituration | Require less mercury for trituration |
| Have larger surface area per volume ratio | Have smaller surface area per volume ratio |
| Have comparatively inferior properties | Have superior properties |

## Low-Copper Amalgam

The process of amalgamation occurs when mercury contacts the surface of silver-tin alloy particles. In this process when the powder particles are triturated the silver and tin in the outer portion of the particles dissolve into mercury forming various compounds such as silver mercury and tin mercury compounds. Mercury has limited solubility for silver (0.035% by weight) and tin (0.6% by weight). Crystals of two binary compounds precipitate into mercury, i.e. $\gamma_1$ and $\gamma_2$ phase. Silver-mercury compound is called as $\gamma_1$ *(gamma-1) phase* which is $Ag_2Hg_3$ and is a *body centered cubic* crystal. Tin-mercury compound is called as $\gamma_2$ *(gamma-2) phase* which is $Sn_{7-8}Hg$ and is *hexagonal* crystals. As the solubility of silver in mercury is much lower than that of tin, the $\gamma_1$ phase precipitates first, and the $\gamma_2$ phase precipitates later. After trituration, $\gamma_1$ and $\gamma_2$ crystals continue to grow as the remaining mercury dissolves in the alloy particles resulting in plastic consistency of the mixture. When mercury dissolves completely the amalgam starts hardening. The reaction rate decreases as unconsumed alloy particles are surrounded and bound together by solid $\gamma_1$ and $\gamma_2$ crystals.

The physical property of the hardened amalgam is influenced by the relative percentages of each of the microstructural phases.

- The more the unconsumed Ag-Sn particles that are retained in the final structure, the stronger the amalgam. The $\gamma$ phase is the strongest.
- The $\gamma_1$ phase is the noblest phase which is resistant to tarnish and corrosion.

- The $\gamma_2$ phase is the weakest phase and is most susceptible to corrosion. Its hardness is about 10% lower than that of $\gamma_1$ phase. The hardness of the phases are in the order of $\gamma > \gamma_1 > \gamma_2$.
- In general, $\gamma$ and pure $\gamma_1$ phases are stable in oral environment. The unconsumed particles only contribute to the overall strength of amalgam if they are bound to the matrix.
- The percentage of $\gamma_1$ phase is 54–56%, unreacted alloys are 27–35% and $\gamma_2$ phase is 11–13% by volume.

### Microstructure of Set Low-copper Amalgam

The set low-copper amalgam consists of unreacted $\gamma$ as core particles which is surrounded by matrix of $\gamma_1$ and $\gamma_2$ phases.

The reaction for low-copper amalgam is expressed in **Figures 15.4A to D and 15.5A and B** .

*Alloy particles ($\beta + \gamma$) + Hg → $\gamma_1$ ($Ag_2Hg3$) + $\gamma_2$ ($Sn_{7-8}Hg$) + unconsumed alloy particles ($\beta + \gamma$).*

### High Copper Amalgam

High copper amalgam alloys are those alloys which contain more than 6% by weight of copper. They are material of choice for restorations because of *superior mechanical properties, corrosion resistance, better marginal integrity and greater clinical longevity*. Two different types of high-copper alloys powders available are:

1. Admixed alloys
2. Single composition alloys or unicomposition alloys.

### Admixed Alloys

Innes and Youdelis (1963) added spherical silver-copper eutectic alloy (71.9 wt% Ag and 28.1 wt% Cu) with low-copper amalgam alloy particles to form admixed alloys. The resulting amalgam from admixed alloys are *more strong, has greater resistance to marginal breakdown and greater clinical performance* than low copper, lathe-cut powder because of increase in residual alloy particles and resultant decrease in matrix. Admixed alloy powders contain 30–55% weight of spherical high-copper powder and 9–20% weight of copper.

When alloy particles are triturated with mercury, silver from silver-copper alloy and silver and tin from silver-tin alloy particles dissolves in mercury. Tin is 170 times more soluble in mercury than copper and silver is 10 times more soluble in mercury than copper. Tin from the solution diffuses to the surface of silver-copper alloy particles to react with copper to form η phase ($Cu_6Sn_5$).

- Gamma-1 phase form simultaneously along with the η phase and surrounds both the η-covered silver copper alloy particles and silver-tin lathe-cut alloy particles

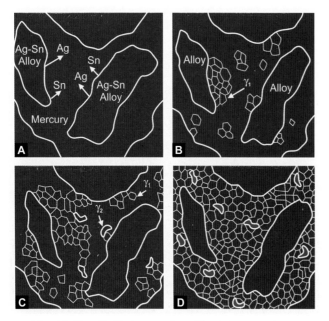

**Figs. 15.4A to D:** Setting reaction of low-copper amalgam.

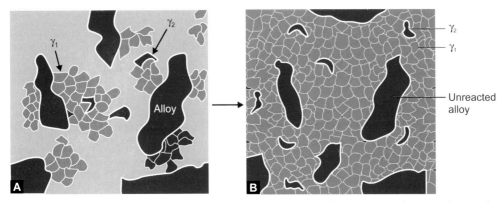

**Figs. 15.5A and B:** Setting reaction of low-copper amalgam: (A) Growth of $\gamma_1$ and $\gamma_2$ crystals; (B) Final set amalgam.

- Gamma-1 phase binds to the unconsumed alloy particles as in the low-copper amalgam.

    Here, $\gamma_2$ phase is completely eliminated although a small portion of $\gamma_2$ phase is formed which is replaced by the $\eta$ phase at the same time.

*Microstructure of set high-copper admixed amalgam:* Set high-copper admixed amalgam consists of unreacted $\gamma$ phase and unreacted Ag-Cu (eutectic) as core particles which are surrounded by halo of $\eta$ ($Cu_6Sn_5$) phase. The matrix is formed by the $\gamma_1$ phase in which the core particles are embedded.

    The reaction of the admixed alloy powder with mercury is expressed in **Figure 15.6**.

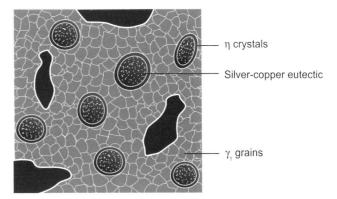

**Fig. 15.6:** Setting reaction of high-copper admixed amalgam.

*Alloy particles ($\beta + \gamma$) + Ag-Cu eutectic + Hg $\rightarrow$ $\gamma_1$ + $\eta$ + unconsumed alloy particles.*

### Single Composition Alloys or Unicomposition Alloys

- Unicomposition alloy particles are atomized particles which have dendritic microstructures with fine lamellae having same chemical composition
- Composition includes Ag, 60 wt%; Sn, 27 wt% and copper 13–30 wt%. Along with this small amounts of Indium or Palladium are added
- On trituration of the alloy particles with mercury, silver and tin from the Ag-Sn phase dissolve in mercury. First $\gamma_1$ phase is precipitated which forms the matrix by binding the partially dissolved alloy particles
- Next $\eta$ phase ($Cu_6Sn_5$) is formed which represents meshes of *rod-like* crystals found dispersed in the matrix and at the surface of the alloy particles
- The $\eta$ crystals are much larger than those formed in the admixed alloys
- The meshed $\eta$ crystals found over the unconsumed alloy particles strengthen the bonding between the alloy particles and $\gamma_1$ crystals
- Whereas the $\eta$ crystals dispersed between the $\gamma_1$ grains tends to interlock them and enhances its resistance to deformation.

*Microstructure of set high-copper single compositional amalgam:* It consists of core particles of unreacted $\gamma$, $\beta$ and $\varepsilon$ are surrounded by rod-shaped mesh of $\eta$ phase. The core particle and the $\eta$ are embedded in the matrix of $\gamma_1$ **(Fig. 15.7)**.

    The reaction of the single composition with mercury is summarized as:

*Ag-Sn-Cu alloy particles + Hg $\rightarrow$ $\gamma_1$ + $\eta$ + unconsumed alloy particles.*

## PROPERTIES

The quality of amalgam is measured by properties listed in ADA specification No 1 (ISO 1559) which emphasize on dimensional change, strength and creep among others.

### Strength

Properly designed and manipulated amalgam restorations possess adequate strength to resist the functional forces especially at the margins. It is found to be one of the strongest directly placed restorative material which is capable of clinically serving for years in the mouth. Although fractures of amalgam restorations occur more commonly at the margins. Amalgam has been found to resist compressive stress better

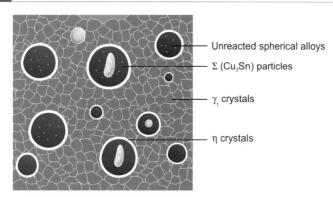

**Fig. 15.7:** Setting reaction of high-copper single composition amalgam.

than the tensile stress. Therefore, the cavity should be designed such that it receives more compressive forces and less tensile forces in function.

## Compressive Strength

- American National Standards Institute (ANSI)/ADA specification No. 1 for amalgam recommends minimum compressive strength after 1 hour to be 80 MPa
- The prepared cavity should be designed to receive maximum compressive forces and minimum tensile or shear forces because amalgam restorations are strongest in compression and weaker in tension and shear

### CLINICAL SIGNIFICANCE

Usually, amalgam fractures at the margins (marginal breakdown) which can lead to corrosion, secondary caries and subsequent clinical failure. Therefore, more conservative approach to replace amalgam restorations with defective margins have been recommended.

- The compressive strength of properly manipulated amalgam should be at least 310 MPa
- The tensile strength of both low-copper and high-copper amalgam ranges between 48 MPa and 70 MPa **(Table 15.5).**

## Tensile Strength

Dental amalgam is much weaker in tension as compared to in compression. The tensile strength of both low and high-copper amalgam ranges from 48 MPa to 64 MPa after 24 hours. The design of the cavity to accept amalgam should be such that it is supported by sound tooth structure to minimize flexion due to tensile stresses.

Factors affecting the strength of amalgam restoration are:

### *Trituration*

- The effect of trituration on strength of amalgam depends on the type of amalgam alloy, time of trituration and the speed of amalgamator
- Overtrituration or undertrituration reduces the strength of both low-and high-copper amalgam
- Maximum strength is achieved when mixing continues till coherent mass of matrix is formed
- Further trituration will leads to cracks in crystals and interfaces lead, thereby reducing its strength.

### *Mercury Content*

- Sufficient Hg mixed, in alloy so that each alloy particle is wetted thoroughly
- If sufficient Hg is not mixed it will lead to dry granular mix resulting in rough, pitted surface of highly reduced strength
- If Hg is in excess then again it will lead to reduction in strength. Higher mercury content promotes formation of gamma-2 phase (weakest phase) even in high copper amalgam. Greater the content of mercury, greater the chance of fracture and corrosion
- Studies on mercury analysis suggest that in large amalgam restorations 2–3% more mercury content is found in the marginal areas as compared to that found in the bulk of the restorations. This is found regardless of the method of condensation of the amalgam.
- Recommended Hg/alloy ratio is 1:1
- The strength of the amalgam is proportional to the amount of unconsumed alloy particles and the volume percentage of the matrix. Greater the amount of unconsumed alloy particles in the matrix, stronger is the mixture.

### *Condensation*

- The amount of condensation pressure and technique of condensation depends on the shape of alloy particles

| Table 15.5: Tensile strength of low-copper and high-copper amalgam. | | | |
|---|---|---|---|
| *Amalgam* | *Compressive strength—1 hour (MPa)* | *Compressive strength—7 days (MPa)* | *Tensile strength (24 hours) MPa* |
| Low copper | 145 | 343 | 60 |
| Admixed high copper | 137 | 431 | 48 |
| Single compositional high Cu | 262 | 510 | 64 |

For lathe-cut alloy increased condensation pressure is required to squeeze out Hg and reduce porosity because the alloy particles are irregularly shaped. Increase condensation pressure leads to decrease porosity and greater strength. This is due to alloy particles been more closely packed resulting in smaller volume of matrix phase

- Spherical alloy when condensed with lighter pressure will provide adequate strength. If greater condensation pressure is applied on spherical alloy particles (high-copper amalgam) the particles tends to slip under pressure making condensation difficult. Therefore, light condensation pressure is applied on spherical particles to gain adequate strength.

### Porosity

- Porosities and voids reduce strength of set amalgam. Porosities results in area of stress concentration leading to corrosion and ultimately fracture of the restoration
- *Causes*: Porosities are caused by reduced plasticity of the mixture, insufficient condensation pressure, insertion of large increments and irregularly-shaped particles
- *Remedy*: Increased condensation pressure reduces porosity and improves adaptation of amalgam at the margins.

### Amalgam Hardening Rate

- Amalgam strength improves with time
- At 20 minutes, the compressive strength of amalgam is only 6% of 1 week strength
- According to ADA specification the compressive strength of amalgam after 1 hour should be at least 80 MPa
- One hour compressive strength of high-copper amalgam is 262 MPa which is much higher than the low-copper amalgam.

---

**CLINICAL SIGNIFICANCE**

After amalgam restoration patient is advised not to bite on hard food for at least 8 hours during which about 70% strength is gained.

---

### Size of the Alloy Particles

Larger size and irregularly-shaped particles have lesser strength as compared to smaller size particles.

### Dimensional Change

- American Dental Association specification No. 1 recommends that amalgam should neither expand

nor contract more than 20 $\mu$m/cm measured at 37°C between 5 minutes and 24 hours after trituration
- Expansion or contraction of amalgam largely depends on its manipulation
- Severe contraction in amalgam restoration can result in microleakage, plaque accumulation and secondary caries
- Similarly, excessive expansion can cause pressure on the pulp resulting in postoperative sensitivity and protrusion of the restoration.

### Theory of Dimensional Change

During setting amalgam undergoes three distinct successive dimensional changes:
- *Stage I*: Initial contraction
  - Initially as the alloy powder and mercury are mixed together, contraction occurs because the particles begin to dissolve and the $\gamma_1$ phase grows
  - Contraction occurs for about 20 minutes from the start of trituration. This contraction is not more than 4.5 $\mu$m. Contraction occurs as long as $\gamma_1$ crystals grow. Studies show that final volume of $\gamma_1$ phase is less than the initial volumes of dissolved alloy powder and mercury.
- *Stage II*: Expansion
  - The growth of $\gamma_1$ phase continues and the particles start impinging upon each other to produce an outward pressure which opposes the contraction in stage I
  - Expansion will be seen if there is sufficient mercury in the mixture.
- *Stage III*: Contraction
  - After a rigid $\gamma_1$ matrix has formed, the growth of $\gamma_1$ crystals cannot force the matrix to expand
  - Instead $\gamma_1$ crystals grow in the interstices containing mercury, and producing a continued reaction.

*Factors influencing contraction are:*
- Reduced Hg/alloy ratio
- Increased condensation pressure
- Size of the particle is small
- Greater trituration time.

Modern amalgam alloys show net contraction whereas earlier formulation of amalgam always showed expansion because:
- Earlier amalgam contained larger alloy particles and they were mixed at higher Hg/alloy ratio
- Earlier hand trituration was used whereas presently high speed mechanical amalgamators are used.

### Delayed Expansion

- In case of moisture contamination of zinc containing low-copper or high-copper amalgam, expansion is observed in restoration which usually occurs after 3–5 days and may continue for months. This expansion can reach values greater than 400 μm

- This type of expansion is called as *delayed expansion or secondary expansion* (**Fig. 15.8**)
- It occurs by reaction of zinc with water producing hydrogen gas
- Hydrogen is produced by electrolytic action involving zinc and water
- The chemical reaction is expressed as:

$$Zn + H_2O \rightarrow ZnO + H_2 \uparrow$$

- $H_2$ does not combine with amalgam
- The hydrogen collects within the restoration, increasing internal pressure to levels high enough to cause the amalgam to creep, thus producing the observed expansion
- Contamination can occur any time during manipulation and insertion
- Severe expansion causes pressure on pulp and results in severe pain
- Pressure centered on the pulp can reach up to 2000 lb/sq inch.

## Creep

- It is a time-dependent plastic deformation of a material under a static or dynamic load
- According to ADA specification No 1 the creep rate should be below 3% (**Table 15.6**)
- Higher the creep rate, greater will be the chances of marginal breakdown of dental amalgam
- Creep rate for low-copper amalgam is 0.8–8% and for high-copper amalgam it is between 0.4% and 1%.

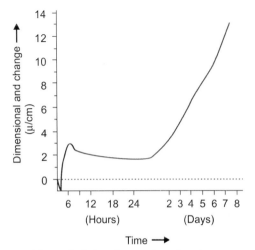

**Fig. 15.8:** Delayed expansion of amalgam.

**Table 15.6:** Comparison of creep rate between low-copper and high-copper amalgam.

| Type of amalgam | Creep % |
| --- | --- |
| Low copper | 2.0% |
| Admixed | 0.4% |
| Single composition | 0.13% |

### Factors Influencing Creep Rates

- *Effect of microstructure on creep rate:*
  - Gamma-1 phase greatly influences the creep rate of low-copper amalgam
  - Creep rates are higher in low-copper amalgam because of the presence of $\gamma_2$ phase and larger $\gamma_1$ volume fractions
  - In cases of high-copper amalgam, the creep rate is much lower as $\gamma_2$ phase is eliminated and $\eta$ phase is present, which acts as barriers to deformation of $\gamma_1$ phase
- *Effect of manipulative variables:*
  - For increased strength of amalgam and reduced creep rate
  - Mercury alloy ratio should be minimized
  - Condensation pressure should be maximum for low copper and admixed amalgam
  - Timing of trituration and condensation should be properly controlled.

## Tarnish and Corrosion

- Dental amalgam restorations show tendency to tarnish and corrode in oral environment
- The degree to which it can occur is greatly influenced by the type of alloy used and the patient's oral environment
- Corrosion usually occurs at the interface of the tooth and restoration
- The space between the restoration and the tooth permits the microleakage of electrolytes and a classic concentration cell process results
- As the restoration ages, the corrosion products formed along the interface of tooth and restoration seals this space making it as self-sealing restoration (**Fig. 15.9**)
- Commonly the corrosion products found along the interface are the *tin chlorides and tin oxides*
- Corrosion products containing copper can also be found in high-copper amalgams

*Factors which increases tarnish and corrosion are:*

- High mercury alloy ratio
- Rough surface texture of the restoration
- Moisture contamination during condensation
- Low-copper amalgam is more susceptible to corrosion due to presence of $\gamma_2$ phase

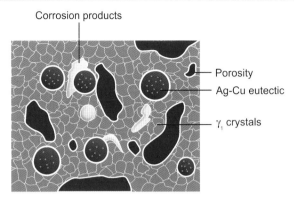

**Fig. 15.9:** Corrosion products in traditional amalgam restoration.

- High-copper amalgam is less prone to corrosion because the presence of $\eta$ phase which is less susceptible to corrosion than the $\gamma_2$ phase.
- Gold restoration placed in contact with amalgam restoration leads to greater corrosion due to large difference in electromotive forces of the two materials
- High-copper amalgam restoration should not be placed adjacent to the low-copper amalgam restoration as they are cathodic with respect to low-copper amalgam.

*Factors which reduce tarnish and corrosion are:*
- Smooth, homogeneous and polished restoration
- Proper mercury alloy ratio
- Proper trituration and condensation
- Avoiding contact of dissimilar metal alloys
- Avoiding moisture contamination.

## Marginal Ditching

- Low-copper dental amalgam has susceptibility to corrosion because of the presence of $\gamma_2$ phase
- The corrosion can compromise the strength and the mercury liberated during the corrosion process reacts with the unreacted $\gamma$ phase and form various reaction products
- These reaction products can cause dimensional change in the restorations and making it prone to fracture especially at the margins **(Fig. 15.10A)**
- This dimensional change occurs in the form of mercuroscopic expansion
- Mercuroscopic expansion is defined as the expansion that occurs when mercury, released by the corrosion of the $\gamma_2$ phase, reacts with the remaining amalgam alloy particles. This will produce an unsupported wedge at the margin of the restoration
- The entire mechanism has been associated with the phenomenon of *marginal ditching*

- The term "mercuroscopic expansion" was originally proposed by *KD Jorgensen (1965)*
- Most common evidence of degradation of low-copper amalgam is marginal fracture
- Combination of brittleness, low tensile strength and electrochemical corrosion leads to marginal fracture
- At some point occlusal stresses of opposing tooth contact creates local fractures producing a ditch at the margin known as "marginal ditching"
- Measured on basis of "Mahler's scale".

### Microleakage in Amalgam Restorations *(Fig. 15.10B)*

- Microleakage occurs when there is marginal gap of around 20 µm between the amalgam restorations and the tooth
- Such microgap can occur due to:
  - Incomplete condensation,
  - High coefficient of thermal expansion of amalgam.
- Lack of corrosion products which are necessary for self-sealing of restoration
- Microleakage can lead to:
  - Marginal fracture of restorations
  - Secondary caries
  - Tooth discoloration
  - Postoperative sensitivity.

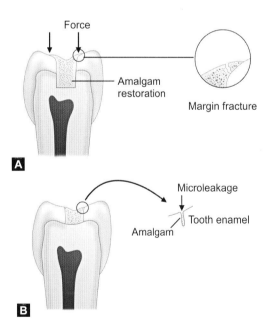

**Figs. 15.10A and B:** (A) Marginal ditching of an amalgam restoration; (B) Microleakage in amalgam restoration.

# FACTORS AFFECTING THE QUALITY OF AMALGAM

*Factors influencing quality of the amalgam restoration controlled by the dentists are:*
- Selection of the alloy
- Mercury-alloy ratio
- Trituration procedure
- Technique employed during condensation
- Marginal integrity
- Anatomical considerations
- Finishing of the final restoration.

    *Factors influencing quality of the amalgam restoration controlled by the manufacturer are:*
- Alloy composition
- Heat treatment of the alloy
- Size and shape of the particles
- Method of manufacturing of the alloy particles
- Surface treatment of the particles
- Mode of supply of alloy particles.

# FACTORS AFFECTING SUCCESS OF AMALGAM RESTORATIONS

Clinical success of amalgam restoration depends on proper cavity design, selection and proper manipulation of the alloy. Modern amalgam restorations which are properly manipulated shows 12–15 years of clinical longevity. Defective restoration is usually due to the fault of the dentist, auxiliary or patient rather than the material.

## Cavity Design

- Amalgam restoration is mechanically retained in the tooth and does not bond chemically to the tooth structure
- The proper cavity design should possess uniform minimum thickness for strength, should have a butt joint form (90° or more) at the margin and should be mechanically retained into the tooth
- The cavity preparation should have vertical walls which converge occlusally to adequately retain amalgam **(Fig. 15.11)**
- Additional retention of amalgam is provided by placing locks, grooves, coves, slots, pins or amalgapins.

## Selection of Materials

### Alloy Particles

- The selected alloy should meet the requirement of ADA specification No. 1.

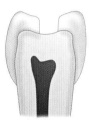

**Fig. 15.11:** Typical amalgam tooth preparation showing occlusal convergence.

- Lathe-cut alloys produce rough irregular surfaces, having large area/volume ratio which require more mercury during trituration
- Spherical alloys are smooth, having more regular surfaces with low area/volume ratio and requires less mercury for trituration
- High-copper alloy which gives maximum strength, high resistance to marginal fracture, low creep and good corrosion resistance are preferred over the low-copper amalgam
- Modern zinc containing high-copper amalgam has shown 90% overall survival after 12 years as compared to non-zinc containing amalgam
- The combined synergistic effect of zinc and copper provides greater corrosion resistance and survivability to the restorations
- Alloys containing more than 0.01% of zinc should be used with caution as it subjected to excessive corrosion and expansion on moisture contamination
- Selection of alloy also depends on the preference of the operator and the assistant
- Factors which affect selection of alloy are: particle size and shape, composition, hardening rate, smoothening of the mix, ease of condensation, ease of finishing and polishing, setting time and operator's choice.

### Mercury

- American Dental Association specification No 6 for dental mercury requires that mercury should be highly pure
- There should be no surface contamination and should contain less than 0.02% nonvolatile residue
- It is the only metal which is liquid at room temperature
- It is volatile at room temperature and has vapor pressure of 20 mg/cubic meter of air
- It is colorless, odorless and tasteless and is difficult to detect
- It is 14 times more denser than water

- It has freezing point of –38.87°C and boiling temperature of 356.9°C
- Lack of purity of mercury adversely affects the physical properties of amalgam
- Pure mercury should be arsenic-free and triple distilled.

## Delivery System of Alloy

- The alloy is available in the form of powder, pellets or pre-proportioned capsules
- Pre-proportioned capsules are most widely used method of dispensing accurate mercury and alloy powder.

## Manipulation of Dental Amalgam

### Mercury Alloy Ratio

- During earlier times, excess mercury was used to attain smooth and plastic mix of amalgam
- But, since excess mercury adversely affects the physical and mechanical properties of amalgam, two techniques were employed to minimize excess of mercury in the final restorations:
  - By squeezing or wringing excess mercury using a squeeze cloth
  - By working each mercury rich amalgam to the top during condensation and then removing this excess mercury
  - However, the modern day concept of reducing the mercury content of the restoration is to reduce the original mercury alloy ratio
  - This method is known as *minimal mercury technique* or *Eames technique*
  - To fulfill the objective of obtaining a coherent and plastic mass after trituration only sufficient mercury should be present in the mixture
  - The recommended mercury alloy ratio is approximately 1:1
  - The mercury alloy ratio varies with different alloy compositions, particle size and shape, heat treatment and condensation techniques
  - The recommended ratio for most lathe-cut alloys is 50% and for spherical alloys, the ratio is close to 42% of mercury.

### Proportioning

- The proportioning of the two components of the amalgam, i.e. alloy and mercury should be accurate
- For accurate proportioning wide variety of mercury and alloy dispensers are available

- Commonly used dispensers are based on volumetric proportioning
- Regardless of the method employed, proper amount of mercury and alloy should always be proportioned before the start of trituration
- Mercury should never be added after trituration.

### Preweight Tablets or Pellets

- Preweighed pellets are convenient way of correctly dispensing the alloy because of their uniformity in weight
- With these tablets an accurate mercury dispenser is all that required
- Mercury dispenser should be held vertically to ensure consistent spills of mercury and should not be tilted at 45° as it leads to altered mercury alloy ratio.

### Pre-proportioned Capsules (*Fig. 15.12*)

- Pre-proportioned disposable capsules with specific quantity of alloy and mercury is widely used in practice currently
- The capsule contains preweight quantity of powder or pellet and mercury
- The mercury and the alloy are physically separated from each other to prevent any amalgamation to occur during storage
- Traditionally available capsules required activation before trituration
- But currently alloys are available in *self-activating capsules* which release mercury into the alloy chamber after first few oscillation of the amalgamator.
  - Advantages
    - ◊ Reliable mercury alloy ratio
    - ◊ Convenient and faster
    - ◊ Eliminates the chances of mercury spills during proportioning.

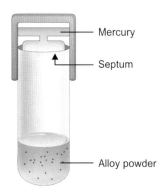

**Fig. 15.12:** Pre-proportioned capsule.

– Disadvantages:
  ◊ Expensive
  ◊ Not possible to make minor adjustment in mercury alloy ratio.

*Trituration*

- *Objective of trituration*:
  – Provide proper amalgamation of alloy and mercury
  – To wet all the surfaces of alloy particles with Hg
  – Attain workable plastic mass
  – To remove the oxide layer from the surface of alloy particles by rubbing
  – To dissolve alloy in Hg for formation of matrix crystals
  – To keep matrix crystals as small as possible.
- *Mechanical trituration:*
  – Traditionally, the alloy and mercury were triturated by hand using mortar and pestle. This is referred to as *hand trituration* (**Fig. 15.13**)
  – Currently mechanical amalgamators are used which standardizes the procedure and saves time (**Fig. 15.14**)
  – A capsule serves as a mortar. A cylindrical metal or plastic piston of smaller diameter than the capsule is inserted into the capsule which serves as the pestle
  – The alloy and mercury are dispensed into the capsule
  – The capsule is secured in the machine and the arms holding the capsule oscillate at high speed after the machine is turned on, to complete trituration
  – Most modern amalgamators have automatic timers to control length of mixing time and have two or more operating speeds

– A wide variety of capsule-pestle combinations are available. Pestles may be plastic or metal and come in variety of sizes, shapes and weights
– In selecting a capsule-pestle combination, the size of pestle is an important consideration
– The diameter and length of the pestle should be considerably less than the comparable dimensions of the capsule
– If the pestle is too large, the resultant mix may not be homogeneous
– Capsules can be reusable or disposable
– Reusable capsules are available with friction fit and screw cap lid. The lid of the capsule should always fit tightly before use
– Disposable capsule should never be reused as there are chances of leakage or fracture of the capsule
– An amalgamator must be used at the speed recommended by the manufacturer
– Spherical alloys require less amalgamation time than the lathe-cut alloys
– Also larger mix requires slightly more amalgamation time than the smaller mixture.

Based on the speed of mixing, amalgamators are of three types:
1. Low speed: 3,200–3,400 cycles/min
2. Medium speed: 3,700–3,800 cycles/min
3. High speed: 4,000–4,400 cycles/min.

*Trituration energy:* Low-copper amalgam require less trituration energy for manipulation as compared to high-copper amalgam. Trituration of amalgam depends on speed and coherence time (TC). Coherence time is defined as minimum time which is required to mix to form a single coherent pellet of amalgam. This time depends on the type of alloy, speed of amalgamator and the size of the mixture.

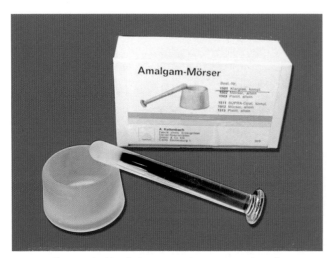

**Fig. 15.13:** Hand trituration using motor and pestle.

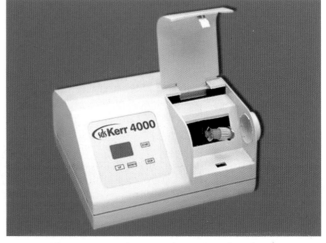

**Fig. 15.14:** Amalgamator for mixing of amalgam.

Factors affecting trituration are:
- Speed or number of unit movement per unit time
- Time required for trituration. Greater the time needed for trituration greater will be amount of trituration energy required
- Amount of thrust—greater the amount of thrust greater will the trituration energy required for mixing
- Weight of the capsule—greater is the weight of the capsule, more will the trituration energy required for mixing
- *Single mixture amalgam* is preferred if less amount of amalgam is required for smaller restoration
- *Double mixture amalgam* is preferred when greater amount of amalgam is required for larger restoration. If more than 4 minutes have elapsed between trituration and condensation then a fresh mixture should be taken because using old mixture will result in weaker amalgam with increased creep.

*Mulling:* Objective of mulling is to improve the homogeneity of the mix and achieve a single consistent mixture. Mulling can be done in two ways:
1. Mixture is enveloped in a dry piece of rubber dam and is vigorously rubbed between thumb of one hand and palm of another hand for 2–5 seconds
2. After mechanical trituration, mix is removed and triturated in pestle-free capsule for 2–3 seconds. This caused the mix to cohere and facilitate easy removal from the capsule.

    The process of mulling should not be done with bare hands because the amalgam can get contaminated and its properties can be adversely affected.

*Advantages:*
- It helps to coat the alloy particles uniformly with mercury
- Helps to remove excess mercury because presence of residual mercury leads to formation of $\gamma_2$ phase which is a weaker phase. At the same time the compressive strength is reduced and the creep rate is increased.

*Consistency of the mixture:* After trituration the resulting mixture should not be granular in appearance, but should have a smooth, shiny appearance and should be coherent. Such an amalgam mixture may be warm when it is removed from the capsule.
- *Normal mixture (Fig.15.15A):*
  - Mixture should be wet and plastic
  - Should have smooth, soft consistency with shiny surface
  - Should have greatest compressive and tensile strength
  - Mixture is warm when removed from the capsule
  - Curved surface should retain luster after polishing.
- *Undertriturated mixture (Fig.15.15B):*
  - Appears dull
  - Crumbly and grainy in consistency
  - Surface appears rough after carving
  - Mixture tends to harden rapidly with excess of mercury
  - Strength is less
  - More prone to tarnish and corrosion.
- *Overtriturated (Fig.15.15C):*
  - Mixture is too plastic to manipulate
  - Difficult to remove from capsule
  - Working time is reduced
  - Can result in higher contraction of the amalgam
  - Increased contraction and increased creep
  - Reduced strength in cases of high-copper amalgam.

### Condensation *(Fig. 15.16)*

- *Objectives:*
  - To adapt amalgam to preparation walls
  - To produce restoration-free of voids
  - To reduce marginal leakage
  - To reduce corrosion by minimizing mercury content in the restoration
  - To enhance strength and reduce creep
  - To compact alloy into the cavity to attain greatest possible density
  - A major objective is to remove any excess mercury from each increment as it is worked to the top by the condensing procedure.

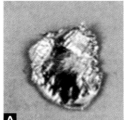 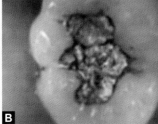 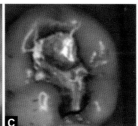

**Figs.15.15A to C:** Diagram to showing consistency of the mix (A) Normal consistency; (B) Undertriturated; and (C) Overtriturated.

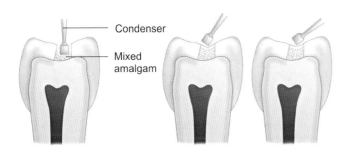

Condenser

Mixed amalgam

**Fig. 15.16:** Process of condensation.

– Once the mixture is ready the process of condensation should begin immediately
– Greater the time elapses between mixing and condensation, the weaker the amalgam. Also, the mercury content and creep of the amalgam is increased
– If partially set amalgam is condensed it often results in fracture and breakup of the matrix
– During condensation, the field of operation should be kept absolutely dry
– Any moisture contamination at this stage especially with zinc containing alloys can result in delayed expansion and related problems of corrosion and loss of strength
– Condensation is usually accomplished within four walls and the floor. If one or more wall is absent, a stainless steel matrix band and retainer is used
– The process of condensation is accomplished either using hand or mechanical instruments.

• *Hand condensation:*
  – A well triturated mixture should never be touched with bare hands as it contains free mercury
  – The mixture is carried to the prepared cavity using an amalgam carrier
  – Smaller increments should be condensed at a time for best results
  – Increment of amalgam when inserted into the prepared cavity is immediately condensed with sufficient pressure to remove voids and to adapt the material to the walls
  – The condenser point is forced into the amalgam mass under hand pressure and is stepped little-by-little toward the cavity walls
  – Condensation is usually started in the center of the restoration
  – The amount of pressure used for condensation depends on the type and shape of alloy particle used
  – After condensation of an increment, the surface should be shiny in appearance

– This shows that sufficient mercury present at the surface to diffuse into the next increment so that each increment bonds to the preceding one
– This process of adding increments is continued till the entire cavity is overfilled
– Any mercury rich material on overfilled cavity is carved.

• *Mechanical condensation:*
  – The procedure and principles of mechanical condensation are the same as those for hand condensation
  – The only difference is that the condensation of amalgam is performed by an automatic device
  – Mechanical condenser either provides impact type of force or uses rapid vibration
  – When using mechanical condenser either of impact or vibratory type the procedure is less fatiguing to the operator
  – Similar clinical results can be obtained using either hand or mechanical condensation
  – The choice of type of method depends on the preference and convenience of the operator.

• *Condensation pressure:*
  – The condensation pressure is influenced by the area of the condenser point and the force exerted by the operator
  – The smaller the condenser, the greater will be the pressure exerted on the amalgam if a given force is applied
  – If the condenser point is too large, sufficient pressure is difficult to generate to condense amalgam properly into the retentive area
  – The average condensation force ranges between 3–4 lb (13.3–17.8N)
  – Although the recommended force for condensation is 15lb (66.7N)
  – The condensation force should ensure maximum density and adaptation to the cavity walls and it should be as great as the alloy allows and is consistent with the patient comfort
  – For non-spherical amalgam, the condensation forces are applied at 45 angulation to cavity wall and floor
  – Large condenser fitting the cavity is used to condense spherical amalgam. Large increment of mixed alloy is used to fill the cavity and then condense with condenser
  – Various shapes of the condenser points are available to provide effective condensation.

## Carving of Restoration

• Once the amalgam has been condensed into the prepared cavity, the restoration is carved to reproduce the proper tooth anatomy **(Fig. 15.17).**

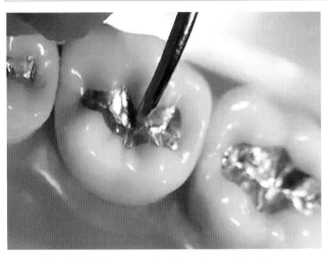

**Fig. 15.17:** Proper carving of amalgam restorations.

- *The objective of carving is:*
    - To simulate the anatomy and natural contour of the tooth rather than to reproduce accurate details
    - To produce restoration with adequate embrasure which is compatible with periodontal tissues
    - To produce restoration which maintains and enhances health and integrity of the periodontium
    - To produce restoration which is not overcontoured or undercontoured.
- Carving should not begin until the amalgam is hard enough to offer resistance to the carving instrument
- It should not be too deep as it will reduce the bulk of amalgam especially from the margins
- Also, it should not be too thin, as it will fracture under masticatory load
- After carving the surface of the restoration should be smoothened by burnishing.

## Burnishing

Burnishing is defined as the process to make shiny or lustrous surface by rubbing and to facilitate marginal adaptation of restorations by rubbing the margin with an instrument.
- *Objectives:*
    - Reduce size and number of voids on the critical surface
    - To adapt amalgam to the cavosurface anatomy.
- *Conditions for the surface for carving:*
    - It is a process of marginal adaptation of amalgam
    - Ball burnisher is commonly used in light strokes from amalgam toward tooth surface
    - Undue pressure and heat generation should be avoided during burnishing.

## Finishing of the Restoration

- Regardless of the alloy, trituration method, and condensation technique employed, the curved surface of the restoration is usually rough
- The surfaces are covered with scratches, pits, and irregularities
- If these defects are not removed by further finishing after the amalgam is completely set, they can result in concentration cell type corrosion
- The final polishing of the amalgam restoration should be done 24 hours after condensation **(Fig. 15.18)**
- The use of dry polishing powders and disks should be avoided as they can easily raise the surface temperature above the 60°C
- This temperature is critical as above this temperature, there are chances of significant release of mercury
- Thus, a wet abrasive powder in paste form should be used for polishing of amalgam restorations.

## MERCURY TOXICITY

- Studies have revealed that mercury penetrates from the restorations to the tooth structure and have often resulted in discoloration of the tooth
- It has also been observed that small amounts of mercury have been released during mastication but chances of toxic reaction from these traces of mercury are insignificant
- However, the most significant contribution of toxicity of mercury is through the vapor phase.
- Metallic mercury vapor can be inhaled and absorbed through the alveoli in the lungs at 80% efficiency.

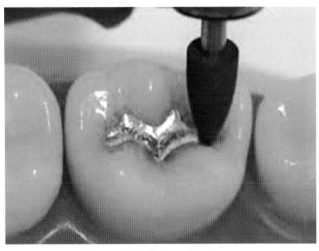

**Fig. 15.18:** Polishing of amalgam.

- Mercury vapors are released during process of trituration, condensation, polishing or removal of old amalgam restorations
- The release of these vapors can be minimized by applying sealant resin for first few days after restoration
- Addition of indium to the alloy particles can reduce vapor pressure of mercury
- The patient's exposure to release of this vapor is minimal during insertion or during function and is well below the *"no effect level"*
- Dentists and their auxiliaries are at primary risk of mercury inhalation as they are exposed daily to mercury intoxication
- The maximum level occupational exposure considered safe is 50 µg of mercury per cubic meter of air per day
- Maximum allowable level of mercury in the blood is 3 µg/L
- Mercury blood levels in patient with amalgam restoration was 0.7 ng/mL as compared to 0.3 ng/mL with patient without amalgam restoration
- Normal daily intake of mercury is 15 µg from food, 1 µg from air and 0.4 µg from water.

### Sources of Mercury Exposure in Dental Operatory

- Amalgam alloy stored for use
- During trituration before hardening
- Amalgam scrap
- During finishing and polishing procedure
- During removal of old amalgam restoration.

## MERCURY HYGIENE

The potential hazards of mercury can be minimized by following certain precautions:
- The operatory should be well ventilated
- All dental personnel and auxiliary should be trained to handle mercury
- Periodic check of dental operatory atmosphere for mercury vapor is mandatory. Dosimeters are used for monitoring
- Floor of the dental operatory should be noncarpeted, nonabsorbent and easy to clean
- Mercury should be stored in well air tight containers
- Any spilled mercury should be cleaned immediately
- Pre-proportioned tightly closed capsules should be used for amalgamation
- Amalgamator with completely closed arm should be used
- All excess mercury, including waste, disposable capsules, and amalgam removed during condensation should be collected and stored in well-sealed containers

- High volume evacuation should be used while finishing or removing amalgam restorations
- All amalgam scrap should be stored in tightly closed container or radiographic fixer solution containing sodium thiosulfate
- To prevent environmental pollution proper disposal through dental vendors is mandatory
- Amalgam scrap and materials contaminated with mercury should not be incinerated or subjected to heat sterilization
- If mercury is spilled it should be cleaned as soon as possible using trap bottles
- If mercury comes in contact with the skin, it should be washed immediately with soap water
- Eye protection, disposable mask and gloves are standard requirement for dental practice
- The use of ultrasonic amalgam condenser should be avoided
- Heating of mercury or amalgam should be avoided.
- Yearly mercury determination of all dental personnel handling mercury should be done.

## BONDED AMALGAM

- The major drawback with nonbonded amalgam is that they do not bond with the tooth structure
- With the development of adhesive systems, bonding of amalgam with the tooth structure was proposed
- Amalgam is strongly hydrophobic, whereas enamel and dentin are hydrophilic
- Bonding system was, therefore, modified with a wetting agent that has the capacity to wet both the hydrophobic and hydrophilic surfaces
- Adhesive system containing (4-methacryloyloxyethy trimellitate anhydride) is used frequently
- The mechanism of bonding an amalgam restoration is similar to that for bonding a composite restoration in some aspects, but different in others
- A bonded amalgam restoration, done properly, seals the prepared tooth structure and strengthens the remaining unprepared tooth structure
- However, the retention gained by bonding may be minimal; consequently, bonded amalgam restorations still require the same tooth preparation as for nonbonded amalgam restorations
- It should also be noted that isolation requirements for a bonded amalgam restoration are the same as for a composite restoration
- Another amalgam technique gaining popularity is the use of light cured adhesive as a sealer under an amalgam restoration

- For this procedure, the prepared tooth structure is etched and primed and the adhesive placed and cured before insertion of amalgam
- This technique seals the tubules very effectively reducing marginal leakage and improving marginal integrity
- The shear bond strength of amalgam to dentin varies between 10 MPa and 14 MPa.

## Advantages

- Slightly increased strength of remaining tooth structure
- Minimal postoperative sensitivity
- Reduced microleakage
- Improved marginal seal
- Elimination of use of retention pins, slots or holes.

## Disadvantages

- Reduced bond strength over period of time
- Technique sensitive
- Costlier than nonbonded amalgam
- Isolation is critical
- No proven long-term clinical benefits.

# GALLIUM ALLOYS

- They are those types of alloy which is formed by the reaction of an alloy powder containing silver-tin-copper with gallium-based liquid containing gallium-indium and tin
- Because of a concern about the possible toxicity of mercury in amalgams, a number of materials have been developed
- Gallium alloys are an example of such a substitute made with silver-tin particles in gallium-indium
- If indium and tin is added appropriately, then melting temperature of gallium can be reduced below the room temperature
- Gallium melts at 28°C
- In this case, gallium-indium has been substituted for mercury in amalgam
- The ADA, in combination with the National Institute on Standards and Technology, has patented a mercury-free direct filling alloy based on silver-coated silver-tin particles that can be self-welded by compaction to create a restoration
- Use of gallium alloys have indicated mixing problems and early moisture sensitivity leading to excessive expansion
- Also, some potential corrosion products tend to accumulate on the intraoral surfaces.

## Composition

### Powder

- Silver: 50%
- Tin: 25.7%
- Copper: 15%
- Palladium: 9%
- Traces: 0.5%.

### Liquid

- Gallium: 65%
- Indium: 18.95%
- Tin: 16%
- Traces: 0.5%.

## Advantages

- Has strength similar to silver amalgam alloys
- Use of mercury is eliminated
- Gallium amalgam expands after trituration leading to better marginal seal
- Setting time of gallium alloy is less
- Creep is adequate
- Physical and mechanical properties similar to high-copper amalgam.

## Disadvantages

- Gallium alloys tends to stick to the instruments, thus handling is difficult
- Corrosion resistance of gallium alloys is less
- Technique sensitive to moisture contamination
- Shows expansion after setting.

# FAILURE OF DENTAL AMALGAM RESTORATIONS (FIG. 15.19)

*Amalgam restoration failures include:*
- Bulk fracture of the restorations
- Pain or sensitivity
- Secondary caries
- Corrosion
- Marginal fracture
- Fracture of the tooth structure forming restorative tooth preparation wall.

*Amalgam restoration failure can be of two types:*
1. *Mechanical failure*:
   - Marginal fracture of restoration
   - Improper manipulation of amalgam
   - Faulty finishing and polishing
   - Incorrect alloy mercury ratio

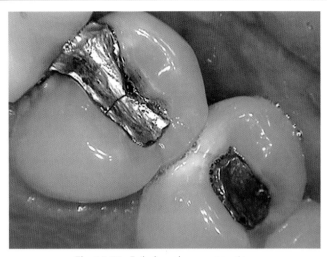

**Fig. 15.19:** Failed amalgam restoration.

– Inadequate tooth preparation
– Bulk fracture of restoration
– Tooth fracture
– Internal stresses due to excessive masticatory stresses
– Discoloration of tooth.

2. *Biologic failure*:
   – Pain after restoration

– Involvement of pulp
– Injury to the periodontium due to proximal overhangs
– Secondary caries due to marginal leakage
– Delayed expansion
– Tarnish and corrosion.

## Causes of Failed Amalgam Restorations

- Improper selection of the case
- Improper cavity design
- Inadequate proximal extension
- Inadequate depth of the preparation
- Undertriturated mixture
- Overtriturated mixture
- Incorrect alloy mercury ratio
- Tarnish and corrosion
- Moisture contamination during manipulation
- Fracture of amalgam due to stress concentration at sharp axiopulpal line angle
- Excessive heat buildup during finishing and polishing
- Improper adaptation of matrix during condensation
- Overhanging margins
- Inappropriate condensation
- Premature contact with opposing tooth
- Presence of $\gamma_2$ phase.

---

# TEST YOURSELF

## Essay Questions

1. Classify dental amalgam. Differentiate between low-copper amalgam and high-copper amalgam.
2. Discuss in detail composition, types, setting reaction and properties of high-copper amalgam.
3. Define trituration. Write in detail about manipulation of dental amalgam.
4. Describe setting reaction of high-copper amalgam.
5. Describe setting reaction of low-copper amalgam.
6. Write in detail about mercury toxicity due to amalgam use.
7. Describe in detail properties of dental amalgam.

## Short Notes

1. Delayed expansion.
2. Mulling.
3. Condensation of amalgam.
4. Mercury hygiene.
5. Microleakage and its significance.

6. Bonded amalgam.
7. Gallium alloys.
8. Eames technique.
9. Marginal ditching.
10. Mercuroscopic expansion.
11. Creep in dental amalgam.

## Multiple Choice Questions

1. In dental amalgam which two elements are main components:
   A. Silver and copper
   B. Copper and tin
   C. Silver and mercury
   D. Mercury and zinc
2. In an amalgam restoration which of the element helps in corrosion resistance the most?
   A. Silver
   B. Mercury
   C. Copper
   D. Iron

3. All instruments used for amalgam restorations should be thoroughly cleaned before autoclaving because:
   A. High temperature will melt the silver component of amalgam and will clog the drain of the autoclave
   B. Steam at high pressure will fuse amalgam to the stainless steel instruments
   C. The amalgam corrosion products are produced when in contact with steam
   d. High temperature will release mercury vapors from the amalgam

4. Compressive strength of dental amalgam is influenced by:
   A. Porosity
   B. Overtrituration
   C. Undertrituration
   D. All of the above

5. Unused amalgam should be:
   A. Placed in the incinerator
   B. Should be stored under water in sealed container
   C. Can be disposed off in general nonmedical waste bin
   D. Should be autoclaved before sending for recycling

6. Dental amalgam is commonly used to restore posterior teeth because:
   A. It is cheap
   B. Easy to manipulate
   C. Has excellent physical properties
   D. All of the above

7. During setting reaction of high-copper amalgam which metal reacts with copper to reduce the formation of gamma-2 phase
   A. Tin
   B. Zinc
   C. Silver
   D. Lead

8. Use of mercury in amalgam has been controversial because of:
   A. Safety concern in patient
   B. Risk to the office personnels
   C. Environmental hazard due to improper disposal of amalgam waste
   D. All of the above

9. Normally mixed amalgam should appear as:
   A. Shiny and soupy
   B. Dry and grainy
   C. As homogenous coalesced mass with slight shine
   D. Liquid-like which can be poured easily

10. Bonding of amalgam at the time of placement of restoration is to:
    A. Seal the margins and reduce microleakage
    B. Increases postoperative sensitivity
    C. Reduces tarnish
    D. Reduces corrosion

11. Which element when reacts with mercury hardens the amalgam?
    A. Copper
    B. Silver
    C. Tin
    D. Zinc

## ANSWERS

| | | | |
|---|---|---|---|
| 1. C | 2. C | 3. D | 4. D |
| 5. B | 6. D | 7. A | 8. D |
| 9. C | 10. A | 11. B | |

## BIBLIOGRAPHY

1. Anusavice KJ. Dental amalgam. Phillips' Science of Dental Materials, 11th edition. St. Louis: Saunders; 2003.
2. Bauer JG. A study of procedures for burnishing amalgam restorations. J Prosthet Dent. 1987;57:669-73.
3. Berry TG, Summitt JB, Chung AK, et al. Amalgam at the new millennium. J Am Dent Assoc. 1998;129:1547-56.
4. Brownawell AM, Berent S, Brent RL, Bruckner JV, Doull J, Gershwin EM, et al. The potential adverse health effects of dental amalgam. Toxicol Rev. 2005;24:1-10.
5. Browning WD, Johnson WW, Gregory PN. Clinical performance of bonded amalgam restorations at 42 months. J Am Dent Assoc. 2000;131:607-11.
6. Craig RG, Powers JM. Amalgam. Restorative Dental Materials, 11th edition. St. Louis: Mosby; 2002.
7. Dodes JE. The amalgam controversy: an evidence based analysis. J Am Dent Assoc. 2001;132:348-56.
8. Duperon DF, Nevile MD, Kasloff Z. Clinical evaluation of corrosion resistance of conventional alloy, spherical-particle alloy and dispersion-phase alloy. J Prosthet Dent. 1971;25:650-6.
9. Eames WB. Preparation and condensation of amalgam with a low mercuryalloy ratio. J Am Dent Assoc. 1959;58:78-83.
10. Greener EH. Amalgam—yesterday, today and tomorrow. Opera Dent. 1979;4:24-35.
11. Innes DBK, Youdelis WW. Dispersion strengthened amalgam. J Can Dent Assoc. 1963;29:587-93.
12. Jorgensen KD. The mechanism of marginal fracture of amalgam fillings. Acta Odontol Scand. 1965;23:347-89.
13. Klausner LH, Green TG, Charbeneau GT. Placement and replacement of amalgam restoration. A challenge for the profession. Oper Dent. 1987;12:105-12.
14. Letzel H, Vrijhoef MM. The influence of polishing on the marginal integrity of amalgam restorations. J Oral Rehabil. 1984;11:89-94.
15. Lloyd CH, Adamson M. The fracture toughness ($K_{IC}$) of amalgam. J Oral Rehabil. 1985;12:59-68.
16. Mahler DB. Research on dental amalgam: 1982-1986. Adv Dent Res. 1988;2:71-82.
17. Mahler DB, Adey JD, Marek M. Creep and corrosion of amalgam. J Dent Res. 1982;61:33-5.
18. Mahler DB, Pham BV, Adey JD. Corrosion sealing of amalgam restorations in vitro. Oper Dent. 2009;34:312-20.

19. Mahler DB, Terkla LG, Van Eysden J, et al. Marginal fracture vs mechanical properties of amalgam. J Dent Res. 1970;49:1452-7.

20 Mandel ID. Amalgam hazards: an assessment of research. J Am Dent Assoc. 1991;122:62-5.

21. May KN, Wilder AD, Leinfelder KF. Burnished amalgam restorations: A two year clinical evaluation. J Prosthet Dent. 1983;49:193-7.

22. Mjor IA. The safe and effective use of dental amalgam. Int Dent J. 1987;37:147-51.

23. Sutow EJ, Jones DW, Hall GC. Correlation of dental amalgam crevice corrosion with clinical ratings. J Dent Res. 1989;68:82-8.

24. Roberson TM, Heymann HO, Swift EJ. Sturdevant's Art and Science of Operative Dentistry: a contemporary approach, 5th edition. St. Louis: Mosby; 2006.

25. Sarkar NK, Park JR. Mechanism of improves corrosion resistance of Zn-containing dental amalgams. J Dent Res. 1988;67:1312-5.

26. Staninec M, Eakle WS, Silverstein S, et al. Bonded amalgam sealants: two-year clinical results. J Am Dent Assoc. 1998;129:323-9.

27. Staninec M. Retention of amalgam restorations: undercuts versus bonding. Quintessence Int. 1989;20:347-51.

28. Walker RS, Wade AG, Iazzetti G, et al. Galvanic interaction between gold and amalgam: Effect of zinc, time and surface treatments. J Am Dent Assoc. 2003;134:1463-7.

# Bonding and Bonding Agents

ADA Specification No. 27; ISO Specification No. 11405:2015

*'Do not confuse motion and progress. A rocking horse keeps moving but does not make any progress.'*
**—Alfred A Montapert**

## INTRODUCTION

One of the primary long-term goals of restorative dentistry is to achieve high strength and durable bond between the tooth structure and the restorative material. This type of bond will promote minimal invasive dentistry and will require adhesive system which will provide strong bond in load-bearing and nonload-bearing areas. This approach benefits by reducing treatment time, retaining restorative material without any form of retention aids, by preserving as much sound tooth structure as possible and by improving the quality of the interface between the restorative material and the tooth walls. Michael Buonocore in 1955, was first to establish the basis for modern adhesive dentistry by describing a technique of bonding acrylic materials with tooth enamel using phosphoric acid. Since then there has been lot of research in the area of adhesive dentistry.

## EVOLUTION OF BONDING

- *1940s (Dr Oscar Hagger):* Concept of adhesion to tooth structure. He developed the first bonding agent called Sevriton Cavity seal
- *1955 (Michael Buonocore):* Father of acid-etching technique. He investigated that phosphoric acid 85% provides superior etching of the tooth enamel

- *1962 (RL Bowen):* First-generation of dentin adhesive. NPG-GMA (N-phenylglycine-glycidyl methacrylate). He first introduced bis-GMA (bisphenol A glycidyl methacrylate) to dentistry
- *1968 (Smith):* Polycarboxylate cement.
- *1972 (Wilson and Kent):* Glass ionomer cement.
- *1978 (Osaco):* Second-generation of dentin adhesive—phosphate ester material, e.g. clearfil Bond system.
- *1979 (Fusayama):* Third-generation of dentin adhesive—application of acid-etching on dentin
- *1982 (Nakabayashi):* Fourth-generation of dentin adhesive—hybrid layer. He described the resin infiltration of dentin collagen as *hybrid layer*
- *1984 (Munksgaard and Asmussen):* Primer
- *1987 (Fusayama):* Fifth-generation of dentin adhesives—total etching and total bonding
- *1991–92 (J Kanca, Gwinnett):* Promoted total etching-total bonding concept in USA. He introduced the dentin wet bonding technique
- *1994 (Barkmeier and Chigira and Watanabe, et al).* Self-etching primer system
- *1997 (Swift-Ferrari-Goracci):* Self-etching adhesives (sixth-generation of dentin adhesives)
- *2000s–2015:* Self-etching and self-adhesive bonding systems popularized.

# INDICATIONS FOR USE OF BONDING AGENTS

- To restore carious or fractured tooth structure
- To alter the shape and color of anterior teeth
- To restore pits and fissure lesions
- To bond all ceramic restorations
- To bond the indirect restorations such as inlays or onlays
- To bond orthodontic brackets
- For better retention of cast crowns or metal ceramic restorations
- To repair fractured composite, porcelain, amalgam or ceramometal restorations
- To desensitize exposed root surfaces
- To bond prefabricated or cast posts
- To seal apical restorations placed during endodontic surgery.

# ADVANTAGES OF BONDING

- Bonds composite resin to tooth enamel and dentin.
- Reduces removal of tooth structure.
- Reduces chances of microleakage or nanoleakage.
- Beneficial in the management of dental hypersensitivity.
- Aids in cusp reinforcement after preparation of the tooth.
- Substantially reinforce remaining tooth enamel or dentin making them less susceptible to fracture.

# CONCEPT OF ADHESION

Adhesion is a process of bonding or attachment of dissimilar materials. Adhesives join two materials when applied to the surfaces to resist debonding and transfer stress across the bonds. The materials to be joined are called as *substrates* or *adherends*. The material used to cause adhesion between two surfaces is called as *Adhesive*. Adhesion is referred to as the bond strength in the dental literature.

## Definition

*Adhesion* is a molecular or atomic attraction between two contacting surfaces promoted by the interfacial force of attraction between the molecules or atoms of two different species.
- *Adhesive:* Those substances that promote adhesion of one material with another.
- *Adhesive bonding:* It is a process of joining two materials by an adhesive agent which hardens on setting.

## Types of Adhesion

- *Chemical adhesion*: Through covalent bonding, hydrogen bonds or polar bonds

- *Mechanical adhesion*: Structural interlocking
- Combination of chemical and mechanical adhesion.

## Requirements for Interface Formation for Adhesion

- The substrate surface should be clean
- Proper wetting of the substrate with adhesive is required Good wetting is ensured by small contact angle and the spreading of the adhesive onto the surface
- There should be intimate adaptation of the material to the substrate without air entrapment
- Should have sufficient physical, mechanical and chemical strength to resist the intraoral forces of debonding
- Adhesive should be well cured under recommended conditions
- Adequate removal of smear layer should be ensured before using adhesive.

## Mechanisms of Adhesion

According to Allen KW (1992), there are four mechanisms of adhesion:

1. *Mechanical adhesion:* It is one of the simplest mechanism of adhesion. Adhesion is achieved when adhesive is interlocked with the irregularities on the surface of substrate or adherend. The resin penetrates these irregularities and forms *resin tags* within the tooth surface and retained micromechanically. For example, adhesion between composite resin and the tooth structure.

2. *Adsorption adhesion:* It is also called as chemisorption method of adhesion. In this type of mechanism, chemical bonding occurs between the adhesive and substrate by primary (ionic and covalent) or secondary (hydrogen bonds, dipole interaction or Van der Waals) valence forces. For example, chemical bonding occurs between the hydroxyapatite crystals or type 1 collagen of tooth structure. Chemical bonding between the glass ionomer cement and the tooth structure.

3. *Diffusion adhesion:* It is the process of interlocking between two mobile molecules such as adhesion between two polymers through diffusion of polymer chains across the interface. By this process substances precipitates on the tooth surface to which resin monomers will bond mechanically or chemically. For example, diffusion of bonding agent within the collagen network of dentin. The rate of diffusion is directly proportional to the concentration gradient of the substance and the temperature.
   The process of diffusion also occurs in solids at molecular level in two ways:
   i. Atoms in the crystalline structure possess energy which is unequal. If this energy is greater than the

bonding energy amongst other atoms, it can move from one location to another within the lattice structure by diffusion

ii. In a crystalline solid structure, there can be space or vacancies at the temperature above absolute zero. Through these vacancies process of diffusion can occurs even in the state of equilibrium. This process is called as *self-diffusion*.

4. *Electrostatic adhesion:* In this type of mechanism electrical double layer is formed at the interface between the metal and the polymer. This type of adhesion does not take place in bonding resins to tooth structure. For example, this type of adhesion occurs between dental plaque and tooth enamel.

## Factors Influencing Adhesion (Fig. 16.1)

### Wetting

Wetting is defined as the relative interfacial tension between a solid substrate and liquid that results in a contact angle of less than 90°. For a strong adhesive joint, good wetting is absolutely essential. This requires the liquid to easily flow over the entire surface and adhere to the substrate. If liquid does not wet the surface of the substrate, adhesion will be poor or negligible. Wetting depends on the *clean* surface and the *surface energy* of the substrate. Cleaner the surface, greater the adhesion. Also, greater the surface energy of the adherend or substrate, greater the adhesion. Metal surfaces which are impurities free possess greater surface energy and will show strong adhesion with liquid adhesives.

### Surface Energy

Surface energy is defined as increase in energy per unit area of the surface. Solids or liquids are made of finite number of atoms or molecules which are bonded by primary or secondary bonds. In solids, the atoms in the lattice arrangement are equally attracted to each other. The interatomic distance between these atoms are equal and the energy is minimal. However, the outermost atoms at the surface of the lattice arrangement are not equally attracted to each other in all directions and their energy is greater. To overcome this energy, greater amount of force will be needed to disrupt the intermolecular bond between the atoms. This energy is called as surface energy. For adhesion, surfaces should be attracted to one another at the interface. In a solid, energy of the surface is more than that of the interior. The increase in energy per unit area of surface is called as *surface energy*. Greater the surface energy of the substrate, greater is the capacity of adhesion.

The energy on the surface per unit area is called as surface energy (in $mJ/m^2$) or surface tension (mN/m). Surface energy of some selected materials are given in **Table 16.1.**

### Contact Angle of Wetting

The extent to which the adhesive wets the surface of the adherend is determined by measuring the contact angle between them. Contact angle is the angle formed at the interface of the adhesive and the adherend. When forces of attraction between molecules of adhesive and that of the substrate is greater than the attraction between the molecules of an adhesive, then the liquid adhesive spreads more broadly over the solid substrate making a smaller contact angle. Smaller contact angle show that the adhesive forces of the interface is stronger than the cohesive forces which holds the molecules of adhesive together. Contact angle therefore indicates the wettability of the adhesive. There is complete wetting at the contact angle of 0° and no

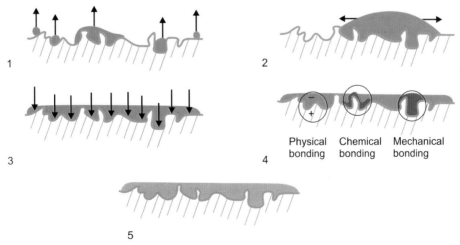

Physical bonding    Chemical bonding    Mechanical bonding

**Fig. 16.1:** Steps in formation of adhesion: (1) Clean surface; (2) Wetting by adhesive; (3) Close adaptation; (4) Good bonding; (5) Adequate curing of adhesive.

**Table 16.1:** Surface energy of some selected materials.

| Materials | Surface energy (mJ/m²) |
|---|---|
| Tooth enamel | 92 |
| Tooth dentin | 87 |
| Gold alloy | 50–54 |
| Ni-Cr alloy | 48 |
| Commercially pure titanium | 50 |
| Acrylic resins | 46–54 |
| Water | 72 at 25°C |
| Mercury | 486 at 25°C |
| Saliva | 53 at 37°C |
| Dentin bonding agent | 34–55 |

**Table 16.2:** Contact angles of probing liquid on some selected solid materials.

| Materials | Contact angle (in degrees) | Probing liquid |
|---|---|---|
| Acrylic denture resin | 75 | Water |
| Feldspathic porcelain | 71 | Water |
| Teflon | 110 | Water |
| Addition silicone | 34–105 | Water |
| Addition silicone (hydrophilic) | 20–78 | Water |
| Condensation silicone | 82–103 | Water |
| Polyether | 30–44 | Water |

wetting occurs at the angle of 180°. The contact angle less than 90° indicates good wetting whereas angle above 90° indicates poor wetting. Therefore, smaller the contact angle, better the wettability and adhesion.

> **CLINICAL SIGNIFICANCE**
>
> The adhesive with smaller contact angle will have better flow into the irregularity on the surface of the adherend. The fluidity of the adhesive affects the extent to which there irregularities are filled.

Contact angle of probing liquids on some selected materials is given **Table 16.2.**

For example, when the mixed gypsum is poured into the elastomeric impression then there should be proper wetting of the impression with the gypsum to ensure good surface quality of the master cast. For this reason, surfactant is first sprayed on the impression before pouring of the cast. Recent impression materials have wetting agent included in the composition by the manufacturer for betting wettability.

### Failure of Adhesion

Failure of adhesion can occur at any of three interfaces, i.e. within the substrate, at the interface between the substrate and adhesive and combination of the two. There are three types of bond failures:
1. *Adhesive failure*: In this type bond failure occurs at the interface of adhesive and the substrate. It can occur due to contamination of the substrate which lead to poor wetting with the adhesive or due to interfacial degradation.
2. *Cohesive failure*: This type of bond failure occurs within the adhesive. It can occur due to high thermal stress.
3. *Combination*: This type of bond failure occurs because of combination of adhesive and cohesive failure.

## SUBSTRATE STRUCTURE

### Structure of Enamel

Enamel is composed of 96% of inorganic matter by weight, 3% of water and 1% of organic material. The inorganic matter consists of hydroxyapatite crystals which are crystalline form of calcium phosphate. The organic material consists of proteins in the form of amelogenins and enamelins. Collectively, they are called as *biological apatite*. Enamel crystals which are hexagonal in structure and are elongated. Enamel crystals are in the form of rods which are arranged in the repetitive pattern called the *head and tail* arrangement. Unsupported enamel rods should be removed during cavity preparation or else there is tendency of dislodgement of the bonding during functional loading.

### Challenges with Bonding to Tooth Enamel and Dentin

- Composition of tooth enamel and dentin is different, i.e. both have different amount of organic and inorganic components
- Bonding agent which bonds with tooth enamel may not bond that well with tooth dentin
- Tooth prepared for bonding to create rough surface may entrap air at the interface
- Isolation of the prepared tooth from saliva, blood, etc.
- There is challenge of fluid exchange through certain components of tooth. Any bonding agent has to compete with water for wetting the tooth surface by displacing or incorporating it.

### Structure of Dentin

Dentin is much more complex than tooth enamel. It is a living tissue which is heterogeneous and consists of 50% volume of inorganic material (hydroxyapatite), 30% volume of organic material (type I collagen) and 20% volume of fluid as compared to enamel which is highly mineralized tissue containing more than 90% volume of hydroxyapatite. Greater proportion of crystals is interspersed among collagen fibers. Lower inorganic content allows greater elastic deformation during functional loading. They contain numerous fluid-filled dentinal tubules which arise from the pulp. Tubules are 0.5–1.5 μm in diameter and are formed at slight angle to the dentinoenamel junction (DEJ). Each dentinal tubule is surrounded by peritubular dentin. Peritubular dentin is surrounded by intertubular dentin which is 9% less mineralized than peritubular dentin.

Intertubular dentin forms the bulk of dentin and contains both organic and inorganic materials. The inorganic component consists of hydroxyapatite crystals which are plate-shaped and are much smaller than the crystals of enamel. The organic component consists of primarily type I collagen which acts as scaffold for mineralization and small amounts of noncollagenous proteins which help in mineralization. Collagen is usually nonsoluble in acid whereas noncollagenous proteins are soluble in acids which are used for etching. After decalcification, noncollagenous proteins are removed from the surface but the dentin matrix remains intact.

### Challenges in Dentin Bonding Substrate

- High fluid content in dentin interferes with bonding
- Fluid present in the dentinal tubules constantly flows outward which reduces the adhesion of resin to the dentin
- Its tubular nature provides a variable area through which dentinal fluid flows to the surface and adversely affects adhesion
- Because of its proximity to the pulp, there is susceptibility of biological effects which the chemicals can cause on the pulp
- Cut dentin surface results in the formation of smear layer which forms smear plugs, which fills the orifice of the dentinal tubules
- Presence of smear layer reduces dentin permeability by 86% thereby drastically reducing adhesion
- Use of vasoconstrictors in the local anesthesia reduces pulpal pressure and fluid flow in the tubules.

### Functions of Bonding Agent

- It seals interface between the tooth enamel or dentin and the restorative material thereby increasing resistance to microleakage decreasing chances of postoperative sensitivity, marginal staining and secondary caries
- It helps in distributing stress along the bonded interfaces

- It resists the separation of the substrate (tooth enamel, dentin, ceramic and composite) from the restorative material.

## ADHESION TO TOOTH STRUCTURE

### Acid Etch Technique

*Etching is defined as the process of increasing the surface reactivity by demineralizing the superficial calcium layer and thus creating the enamel tags.*

Acid etch technique was first introduced by *Michael Buonocore* in 1955. Phosphoric acid used by him as surface conditioning agent is still widely used as an etchant for bonding enamel and dentin. This technique is the most effective way of improving micromechanical bonding and marginal seal between the enamel and the resin. It is a simple, conservative and effective means of bonding resin to the tooth surface.

### Mechanism of Action

After tooth or cavity preparation, smear layer is formed on the surface of the tooth. It consists of entirely hydroxyapatite debris from high speed cutting during tooth preparation. When an etchant is applied to the tooth surface, it dissolves the smear layer and penetrates it (*see* **Fig. 16.4**). There is preferential dissolution of hydroxyapatite crystals from enamel and dentin to form microporous surface topography.

### Acid Treatment of Enamel

It depends on orientation of enamel crystals and rods. After removal of smear layer by acid etchant, there is differential dissolution of enamel crystals in each prism. The etched surface gives a *frosted* appearance. Scanning electron microscopic view of enamel bonding agent applied over the etched enamel shows cup-shaped macrotags and numerous fine microtags **(Fig. 16.2).**

### Acid Treatment of Dentin

The concept of etching of dentin gained popularity when Fusayama introduced the total-etch technique in 1979. His study claimed that etching with 37% phosphoric acid etched both the enamel and dentin simultaneously and has increased retention of the resin. Another study by *Nakabayashi* et al. (1984) stated that hydrophilic resins can infiltrate the acid demineralized dentin and can produce a strong resin dentin layer with numerous micromechanical interlocking called the *hybrid layer*. This technique in which the tooth is etched and then rinsed to remove acid is called as *total etch technique* or *etch and rinse technique.*

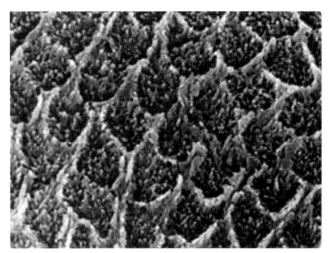

**Fig. 16.2:** Surface of enamel after etching with 37% phosphoric acid.

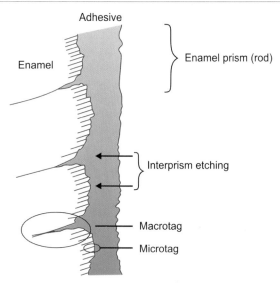

**Fig. 16.3:** Acid etching technique.

Acid etching of dentin with phosphoric acid first dissolves the smear layer and then exposes collagen, increasing dentin permeability and chemically modifies the surface to form a microporous surface. The microporous surface is composed of a complex network of collagen fibrils which are devoid of any mineral content and has significant amount of water containing displaced hydroxyapatite crystals. Also, during etching of dentin surface, acid soluble phosphoproteins are removed which are implicated in mineralization of collagen surfaces.

Etching of tooth surface increases total surface energy and creates contact angle which is effectively as low as zero. This enables the primer to readily wet the surface and penetrates the microporous surface. In dentin, it diffuses through the surface of demineralized region and entangles collagen fibers on polymerization. Resin copolymerizes with primer which has penetrated the micropores forming resin tags on polymerization. Resin tags are 6 µm in diameter and 10–20 µm in length and produces mechanical bond to enamel **(Figs 16.3 and 16.4).**

- *Different concentrations of phosphoric acid:*
  - *Buonocore:* 85% phosphoric acid
  - *Gwinnett:* 50% phosphoric acid—results in the formation of monocalcium phosphate monohydrate precipitate which can be easily rinsed off
  - Concentration 27% phosphoric acid results in formation of dicalcium phosphate monohydrate precipitate which cannot be easily removed and consequently interfere with adhesion
  - *Silver stone:* 30–40% phosphoric acid

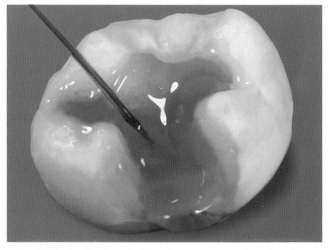

**Fig. 16.4:** Application of acid etchant on prepared tooth surface.

  - Current phosphoric acid gel: 37%
  - Concentrations greater than 50% results in the formation of monocalcium phosphate monohydrate which reduces further dissolution.
- *Etching time:*
  - Current etching time for most etching gels are 15 seconds
  - Greater etching time is required for teeth with greater fluoride content
  - Shorter etching time of 15 seconds results in acceptable bond strength which is comparable to etch time of 60 seconds.

## Classification of Micromorphologic Patterns of Enamel Etching

- *Type 1 (preferentially prism center etching):* Dissolution of enamel prism cores without dissolution of prism peripheries. The resulting tags are *cone* shaped
- *Type 2 (preferential prism periphery etching):* Dissolution of interprismatic enamel leaving the prism cores intact. The resulting tags are *cup*-shaped
- *Type 3 (mixed pattern):* Etching is less distinct than the other two patterns. The resulting area bears no resemblance to enamel prism.

### Procedure of Acid Etching (Figs. 16.5A to D)

- Tooth is cleaned and polished with pumice paste
- The acid etchant is applied onto the cleaned tooth surface for 15 seconds. Short etching time produces acceptable bond strength, reduces treatment time and conserves enamel
- The acid rinsed with stream of water for about 20 seconds and the tooth enamel is completely dried
- The dried enamel surface will appear *frosty white,* denoting a proper etching treatment **(Fig. 16.6)**
- After dentin is etched it should not be dried aggressively post-rinsing because it can lead to formation of impermeable collapsed collagen fibers which can cause bond failure
- When dentin is etched in total-etch technique, dentin bonding agent and primer is used which is compatible with both moist enamel and moist dentin

- Surface should be kept clean and dry before bonding agent is applied for sound mechanical bond. Etching increases the surface energy of the tooth enamel and reduces the contact angle to almost 0° thereby increasing the wettability
- Any contamination at this stage will result in reduced bond strength
- If contamination occurs with blood or saliva or oil through compressor line, the contaminant is removed and the tooth surface is again etched for 10 seconds before proceeding with the procedure.

*Bond strength:* Bond strength to etched enamel range between 15 MPa and 25 MPa

### Advantages of Enamel Adhesion

- Increased bond strength
- Adequate retention
- Prevent microleakage
- Cuspal reinforcement
- Less susceptible to fracture.

## DENTIN BONDING AGENT

### Definition

*A material used to promote adhesion or cohesion between two different substances or between a material and natural tooth structures.* —*GPT 8th Edition*

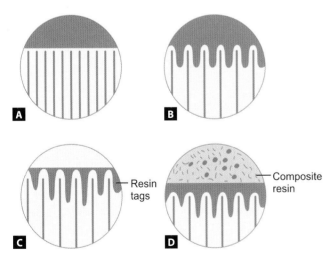

**Figs. 16.5A to D:** Procedure of acid etching: (A) Unetched enamel rods; (B) Etched enamel rods; (C) Enamel boding agent forming resin tags; (D) Composite resin bonded micromechanically.

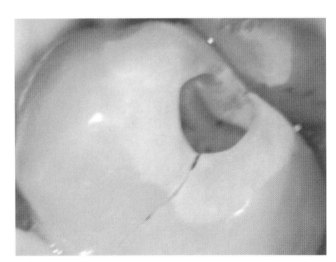

**Fig. 16.6:** Frosty white appearance of tooth enamel after etching.

## Ideal Requirements

- Should provide excellent bond strength
- Should provide immediate and durable bond
- Should adequately remove smear layer from the tooth substrate
- Should allow good wetting
- Should permit polymerization with tooth structure and copolymerization with composite resin matrix
- Should be able to maintain or reconstitute dentin collagen matrix
- Should prevent microleakage or nanoleakage
- Should be biocompatible and nonirritating
- Should be economical
- Should be easy to manipulate
- Should have high early strength in order to permit finishing and polishing
- Should provide strong durable bond with substrate and tooth structure
- Should ensure efficient monomer diffusion and penetration.

*Types of bonding observed in dentin bonding agents:*
- Micromechanical interlocking, chemical bonding with the tooth substrate
- Copolymerization with the composite resin matrix.

## Composition

*Bonding agents consists of:*
- Etchant
- Primers
- Adhesive
- Initiators and accelerators
- Fillers
- Other ingredients.

### Etchant or Conditioners

- It is defined as *an agent that is capable of etching a surface* ——*GPT 8th Edition*
- It is commonly used etchant is 37% *phosphoric acid* which is supplied in the form of gels
- Other materials used as etchant are maleic acid, tartaric acid, hydrofluoric acid, ethylenediamine-tetraacetic acid (EDTA), citric acid, polyacrylic acid, etc.
- *Fusayama et al. (1979)* concluded from their study that 37% phosphoric acid substantially improved the retention of the restoration and also did not harm the pulp
- Concentration of phosphoric acid more than 50% leads to formation of monocalcium phosphate monohydrate on the etched surface which inhibits further removal or dissolution of the smear layer

- Acid etchants are supplied in the form of gel which are formed by adding small amounts of microfillers or cellulose thickening agents. Colloidal silica can also be added to form acidic gel
- Etchant aids in removing the smear layer and creating micropores which allow infiltration of the resin monomers to allow subsequent curing.

### CLINICAL SIGNIFICANCE
It should be ensured during etching that air bubble is not incorporated because etching will not occur in the area of air pocket.

### Primers

- *It is a hydrophilic, low viscosity resin which permits adhesion to the substrate such as enamel or dentin*
- Primers are bi- or multifunctional molecules with chemical termination group that reacts with adherends. It has an adhesive group at one end to react with tooth enamel or dentin and polymerizable group at the other end to cross-link with resin overlayers
- After tooth etching when the surface is dried, the demineralized collagen network readily collapses. In order to maintain expanded collagen network without water for the infiltration of hydrophobic adhesive monomer, primer is required
- The adhesive and polymerizable layers are separated by a spacer which determines the properties of the primer including the solubility and wetting
- They are hydrophilic monomers dissolved in a solvent such as acetone, water or combination of ethanol and water
- In self-etching bonding agents, the primer which is acidic in nature contains carboxylic acid groups
- The primary function of the primer is to wet the surface and penetrate microporosities
- Commonly used primers are N-(4-tolyl)glycine-glycidyl methacrylate (NTG-GMA), hydroxyethyl methacrylate (HEMA), 4-methacryloyloxyethyl trimellitate anhydride (4-META) monomers dissolved into organic solvents.
- Some primers used in fourth- and fifth-generation bonding agents are solvent free
- Primers have different evaporation rates, drying patterns and penetration characteristics which influence the bond strength
- If the primer can both etch and prime at the same time then it is called as *self-etching primer.* In such primers acidic monomers are used. For example, HEMA-phosphate, phenyl-P, 10-MDP (10-methacryloyloxydecyl dihydrogen phosphate) and 4-META.

- Early dentin bonding agent used silane coupling agent instead of primers. These coupling agents were similar to the one which were used to bond inorganic fillers to the resin matric of composite resins. The coupling agents were based on M-R-X concept.

## What is M-R-X Concept?

**M-R-X** generically represent the silane coupling agent.
- **M:** It is an unsaturated methacrylate group or groups which can copolymerize with other monomers of the resin composite or resin cement
- **R:** It is a spacer which gives flexibility and mobility for the M and X groups, thereby increasing the reactivity of the groups
- **X:** It is a group which is capable of reacting chemically with the silica material such as glass and silicate fillers particles in composite resins, porcelain or with calcium ions in dental hard tissues.

    **M-R-X** concept was first used in the first dentin bonding system called as Sevriton (DeTrey of Amalgamated Dental which is now called Dentsply DeTrey, Germany).

    During bonding with dentin, the methacrylate group of the M-R-X molecule reacts with the resin matrix of the composite material and form a chemical bond between the composite and the tooth structure. The $Ca^{++}$ ions within the hydroxyapatite mineral phase of dentin chelates with the phosphate and the carboxylic groups.

## Adhesive

The rationale behind using adhesives in dentin bonding is to occupy the interfibrillar space of the collagen network forming the hybrid layer and the resin tags which on polymerization provide the micromechanical retention. Apart from this, it should also prevent leakage of fluid along the interface of tooth and the restorative material. The adhesives should be hydrophobic in order to resist permeation of the fluids along the intermediate layer. However, they require certain amount of hydrophilic component to allow diffusion into the hydrophilic primer wetted dentin surface. Usually adhesives are composed of resins of hydrophobic dimethacrylate oligomers which are compatible to monomers used in primers. These hydrophobic dimethacrylates are bisphenol A-glycidyl methacrylate (Bis-GMA), triethylene glycol dimethacrylate (TEGDMA), urethane dimethacrylates and small amount of hydrophilic monomer such as HEMA. The dimethacrylates show high bond strength but inevitability absorbs water and swells. Recent research reveals that carbamides are more hydrolytically stable than ester groups. For this reasons methacrylates have been replaced by methacrylamides.

## Solvents

The primers and the adhesives should have low viscosity to flow into the resin tags. The low viscosity is partly because of dissolution of the monomers in the solvent. The most commonly used solvents are water, ethanol and acetone. Apart from improving wetting of the dentin surface, solvents also contributes to the improve bond adhesion. The function of water is to re-expand the collapsed collagen network and ionize the acidic monomers. Ethanol is used in conjunction with water as a cosolvent. This water alcohol mixture is called as "azeotropic" as they form hydrogen bonds between the water and ethanol molecules resulting in better evaporation of the water-ethanol aggregates as compared to pure water. Although acetone has four times higher vapor pressure than ethanol but it is highly volatile in comparison. High volatility of acetone reduces the shelf life of acetone containing adhesives by higher rate of evaporation of the solvent. Ethanol and acetone containing solvents have better miscibility with relatively hydrophobic monomers.

## Initiators and Accelerators

Mostly bonding agents are light cured and contains activators such as camphorquinone and an initiator such as organic amine. In dual cure initiator system, the self-cure initiator component is benzoyl peroxide.

## Fillers

Most bonding agents are unfilled but some may contain fillers ranging between 0.5% and 40% by weight. Filler particles include microfillers called as "nanofillers". Filled bonding agents produce higher bond strength. Role of fillers as strengthening agent in adhesive is debatable as it is not clear whether these filler particles actually penetrate into the demineralized collagen networks. The reason being the interfibrillar space between the collagen networks is in the range of 20 nm whereas the size of filler particles is in the range of 40 nm.

## Other Ingredients

- May contain glutaraldehyde as desensitizer
- The adhesive marketed by 3M ESPE (Adper Prompt, Single Bond, Scotchbond Multipurpose) contains polyalkenoic copolymer to provide better moisture stability
- Fluorides are added to prevent secondary caries
- Benzalkonium chloride and chlorhexidine is added to prevent collagen degradation

- Component such as parabene, 12-methacryloyloxy-dodecylpyridinium bromide are added as antimicrobials in the monomer.

# PROPERTIES OF DENTIN BONDING AGENTS

## Bond Strength

- The efficacy of dentin bonding agents is usually evaluated by measuring its bond strength. There are various tests available to measure the bond strength of adhesives
- Factors which can show variable results during measuring of the bond strengths are: Amount of water content, presence or absence of smear layer, dentin permeability, orientation of the dentinal tubules relative to the surface and method employed to measure the bond strength
- Dentin bonding agent with bond strength of 20 MPa is considered as optimal.

### Classification of Bond Strength Testing Methods

Based on the size of the bonded area, bond strengths can be tested as:
1. Macrobond strength testing method
2. Microbond strength testing method.

- *Macrobond strength testing method*: Macrobond strength can be measured under shear or tensile or push or pull method
  - *Macroshear bond testing*: It is one of the most commonly used testing method for measuring the macrobond strength. In this test, a composite cylinder with a diameter of about 3–4 mm is polymerized on a flat ground enamel or dentin surface after applying the dentin bonding agent. Testing can be done immediately or after 24 hours of bonding or after several months in water storage at 37°C. Shear force is applied parallel to the tooth surface in order to shear the composite cylinder
  - *Pullout testing*: In this testing also shear force is applied. Benefit with this testing is that both bond strength and marginal adaptation using scanning electron microscope (SEM) can be evaluated using same specimen. However, its disadvantage is that during water storage, the composite specimen can swell inducing significant amount of friction which can actually misinterpret the adhesive performance
  - *Macrotensile bond testing*: This testing is similar to macroshear bond testing except tensile force component is used to assess bond strength.

- *Microbond strength testing method*: One distinct advantage of microbond strength testing is the ability to evaluate the effect of local tooth structure on the bond strength and depth profiling of the different substrates. To measure bond strength with microbond testing both shear and tensile forces are used.
  - *Microshear bond testing*: This method is useful when brittle substrates are used. Here shear force is applied at the tooth and adhesive interface. The Finite element analysis shows that the results obtained are influenced by highly nonuniform stress distribution which can underestimate the local stresses causing fracture of the specimen
  - *Microtensile bond testing*: This type of testing is one of the most acceptable testing currently used to measure the bond strength of the dentin bonding agents.

*Advantages of microtensile testing method:*
- More adhesive failure and less cohesive failure
- Higher initial bond strengths
- Allows measurement of local bond strength
- Allows testing of bonding of the irregular surfaces
- Allows testing of very small areas
- Facilitates SEM analysis of the failed bonds.

*Disadvantages of microtensile testing method:*
- Technique sensitive
- Difficult to measure bond strength less than 5 MPa
- Require special equipment
- Size of sample is small which can dehydrate easily.

## Microleakage

The degree of microleakage is measured by penetrating tracers and staining agents at the restoration tooth interface. Recent bonding agents show greater resistance to microleakage and better bond strength.

## Aging Effect

It is important to study the aging effect on the bond strength to predict durability of the bonding agent clinically. This is done by using various aging tests. Studies reveal that three step bonding agents show little or no change in the bond strength as compared to two-step bonding agents which show significant decrease in the bond strength over a period of 4–5 years. The durability of the bond can greatly increase if the good bonding occurs at the peripheral etched enamel which seals the resin tooth interface from leakage. Studies with transmission electron microscope (TEM) have shown that degradation of the hybrid layer is one of the primary reasons for aging of the bond.

# SMEAR LAYER

As mentioned before, cut dentin surface involves the formation of smear layer which blocks the orifice of dentinal tubules by smear plugs. Presence of smear layer reduces permeability of dentin by 86%, thereby reducing adhesion. Smear layer is briefly discussed in the following section:

## Definition

*It is a tenacious deposit of microscopic debris which covers the tooth enamel and dentin after tooth preparation.* It can also be described as poorly adherent layer of ground dentin which is produced by cutting dentin surface.

The term *smear layer* was coined by Boyde, Switsur and Stewart (1963). It consists of two separate layers, a superficial layer and loosely attached layer to the underlying dentin. Clinically produced smear layers have an average depth of 1–5 mm. When tooth structure is prepared by a bur, residual organic or inorganic components form the smear layer. The smear layer fills the orifice of dentinal tubules to from *smear plugs* **(Figs. 16.7 and 16.8).**

### Components of Smear Layer

Smear layer consists of both organic and inorganic components.
- *Inorganic component:* It contains tooth structure and nonspecific inorganic debris
- *Organic components* contain:
    - Heat coagulated proteins such as gelatin formed by the deterioration of collagen heated during tooth preparation
    - Nonviable or viable pulp tissue
    - Odontoblastic processes
    - Quality of saliva
    - Some blood cells
    - Microorganisms.

*Factors affecting the depth of smear layer are:*
- Dry or wet cutting of the dentin
- The type of instrument used
- The amount and chemical used for irrigation.

### Role of Smear Layer in Dentin Bonding

Smear layer consists of two layers:
1. *Solid phase:* Made up of cutting debris. Primarily denatured collagens
2. *Liquid phase:* Made up of tortuous fluid-filled channels around the cutting debris.
    - Smear layer, may also be a deterrent to the bonding process, since it may serve as a barrier to the penetration of resin to the underlying dentin substrate.
    - The removal of smear layer **(Fig. 16.9)** and demineralization of dentin matrix may facilitate bonding through a number of mechanisms like exposed collagen promotes micromechanical bonding to resin by providing a framework.

*Agents used for smear layer removal are:*
- About 37% phosphoric acid
- Polyacrylic acid
- Chelating agents, EDTA
- Maleic acid
- Citric acid.

# HYBRIDIZATION THEORY

This theory was first proposed by *Nakabayashi* (1982) and it is the most commonly accepted theory for adhesion to dentin. Demineralization of superficial dentin by acid etching exposes collagen fibril network having inter- and

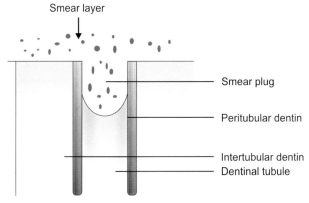

Smear layer

Smear plug

Peritubular dentin

Intertubular dentin
Dentinal tubule

**Fig. 16.7:** Smear layer.

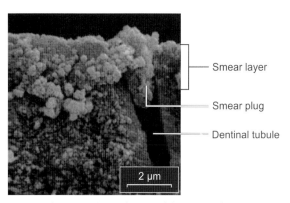

Smear layer

Smear plug

Dentinal tubule

2 μm

**Fig. 16.8:** Smear layer and the smear plugs.

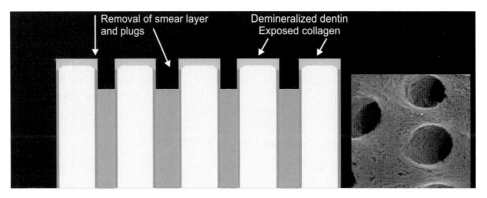

**Fig. 16.9:** Removal of smear layer.

intrafibrillar microporosities. When low viscosity monomers are placed in contact of this surface it diffuses into the demineralized region to form resin-dentin interdiffusion zone. Polymerization of this zone forms a hybrid zone of resin-reinforced dentin. Formation of this hybrid layer is said to be the primary bonding mechanisms for most of the adhesive systems.

## Classification of Bonding Agents

- *Based on the chronology of development dentin bonding agents (Fig. 16.10)*:
  - First-generation bonding agent
  - Second-generation bonding agent
  - Third-generation bonding agent
  - Fourth-generation bonding agent
  - Fifth-generation bonding agent
  - Sixth-generation bonding agent
  - Seventh-generation bonding agent.
- *Based on the type of substrate*:
  - Enamel bonding agent
  - Dentin bonding agent.
- *Based on the interaction with the smear layer*:
  - Smear layer modifying agents
  - Smear layer removing agents
  - Smear layer dissolving agents.
- *Based on number of clinical steps and mechanism of adhesion (according to Van Meerbeek 2003)*:
  - *Etch and rinse adhesives*:
    - Fourth-generation three-step adhesive: Conditioner, primer and adhesive
    - Fifth-generation two-step adhesive: Conditioner, combined primer and adhesive resin.

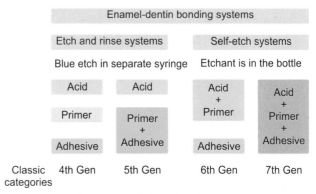

**Fig. 16.10:** Different enamel-dentin bonding agents generations.

- *Self-etch adhesives*:
  - Sixth-generation two-step: Self-etching primer and adhesive resin
  - Seventh-generation one-step: Self-etching primer/adhesive two components; self-etching primer one components.

### First-generation Dentin Bonding Agents

- Early dentin bonding agents were based on application of silane coupling agents such as glycerophosphoric acid dimethacrylate which is used to provide bifunctional molecule
- The hydrophilic phosphate part reacted with calcium ions of the hydroxyapatite
- The hydrophobic methacrylate groups bonded to the acrylic resin (unfilled resins)
- N-phenylglycine-glycidyl methacrylate, a surface active comonomer was the basis of first commercially available dentin bonding agent.

- N-phenylglycine-glycidyl portion chelate with calcium in dentin to form a water resistance chemical bond
- Mechanism of bonding is due to deep penetration of the resin tags into the exposed dentinal tubules after etching and chelating component which bonds to the calcium component of dentin
- So they form a stronger bond with enamel rather than dentin
- First commercial dentinal adhesives, e.g. Crevident-SS white (1965).

### Disadvantages

- First-generation bonding agents ignored the smear layer.
- They had very *low bond strength* 2–3 MPa
- The bond strength was not durable and individual component lacked stability during storage.

### Second-generation Dentin Bonding Agents

- Introduced in 1978, commercial product being Clearfil bond system F, e.g. Clearfil Bond, Scotchbond, Bondite and Prisma Universal Bond
- It was composed of phosphate ester material [phenyl P and hydroxyethyl methacrylate (HEMA)] dissolved in ethanol
- Bonding was due to polar interaction between positively charged $Ca^{++}$ ions present in the smear layer and the negatively charged phosphate ions in the resin matrix
- The resins were devoid of hydrophilic group and had large contact angles on intrinsically moist surfaces. Smear layer was the weakest link because of its loose attachment to the dentin surface
- These bonding agents did not properly wet the dentin and could not penetrate the entire depth of smear layer
- Performance of second-generation adhesives was unacceptable after six months
- Bonding material showed tendency to peel from the dentin surface after water storage indicating that the interface between dentin and some types of chlorophosphate ester-based material was unstable
- *Three types are available:*
    1. Etched tubule dentin bonding agent.
    2. Phosphate ester dentin bonding agent.
    3. Polyurethane dentin bonding agent.

### Disadvantages

- Very low bond strength of 1–5 MPa
- In vitro performance clinically unacceptable.

### Third-generation Dentin Bonding Agents

- Two-components primer and adhesive system were introduced
- Alteration or removal of the smear layer is done before bonding
- Conditioning agents included HEMA solution of maleic acid, 2% aqueous nitric acid, 10% citric acid and aqueous EDTA
- This type dentin adhesive was based on use of acid group to react with $Ca^{++}$ ions and a methacrylate group to copolymerize with unfilled resin which was applied before placing the composite resin.

*Two approaches were employed:*
1. Modifying the smear layer to improve its properties
2. Removal of smear layer without disturbing the smear plugs which occluded the dentinal tubules.

### Involves Four Steps

1. Etching with an acid conditioner to remove smear layer
2. Priming with a bifunctional resin in a volatile solvent
3. Bonding with an unfilled or partially filled resin
4. Placement of resin-based composite.

### Advantages

- High bond strength 8–15 Mpa
- Reduced chances of microleakage
- Forms strong bond to wet and dry dentine
- Requirement for retention in the tooth preparation is reduced.

### Disadvantages

- Bond strength reduced over a period of time
- Chances of microleakage increases with time.

*Examples of third-generation bonding agents:*
- *Tenure (oxalate system)*: Acid solution of ferric oxalate to alter smear layer
- *GLUMA*: Mechanical bond to dentin chemical bond to collagen
- *Scotchbond II*: Primer is an aqueous solution of HEMA acidified with maleic acid.

### Fourth-generation Dentin Bonding Agents (Fig. 16.11)

- Introduced in 1990s called as *total-etch technique or etch and rinse technique*
- Concept was proposed by *Fusayama T* (1979)
- Based on the removal of smear layer and bonding of resin to the dentin substrate
- Application of conditioner to the dentin results in partial or total removal of the smear layer. It is called total etch

**4th Generation (3 Steps)**
1. Etchant
2. Primer
3. Adhesive

— Total etch
— Formation of hybrid layer
— Acceptable bond strength (17–25 Mpa)

• Compobond LCM
• Scotchbond MP
• Syntac

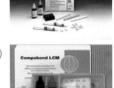

**Fig. 16.11:** Fourth-generation bonding agents.

as it involves simultaneous application of an acid to enamel and dentin
• The acid demineralizes intertubular and peritubular dentin exposing the collagen fibers
• Dentin is demineralized up to depth of 7.5 µm depending on the type, amount of acid used and time of application
• When primer and bonding agents are applied to the etched dentin it results in the formation of resin-dentin intertubular zone or *hybrid layer.*

### Components of Fourth-generation Bonding Agents

1. *Conditioner (etchant):* Commonly used acids are 37% phosphoric acid, nitric acid, maleic acid, oxalic acid, hydrochloric acid and citric acid. They aid in removal of the smear layer
2. *Primer:* It consists of monomers like HEMA (2-hydroxyethyl methacrylate) and 4-META dissolved in acetone or ethanol. They enhance wettability of the dentin surface and help in binding between the dentin and resin and encourage monomer infiltration of demineralized peritubular and intertubular dentin
3. *Adhesives:* It is a low viscosity semifilled or unfilled resin which flows easily and combines with the monomers to

form a resin reinforced hybrid layer and resin tags to seal the dentine tubules.

### Steps Involved (**Figs. 16.12A to D**)

• Simultaneously etch dentin and enamel with conditioner for 15 seconds
• Rinse to remove etchant and dissolved tooth minerals
• Dry with air to ensure adequate etching
• Slightly moisten the surface before applying the primer. Care is taken so that the collagen mesh is not desiccated. Desiccation will lead to collapse of collagen network and form dense film which is difficult to infiltrate with the primer. The hydrophilic primer penetrates the collagen network when applied on moist dentin surface. Primer is then cured adequately
• Dry to remove primer solvent
• Adhesive is then applied to enamel and dentin and is cured
• Then composite resin is applied over the adhesive and then cured.

### Advantages

• Ability to bond to both enamel and dentin
• Results in increased bond strength of 17–30 MPa
• Bonds to moist dentin.
Examples of fourth-generation bonding agents:
• All Bond 2 (Bisco)
• Optibond FL (Kerr)
• Scotchbond Multipurpose (3M).

### Fifth-generation Dentin Bonding Agents (**Fig. 16.13**)

• Referred as *one bottle, total etch bonding agents*
• In this type, the primer and bonding agents are combined in a single bottle but a separate etching step is required
• This makes the bonding system simpler and faster as compared to fourth-generation bonding agents.

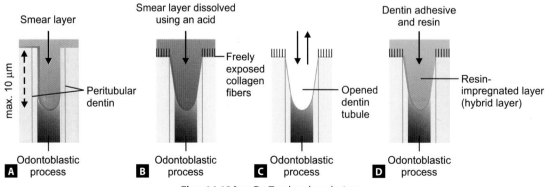

**Figs. 16.12A to D:** Total-etch technique.

5th Generation (2 Steps)
1. Etchant
2. Single component
(Primer + Adhesive)

— Total etch (E and D)
— Wet bonding
— Formation of hybrid layer
— Acceptable bond strength (20–24 MPa)

• Exite
• Single-bond
• One-step

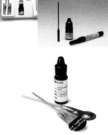

**Fig. 16.13:** Fifth-generation bonding agent.

## Advantages

- Higher bond strength
- Easy to use
- Reduced number of steps
- Less technique sensitive
- Faster and simpler
- Reduced postoperative sensitivity.

## Disadvantages

Less bond strength than fourth-generation bonding agents.

## Composition

1. Acid etching agent: Thirty-seven percent phosphoric acid.
2. Primer and bonding agent in one bottle.

Examples of fifth-generation bonding agents are:
- One step plus (Bisco)
- Prime and bond NT (Denstply)

- Adper single bond plus (3M)
- Optibond SOLO plus (Kerr)
- Excite (Ivoclar Vivadent).

## Sixth-generation Dentin Bonding Agents

- These are also called as self-etching-primer system
- Sixth-generation bonding agents are divided into two types:
  - Type I: Self-etching primer
    - Available in two bottles-primer and adhesive
    - Primer is applied before the adhesive
    - Water is used as solvent in these systems. Water aids in ionization of the primer. Water-based adhesives have lower strength than acetone-based adhesives because water inhibits polymerization of the adhesive monomers, e.g. Clearfil SE bond.
  - Type II: Self-etching adhesives (all-in-one)
    - Supplied in two bottles-primer and adhesive
    - A drop from each is mixed and then applied to the tooth surface
    - They use polymerizable acidic monomers to simultaneously demineralize and prime tooth surfaces, e.g. Adper Prompt L-Pop, Xeno III.
- Self-etching primers are acidic primers which include a phosphonated resin molecule which etch and prime together. Here the etching step is eliminated
- Mechanism of bonding is based on simultaneous etching and priming of enamel and dentin incorporating smear plugs into the resin tags **(Fig. 16.14)**
- Rinsing and drying step is eliminated thereby reducing the chances of overdrying and overwetting.

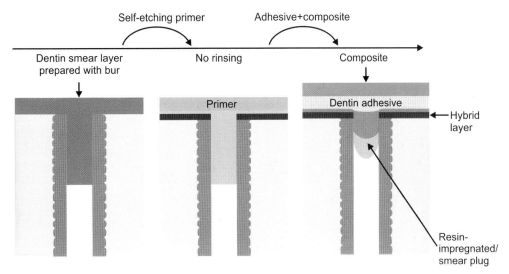

**Fig. 16.14:** Mechanism of bonding in sixth-generation bonding agents.

- Water is integral part of this system as it is required to ionize the acidic monomers and demineralize the dental hard tissues
- They do not etch enamel as well as the dentin
- Self-etching primers are classified according to acidity as mild, moderate and severe
- Mild self-etching primers provide excellent dentin bond strength and poor enamel bonds
- While severe or aggressive self-etching primer provide excellent enamel bond strength and poor dentin bond strength.

### Advantages

- Reduced postoperative sensitivity
- Faster and less technique sensitive
- Lesser number of steps involved.

### Disadvantages

- May require refrigeration
- As they have acidic solution storage is difficult
- Promote water sorption.

### Seventh-generation Dentin Bonding Agents (Fig. 16.15)

- Seventh-generation bonding agents introduced in the early 2000s
- Also called as self-etching adhesives or all-in-one. Separate etching and mixing steps are eliminated in this system
- They contain acidic primers and adhesive monomers in a single bottle. They can etch, prime and bond in a single application. Acidic monomer in this system contains a polymerizable group which copolymerizes with other monomers and subsequently added bonded resins
- The acidic primer helps in demineralizing the smear layer which is used as a bonding substrate. The smear layer is not rinsed because it is part of the *hybrid layer*. This layer is approximately 0.5–5 μm. With this the collagen is exposed and is penetrated by hydrophilic monomer which polymerizes along with the primer

- In this technique as water is used as a solvent drying or wetting of the dentin surface is less critical in comparison to bonding agents with ethanol or acetone solvents
- The adhesive tends to behave as semipermeable membranes which results in hydrolytic degradation of resin-dentin interface
- They are available both as light cured and dual cured products. Although in dual cure formulation separate catalyst is required during mixing
- They should be refrigerated to maintain stability during storage. Increased storage or increase in temperature reduces its stability
- Chances of voids, potential marginal leakage, and postoperative sensitivity is reduced
- Clinical performance of bonding agents is based on the amount of bond strength with enamel and dentin
- The bond strength for enamel and dentin are 19 MPa-32 MPa and 18 MPa-28 MPa, respectively which is comparable to bond strengths of other generation bonding agents
- This bonding agent is found to be incompatible with self-cured composites as the acidic primer tends to interfere with the curing process of these resins
- Usually light cured bonding agents are advised for bonding direct resin composites and ceramic veneers
- This adhesive tends to behave as semipermeable membranes which results in hydrolytic degradation of resin-dentin interface
- This generation bonding agents have shown disinfecting and desensitizing properties, e.g. G bond and i bond.

### Other Clinical Applications of Dental Adhesives

#### Glass Ionomer Restoratives

Glass ionomer materials are already discussed in chapter on dental cements. These materials show chemical bonding to the tooth structure. They have high fluoride releasing capacity and are very useful for patient having high caries index. They are translucent and are used as esthetic filling material in class V lesions (*see* page 310, Chapter 18).

### Desensitization

Dentin hypersensitivity is one of the common clinical conditions which at times are difficult to treat. It is best explained by the hydrodynamic theory. Patient often complains of discomfort when teeth are subjected to temperature changes, chemical erosion, mechanical

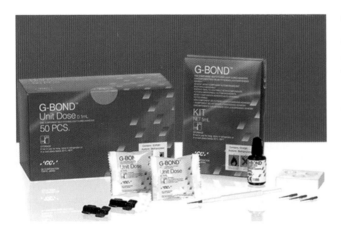

**Fig. 16.15:** Seventh-generation bonding agent.

abrasion, tactile stimulation and osmotic gradients. The cervical portion of the tooth is the most common site of hypersensitivity. Dentin hypersensitivity is common in patient with gingival recession and root surface exposure.

Dentin bonding agents are used to treat hypersensitive root surfaces. Reduction of sensitivity is due to the formation of resin tags and a hybrid layer on application of dentin bonding agents. Occlusion of dentinal tubules on using dentin bonding agents reduces sensitivity. Other methods of treating hypersensitivity include use of desensitizing paste, $CO_2$ laser application, antibacterial agents, fluoride rinses, fluoride varnishes, calcium phosphates, potassium nitrate and oxalates (*see* page 501, Chapter 28).

## Bonded Amalgam Restorations

To reduce microleakage in amalgam restorations, resin based adhesives are used to bond amalgam restorations. The attachment of adhesive to amalgam may be because of mechanical bonding of the uncured adhesive material with setting amalgam mix during condensation of amalgam. Shear bond strength between the adhesive and amalgam is shown to be 10–14 MPa with some currently used adhesive systems.

Use of dental bonding agents below amalgam reduces microleakage and improves marginal integrity of the restoration. It has also shown to improve the fracture resistance of the residual tooth structure under amalgam restorations (*see* page 234, Chapter 15).

## Indirect Adhesive Restorations

Indirect ceramic and resin based restorations are bonded with the help of universal adhesive systems. Resin cements along with these universal adhesive system provides a durable bonding of the indirect restorations. The internal surfaces of ceramic restorations are often etched with 6–10% hydrofluoric acid for 1–2 minutes except for aluminous core and zirconia core ceramics. The hydrofluoric acid is then rinsed off for 2 minutes and the surface is dried using three way air syringe. A silane coupling agent is applied on the etched surface and air dried. The coupling agent acts as primer as it modifies the surface characteristics of the etched ceramic surface. The use of silane coupler increases the bond strength between resin cement and ceramic by 25%. Indirect composite restorations can also be bonded using universal adhesive system. Benefit of indirect composite restoration is that polymerization shrinkage occurs outside the mouth.

# TEST YOURSELF

## Essay Questions

1. Classify dentin bonding agents. Discuss the etch and rinse technique.
2. Describe the acid-etch technique.
3. Describe the patterns of etching seen in the enamel.
4. Discuss the self-etch bonding systems.
5. Discuss the self-adhesive system.
6. Discuss in detail the composition of dentin bonding systems.

## Short Notes

1. Hybrid layer.
2. Role of primers in bonding.
3. Challenges in bonding to dentin.
4. Principles of adhesion.
5. Wetting.
6. Contact angle.
7. Application of bonding agents.

## Multiple Choice Questions

1. Most commonly used acid to etch tooth surface during bonding is:
   A. Citric
   B. Phosphoric acid
   C. Hydrochloric acid
   D. Hydrofluoric acid
2. Smear layer:
   A. Is necessary for bonding
   B. Is tenacious layer of cut tooth debris and contaminants from the saliva
   C. Is easily removed by rinsing with water
   D. Is left on the surface of dentin when bonding agent is applied
3. Adhesion to dentin:
   A. Is accomplished when the dentin is kept moist after etching
   B. Is best when the dentin surface is etched with 35% phosphoric acid for 30 seconds

C. Is inhibited by the formation of hybrid layer

D. Is stronger when the dentin is dried after etching

4. Hypersensitivity to dentin can be caused by:

A. Opened dentinal tubules

B. Changes in pressure within the dentinal tubules

C. Stimulation of odontoblastic processes within the dentinal tubules

D. Desiccation of the etched surface

E. All of the above

5. Bonding to enamel is not:

A. Achieved by micromechanical retention

B. Achieved by chemical retention

C. Achieved by resin tags penetrating irregularities on the enamel surface

D. Stronger than bonding to dentin

6. Good adhesion is possible by which of the following:

A. Saliva or blood on the etched tooth surface

B. Oil from the handpiece

C. Moist dentin after rinsing of the etched surface and drying it lightly

D. Eugenol containing temporary cements

7. The primary constituent of dentin bonding agents is:

A. HEMA

B. bis-GMA

C. Methyl methacrylate

D. 37% phosphoric acid

8. Clinical significance of smear layer is:

A. Provides calcium for adhesion to composites

B. Increases wetting action of the bonding agents

C. Bonded to the tooth structure and prevents composite adhesion

D. All of the above

## ANSWERS

| | | | |
|---|---|---|---|
| 1. B | 2. B | 3. A | 4. E |
| 5. B | 6. C | 7. A | 8. C |

## BIBLIOGRAPHY

1. Akpata ES, Behbehani J. Effect of bonding systems on postoperative sensitivity from posterior composites. Am J Dent. 2006;19:151-4.

2. Anusavice KJ. Phillip's science of dental materials, 11th edition. St. Louis: Saunders; 2003.

3. Asmussen E, Munksgaard EC. Bonding of restorative resins to dentin: status of dentine adhesives and impact on cavity design and filling techniques. Int Dent J. 1988;38:97-104.

4. Bowen RL, Eichmiller FC, Marjenhoff WA, et al. Adhesive bonding of composites. J Am Coll Dent. 1989;56:10-3.

5. Buonocore MG. A simple method of increasing the adhesion of acrylic filling materials to the enamel surfaces. J Dent Res. 1955;34:849-53.

6. Buonocore MG. The use of adhesives in dentistry. Springfield, IL: Charles C Thomas; 1975.

7. Cardoso MV, de Almeida Neves A, Mine A, Coutinho E, Van Landuyt K, De Munck J, et al. Current aspects on bonding effectiveness and stability in adhesive dentistry. Aust Dent J. 2011;56:31-44.

8. Consensus development conference statement on dental sealants and the prevention of tooth decay. National Institutes of Health. J Am Dent Assoc. 1984;108:233-6.

9. Douglas WH. Clinical status of dentine bonding agents. J Dent. 1989;17:209-15.

10. Fusayama T, Nakamura M, Kurosaki M, et al. Non-pressure adhesion of a new adhesive restorative resin. J Dent Res. 1979;58:1364-70.

11. Gilpatrick RQ, Ross JA, Simonsen RJ. Resin to enamel bond strength with various etching times. Quintessence Int. 1991;22:47-9.

12. Gwinnett AJ, Kanca J. Micromorphology of the bonded dentin interface and its relationship to bond strength. Am J Dent. 1992;5:73-7.

13. Gwinnett AJ, Tay FR, Pang KM, Wei SH. Quantitative contribution of the collagen network in dentin hybridization. Am J Dent. 1996;9:140-4.

14. Haller B. Which self-etch bonding systems are suitable for which clinical indications? Quintessence Int. 2013;44:645-61.

15. Houpt M, Fuks A, Eidelman E. The preventive resin (composite resin/sealant) restoration: nine-year results. Quintessence Int. 1994;25:155-9.

16. Ikemura K, Endo T. A review of our development of dental adhesives—effects of radical polymerization initiators and adhesive monomers on adhesion. Dent Mater J. 2010;29:109-21.

17. Kamada K, Yoshida K, Taira Y, et al. Shear bond strengths of four resin bonding systems to two silica-based machinable ceramic materials. Dent Mater J. 2006;25:621-5.

18. Liu Y, Tjäderhane L, Breschi L, Mazzoni A, Li N, Mao J, et al. Limitations in bonding to dentin and experimental strategies to prevent bond degradation. J Dent Res. 2011;90:953-68.

19. Marshall SJ, Bayne SC, Baier R, et al. A review of adhesion science. Dent Mater. 2010;26:e11-6.

20. Mertz-Fairhurst EJ, Curtis JW Jr, Ergle JW, Rueggeberg FA, Adair SM. Ultraconservative and cariostatic sealed restorations: results at year 10. J Am Dent Assoc. 1998;129:55-66.

21. Miguez PA, Castro PS, Nunes MF, et al. Effect of acid etching on the enamel bond of two self-etching systems. J Adhes Dent. 2003;5:107-12.

22. Miranda C, Prates LH, Vieira Ride S, et al. Shear bond strength of different adhesive systems to primary dentin and enamel. J Clin Pediatr Dent. 2006;31:35-40.

23. Mohan B, Kandaswamy D. A confocal microscopic evaluation of resin-dentin interface using adhesive systems with three different solvents bonded to dry and moist dentin: an in-vitro study. Quintessence Int. 2005;36:511-21.

24. Moszer N, Salz U, Zimmerman J. Chemical aspects of self-etching enamel dentin adhesives: a systematic review. Dent Mater. 2005;21:895-910.

25. Nakabayashi N, Kojima K, Masuhara E. The promotion of adhesion by the infiltration of monomers into tooth substrates. J Biomed Mater Res. 1982;16:265-73.

26. Nakabayashi N, Nakamura M, Yasuda N. Hybrid layer as dentin bonding mechanism. J Esthet Dent. 1991;3:133-8.

27. Nakabayashi N, Takarada K. The effect of HEMA on bonding to dentin. Dent Mater. 1992;8:125-30.

28. Overton JD, Vance RI. Effect of adhesive volume on the bond strength of bonded complex amalgam restorations. Am J Dent. 2005;18:320-22.

29. Pashley D, Tay FR. Aggressiveness of contemporary self-etching adhesives. Dent Mater. 2001;17:430-44.

30. Pashley DH, Carvalho RM, Sano H, Nakajima M, Yoshiyama M, Shono Y, et al. The microtensile bond test: a review. J Adhes Dent. 1999;1:299-309.

31. Perdigão J. Dentin bonding-variables related to the clinical situation and the substrate treatment. Dent Mater. 2010;26:e24-37.

32. Perdigao J, Geraldeli S, Hodges JS. Total etch versus self-etch adhesive: effect on postoperative sensitivity. J Am Dent Assoc. 2003;134:1621-9.

33. Perdigao J, Geraldeli S. Bonding characteristics of self-etching adhesives to intact versus prepared enamel. J Esthet Restor Dent. 2003;15:32-41.

34. Perdigao J, Swift EJ, Lopes GC. Effects of repeated use on bond strength of one bottle adhesive. Quintessence Int. 1999;30:819-23.

35. Roberson T, Heymann H, Swift EJ. Sturdevant's Art and Science of Operative Dentistry, 5th edition. Philadelphia: Mosby; 2006.

36. Salz U, Zimmermann J, Zeuner F, et al. Hydrolytic stability of self-etching adhesive systems. J Adhes Dent. 2005;7:107-16.

37. Simonsen RJ. Retention and effectiveness of dental sealant after 15 years. J Am Dent Assoc. 1991;122:34-42.

38. Spencer P, Wang Y, Walker MP, et al. Interfacial chemistry of the dentin/adhesive bond. J Dent Res. 2000;79:1458-63.

39. Stangel I, Eliis TH, Sacher E. Adhesion to tooth structure mediated by contemporary bonding systems. Dent Clin N Am. 2007;51:677-94.

40. Turkan SL. Clinical evaluation of a self-etching and a one bottle adhesive system in two years. J Dent. 2003;31:527-34.

41. Van Meerbeek B, De Munck J, Yoshida Y, Inoue S, Vargas M, Vijay P, et al. Buonocore memorial lecture: Adhesion to enamel and dentin: current status and future challenges. Oper Dent. 2003;28:215-35.

42. Vaught RL. Mechanical versus chemical retention for restoring complex restorations: what is the evidence? J Dent Edu. 2007;71:1356-62.

# Composite Restorative Materials

ADA Specification No. 27

*'It is better to preserve than to repair, better repair than to restore, better to restore than to reconstruct.'*

**—AN Didron**

## INTRODUCTION

Silicate cements were the first tooth-colored materials, which were available for cavity restorations at the start of the 20th century. The drawbacks of this material were high-acidic pH, loss of translucency, loss of mechanical properties, surface crazing and severe erosion with time. These materials were replaced by acrylic resins in 1940s and 1950s as they were tooth colored, insoluble in oral fluids, easy to manipulate and having low cost. But, their major drawbacks were relatively poor wear resistance and high-polymerization shrinkage leading to microleakage and staining. A major breakthrough in the field of direct tooth-colored restorative material was made by Dr RL Bowen in 1962 when he introduced the composite material and called it *Bowen's resin*. This resin material was made of bisphenol-A glycidyl dimethacrylate (BIS-GMA)—a dimethacrylate resin—which was made to bond with resin matrix and filler particles by organosilane-coupling agent. The materials used as esthetic restorations are silicate cements, acrylic resins, glass ionomers, composites and fused porcelain. Currently, composite resins are most commonly used direct-esthetic restorative material to restore anterior and posterior teeth. In this chapter, composite material is discussed in detail.

## DEFINITION

Composite material is defined as:
*A highly cross-linked polymeric material reinforced by a dispersion of amorphous silica, glass, crystalline, or organic resin filler particles and/or short fibers bonded to the matrix by a coupling agent.*

**—GPT 8th Edition**

## EVOLUTION OF COMPOSITE RESIN MATERIAL

- *1871*: Silicate cement were introduced
- *1930*: Polymethyl methacrylate (PMMA) was first used as denture base resins
- *1951*: Inorganic fillers were added to the direct-filling materials
- *1938*: *Paffenbarger et al.* stated that silicate cements were prone to acidic decay and required replacement after 4–5 years
- *1953*: *Paffenbarger* suggested the use of filler to reduce the coefficient of thermal expansion (CTE) of these resins
- *1955*: *Dr Michael Buonocore,* introduced the *acid-etch technique*
- *1956*: *Dr RL Bowen* developed the BIS-GMA (Bowen resin) and silanized inorganic filler
- *1962*: *Silane-coupling agents* were introduced
- *1968*: *Polymeric coating was developed on the fillers*
- *1972*: Silica, barium oxide, boric oxide and aluminum oxide were added to yield radiopacity by *Bowen and Cleek*
- *1973–74*: *Silverstone* and *Chow* and *Brown* worked on the "acid-etch technique" to figure out the correct concentration of phosphoric acid used

- *1973*: Ultraviolet (UV)-cured dimethacrylate composite resins
- *1976:* Microfilled composites were first introduced
- *1977:* Visible light-cured dimethacrylate composite resins were introduced
- *1980*: *Fusayama* made significant contribution in the area of adhesive bonding agents
- 1989: Midhybrid composites were introduced
- *1995*: *Compomers* were introduced
- *1996*: Flowable composites were developed
- *1997*: Packable composites were introduced
- *1998*: Fiber-reinforced, ion releasing composites and ormocers were developed
- *2002*: Minihybrid composites were introduced
- *2005*: Low-shrinkage composites were developed
- *2009*: Nanofilled and nanohybrid composites were marketed
- *2011*: Bulk fill composites and universal adhesives were first introduced.

## APPLICATIONS AND USES

- For restorations of mild-to-moderate Class I and Class II tooth preparations
- Restoration of Class III, IV and V preparations of teeth especially when esthetics is important
- Restoration of Class VI preparations of teeth where high-occlusal stress is not present
- Core buildup for grossly damaged teeth
- As a pit and fissure sealant and in preventive resin restorations (PRR)
- To restore erosion or abrasion defects in cervical areas of premolars, canines and incisors
- For restoration of hypoplastic defects on the facial or lingual areas
- Esthetics enhancement procedures like partial and full veneers, tooth discolorations and diastema closures
- For cementation of indirect restorations like inlays, onlays and crown
- For repair of fractured ceramic crowns
- For bonding orthodontic appliances.

## CONTRAINDICATIONS

- If isolation of the operating site is difficult
- Where there is presence of high-occlusal forces
- Should not be used where indirect restorations is indicated
- Class V lesions where esthetics is not of prime concern
- When lesions are extending to the root surface and are located subgingivally

- Patients having high-caries index and poor-oral hygiene.

### Advantages

- Shows high esthetics
- Requires minimal tooth preparation therefore, maximum preservation of tooth structure
- Tooth preparation is less complex as compared to amalgam
- Possess low-thermal conductivity and shows bonding with enamel and dentin
- Finishing and polishing can be done immediately after curing the restorations
- Repair rather replacement of the restoration is possible
- Have extended working time and are therefore, easy to manipulate
- No galvanism, as it does not contain any metal.

### Disadvantages

- Polymerization shrinkage leads to gap formation on the margin resulting in secondary caries and staining
- More difficult and time consuming
- More expensive than amalgam restoration
- Requires isolation and has multiple steps
- Is more technique sensitive than other restorative material
- Establishing proximal contacts and contours and finishing is difficult
- Has low-wear resistance
- Postoperative sensitivity can result due to polymerization shrinkage
- In large preparations, composites may not last as long as amalgam fillings.

## IDEAL REQUIREMENTS

- Should have CTE closer to that of enamel
- Should not absorb water
- Should have minimum or no polymerization shrinkage
- Should have good wear resistant
- Should have smooth surface texture
- Should be radiopaque
- Should have higher modulus of elasticity
- Should be less soluble in oral fluids.

## COMPOSITION

Basically, composite restorative material consists of the continuous polymeric or resin matrix in which inorganic filler material is dispersed.

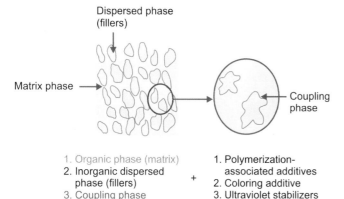

1. Organic phase (matrix)
2. Inorganic dispersed phase (fillers)     +
3. Coupling phase

1. Polymerization-associated additives
2. Coloring additive
3. Ultraviolet stabilizers
4. Radiopacifiers

**Fig. 17.1:** Components of composite resin.

Dental composite resins are complex materials and contain **(Fig. 17.1):**

- *Matrix*: An organic resin component that forms a continuous phase and binds to the filler particles
- *Inorganic filler*: Reinforcing particles and fibers, which are dispersed in the matrix
- *Coupling (interfacial) agent*: It helps in adhesion between the resin matrix and the filler particles
- *Activator-initiator system*: To activate the setting mechanism
- *Coloring pigments*: Added to match the shade of the tooth structure
- *Polymerization inhibitors*: Extends storage life and increases the working time for chemically activated resin
- *UV stabilizers*: Improves color stability.

## Resin Component—Matrix

Composite resins vary in their resin component but all the variations are diacrylates. These resin matrix results in highly cross-linked polymers, which improve strength and rigidity of composites and sealants. Cross-linking greatly improves modulus and reduces its solubility. The formed matrix is a continuous phase in which the reinforcing filler is dispersed. Most of the composite used in dentistry consists of combination of aliphatic or aromatic dimethacrylate monomers.

- *Bisphenol-A glycidyl dimethacrylate*: It is a high-viscosity aromatic monomer synthesized by *Bowen* in the USA in 1960s. Its primary drawback is that it does not bond to tooth structure effectively and has high-water sorption. It requires highly fluid monomers to dilute BIS-GMA. Triethylene glycol dimethacrylate (TEGDMA) is added to significantly reduce the viscosity of BIS-GMA and to allow increased filler loadings
- *Urethane dimethacrylate (UDMA)*: Oligomeric compounds have either partially or completely replaced BIS-GMA

- *Triethylene glycol dimethacrylate*: They are low-viscosity diluent monomers, which are incorporated to reduce viscosity of resin paste and facilitate in clinical handling. They also produce extensive cross-linking among polymer chains resulting in resin matrix, which is rigid and is resistant to softening with heat or solvents such as alcohol. Drawbacks of adding these monomers are that they increase polymerization shrinkage, increase flexibility and reduce abrasion resistance of composites. More the quantity of these monomers, greater will be polymerization shrinkage and there will be greater tendency for marginal leakage. Presently, all commercially available composites have vinyl monomers, which polymerize using free radical initiators. Other monomers used are *EGDMA* (ethylene glycol dimethacrylate) and *HEMA* (hydroxyethyl methacrylate).

## Filler Particle

Addition of filler particles to the resin matrix significantly improves its properties. Inorganic filler particles comprise of 30–70% by volume or 50–85% by weight of total composites. Smaller filler particles are obtained through hydrolysis or precipitation to form fumed or pyrolytic silica, which ranges from 0.06 μm to 0.1 μm. The first generation composites consisted of quartz filler particles. These were chemically inert but were very hard. These particles were very difficult to grind and had tendency to abrade the opposing natural tooth. Currently, filler particles include borosilicates, fused quartz, aluminum silicate, ytterbium fluoride or lithium aluminum silicate glasses. Barium, strontium, zirconium and zinc glasses can be added to provide radiopacity. Instead of crystalline quartz, amorphous silica is preferred as they have composition and refractive index similar to the quartz but are not that hard and can be easily polished.

### Latest Trend

Recently, *solution-gel procedure* is introduced for forming filler particles. In this process, the silicate precursors are polymerized to form particles in the range of nm, which are mostly monodispersed particles. This helps in producing different particle sizes, which are blended to optimize the packing efficiency and filler-loading capacity of the composites. It allows the production of nanocomposites, which approach the size of the polymer matrix molecules.

### Advantages

- Filler particles *improves mechanical properties such as compressive strength, modulus of elasticity, hardness and wear resistance*—when the volume fraction of the filler particles approaches approximately 70%, the abrasion resistance and the fraction resistance are greatly improved thereby increasing the clinical durability and longevity

- *Reduction in coefficient of thermal expansion and contraction*—increased filler content decreases the overall CTE. When the filler content is increased, the reduction in the CTE approaches that of the tooth structure and less interfacial stress is produced
- *Workability is improved by increasing viscosity*—addition of fillers increases the viscosity of the composite resin. Greater the filler content, greater will be the viscosity. Factors affecting the clinical manipulation and handling of the composite resins are the size and shape of filler particles, their consistency and the filler loading. The adequate amount of filler content provides control of workability of the composite resin. It allows ease in building proximal contact, carving occlusal anatomy and helps in minimizing voids
- *Reduction in water sorption, softening and staining*—greater the filler content, lesser is the water sorption. Less water sorption provides greater resistance to staining
- *Reduces the polymerization shrinkage*—greater amount of filler loading reduces the polymerization shrinkage in proportion of filler volume fraction. Although, polymerization shrinkage cannot be eliminated completely, it usually varies from 1 to 4% by volume among different commercial products
- *Less heat evolved during polymerization*
- *Gives radiopacity, if barium or strontium glasses or other heavy metal glass is used.* Radiopacity helps in detecting secondary caries, proximal wear and marginal leakage by providing radiographic contrast. Composite resins are inherently radiolucent therefore adding radiopaque salts improves radiopacity and is helpful in providing diagnostic contrast.

### Factors Influencing Role of Filler in Composition

- Amount of filler added in the resin is mainly influenced by the total filler surface area
- Size of particles and its distribution
- Index of refraction—should be adequate to achieve sufficient translucency
- Radiopacity
- Hardness of the filler particles.

### Types of Fillers

- Ground quartz
- Colloidal silica
- Glasses or ceramic-containing heavy metal
- Radiopaque silicates.

### Quartz

Obtained by grinding/milling quartz used in conventional composites. They are hard, chemically inert, and difficult to polish and has tendency to abrade opposing tooth. Particle size ranges between 0.1 μm and 100 μm. It has been used as reinforcing filler in the earlier dental composites. It is chemically inert and very hard, which is difficult to grind and polish.

### Colloidal Silica

Also called as *microfiller*. They are obtained by a pyrolytic or precipitation process. The process consists of silicon compound, which is burned in an $O_2$ or $H_2$ atmosphere to produce a macromolecule chain of $SiO_2$. The size of these particles is 0.04 μm. Colloidal silica particles have a large surface area (50–400 $m^2$/g) thus even small amount of filler thickens the resin because silica surface forms polar bonds with the monomer, which inhibits its flow and increases its viscosity.

### Radiopaque Silicates

By adding glasses and ceramics-containing heavy metals such as barium, strontium and zirconium filler particles are made radiopaque. The glasses have indices of refraction of about 1.5, which match that of the resins.

**CLINICAL SIGNIFICANCE**

The refractive index of the filler particles should match that of the tooth structure in order to achieve optimal esthetics. The refractive index of BIS-GMA and TEGDMA is 1.55 and 1.46, respectively. When both these components are mixed in equal proportions they result in refractive index of 1.5, which is capable of providing adequate translucency.

*Nanofillers:* Nanofillers are filler components, which are manufactured using nanotechnology and are different from the conventional fillers. When manufacturing conventional filler particles large quartz, glasses or ceramic particles are milled to smaller particle sizes. The conventional filler particles cannot be milled less than 100-nm size. On the other hand, nanofillers are monodispersed, nonaggregated and nonagglomerated silica nanoparticles, which are in the range of 20–75-nm sizes. These filler particles are capable of high-filler loading of up to 79.5%. The reduced filler particle size of nanofillers permits an increased interfacial area between the matrix and the fillers leading to better dispersion. These filler particles provide increased flexural strength and surface microhardness. They also provide better optical properties and better esthetics than conventional composites. Nanofillers, which consist of primary zirconia-silica particles of sizes 2–20 nm, are spheroidal particles having average size of 0.6 μm are called as nanoclusters.

## Coupling Agent

A coupling agent is used to produce a strong bond between the filler particles and the resin matrix. It is a difunctional surface—active silane material, which reacts with the surface of filler particles and organic matrix to provide adhesion between the two surfaces. The need for coupling agent is due to the fact that the filler particles are not soluble in resin matrix because the resins are hydrophobic in nature whereas the silica-based filler particles are hydrophilic in nature due to surface layer of the hydroxyl groups bound to the silica. The coupling agent is incorporated to address this issue as the silanes have hydroxyl and methacrylate groups on either ends. The hydroxyl group reacts with the hydroxyl group of the filler by a condensation reaction between the silica glass particles and the silane. Likewise methacrylate group of the silane reacts with the resin matrix forming a bond between it and the resin matrix. Thus, a bond between the filler particles and the resin matrix through the coupling agent allows distribution of stress produced during function. Good adhesion helps in improving the physical and mechanical properties and inhibits leaching at the resin-filler interface. It also reduces surface wear of the filler particles.

Most commonly used coupling agent is $\gamma$-methacryloxy-propyltrimethoxysilane (organosilane). The methacrylate group of organosilane forms covalent bond with the resin when it is cured. Other coupling agents used are:

- Zirconates
- Titanates.

*Advantages*

- It increases bonding between the filler particles and matrix
- It increases wear resistance
- It allows transfer of stress from more flexible polymer to stiffer filler particles
- It provides bond between the two phases of composite resins.

## Activator-Initiator Systems

Visible *light-activated systems:* Single paste contains a two-component initiator system comprising a photosensitizer and a tertiary amine. The photosensitive diketone, usually 0.2–0.7% camphorquinone, absorbs the radiant energy of wavelength approximately 470 nm (blue light). The amine initiators used are dimethylaminoethyl methacrylate (DMAEMA). The diketone combines with the amine to form a complex that breaks-down to release free radicals, which then initiate polymerization of the resin. Initially, UV light was used as light source to initiate free radicals but now UV light curing composites are replaced by visible light-activated composites. Light-cured composites are more widely used than the chemically cured composites because of improved depth of cure and controlled working time.

## Chemically Activated Systems

Supplied in two pastes system, one paste contains an initiator, benzoyl peroxide, and the other paste a tertiary aromatic amine accelerator (N, N dimethyl P-toluidine). Combination of the two pastes will yield free radicals, which initiate polymerization of the resin. These materials are mainly used for large restorations and core buildup where light curing is not possible.

## Other Systems

Dual-activated composites have both a light activated and a chemically activated initiating systems and are packaged as two pastes. The light activation mechanism is used to initiate polymerization and the chemical activation is relied upon to continue and complete the setting reaction.

## Inhibitors

To minimize or prevent spontaneous polymerization of monomers inhibitors are added to the resin systems. These inhibitors have a strong reactivity potential with the free radicals. They inhibit chain propagation by terminating the ability of the free radical to initiate polymerization process. Butylated hydroxytoluene (BHT) is used in a concentration of 0.01 wt% as inhibitor.

*Advantages*

- It extends storage life of resins
- It ensures sufficient working time.

## Optical Modifiers

To match the appearance of teeth, dental composites must have coloration (shading) and translucency that can simulate tooth structures (i.e. dentin and enamel), shading is achieved by adding different pigments. The translucency and opacity are balanced as required to simulate dentin and enamel. Optical modifiers have the ability to affect the light transmission through the resin during polymerization. Darker shades with greater opacities require greater curing time or are applied in thinner layer for complete polymerization.

The optical modifiers usually used are metal oxides like titanium oxide, aluminum oxide and even the sulfides. These are added in minute amounts 0.001–0.007 wt% as they are effective opacifiers. Optical modifiers and opacifiers affect the light-transmitting ability of the composite resins. Darker shade resins transmit less light than the lighter shade resins. To avoid this, darker shade resins should be cured in thinner layers as compared to the lighter shade resins to ensure optimal polymerization.

*Color pigments are metal oxides used for staining:*
- Cadmium/gold—yellow
- Nickel—gray
- Ferric—red
- Copper—green
- Tin—brown.

*Ultraviolet stabilizers:* To prevent discoloration with age of composites, compound is incorporated, which absorbs electromagnetic radiation. It also improves color stability, e.g. 2-hydroxy-4 methoxybenzophenone.

## Classification of Composite Restorative Materials

1. According to Sturdevant:
   I.  On the basis of matrix composition:
       - BIS-GMA based
       - UDMA based
       - Silorane based.
   II. On the basis of polymerization method:
       - *Self-cured or chemically cured or two component systems*: Amine accelerators were used to increase polymerization rates
       - *Ultraviolet light curing*: UV light is used which initiate polymerization. UV light curing units were of limited reliability and presented safety problems
       - *Visible light curing*: Most popular today, but their success depends on the access of high-intensity light to cure the matrix material
       - *Dual curing*: Combining self-curing and light curing. The self-curing rate is slow and is designed to cure only those portions that are not adequately light-cured
       - *Staged curing*: By filtering the light from the curing unit during an initial cure, it is possible to produce a soft, partially cured material that can be easily finished.
   III. On the basis of size of filler particles **(Fig. 17.2)**:
       - Megafill-contains megafillers—very large individual filler particle
       - Macrofill-contains macrofillers (10–100 μm)
       - Midfill-contains midfillers (1–10 μm)
       - Minifill-contains minifillers (0.1–1 μm)
       - Microfill-contains microfillers (0.01–0.1 μm)
       - Nanofill-contains nanofillers (0.005–0.01 μm).
2. *Lutz and Phillips classification (1983)*: Based on the filler particle size and distribution:
   - *Type 1: macrofilled composite resin*: Referred to as "conventional" or "traditional" composite

   - *Type 2: microfilled composite resin*: Fillers are amorphous silica particles of 0.04 μm average diameter
   - *Type 3: hybrid composite resin*: Often known as "small-particle composites". They are combination of macrofiller and microfiller particles. They are probably the most commonly used composite resins.
3. *Willems classification (1992)*: Based on morphological and mechanical characteristics. The properties considered are the size and percentage of filler particles, modulus of elasticity, compressive strength and surface roughness.
   - Densified composites; midway filled—(<60% volume filler particles):
       - Ultrafine (particle size <3 μm)
       - Fine (particle size >3 μm).
   - Densified composites; compact filled—(>60% volume filler particles):
       - Ultrafine (particle size <3 μm)
       - Fine (particle size >3 μm).
   - Homogeneous microfine composites
   - Heterogeneous macrofine composites
   - Miscellaneous composites—combination of densified and microfilled composites
   - Traditional composites
   - Fiber-reinforced composites.
4. *According to Phillips*: Based on the basis of particle size and size distribution **(Table 17.1)**
5. On the basis of mode of curing:
   - Instant cure
   - Soft cure
   - Stepped cure
   - Oscillating cure
   - Delayed cure
   - Ramped cure.
6. On the basis of ISO specification for composite resins:
   - *Class I*—self-curing resins, which polymerize by mixing an initiator and an activator
   - *Class II*—resins, which polymerize by applying energy from the external source such as visible light or heat. It can be subdivided into:
       - *Class II group A*—resins, which require energy application intraorally for polymerization
       - *Class II group B*—resins, which require energy to be applied extraorally. These resins consist of indirect composite materials for fabrication of inlays and onlays.
   - *Class III*—resins, which are dual cured, i.e. have self-curing component (internally) and light-curing component (externally).

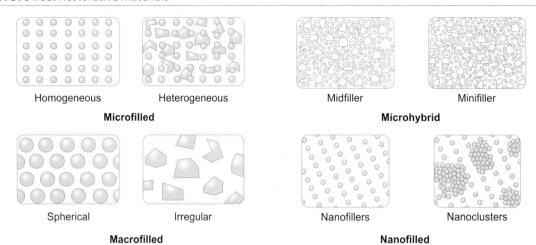

**Fig. 17.2:** Classification of composite based on particle size.

**Table 17.1:** Basis of particle size and size distribution.

| Category | Particle size | Indications |
|---|---|---|
| Traditional (large particles) | 1–50 µm glass | Used in high-stress areas |
| Hybrid (large particles) | 1–20 µm glass, 0.04 µm silica | High-stress area, which requires high polish, in Class I, II, III, IV restorations |
| Hybrid (midfiller) | 0.1–10 µm glass, 0.04 µm silica | In Class III, IV restorations requiring high polishability |
| Hybrid (minifiller) | 0.1–2 µm glass, 0.04 µm silica | Moderate stress area in Class III, IV restorations |
| Packable composites | Midfiller/minifiller hybrid with lower filler ratio | Restorations requiring increased condensability |
| Flowable composites | Midfiller with finer particles | Restorations requiring better flow |
| Homogeneous microfill | 0.04 µm silica | Low-stress area requiring high polishability |
| Heterogeneous microfill | 0.04 µm silica, prepolymerized resins | Low-stress area where reduced polymerization shrinkage is needed |

## CURING OF DENTAL COMPOSITES

*Curing or polymerization is defined as forming of a compound by joining together of molecules of small molecular weights into a compound of large molecular weight.*

—*GPT 8th Edition*

Polymerization is a process of joining small-molecular weight monomers to form long chain, high-molecular weight molecules called as polymers. This chemical reaction is made possible because of initiators and activators. Both these components start the chemical reaction by linking the molecules to form high-molecular weight polymers. This linking process is called as *addition polymerization*. Likewise, when side groups of polymers share their molecules to from covalent bonds by linking the chains together it is called as *crosslinking*. Crosslinked polymers are much stronger and tougher than the linear chain-linked polymers.

## Methods of Curing

### Chemically Activated System

Supplied as two paste system—*base paste* contains benzoyl peroxide initiator and *catalyst paste* contains tertiary amine activator (N, N-dimethyl-p-toluidine).

The initiator and accelerator must be kept separately until just before mixing. When both base paste and catalyst paste are mixed together in equal amounts then polymerization reaction is initiated. The tertiary amine activator reacts with the benzoyl peroxide initiator to release free radicals, which initiate polymerization reaction. Since working time cannot be controlled, the mixture should be placed and contoured quickly. Air entrapment during mixing is unavoidable and therefore it can lead to formation of pores and trap oxygen. Pores can weaken the structure and oxygen is found to inhibit polymerization reaction.

Trapped oxygen lead to the formation of oxygen-inhibited layer. During the initial stage of polymerization, the trapped oxygen reacts with the free radicals faster than the monomer. This reaction forms a layer of unpolymerized surface layer. The thickness of this unpolymerized layer is influenced by viscosity of the resin, type of initiating system used and the solubility of the oxygen in the monomer.

The reaction in chemically cured resins can be summarized as:

Diacrylate monomer (in both pastes) + accelerator base paste + initiator catalyst paste → Crosslinked polymers

*Advantages*
- No equipment required, manipulation is easy
- Long-term storage stability
- By varying proportions, working and setting time can be manipulated
- Degree of polymerization is equal throughout the mixture
- Marginal stress buildup during polymerization is less as compared to the light cure resins.

*Disadvantages*
- Air entrapment during mixing is inevitable and can cause porosity that leads to weakening of the mixture
- Working time of the mixture cannot be controlled
- Color instability
- Difficult to mix evenly causing unequal degree of polymerization.

*Uses:* For large core buildups and for those restorations which cannot be readily cured by light source.

### Light-activated System

*Ultraviolet light-activated system:* These were initially used systems, where UV light was used to initiate free radicals.
- *Drawbacks*—it had limitation in polymerization of thicker sections and lacked penetration through the tooth structure.

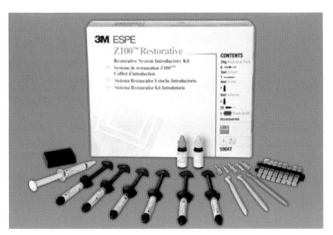

**Fig. 17.3:** Light-activated composite curing system.

*Visible light-activated systems:* Have replaced UV light-activated system, as they have greatly improved depth of cure and a controlled working time **(Fig. 17.3)**.
- They are supplied as single paste system in a lightproof syringe. It contains the photoinitiator, which is camphorquinone 0.25% and amine accelerator, which is diethyl-amino-ethyl methacrylate. When these components are exposed to light of wavelength 468 nm, the photoinitiators are activated, which interact with the amine to form free radicals, which initiate polymerization
- Camphorquinone is commonly used photoinitiator, which absorbs blue light with wavelengths between 400 nm and 500 nm. 0.25% by weight of camphorquinone is required for the reaction
- Amine initiator such as DMAEMA is required to interact with camphorquinone (photoinitiator).
  The reaction in light cure resins is summarized as:

Diacrylate monomer + photoinitiator + visible light (468 nm) → Crosslinked resin

### Benefits Over Chemical Cure Composites (Table 17.2)
- Mixing is not needed and thus it improves strength and reduces staining and porosity
- Aliphatic amines are used, which enhance color stability
- Working time can be controlled by the clinician as polymerization only takes place on exposure to light
- Addition in increments allows incorporation of multiple shade in single restoration
- Addition in increments also compensate for polymerization shrinkage within each increment.

### Drawbacks Over Chemical Cure Composites
- Limited curing depth of 2 mm or less, therefore the composite should be added in increments
- Relatively poor accessibility in posterior or interproximal regions
- Variable exposure times depending on the type of shade, darker shades require longer exposure time
- Sensitive to room illumination as skin or crust may form on opened composite syringe
- Requires special light curing unit
- Darker shades requires longer exposure time
- Polymerization is influenced by addition of UV absorbers, fluorescent dyes or inhibitors, which absorbs light and prevent reaction
- Protective glasses are required for the clinician when working with light curing units
- Technique sensitive and clinician requires proper training
- Some light curing unit generates heat, which can cause discomfort to patient.

**Table 17.2:** Comparison between light cure and chemical cure resins.

| Light cure resins | Chemical/self-cure resins |
|---|---|
| Light of correct wavelength is required for activation | Activation by peroxide amine system |
| Polymerization is toward the source of light in the center | Polymerization occurs throughout the bulk of resins |
| Working time under control of operator | Working time cannot be controlled by operator |
| Polymerization shrinkage occurs toward the source of light | Shrinkage occurs toward the center of the bulk |
| Supplied as single component system | Supplied as two component system |
| Less polymerization shrinkage | More shrinkage |
| Greater wear resistance | Less wear resistance |
| Excellent esthetics | Esthetics less |
| Less chances of air entrapment during manipulation | Greater chances of air entrapment during manipulation |
| Greater color stability | Less color stability |

## CURING LAMPS

These are handheld devices, which are capable of emitting light. They consist of small and rigid light guide, which is made of fused optical fibers. Some of the curing lamps have power source connected to the dental handpiece with flexible liquid-filled light guide. Usually, the curing lamps are filtered to transmit light only in visible range (400–500 nm) activate the photoinitiator, camphorquinone in light cure resins. When the free radicals are released, polymerization of light cure resins begins. The factors, which influence the polymerization process, are wavelength, intensity and time of exposure of the light emitted from the curing lamp.

For maximum curing, radiant energy of 16,000 mJ/cm$^2$ is required to cure 2-mm thick layer of resin. If a lamp-emitting 400 mW/cm$^2$ is exposed for 40 seconds then this energy is delivered. For exposure of 20 seconds, lamp should emit 800 mW/cm$^2$ to deliver 16,000 mJ/cm$^2$. Therefore, if the power density of the lamp is increased, its degree and rate of curing also increases. Although, using a high-intensity curing light for faster curing can result in increased shrinkage stress buildup. One of the most commonly used curing lamps is a quartz bulb with tungsten filament. Other lamps are also available for photoinitiation of the composite resin.

### Types of Lamps used for Curing

1. *LED lamps:* These are *light-emitting diodes,* which emit radiation only in the blue part of the visible spectrum between 440 nm and 480 nm. They use junctions of doped semiconductors, which are based on gallium nitride to emit blue light. This range matches the photoabsorption range of photosensitizer such as camphorquinone. They do not require filters **(Fig. 17.4)**.
   - *Benefits:* Require low wattage, can be battery operated, do not generate heat, do not require a cooling fan and have long lifespan
   - *Drawback:* Produce lowest intensity radiation.
2. *QTH lamps*—mean *quartz-tungsten-halogen* lamps. They are one of the earliest and most common forms of light cure systems, which use quartz bulb with a tungsten filament. The light source emits white light, which is filtered to remove heat and all wavelengths except those in the violet-blue range between 400 nm and 500 nm. The intensity of bulb reduces with use and therefore, calibration meter is required to measure the output intensity. QTH lamps emit radiant power density in the range of 300–1,200 mW/cm$^2$ in the violet blue spectrum. The intensity of light from these lamps is not uniform for all areas of the light tip, i.e. it is greatest in the center of the tip. The intensity is also reduced, if the distance from the source is increased. Protective eye device are used to filter the visible light beam to facilitate the operator to directly visualize the curing procedure. Direct observation of the tip should be avoided, as it may cause retinal damage to the eyes **(Fig. 17.5)**.

*Factors influencing reduction of intensity of light from QTH lamps:*
- Light tip is chipped off
- Resin is deposited on the light tip
- Distance of the tip to resin is increased
- Lack of uniformity across the light tip
- Burn out of the bulb filament
- Change in line voltage.

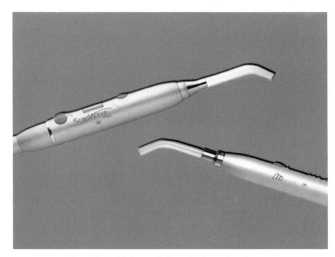

**Fig. 17.4:** Light emitting diode curing lamps.

3. *PAC lamps*: These are *plasma arc curing* lamps, which use xenon gas ionization to produce plasma. High-intensity light is obtained by plasma that forms between two tungsten electrodes under pressure. The high-intensity white light is filtered to remove heat and to allow blue light to be emitted. This violet-blue region matches the photoabsorption range of camphorquinone. PAC lamps can cure composite resins with photoinitiators other than that of camphorquinone as in these devices light intensity light is obtained at the lower wavelength. Exposure from PAC light for 10 seconds is equivalent to 40 seconds exposure from QTH lamps. Therefore, use of PAC lamps saves time in procedures which require multiple exposures **(Fig. 17.6)**

4. *Argon laser lamp*: These lamps have highest intensity and emit at a single wavelength of 490 nm. These laser lamps are designed to emit light in only blue spectrum, which lies in the photoabsorption range of camphorquinone. Therefore, they do not require filters.

## Dual-cure Resins

Dual-cure resins are beneficial in situations, where adequate light penetration is not there. It consists of chemical curing and visible curing components in the same resins. The two paste systems contain initiator and activator of both light curing and chemical curing resins. When two pastes are mixed and placed into the tooth, the light curing initiates the chemical polymerization reaction by initiating tertiary amine and camphorquinone combination. On the other hand, the chemical curing is promoted by tertiary amine and benzoyl peroxide combination in the areas, which are not cured by light to ensure complete polymerization of the resin. Dual-cure resin systems are prone to porosity and air inhibition.

Alternately, chemical or light cure resins are used to produce tooth inlay directly over the tooth or over the die. This inlay is directly cured over the tooth or on the die. This cured inlay is then transferred to an oven for additional heat or light curing. Once curing is completed, inlay is cemented on the tooth with resin-based composite **(Fig. 17.7).**

## CURING DEPTH, DEGREE OF CONVERSION AND EXPOSURE TIME

As the distance between tip of the light source and the surface of the resin increases, there is decrease in the intensity of the light. To achieve optimal polymerization of the composite resin, it is important to understand factors such as depth of cure, degree of conversion (DC) and the exposure time.

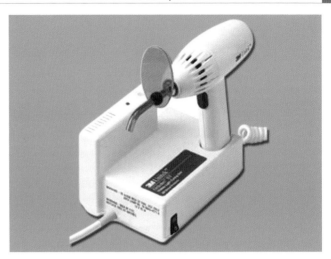

**Fig. 17.5:** Quartz-tungsten-halogen curing lamp.

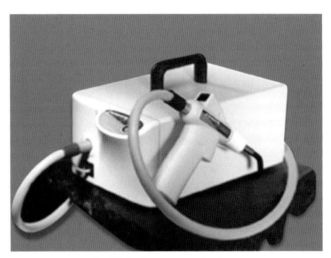

**Fig. 17.6:** Plasma arc curing lamp.

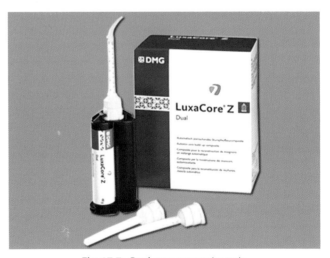

**Fig. 17.7:** Dual-cure composite resin.

Currently used light cure units have increased light intensities (more than 1,000 mW/cm$^2$) and therefore have greater depth of cure and reduced exposure time. The curing light source should be held at the distance not greater than 1 mm from the surface of the resin. Increasing the distance between the light source and the resin will reduce the light output. Curing light's output intensity should be regularly checked and the clinician should place the light tip perpendicular to the restorative resin. The light tip should be maintained at the same distance and position at the time of exposure. Curing angle of 90°, the light source and the resin is critical, as it delivers maximum light intensity at this angle. For optimal polymerization, the light intensity should provide adequate radiant energy influx (about 16 J/cm$^2$).

## Depth of Cure

It is relevant to the light-cured composite resins. Penetration of light through light-activated resins depends on number of factors. These factors can be composite resin related or light related. The composite resin-related factors include filler particle size, translucency, shade of the resin and distribution and concentration of the filler particles; whereas light-related factors include light intensity, exposure time, irradiance and spectral distribution. Light irradiance is equal to power (energy/time) per unit area. Better irradiance improves the penetration of the light through the restorative resins. Again, greater the intensity of light, more photon will be available for absorption by the photosensitizers such as camphorquinone. These will react with the tertiary amines to form free radicals to initiate polymerization of the resins. The surface of the resins shows better polymerization than the deeper layers because of attenuation of light reducing the amount of polymerization. Therefore, curing depth should be limited to 2–3 mm of the resin and the restoration should be cured in increments.

## Degree of Conversion

During the polymerization reaction of the composite resin, the number of carbon double bonds converted into single bond shows the number of monomers taking part in the reaction. Even at the end of polymerization reaction not all the monomer particles are converted into the polymers. The reaction keeps occurring indefinitely. DC shows the percentage of carbon double bonds of methacrylate monomer that is converted into single bonds during the polymerization of the resin. More the DC of the resin, better are its properties such as strength, wear resistance and durability. It is observed that DC for BIS-GMA-based composites is about 50–60% meaning this percentage of methacrylate monomers have been converted into the polymers. Although, this does not mean that the remaining

40–50% of monomer is left unreacted in the resin. Actually this left monomer can covalently bond to one of the two methacrylate group per dimethacrylate molecule of the polymer resin to form the pendant group.

Factors influencing DC are:
- Composition of resin
- Light transmission through the resin material
- Amount of initiator, inhibitor or activator
- Type and amount of filler particles.

### CLINICAL SIGNIFICANCE

The total degree of conversion between the chemically activated and light-activated composite resin having same monomer composition is similar. DC for both types of resins is around 50–70%. Also, there is not much of significant difference in polymerization shrinkage of comparable light-activated resins and chemically activated resins. However, polymerization shrinkage in light-activated resins can cause greater stress buildup and marginal leakage resulting in secondary caries, postoperative sensitivity and staining **(Fig. 17.8)**.

## PROPERTIES

### Thermal Properties

The CTE of composites is approximately three to four times higher than that of tooth enamel and dentin. This results in greater thermal expansion and contraction of composite resin as compared to the tooth structure. Thermal stresses place additional strain at the tooth resin interface, which adds to the detrimental effect of polymerization shrinkage. Thermal changes can lead to material fatigue and early bond failure leading to formation of gap between the tooth and the resin. This gap can result in microleakage. This gap formation can be reduced by increasing filler content with lower CTE in the composition. The linear CTE of composite resins varies between 25–38 × 10$^{-6}$/°C and 55–68 × 10$^{-6}$/°C.

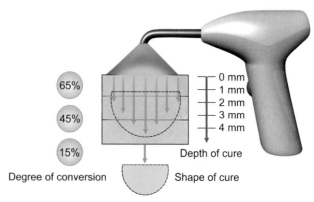

**Fig. 17.8:** Degree of conversion and depth of cure.

## Water Sorption

The property of water sorption can lower the modulus of elasticity and improve the flow rate by increasing the effective free volume for chain segment motions. It was initially suggested that water sorption can compensate for polymerization shrinkage. But polymerization shrinkage and stress development is instantaneous whereas water sorption is a gradual process taking months to approach equilibrium. Therefore, water sorption cannot compensate for polymerization shrinkage. The matrix resin tends to absorb water resulting in swelling. This swelling is not adequate to counteract polymerization shrinkage. The absorption of water by composite resin is correlated with reduction in surface hardness and wear resistance. Microfilled composites have greater water sorption values ($26$–$30$ µmg/mm$^3$) because of their larger volume fraction of matrix in comparison to the hybrid composites ($5$–$17$ µmg/mm$^3$). This makes them more susceptible to discoloration by water-soluble stains.

*Factors influencing greater water sorption of the composite resin:*

- Unpolymerized resins have greater susceptibility to water sorption
- Air voids incorporated during mixing or placing the resin
- Weakening of the coupling bond between the matrix and resin makes the interface more susceptible to water sorption.

## Solubility

Incomplete polymerization of the composite resin especially in the deep restoration due to inadequate light intensity and duration leads to greater susceptibility to solubility of the resin matrix. The unpolymerized resin shows increased amount of solubility as the inorganic ions present in the fillers tend to leach into the surrounding environment and contribute to the breakdown of the restoration. The hydrolysis of the restorative resin is explained as—when the wet environment (like saliva) adds with cyclic loading due to mastication and abrasion there is reduction of the surface energy leading to the weakening of the coupling bond between the matrix and the filler particles resulting in its breakdown at the interface. Water solubility of composites varies between $0.01$ mg/cm$^2$ and $0.06$ mg/cm$^2$. Adequate polymerization of the composite resin is critical in light-cured resins. If the resins are inadequately polymerized, it will show greater water sorption, solubility and earlier color instability.

## Color Stability

Longevity of the composite resin is assessed by how long the restoration retains its color and finish. Compared to the earlier composite resins, recent advances in composite resins are more resistant to discoloration. Discoloration can be of three types:
1. Marginal
2. Surface
3. Bulk.

### Marginal Discoloration

This type of discoloration usually occurs due to improper adaptation of the resins at the margins of the cavity or can be due to polymerization shrinkage stresses, which leads to breakage of interfacial bond between the resin and the wall of the cavity. The gap, which forms at the margins leads to discoloration. This type of discoloration can be avoided by properly adapting the resin at the cavity walls and applying unfilled resins after finishing and polishing of the restoration to fill and improve the marginal adaption.

### Surface Discoloration

This type of discoloration occurs because of surface roughness of the composite restoration. Composite resins with large filler size particles are more susceptible to surface discoloration. Proper finishing and polishing procedure of the composite restoration is recommended by using graded abrasives. If an air void is trapped during restoration, it may appear as dark spot once the resin wears with use.

### Bulk Discoloration

This type of discoloration is more common in self-cure resins due to chemical degradation of the components of the resin matrix. This degradation can cause absorption of fluids from the oral cavity and ultimately discoloration over a period of time.

Self-cure resins have inferior color stability as compared to light-cure resins because of the presence of tertiary amine accelerators, which form colored products on oxidation. If composites are placed in artificial aging conditions, they are found to be susceptible to staining. Recently introduced nanocomposites can be finished and polished to high luster to deliver high-quality esthetic restorations, which show greater resistance to discoloration.

## Radiopacity

Radiopacity in composite resins is imparted by adding certain glass fillers such as barium, strontium and zirconium. Radiopacity acts as valuable diagnostic aid in detecting secondary caries, poor proximal contacts and wear of proximal surfaces. Although, all composite resins are not radiopaque certain resins such as flowable composites are radiolucent. Radiolucent restoration makes it difficult, if not impossible to detect caries. Radiopacity is imparted to the composite resins by including heavy metals such as barium, strontium and zirconia in their composition. These glass fillers have same refractive index as that of the resins. Drawback of using barium to provide radiopacity is that it found to be less chemically inert that quartz fillers in aqueous medium.

### Wear Resistance

Wear of composites is a complex phenomenon, which is due to number of intrinsic and extrinsic factors. Composite resins have lower resistance to wear because softer matrix resin wears more rapidly than the harder filler particles. This leads to exposure of filler particles on the surface which is susceptible to fracture. Due to this reason, initially the use of composite resins was confined to restoration of anterior teeth and was seldom used in posterior teeth. Recently, high-wear resistant composite resins are developed, which are commonly used in the posterior teeth as well.

Wearing in composites can be of two types—(1) abrasive wear and (2) erosive wear. Abrasive wear of composite resin occurs due to chewing and tooth brushing and erosive wear occurs due to degradation of composite in oral fluids.

#### Factors Contributing to Wear of Composite Resins

- *Filler particles*: Wear resistance is directly proportional to the filler content. Studies show that greater the filler content, more the fracture toughness and therefore, greater wear resistance. Higher particle-filled composites show greater wear resistance than microfilled composites
- *Filler particle size*: Wear resistance can be improved by reducing the size of the filler particles. Larger size filler particles transmit greater stress to the matrix resins forming microcracks as compared to smaller filler particles, which transmit less stress to the matrix resin. Filler particle size less than 1 µm, which are well-bound to the matrix are more wear resistant than the larger filler composite resins. Composites with softer filler particles with hardness similar to tooth enamel result in reduced tooth wear
- *Location of the restoration*: More distal or posterior the composite restoration, greater the amount of wear
- *Porosity*: Greater the amount of internal porosities, especially in the stress-bearing areas, greater the amount of wear
- *Degree of polymerization*: Greater the amount of polymerization, greater is the wear resistance. Therefore, heat-cured resins have greater wear resistance than the self-cured resins.

- *Coupling agent*: If silane coupling agent is absent at the matrix filler interface, the wear resistance reduces to almost half
- *Finishing and polishing*: Wear resistance is reduced, if composite restoration is finished with the help of carbide or diamond finishing bur. This is due to heat generation during finishing and polishing procedure. Use of low-viscosity unfilled resin over the composite decreases wear resistance by 50%
- *Type of restoration*: Larger restorations wear more than the smaller restorations.
  - *Parafunctional habits*: There is greater wear of composite restorations in patients having parafunctional habit such as bruxism as compared to normal chewing habit. Posterior composites should be avoided in such patients.

#### Mechanism of Wearing in Composite Resins

There are two mechanisms of wear in composite resins:
1. *Two-body wear*: This mechanism is based on direct contact of the opposing tooth or proximal surface to the composite restoration. Here the small area of restoration is exposed to high amount of stress from the opposing cusp.
2. *Three-body wear*: In this mechanism, there is wear in the noncontacting area due to mostly food particles, which are forced between the two occlusal surfaces. One occlusal surface being the composite restoration and other being the tooth surface. This type of wear can be influenced by number of factors such as toughness, porosity, filler content, silane coupling agent stability and types of filler particles in the composite resin.

### Setting Reaction

Setting or hardening of composite resin begins through rapid free radical polymerization reaction. In this reaction, the monomer component of the composite resin is transformed into crosslinked polymer matrix in 15–30 seconds. This rapid reaction is called as *"Snap-set"*, which means that viscosity of the resin increases rapidly after the hardening process begins but the handling consistency remains same throughout the working time. The working time for self-cure resin is about 2 minutes. The polymerization reaction although does not even complete within several hours but after the setting reaction, the composite resin becomes sufficiently hard, so that it can be finished and polished. Setting time of composite resins is determined by controlling amounts of initiators and accelerators by the manufacturer. Chemically activated resins or self-cure resins have setting time ranging from 3 minutes to 5 minutes from the start of mixing. Polymerization of composite is not complete after 24 hours and it is found that about 25–45% of double bonds remain unreacted. Although polymerization reaction continues, the composite restoration can be finished and polished after initial setting.

In cases of light-activated resins or light cure resins, setting time depends on intensity and penetration of the light beam. In these resins, 75% of polymerization is complete after 10 minutes of light exposure and it continues further till the period of at least 24 hours.

## Biocompatibility

All the major component of composites such as BIS-GMA, TEGMA or UDMA are found to be cytotoxic in nature when used in pure form. Biological effects of cured composite depend on the actual release of these components from the composite. The quantity of components release depends on the type of composite, the method and efficiency of the cure. Dentin barrier such as application of dentin-bonding agent or cavity base usually reduces the ability of these components to reach the pulp.

Bisphenol A (BPA), which is precursor of BIS-GMA is found to be a xenoestrogenic and having antiandrogenic activities. BPA is capable of causing reproductive anomalies especially in the development stages of the fetus. Its effect on human beings is still debatable and is unclear. Estrogenicity of component in resin is associated with BPA and BPA-dimethacrylate monomers, which is found in the monomers of the base paste of dental sealants. Studies suggest that when BPA and BPA-dimethacrylate monomers were applied to the cancer cells there was reduced cell proliferation and DNA synthesis.

Composite materials should never be used as direct pulp capping agent, as it poses greater risk of adverse biological response to the pulp. Inadequately, cured composites at the cavity floor can act as reservoir of diffusible components, which can induce long-term pulpal effects. Another cause can be when a clinician attempts to cure thick layer of resin or the exposure of the light is not sufficient. There have been no studies to prove the effects of released components on the pulp. HEMA is hydrophilic and is strongly allergic. It has been shown that HEMA is able to transverse dentinal tubules and appear in the pulpal tissue leading to allergic responses. Clinician or personnel who handle uncured composite regularly may exhibit signs of contact allergy to composites.

Clinical and laboratory evidence show that tissue cells respond less favorably to composite resin than to glass ionomer. Incompletely cured resin, particularly in those materials with low-filler content, appears to be a tissue irritant. Composite resins should be highly polished as rough surfaces will lead to plaque accumulation.

## Microleakage

Polymerization shrinkage of composite resin after curing can subsequently result in marginal leakage. The material has tendency to contract from the gingival margin during curing due to polymerization shrinkage. This contraction results in the formation of a gap between the restoration and the tooth. The gap so formed leads to marginal leakage. It allows bacterial ingrowth and can cause secondary caries or adverse pulp reaction. Microleakage can also result in problems of staining and discoloration of composites and sensitivity of the tooth. This is one of the major problems with Class II and Class V restorations. In restorations, which extend onto the root surface, it is beneficial to place a lining of resin-modified glass ionomer before placement of composite to reduce the risk of microleakage **(Fig. 17.9).**

## POLYMERIZATION SHRINKAGE

Composite resins undergo a substantial amount of polymerization shrinkage during setting and it may affect the adhesion between the restoration and the tooth. This phenomenon cannot be avoided but can be minimized by following a proper technique. Polymerization shrinkage in hybrid composites is only 0.6–1.4%; whereas in microfilled composites, it is 2–3%. It creates stresses as high as 13 MPa between the composite and the tooth structure. These stresses can severely affect the adhesion between the resin and tooth structure leading to microleakage. If the stress exceeds the tensile strength of the enamel, it can result in fracture of enamel along the interface. Polymerization shrinkage is greatest in region where curing is done most rapidly.

In chemically activated resins or self-cure resins, polymerization reaction occurs rapidly in the center, as it is insulated from all the sides and the heat generated during the reaction accelerates the chemical reaction. The contraction occurs more slowly and evenly with a tendency to draw toward the center of the restoration in chemically cured composites. This contraction toward the

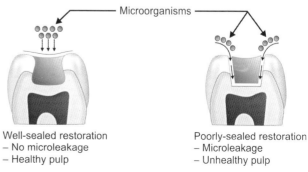

**Fig. 17.9:** Microleakage in composite restorations.

center highlights the importance of concept of adhesion of composite resins to the tooth structure.

Polymerization shrinkage in light cure resins occurs similar to the self-cure resins except that the contraction occurs fastest in area closest to the activator. Polymerization shrinkage occurs toward the light source and tends to pull away the resin away from the tooth structure. In cases of light cure composites, net effect of contraction can be reduced by adding and curing composites in increments. Use of glass ionomer cement (GIC) as base can reduce the amount of shrinkage, as the quantity of composite required will be less **(Fig. 17.10).**

The amount and quality of light directed on the composite resins influence the degree of polymerization. Duration of exposure of light is critical for polymerization reaction. Shorter exposure of light will produce less polymerization than longer exposure. Accepted time for light exposure is 40 seconds, although 60 seconds of exposure will result in better polymerization. However, exposure time of more than a minute does not significantly improve polymerization of the resin.

---

**CLINICAL SIGNIFICANCE**

The effect of polymerization shrinkage can be minimized by curing composite resin in small increments not more than 2 mm and providing adequate exposure of light. Another way of managing polymerization shrinkage is by placing indirect restoration.

---

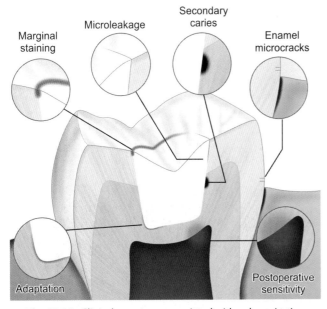

**Fig. 17.10:** Clinical symptoms associated with polymerization shrinkage of composite restorations.

## Configuration Factor or C-factor

It is related to the geometry of cavity preparation and is represented by a ratio between the bonded surface area of the resin-based composite to the unbonded surface or free surface area.

$$C-factor = \frac{Bonded\ surface}{Unbonded\ surface}$$

Configuration or C-factor was first advocated by AJ Feilzer et al. in 1987. Greater the value of the C-factor, larger will be the effect of residual polymerization. Also, higher the C-factor, greater are the chances of disruption of the bond from the polymerization effects. Higher C-factor means that there is less unbonded surface, which is available and therefore there is less flow of composite resin over this area resulting in greater interfacial stress and polymerization shrinkage. Stress can cause interface breakdown, gap formation and microleakage. On the other hand, when the C-factor is low, i.e. a smaller ratio occurs between the bonded and unbonded or free surface, composite resin easily flows over the larger unbonded surface undergoing polymerization resulting in less stress caused during polymerization shrinkage.

## C-Factors in Different Preparations

- Class I and Class V preparation have five bonded surface and one unbonded surface are at the greatest risk as the C-factor is 5/1 = 5
- Class II preparation has four-bonded surface and two unbonded surface, so the C-factor is 4/2 = 2
- Class III preparation has three bonded surface and three unbonded surface and has C-factor as 3/3 = 1
- Class IV preparation has one bonded surface and four unbonded surface and has C-factor as 1/4 = 0.25. Therefore, it is at low risk of effects of polymerization shrinkage **(Fig. 17.11).**

*Polymerization shrinkage can be minimized by using:*
- *Soft-start polymerization instead of high-intensity curing:* In this technique, curing begins with low intensity and ends with high intensity. This allows slow initial polymerization and greater level of stress relaxation in the early stages and ends at the maximum intensity once the gel point is achieved. With such approach, highest level of DC is achieved after maximum of internal stress is relaxed. Curing lamps are available, which provide soft-start exposure sequences

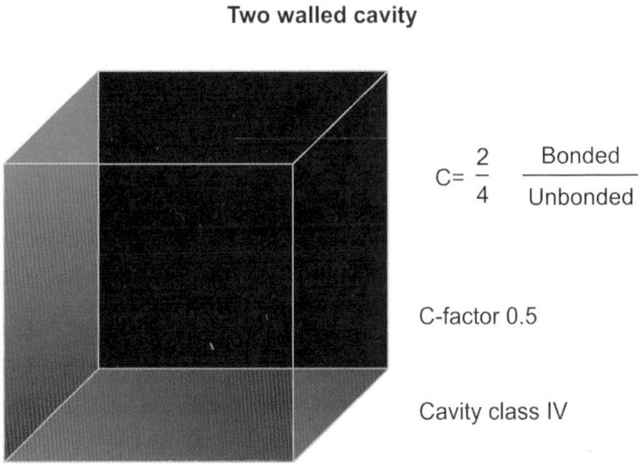

Two walled cavity

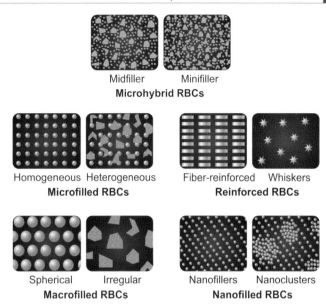

$$C = \frac{2}{4} \quad \frac{\text{Bonded}}{\text{Unbonded}}$$

C-factor 0.5

Cavity class IV

**Fig. 17.11:** Configuration factor for class IV cavity preparation.

- *Resins added and cured in increments*: Using layering technique can reduce polymerization stress by minimizing C-factor. In this technique, the restoration is built up in increments, i.e. curing one layer at a time. This effectively reduces polymerization stress by minimizing the C-factor. Adding small increments in thin layers reduces the bonded surface area and maximizes the unbonded surface area thereby reducing the C-factor. Layering technique addresses the depth of cure and residual stress concentration issues but increases time of curing the restoration
- *By using stress-breaking liner such as dentinal adhesive*
- *Ramped curing and delayed curing*—are two methods employed to reduce stress buildup during polymerization. In ramped curing method, the intensity of the light is increased gradually during the exposure. This ramping is achieved by using stepwise, linear or exponential modes. In the method of delayed curing, the composite restoration is initially cured with low-intensity light for a few seconds to achieve initial hardening. Then the clinician removes excess material by sculpting to proper contour and adjusting the occlusion. After the correction, he applies second exposure of high-intensity light for the final curing of resin.

## TYPES OF COMPOSITES (FIG. 17.12)

### Macrofilled Composites

Macrofilled composite also called as *traditional* or *conventional* composites. These composites were developed in early 1970s and were modified over a period of time.

### Composition

Inorganic filler particles in the form of *finely ground amorphous silica and quartz*. Filler particles are surrounded

Midfiller        Minifiller
**Microhybrid RBCs**

Homogeneous  Heterogeneous          Fiber-reinforced   Whiskers
**Microfilled RBCs**                    **Reinforced RBCs**

Spherical        Irregular            Nanofillers    Nanoclusters
**Macrofilled RBCs**                    **Nanofilled RBCs**

**Fig. 17.12:** Types of composite resins
*Abbreviation:* RBCs, resin-based composites.

by the resin matrix. Average size of the particles is 8–12 μm, although particles can be as large as 50 μm. Fillers usually comprise 70–80% by weight of composite **(Figs. 17.13A to C)**.

### Properties

- Macrofilled composites have improved properties than the unfilled resins
- *Compressive strength*—250–300 MPa
- *Tensile strength*—50–65 Mpa
- *Modulus of elasticity*—8–15 GPa
- *Coefficient of thermal expansion*—25–35 ppm/°C
- *Water sorption*—0.5–0.7 mg/cm$^2$
- *Knoop hardness*—55 KHN
- *Radiopacity*—2–3 mm Al
- *Esthetics*—polishing results in rough surface and it is due to faster wear of the resin matrix than the filler particles.

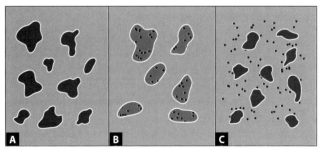

**Figs. 17.13A to C:** Types of filler particles; (A) Conventional; (B) Microfilled; (C) Hybrid.

**CLINICAL SIGNIFICANCE**
- Greater surface roughness due to abrasive wear of the soft resin matrix exposing the wear resistant resin particles
- Polishing results rougher finish
- More susceptible to discoloration and extrinsic staining due to rough surface, which retains stains
- Poor-wear resistance.

### Microfilled Composites

They were first developed in the late 1970s to overcome the problems of surface roughening and low translucency of macrofilled and small particle composites. Here, colloidal silica particles are used as inorganic filler.

#### Composition

Inorganic filler particles are in the form of *colloidal silica particles* in the range of 0.01–0.1 μm. The size of these filler particles was much smaller than those of macrofilled composites. Several small filler particles have larger surface area than a single large particle and therefore it was very difficult to load large volume of microfillers in the resin matrix. The volume of fillers in microfilled composites was only 35–50% as opposed to 70–85% in other composites. Lower volume of filler resulted in composite with poor mechanical properties. In order to improve properties attempt was made to increase the volume of filler particles. Initially, there was a limitation in adding the amount of filler because of the high-surface area to volume ratio of the filler thereby greatly increasing the viscosity. Although numbers of methods are used to increase the filler loading but the most common method is through the use of prepolymerized particles.

*Prepolymerized filler particles* are obtained by mixing 60–70% by weight of silane-treated colloidal silica to a monomer at a slightly raised temperature. This combination is polymerized at an increased temperature and pressure using benzoyl peroxide. After complete polymerization, the material is freezed and then ground to fine particles in the range of 1–200 μm. The prepolymerized particles are called as *organic fillers*. This term is a misnomer as they contain high percentage of inorganic fillers. Although prepolymerized particles allow higher filler loadings but they cannot bond to the matrix phase using silane coupling agents. For this, matrix monomers diffuse into the filler particles to form micromechanical interlocks to result in *interfacial bonding*. These organic fillers permit the greater amount of filler content, thereby reducing polymerization shrinkage **(Figs. 17.14A and B)**.

Alternately, microfillers were clumped together by heating them or by condensing them into large particles to increase the filler volume.

#### Properties

- Microfilled composites are highly esthetic restorative composites but their properties are inferior to those of traditional composites. This is due to the fact that 40–60% by volume of microfilled composites are made of resin matrix, which can result in greater water sorption, greater coefficient of thermal expansion and reduced elastic modulus
- *Compressive strength*—250–350 MPa
- *Tensile strength*—30–50 MPa have reduced tensile strength because of weak bond of prepolymerized particles to the clinically cured resin matrix.

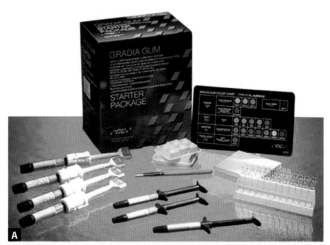

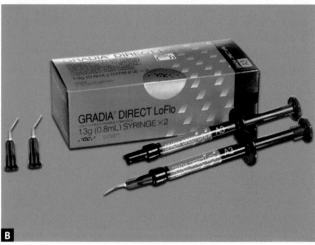

**Figs. 17.14A and B:** Microfilled composite resin.

- *Modulus of elasticity*—3–6 GPa—reduced modulus of elasticity, greater CTE and water sorption are due to the presence of larger amount of resin as compared to the inorganic fillers
- *Coefficient of thermal expansion*—50–60 ppm/°C
- *Water sorption*—1.4–1.7 mg/cm$^2$
- *Knoop hardness*—25–35 KHN
- *Curing shrinkage*—2–3%
- *Radiopacity*—0.5–2 mm Al
- *Esthetics*—greater resin content and presence of microfillers are responsible for improved surface finish.

---

**CLINICAL SIGNIFICANCE**

- Material of choice for esthetic restorations of anterior teeth especially in nonstress-bearing areas (Class III and Class V)
- Material of choice for restoring subgingival areas because of their smooth surface
- As composite veneering material in patient without parafunctional habits
- Class V restorations, small Class I restorations and Class III restorations
- The use of these materials should not be used in stress-bearing areas (Class II and Class IV), as they have inferior properties and have greater susceptibility to fracture
- Diamond burs should be preferred over tungsten carbide burs for trimming composite to reduce the risk of chipping.

---

### Disadvantages

- Weak bond between the composite particles and the resin matrix resulting in chipping of the material. Due to this shortcoming, the microfilled composites are used mostly in the nonstress-bearing areas
- Physical and mechanical properties are inferior to traditional composites.

### Small Particle-filled Composites

These composites were developed to improve the surface smoothness and enhance the physical and mechanical properties of traditional composites.

### Composition

- Inorganic fillers are ground to the size of range between 0.5 μm and 3.0 μm. Broad distributions in the particle size permit high-filler loading of small particle-filled (SPF) composites
- Contain 80–90% by weight of inorganic fillers. These inorganic fillers can be either amorphous silica or

glasses, which contains heavy metal for radiopacity. Colloidal silica is added 5% by weight to adjust the viscosity of the paste to facilitate in packing into the cavity
- Matrix resin of the SPF composites is similar to the traditional and microfilled composites.

### Properties

- As they have greater filler content, they have superior physical and mechanical properties
- *Compressive strength*—350–400 MPa
- *Tensile strength*—75–90 MPa greater than the traditional composites and about double than the microfilled composites
- *Modulus of elasticity*—15–20 GPa
- *Coefficient of thermal expansion*—19–26 ppm/°C
- *Water sorption*—0.5–0.6 mg/cm$^2$
- *Knoop hardness*—50–60 KHN
- *Curing shrinkage*—2–3% by volume
- *Radiopacity*—since they contain heavy metal glasses in fillers, they are radiopaque. This property aids in the diagnosis of *secondary caries* in the posterior teeth. But these heavy metal glass filler are softer and tend to wear and deteriorate with time reducing the durability of the restoration
- Has greater wear resistance and reduced polymerization shrinkage.

---

**CLINICAL SIGNIFICANCE**

- Small particle-filled composites are indicated in high stress and abrasion-prone restorations of Class IV and Class II
- They have relatively smooth surface but is less than microfilled composites.

---

### Hybrid Composites

Currently, majority of the composites used are the hybrid composites. This type of composite was developed to provide better surface smoothness and esthetics than the small particles without compromising on the mechanical properties **(Fig. 17.15)**.

### Composition

- Contains two types of filler particles namely—(1) colloidal silica and (2) ground particles of glass-containing heavy metals
- Filler particles contain submicron particles of size 0.04 μm and small particles of size 1–4 μm. Microhybrid composites contain mixture of small particles (0.5–3 μm) and microfine filler particles (0.04 μm)

- Total filler content is 75–80% by weight of which colloidal silica constitutes 10–20% by weight of the total filler content
- Combination of different sizes of filler particles improves the properties and polishability of composite materials.

## Properties

The properties of hybrid composites range between the traditional and the SPF composites. Recently, microhybrid composites are introduced, which blend submicron particles (0.04 μm) and the small particles of 0.1–1 μm. This blending improves the handling characteristics and good polishability. This has provided clinical flexibility to be used in both anterior and posterior regions.

- *Compressive strength*—300–350 MPa
- *Tensile strength*—40–50 MPa
- *Modulus of elasticity*—11–15 GPa
- *Coefficient of thermal expansion*—30–40 ppm/°C
- *Water sorption*—0.5–0.7 mg/cm$^2$
- *Knoop hardness*—50–60 KHN
- *Curing shrinkage*—2–3% by volume
- *Radiopacity*—2–4 mm Al, as they have heavy metal atoms, they aid in the radiographic detection of secondary caries.

### CLINICAL SIGNIFICANCE

- Material of choice for Class III and Class IV restorations in anterior region
- Can also be used in posterior load-bearing areas.

## Nanohybrid Composites

These are recently introduced microfilled hybrids, which uses the nanofiller technology of using the filler size and increasing the filler loading. Nanofiller particles are monodispersed, nonaggregated and nonagglomerated silica nanoparticles, which are in the range of 20–75 nm. Nanoparticles are discrete particles, which develop into three-dimensional macromolecule chain, which have minimal effect on viscosity. These composites can be treated as first universal composites, which combine the properties of microfilled composites (handling and polishability) and macrofilled composites (wear resistance).

Nanosized or near-nanosized fillers are produced by solution-gel processing of silica, polyhedral oligomeric silsesquioxanes (POSS) or metal-oxide nanoparticles. As these particles can be easily agglomerated, a wider range of filler sizes is possible and high-filler levels are generated **(Fig. 17.16)**. Nanohybrid and nanofilled resins are two types of composites called as nanocomposites. Nanohybrid consists of mixture of two or more range of filler particles where at least one is nanoparticle size. If the filler particle size is more than 100 nm, these particles will scatter visible light and will reduce the translucency and reduce depth of cure of the composites. Therefore, all nanocomposites should have filler particle size strictly below 100 nm. Some available nanocomposites are—Tetric N-Ceram (Ivoclar Vivadent), Herculite Ultra (Kerr/Sybron) and Filtek Z350XT (3M ESPE).

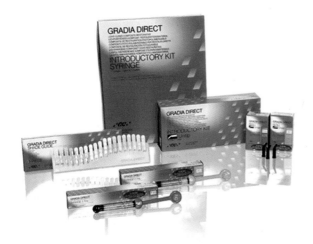

**Fig. 17.15:** Hybrid composite resin.

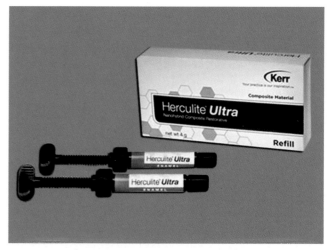

**Fig. 17.16:** Nanohybrid composite resin kit.

## Composition

They contain nanometer-sized filler particles in the range of 0.005–0.01 μm throughout the resin matrix. They are combined with more conventional type of filler technology.

> **CLINICAL SIGNIFICANCE**
>
> Nanofilled composites can be used in both anterior and posterior regions. They have slightly better polishability because of the smaller particle size. Higher filler levels can result in good physical properties and esthetics. Nanofilled composites are not as strong as hybrid composites. Therefore to improve mechanical properties two or more filler particles are incorporated.

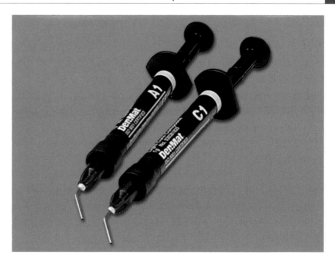

**Fig. 17.17:** Flowable composite resin.

## Advantages

- Improved mechanical properties
- Can be finished and polished to high luster
- Less biodegradation of material with time
- Reduced polymerization shrinkage because of reduced particle size
- Reduced marginal leakage, discoloration and postoperative sensitivity.

### Flowable Composites

These are lightly filled low-viscosity composites, which were developed to be used in areas of limited accessibility. As the filler content is low, these materials flow easily, spread uniformly and have good adaptation to the cavity walls. Flowable composites exhibit higher polymerization shrinkage and lower wear resistance than the microhybrid composites. They should always be placed in thin layers because of higher shrinkage **(Fig. 17.17).**

## Composition

They are composed of traditional composite resins with filler loading reduced to 30–55% volume as compared to 57–72% volume of traditional hybrid composite resin. The size of the filler particles varies between 0.6 μm and 1.0 μm.

## Properties

- *Flexural strength*—70–120 MPa
- *Modulus of elasticity*—4–8 GPa
- *Polymerization shrinkage*—3–5% volume
- *Radiopacity*—1–4 mm Al.

> **CLINICAL SIGNIFICANCE**
>
> - Flowable composites are recommended in small Class I restorations as pit and fissure sealants
> - They are used in Class V restorations and abrasion/abfraction lesions, as they have low modulus of elasticity and low viscosity. As their elastic modulus is closer to the tooth structure, they can flex with the tooth in areas of stress. They are placed directly into the prepared cavity through small needles from the syringe. Because of their low-viscosity they easily flow into the irregularities created by diamond bur
> - Can be used as marginal repair materials
> - Can be used thin layer liner in large Class II restorations because they adapt well and have low-elastic modulus, which allows them to cushion against stresses created by polymerization shrinkage or heavy masticatory forces
> - Are indicated in areas of limited accessibility, which are exposed to minimal wear
> Useful as Class I restoration in gingival areas.

## Advantages

- Ease to use and handle
- Good wettability
- Excellent adaptation
- Greater flexibility due to low-elastic modulus.

## Disadvantages

- High-polymerization shrinkage
- Low-wear resistance
- Low strength
- Inferior mechanical properties.

## Packable Composites

Packable or condensable composites were introduced in the late 1990s to provide a resin material, which could be used like amalgam. These composites have higher viscosity and are condensed into the cavity similar to amalgam. They are type of hybrid composite, which were developed to accomplish two goals namely easy restoration of the proximal contact and similar handling properties as amalgam. Some of the packable composites are based on the newly introduced concept called PRIMM (polymer rigid inorganic matrix material). This system consists of a resin and a ceramic component. The fillers are incorporated as a continuous network or scaffold of ceramic fibers **(Fig. 17.18).**

### Composition

- They consist of fibrous, elongated filler particles of size 100 µm and textured surfaces that interlock and resist flow causing the uncured resin to be stiff and resistant to slumping.
- The inorganic filler content is 65–81% by weight. They have higher filler content than the hybrid composites.

### Properties

- Tensile strength is 40–45 MPa
- Modulus of elasticity is 3–13 GPa
- The uncured resin remains stiff and resistant to slumping but yet can be molded by pluggers.
- Rough surfaces and fibrous fillers produce the packable consistency.

- Packable composites have not presented with any advantage over the hybrid composite for restoring the posterior teeth
- Physical and mechanical properties of these composites are similar to traditional hybrid composites. They have been shown to have reduced wear resistance
- As long-term clinical studies are not available to determine its longevity. They are used in posterior teeth in areas of high-functional loading as they are stronger and more wear resistant.

### Indications

- Restoration in stress-bearing areas
- Class II restorations, as they allow easier development of proximal contacts.

### Advantages

- Can be condensed similar to amalgam **(Fig. 17.19).** They are not truly condensed but are packed into the prepared cavity
- Greater ease in establishing proximal contact
- Provide better reproduction of occlusal anatomy
- Owing to greater filler content they show less polymerization shrinkage
- Physical and mechanical properties similar to hybrid composites.

### Disadvantages

- Difficult in handling
- More time consuming than amalgam

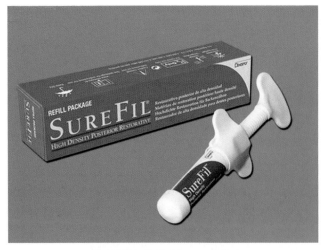

**Fig. 17.18:** Packable composite.

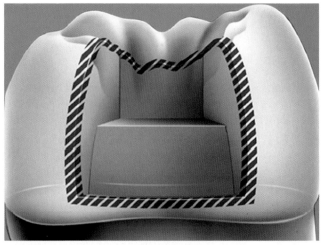

**Fig. 17.19:** Packable composite packed into prepared cavity similar to amalgam.

- Poor esthetics because of rough surface
- No long-term clinical studies to support the material.

## Compomers

These are polyacid modified resin composites having filler content derived from both composites and glass ionomers. These materials are low-fluoride releasing composites, which contain vinyl groups and can be light cured.

For example, Hytac (ESPE), Compoglass (Ivoclar Vivadent), Dyract (Dentsply), F2000 (3M–ESPE) **(Fig. 17.20).**

## Setting Reaction

Reaction of glass ionomer within the compomer requires oral fluids to diffuse into the composite. Fluoride is able to diffuse out of the composite after the fluids swell the composite and expose the polymer network. This released fluoride is less as compared to conventional GIC or resin-modified GIC.

The fluoride release capacity and properties vary between different brands of materials. Hytac has lower fluoride release and superior properties simulating resin composites whereas Dyract, Compoglass, F2000 simulates resin modified GIC.

## Composition

They are composed of polyacid-modified monomers having fluoride-releasing silicate glasses. The filler content ranges between 42% and 67% by volume and the average filler particle size is 0.8–5 μm. It is packaged in single paste in form of Compules and syringes.

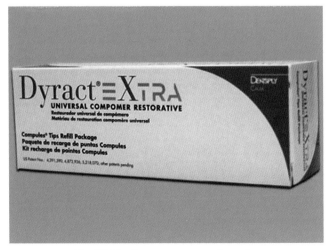

**Fig. 17.20:** Compomer restorative resin.

## Properties

- *Compressive strength*—180–250 MPa
- *Elastic modulus*—6–7 GPa
- *Flexural strength*—65–125 MPa.

Fluoride release capacity is less than GIC and resin-modified GIC. Also, they do not recharge after fluoride treatment.

### CLINICAL SIGNIFICANCE

- Patient with medium risk of caries as fluoride release is less
- For improving the bond strength, etching and bonding is advised.

## "Smart" Composites

This type of composite was introduced in 1998 with the concept that a restorative material will react with the oral environment to fight recurrent caries. When acidity of the area around the restoration increased these "Smart" composite would release fluoride, calcium and hydroxyl ions in order to counteract the acids released by bacterial byproducts. Bacteria in the plaque would release acid as a byproduct of their metabolism of sugar or cooked starch to demineralize the tooth. These composite further would aid in remineralizing the tooth structure. However, there are no long-term clinical studies to confirm the effectiveness of the material.

## Core Buildup Composites

These composites have high-filler content to improve strength and are used in badly broken down teeth. These materials replace tooth structure lost due to caries or trauma and help in building adequate structure, which can retain crown. Core buildup composites can be light-cured, self-cured or dual-cured.

### Requirements for Core Buildup Composites

- Should have low-polymerization shrinkage stress to reduce microleakage
- Should have good compressive strength and wear resistance
- Should show improved depth of cure of at least 4 mm. These materials are often translucent and are highly conducive to light transmission
- Should have good flow to allow easy adaptation to the cavity walls
- Should bond well to the tooth structure in order to minimize microleakage.

Tooth-colored core buildup material is indicated when all ceramic crown need to be placed over the core. Amalgam buildup of badly broken teeth will have unesthetic appearance below the all ceramic crown.

Some of the core buildup materials are Surefil SDR, EvoCeram Bulk Fill, Tetric EvoCeram Bulk Fill.

### Provisional Restorative Composites

Composite materials are used to overcome the drawback of acrylic provisional material. These materials can be self-cured, light-cured or dual-cured. Self-cured material can be automixed or hand mixed and can be used with any type of matrix. After curing, it becomes difficult to remove from undercut area. Light-cured material requires clear plastic template and there is difficulty to completely cure in deep areas. Dual cure material requires additional time to light cure after chemical cure. They can be easily removed from the undercut area when they attain putty like consistency and extra material can be trimmed and finally cured with light.

### Uses

They are often used to fabricate provisional onlays, crowns and small-span bridges. Their use in long-span bridges should be avoided because of their brittleness especially if used in patient with parafunctional habits.

### Advantages

- Low shrinkage and less heat release during curing
- Good strength and good hardness
- Less wear
- Biocompatible
- Can be repaired easily with flowable composite.

### Disadvantages

- Increase in cost
- Brittle and should not be used for long-span bridges
- Color shades are limited.

### Composites for Posterior Restorations

Posterior composites *are hybrid resin composites designed for use in posterior areas, where a stiffer consistency facilitates condensation in posterior teeth.*

*Posterior composites used are:*
- Hybrid composites
- Packable composites
- Nanofilled composites
- Silorane-based posterior restorations.

### Criteria for Selection of Posterior Composite

Composite should be used in posterior region instead of amalgam, if there is high demand from patient due to esthetic reasons. There are very few advantages of using composites in posterior region. One distinct advantage is conservation of tooth structure as in composite restoration mechanical undercuts are not required for retention, which is a requirement in amalgam restoration.

### Selection Criteria

- Microfilled composites are resin of choice to restore smooth surface carious lesion in Class III and Class V
- Small particle composites have excellent esthetics and durability, and can be used in all anterior region
- Hybrid composites can be used in high-stress region where esthetic requirements are high
- Nanocomposites have increased filler loading and have better mechanical properties
- Packable composites are used in high stress and wear-prone posterior region
- Composite restoration should be avoided in large restoration exceeding one-third of buccolingual width of the tooth or cuspal coverage of fractured tooth
- Masticatory load should be borne by the sound tooth structure and should be avoided on the resin
- Posterior composites should not be used in patient with parafunctional habits such as bruxism.

### Silorane-based Posterior Restorations

This type of posterior composite has uniqueness in reducing polymerization shrinkage, thereby minimizing microleakage and postoperative sensitivity. The polymerization shrinkage is less than 1% in comparison to other materials. They contain fine particles silane-coated quartz fillers with yttrium fluoride to enhance radiopacity. They have tetrafunctional "silorane" monomers, which use ring-opening polymerization. They utilize combination of epoxy functionality along with siloxane units, which when cured result in low shrinkage.

The physical and mechanical properties of this material have been found to be similar to other microhybrid composites **(Fig. 17.21).**

### Fiber-reinforced Composites

These composites include fibers having diameter of 5–10 μm and effective lengths of 20–40 μm. The main advantage is that they have excellent strength in the primary fiber direction. It is difficult to pack the fibers or orient their direction efficiently. Small additions of fibers to regular fillers are effective in improving properties. The limiting factor is that fibers may be used only with

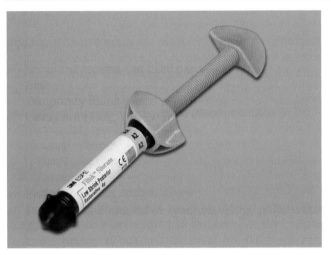

**Fig. 17.21:** Silorane-based posterior composite resin.

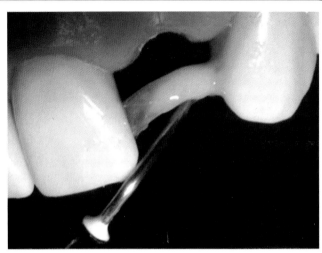

**Fig. 17.22:** Fiber-reinforced composite.

dimensions greater than 1 μm because of the concerns for carcinogenicity of submicron fibers such as asbestos **(Fig. 17.22).** These fibers are surface treated to improve their adhesion to the overlying composite and are incorporated into the resin matrix during fabrication and before curing. For example, Ribbond and TESCERA (Bisco).

### Advantages

- Greater flexural strength
- Increased fracture resistance.

## CLINICAL MANIPULATION

### Preoperative Evaluation

Operating site is cleaned using pumice slurry to remove plaque, calculus and superficial stains to improve bonding. Local anesthesia can be given, as it makes the procedure pleasant, time saving and reduces salivation. The best type of resin composite for the restoration should be chosen. For posterior teeth, composites with good mechanical properties and for anterior teeth, composites with good esthetics are chosen. For cervical lesions highly polishable composites are selected. Appropriate shade is selected for use in the area of interest.

### Guidelines for Tooth Preparation

- It is limited to the extent of the defect and removal of all fault, old material or friable tooth structure
- Proximal contact clearance is not necessary unless it is required to facilitate proximal matrix placement
- To facilitate bonding the tooth surface is made rough using diamond abrasives

- Pulpal and axial walls need not be flat
- Enamel bevel is given to increase the surface area for etching and bonding
- Cavosurface presents on the root surfaces are made with a butt joint.

### Acid Etching

The prepared tooth surface is etched with 37% phosphoric acid for 15 seconds and rinsed. Etched surface should not be contaminated by mouth fluids. If it happens, reapply the etchant for 10 seconds. The etched enamel surface should be dried to examine for a *frosted, matte* appearance to confirm proper enamel etching **(Fig. 17.23).**

### Application of Bonding Resin

The adhesive or bonding agent is applied over the etched surface and cured following the manufacturer's instructions.

### Use of Cavity Liners

If the preparation is conservative, liner is not required in addition to adhesive agent. In deeper preparations, however, calcium hydroxide or a glass-ionomer liner may be useful. Zinc oxide eugenol should not be used as liner below composite restoration as it inhibits its polymerization.

### Advantages of Glass-ionomer Liners under Posterior Resin Composite Restoration

- Glass-ionomer materials bond to both tooth structure and overlying resin composite
- It releases fluoride reducing the incidence of secondary caries

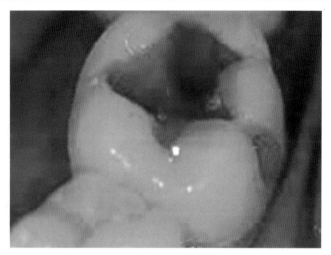

**Fig. 17.23:** Acid etchant applied over the prepared cavity.

- It improves marginal integrity and reduces marginal leakage
- It reinforces the preparation walls by adhering to dentin and minimizes cuspal deformation under load
- Glass-ionomer liners reduce the rise in pulpal temperature associated with application of the curing light during incremental insertion procedures and thereby reduce postoperative sensitivity.

### Bonded-base Technique: Sandwich Technique

If the gingival margin of a Class II preparation is in enamel but within 1 mm of the cementoenamel junction, or if it is in dentin, an RMGI (resin-modified glass ionomer) restorative material should be placed as the initial increment in the proximal box. This technique is known as the *bonded-base or open sandwich technique*, if the gingival glass-ionomer increment comes in contact with the external environment. If it is covered by composite, then it is called as the *closed sandwich technique*.

*Advantages*
- Reduces marginal leakage
- Has good antibacterial activity
- Clinical performance is improved
- Has a chance of reduced postoperative sensitivity and reduced *in vivo* demineralization adjacent to the gingival margin.

### Resin Composite Placement

- Teflon-coated hand instruments are used. Low-viscosity composites available in the form of syringe are convenient. Composite gun is also available for use
- *Self-cured composites* not used extensively. For their mixing, the accelerator and base pastes are mixed on a mixing pad for 30 seconds and applied immediately to the etched and primed tooth surface. If two or more increments are required, then they are packed within 1 minute. The matrix is held for 3 minutes as such without any light curing
- *Light-cured composites* are most commonly used because of less discoloration, less porosity and easy placement.

### Incremental Technique

Light-cured resin composite should be placed in successive, laminated increments. *Rationale for this is*:
- To ensure proper curing and to reduce excessive polymerization shrinkage
- It increases marginal adaptation and reduces gap formation
- Less marginal leakage
- Reduces cuspal deformation as the cusps become more resistant to subsequent fracture
- Minimizes postoperative sensitivity
- *C-factor* decreases leading to increased bond strength.

### First Increment

Resin composites should be handled with caution at the gingival margin, as there is tendency for microleakage to occur in that area. After ensuring proper isolation, first increment of thickness 1.0 mm is placed against the gingival wall. A thin first layer will ensure proper light penetration throughout the increment and is cured for 20 seconds. Composite resin can also be injected using syringe tip. It significantly reduces voids adjacent to the preparation walls compared to placing material with a plastic instrument **(Fig. 17.24).**

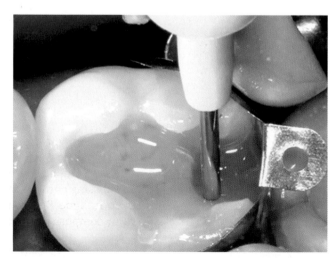

**Fig. 17.24:** First increment is injected against the gingival wall.

## Additional Increments

Subsequent increments are placed in thickness of around 2.0 mm. An oblique layering technique is used whenever access allows and the restoration should be cured from the facial and lingual aspects after removal of the matrix.

*The different designs for increment placements are:*
- Horizontal layering
- Vertical layering
- U-shaped layering
- Oblique layering
- Three increment design.

For proximal contact area buildup—after the proximal box has been filled to the level of the pulpal floor, the proximal box and occlusal preparations can be incrementally filled and cured simultaneously. Additional curing of 20 seconds from facial and lingual side is also done for complete polymerization.

## Alternative Techniques

A conical light-curing tip can be used. The proximal box is filled with composite just gingival to the contact area, and the conical tip is wedged into the resin composite. The cone is used to apply pressure to the matrix band and push it against the adjacent tooth during curing. Subsequent increments restore the cone-shaped gap formed by the tip. This ensures adequate interproximal contact and minimizes the thickness of resin composite that the light must penetrate.

## Final Increment

Careful control of the final increment will minimize the amount of finishing. A rounded, cone-shaped instrument (e.g. PKT3), slightly moistened with resin adhesive or a low-viscosity resin specifically designed to prevent sticking of resin composite to the instrument, may be used to shape and form the occlusal surface before curing. The use of an occlusal stent can reduce finishing of resin composite restorations. Another method for replacing occlusal anatomy and reducing finishing is called the *successive cusp buildup technique*. With this procedure, incremental resin composite placement is accomplished but the clinician stops the oblique layer placement and cure at a point judged to be the base of the pit and fissure anatomy for the final restoration. The final increments of resin composite are positioned and adapted to replace the missing portions of the inner inclines of the cusps, one cusp at a time. Because of their stiffer viscosity, packable resin composites work well in this situation.

The packable resin composite can be adapted and shaped without slumping prior to curing. As each cusp is

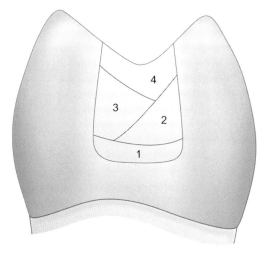

**Fig. 17.25:** Increment placement of composite resin.

replaced with resin composite, it is briefly cured (5 seconds) to set the material in place. It is not necessary to fully cure each increment at this point, since the entire occlusal surface, and therefore all preceding increments will be irradiated after the final cusp is replaced with resin composite and is irradiated for the full-curing time. This technique has been shown to provide enhanced occlusal anatomy, thereby reducing subsequent finishing **(Fig. 17.25).**

## Finishing

Finishing and polishing procedures of composite restorations is an important step. Rough composite restoration can lead to secondary caries, inflammation of gingival and surface staining of the restorations. The smoothest surface can be obtained, if unfinished resin composite is cured against a smooth matrix. This reduces porosities and oxygen-inhibited layer **(Fig. 17.26).**

Three factors influence finishing and polishing of the composite restorations. These are:
1. *Environment*: The finishing and polishing procedure can be performed in either dry or wet field. Dry field allows better visualization but increase the chances of marginal leakage due to heat production. Moist field is recommended as reduces heat generation and marginal leakage.
2. *Delayed finishing*: Early finishing of resin composite (3 minutes after placement) has been shown to significantly increase microleakage. Therefore, finishing should be delayed as long as is practical to minimize adverse effects. Delayed finishing for 10–15 minutes will allow approximately 70% of maximal polymerization to occur during the dark-curing phase following application of the curing light.

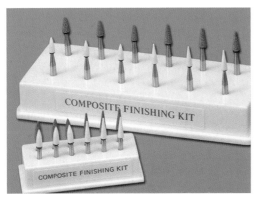

**Fig. 17.26:** Composite polishing kit.

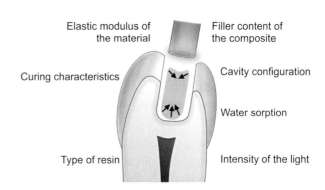

**Fig. 17.27:** Factors influencing success of composite restorations.

3. *Type of material used*: Course to ultrafine aluminum oxide disks provides the best surface with minimal trauma. Other finishing materials are fine and extrafine polishing pastes, silicone-based systems, silicon carbide-impregnated polishing brushes and points.

### Pulse Delay Technique

With this technique, the final increment is cured for a brief period (3–5 seconds) at low irradiance (150 mW/cm$^2$) to initiate the curing reaction at a reduced rate. After 3–5 minutes, the composite is again cured with a high level of irradiance. During the interim between the two curing periods, the occlusal surface is shaped and finished. The effects of manipulating this incompletely cured resin composite on physical properties and clinical performance is not known. Coarse diamond instruments are used to remove gross excess. The composite material can then be finished and blended to the tooth with successively finer grits of polishing points, cups or disks. Aluminum oxide disks, used in series from coarse to very fine, tend to render some of the smoothest finishes to resin composite. Finishing strips coated with aluminum oxide particles can be used to finish proximal surfaces. A final high polish may be accomplished using a rubber prophylaxis cup with aluminum oxide or diamond-polishing pastes.

### Rebonding and Final Cure or Glazing

It is widely reported that finishing procedures produce microcracks and remove the highly polymerized surface of the restorations. Surface sealer or low-viscosity resin with little or no filler is used to fill the surface porosities and seal the microcracks. Rebonding improves marginal integrity of resin composite restorations, reduces microleakage and marginal staining, improves esthetics, creates smooth glassy surface and fills surface porosity **(Fig. 17.27).**

## REPAIRING OF COMPOSITE RESTORATIONS

Repair of composite restoration is done, if the defect is localized. These defects can be in the form of marginal defects, discoloration and secondary caries. The rationale of repairing composite restoration is to preserve the tooth structure and to reduce the potential harmful effects on the pulp. The areas, which are easily accessible, are roughened with a diamond, etched, primed and adhesive is applied and composite is inserted and cured. If the areas are not easily accessible, the preparation is done to expose the area of interest. In certain cases, matrix band may be used to contour the resin.

If a void is detected before contouring of composite, additional resin is added immediately.

For adequate repair of composite restorations, the surface is roughened etched and adhesive is applied before adding resin to obtain adequate bond. Flowable composites are commonly used to repair composite because of their low viscosity and wetting.

*Factors influencing bond strength of repair resin are:*
- Viscosity of adhesive
- Age of the existing resin
- Type and concentration of fillers
- Voids
- Compositing of the resin
- Type of burs used.

## TROUBLESHOOTING AND ITS MANAGEMENT

### Pain Due to Pressure

*Causes*

Presence of small air bubble in restoration. So, with occlusal stress, due to resiliency of dentin, air bubble is pressed and enters the exposed dentinal tubules. It leads to pressing of nerve endings resulting in pain.

### Management

New restoration is recommended.

### Poor Isolation of the Operating Field

#### Causes

Rubber dam not used or leaking rubber dam is used, cotton roll isolation is inadequate, proper technique not used, deep gingival preparation which cannot be isolated.

#### Management

- Use of proper technique
- Matrix band can be used to isolate the preparation
- Nonbonded restorative material can be used
- If area is contaminated, then bonding procedure should be repeated.

### Incorrect Shade

#### Causes

Inappropriate shade selection, dry tooth, wrong shade selection, shade tab not matching the actual composite shade.

#### Management

- Natural light should be used for shade selection
- Different zones require different shades
- Shade selection is done when the tooth surface is moist.

### White Line Around the Margin of Restoration

#### Causes

Improper contouring, inadequate etching or bonding, using high-intensity light-curing technique.

#### Management

Re-etch, prime and bond the area:
- Proper finishing is required
- Conservatively remove defects and restore
- Adequate etching
- Slow start polymerization.

### Poor Surface of Restoration

#### Causes

Poor technique, deep gingival preparation, isolation difficult, repeated etching and priming.

### Management

- Better technique
- Use of matrix
- Microfilled restorative material.

### Voids

#### Causes

Faulty mixing of self-cured composites, space left between increments and composite with larger filler particles.

#### Management

Proper technique and repair by addition of microfilled composites.

### Open Contacts

#### Causes

Improper contoured or thick matrix band, improper wedge and movement of matrix band.

#### Management

Thin matrix band held properly and correct wedging.

### Improper Contouring and Finishing

#### Causes

Improper contoured or thick matrix band, improper wedge, movement of matrix band, undercontoured or overcontoured restoration and inadequate tooth form.

#### Management

Proper matrix and proper instrumentation.

### Poor Retention

#### Causes

Inadequate tooth preparation, operative site contamination and poor-bonding technique.

#### Management

Secondary retentive features, proper isolation and using one system bonding systems.

### Fracture of the Restoration

*Causes*

Incomplete etching or washing of the acid and wrong application of bonding agent.

*Management*

Correct application of composite resins.

### Postoperative Sensitivity

*Causes*

Overetching, inadequate isolation, contamination of composite restoration, inadequate curing of composite and inadequate pulp protection.

*Management*

Proper etching, curing, pulpal protection and isolation.

### Recurrent Caries

*Cause*

Caries left in the cavity.

*Management*

Proper caries removal.

## INDIRECT RESIN COMPOSITES

Indirect composite resins are restorative materials, which are used to fabricate restoration outside the mouth using indirect method. Mostly indirect restorations are fabricated on a replica of the prepared tooth in the dental laboratory. The restoration can also be fabricated chairside using computer-aided design and computer-aided manufacturing (CAD-CAM) systems or can be milled in the laboratory using additive or subtractive technology **(Fig. 17.28).**

### Rationale

There are certain disadvantages of using composite resins directly in the patient's mouth for restoring teeth. These disadvantages are:
- *Polymerization shrinkage*—leads to gap formation and microleakage. Effect is less in indirect resin composite (IRC) as curing takes place outside the mouth
- *Degree of conversion*—composite resin does not completely undergo polymerization. DC of direct

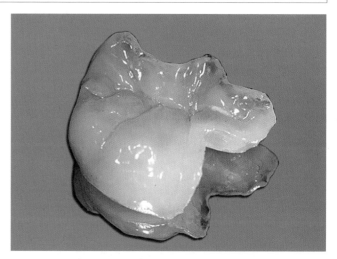

**Fig. 17.28:** Indirect resin composite onlay.

composite resin varies between 55% and 65%, whereas in IRC, it increases to 75–81%
- *Depth of cure*—effective depth of cure of direct composite resin in deeper layers is questionable especially depth of more than 4 mm
- *Wear*—direct composite exhibits excessive wear in region of high-occlusal stress. IRC have better wear resistance
- *Contour and contact*—it is challenging to achieve proper contact and contour with direct composite resin. IRC has better contact and contour, as it can be controlled in the laboratory.

### Indications

- Inlays and onlays
- Laminate veneers
- Implant supported restorations
- Full veneer crowns
- Jacket crowns
- Fiber-reinforced bridges.

### Contraindications

- Patient with temporomandibular joint (TMJ) problems
- Patient with parafunctional habits
- Difficulty in achieving isolation.

### Advantages

- *Control of polymerization shrinkage*—in IRC, since the polymerization takes place outside the mouth, it results in slightly smaller restoration than the preparation. This space between the indirect restoration and tooth is filled by thin layer of luting cement

- *Secondary polymerization*—apart from polymerization with light, the indirect restoration under polymerization by heat, intense light and pressure. This greatly improves strength and hardness of the restoration
- *Properties*—improved mechanical and physical properties
- *Esthetics*—better esthetics as the restoration can be well polished in the laboratory
- *Contact and contours*—better control over contact and contours of the restoration
- *Repair*—can be easily repaired with light cure composites.

## Disadvantages

- Expensive—additional cost due to laboratory procedure
- Less conservative—may require more tooth removal
- The final restoration is difficult to modify or improve at the chairside
- Thin layer of luting cement can undergo shrinkage at the tooth-restoration interface.

### Classification of Indirect Composite Resins

Based on type of filler content and generation of use:
- Based on type of filler:
  - Microfilled composite
  - Fine hybrid composite
  - Coarse hybrid composite.
- Based on the generation:
  - First-generation materials (early 1980s)
  - Second-generation materials (early 1990s).

### First-generation Indirect Resin Composites

These resin materials were introduced in early 1980s and were first developed by Mormann et al. and Touati et al. They were light-cured materials, which were similar to direct composite resin. For example, SR-Isosit inlay system, Brilliant Coltene, Concept (Ivoclar), Dentocolo (Kulzer), Visio Gem (3M ESPE) **(Fig. 17.29)**.

### Second-generation Indirect Resin Composite

These resin materials were introduced in 1990s, which differed in their composition from the first-generation materials. They were composed of microhybrid ceramic fillers with a diameter of 0.04–1 µm. The filler content was 70–80% by weight and the resin matrix was about 33%. The inorganic content was almost twice than the organic matrix. For example, Artglass (Kulzer), Cristobal plus (Dentsply), BelleGlass HP (Kerr Lab corporation).

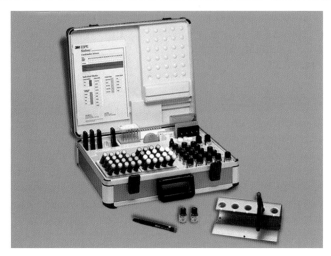

**Fig. 17.29:** Indirect laboratory composite.

### Current Generation of Indirect Resin Composites

1. Sculpture Plus Nanohybrid Composite (Pentron Lab Technologies)
2. Gradia Light Cured Microceramic Composite (GC America)
3. TESCERA ATL (Bisco).

Current generation of IRC has greater amount of inorganic microfillers than earlier resins. These materials are available in three forms mimicking different part of tooth structure, i.e. dentin, body and incisal. All the three forms differ slightly in their composition of matrix and fillers. The body and incisal forms consist of reinforced microfill with nanoparticles as fillers. Apart from the nanoparticles, large *"reinforcement"* particles are added to these resins to further improve its strength. These reinforcement particles act as *crack arrestor* and hence they are also referred to as "reinforced microfill". These composite resins have improved physical and mechanical properties and exhibit improved polishability and wear resistance.

## RECENT ADVANCES IN COMPOSITE RESINS

### Organically Modified Ceramic Oligomers (Ormocer)

Ormocer means organically modified ceramic oligomers. These resins are hybrid structures, which contain combination of inorganic and organic copolymers. There exists large spacing between crosslinks on curing. This results in less polymerization shrinkage, whereas the inorganic network with its glasslike structure improves abrasion resistance and has low-water sorption.

Ormocer resins provide distinct advantages such as reduced polymerization shrinkage, excellent biocompatibility, easy manipulation and excellent esthetics **(Fig. 17.30)**.

### Polyhedral Oligomeric Silsesquioxane

These are 12-sided silane molecule, which copolymerizes with different monomers. It is molecule-sized hybrid organic-inorganic oligomeric compound, which disperses homogenously in compatible monomers and on curing results in crosslinked network. These resins can provide with restorations, which can be polished to high luster and also retain polishability for longer duration. Apart from this, they have excellent wear resistance and mechanical properties. For example, Artiste Nano-Hybrid Composite (Pentron Clinical) **(Fig. 17.31)**.

### Polycarbonate Dimethacrylate

This type of resin, when cured, results in polyester, which uses carbonate links to connect the methacrylate to the central part of the monomer. This type of composite resin has properties similar to packable composite. Amalgam-like composite can be light cured in bulk segments without resulting in high-residual shrinkage stress. For example, Alert (Pentron Clinical Technologies) **(Fig. 17.32)**.

### Dimethacrylate with Bulk Space-filling Central Group

This type of resin contains bulky space-filling dimethacrylate monomer (4,8-dimethacryloxy methylene-tricyclodecane). It produces less residual stress on polymerization. For example, Venus diamond (Kulzer) **(Fig. 17.33)**.

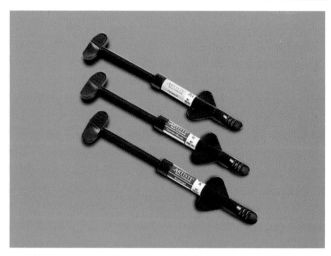

**Fig. 17.31:** Artiste Nano-Hybrid composite (Pentron Clinical).

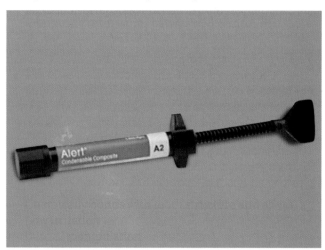

**Fig. 17.32:** Alert composite (Pentron Clinical).

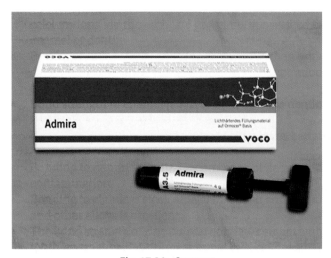

**Fig. 17.30:** Ormocer.

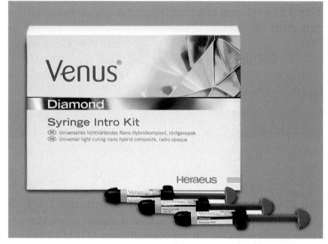

**Fig. 17.33:** Composite based on dimethacrylate with bulk space-filling central group.

# TEST YOURSELF

## Essay Questions

1. Classify composite resins. Discuss manipulation of composite resins in detail.
2. What do you mean by polymerization shrinkage. Discuss in detail in relation to composite resins.
3. Discuss the composition of composite resins.
4. Classify composite resins. Write its composition and describe the role of fillers in composite resin. Add a note on visible light-activated resins.

## Short Notes

1. Polymerization shrinkage.
2. Hybrid composites.
3. Nanocomposites.
4. Flowable composites.
5. Packable composite.
6. Configuration factor.
7. Indirect resin composites.
8. Recent advances in composites.
9. Curing lamps.
10. Soft-start polymerization.
11. Preventive resin restorations.
12. Repair of composite.
13. Low-shrink composites.
14. Core buildup composites.
15. Curing systems for composites.

## Multiple Choice Questions

1. Activation of visible light-cured composites is achieved by:
   A. P-toluidine
   B. Benzoyl peroxide
   C. Camphorquinone
   D. Bisphenol A
2. Most commonly used pit and fissure sealants are:
   A. Unfilled acrylic resins
   B. Polyurethane
   C. BIS-GMA
   D. Filled resins
3. Polymerization shrinkage of composite resin:
   A. Greater than 10% of the volume
   B. Has no effect on the final restoration
   C. Can be reduced by placing and curing resin in increments
   D. Restoration should be repeated

4. Composite resins are classified based on:
   A. Strength
   B. Polishability
   C. Resin content
   D. Filler particle size
5. To improve wear resistance the composite resin should:
   A. Have larger filler particles
   B. Have higher polish
   C. Be light-cured
   D. Have higher filler content
6. Compomer restorative materials:
   A. Release as much fluoride as glass-ionomer cement
   B. Are self-cure resins
   C. Similar to composite resin in their makeup than glass ionomers
   D. Similar to glass ionomers and do not require separate bonding agents
7. Silane coupling agent in composite resins helps:
   A. In sticking of various increment
   B. To reduce oxygen-inhibited layer
   C. Composite retain its layer
   D. To improve bond between the filler particles and the resin matrix
8. Which type of composite resin can be polished to high luster:
   A. Small-sized hybrid
   B. Microfilled
   C. Mid-sized hybrid
   D. Macrofilled
9. Light cure composites when compared to self-cure composites are:
   A. Contain resin, filler and initiator
   B. Should be polished after 24 hours
   C. Shrink when they harden in the mouth
   D. Dentist can take 10 minutes to place them in cavity
10. For curing light cure composites, which should not be done:
    A. Using special eyewear with orange filters
    B. Exposure duration of light for 40–60 seconds
    C. Light cure tip should be held 1 cm away
    D. Placing composite in increments of 1–2 mm

## ANSWERS

| | | | |
|---|---|---|---|
| 1. C | 2. C | 3. C | 4. D |
| 5. D | 6. C | 7. D | 8. B |
| 9. D | 10. C | | |

# BIBLIOGRAPHY

1. Bayne S, Thompson JY, Swift EJ. A characterization of first generation flowable composites. J Am Dent Assoc. 1998;129:567-77.

2. Boaro LC, Goncalves F, Guimaraes TC, Ferracane JL, Versluis A, Braga RR. Polymerization stress, shrinkage and elastic modulus of current low-shrinkage restorative composites. Dent Mater. 2010;26:1144-50.

3. Bowen RL. Properties of a silica reinforced polymer for dental restorations. J Am Dent Assoc. 1963;66:57.

4. Boyer DB, Chan KC, Reinhardt JW. Build up and repair of light cured composites: bond strength. J Dent Res. 1984;63:1241.

5. Chen MH. Update on dental nanocomposites. J Dent Res. 2010;89:549-60.

6. Chen RCS, Chan DCN, Chan KC. A quantitative study of finishing and polishing techniques for a composite. J Prosthet Dent. 1988;59:291-8.

7. Chiche GJ, Aoshima H. Smile design: a guide for clinician, ceramist and patient. Chicago: Quintessence Publishing co, Inc; 2004.

8. Choi KK, Condon JR, Ferracane JL. The effects of adhesive thickness on polymerization contraction stress of composites. J Dent Res. 2000;79:812.

9. Cobb DS, Mac Gregor KM, Vargas MA, et al. The physical properties of packable and conventional posterior resin-based composites: a comparison. J Am Dent Assoc. 2000;131:1610-5.

10. Condon JR, Ferracane JL. In vitro wear of composites with the varied cure, filler level, and filler treatment. J Dent Res. 1997;76:1405.

11. DeShepper EJ, Tate WH, Powers JM. Bond strength of resin cements to microfilled composites. J Dent. 1993;6:235-8.

12. Drummond JL. Degradation, fatigue and failure of resin dental composite materials. J Dent Res. 2008;87:710-9.

13. Feilzer AJ, de Gee AJ, Davidson CL. Quantitative determination of stress reduction by flow in composite restorations. Dent Mater. 1990;6:1636.

14. Ferracane JL, Mitchem JC, Condon JR, et al. Wear and marginal breakdown of composites with various degrees of cure. J Dent Res. 1997;76:1508.

15. Ferracane JL. Resin composite—state of the art. Dent Mater. 2011;27:29-38.

16. Gwinnett AJ, Kanca JA. Micromorphology of the bonded dentin interface and its relationship to bond strength. Am J Dent. 1992;5:73-7.

17. Jain P, Belcher M. Microleakage of class II resin based composite restorations with flowable composite in the proximal box. Am J Dent. 2000;13:235-8.

18. Kejiei I, Lutz F. Marginal adaptation of class V restorations using different restorative techniques. J Dent. 1991;19:24-32.

19. Lambrechts P, Braem M, Vanherle G. Evaluation of clinical performance for posterior composite resins and dentin adhesives. J Oper Dent. 1987;12:53.

20. Leevailoj C, Cochran MA, Matis BA, et al. Microleakage of posterior packable resin composites with and without flowable liners. Oper Dent. 2001;26:302-7.

21. Leinfelder KF, Bayne SC, Swift EJ Jr. Packable composites: overview and technical considerations. J Esthet Restor Dent. 1999;11:234-49.

22. Leinfelder KF, Taylor DF, Barkmeir WW, et al. Quantitative wear measurement of posterior composite resins. Dent Mater. 1986;2:198-201.

23. Lutz F, Phillips RW. A classification and evaluation of composite resin systems. J Prosthet Dent. 1983;50:480.

24. Malhotra N, Mala K. Light curing considerations for resin based composite materials: a review. Part I. Compend Contin Educ Dent. 2010;31:498-505.

25. Manhart J, Chen HV, Hickel R. The suitability of packable resin-based composites for posterior restorations. J Am Dent Assoc. 2001;132:639-45.

26. Manhart J, Chen HY, Hamm G, et al. Review of the clinical survival of direct and indirect restorations in posterior teeth of the permanent dentition. Oper Dent. 2004;29:481-508.

27. Murchison DF, Roeters J, Vargas MA, et al. Direct anterior restorations. In: Summit JB, Robbins JW, Hilton TJ, Schwartz RS, Santos JD Jr. (Eds). Fundamentals of Operative Dentistry: A Contemporary Approach, 3rd edition. Hanover Park: Quintessence Publishing Co, Inc; 2006. pp. 261-88.

28. Oysaed H, Ruyter IE. Water sorption and filler characteristics of composites for use in posterior teeth. J Dent Res. 1986;65:1315.

29. Perry R, Kugel G, Kunzelmann KH, et al. Composite restoration wear analysis: conventional methods vs three dimensional laser digitizer. J Am Dent Assoc. 2000;131:1472.

30. Peutzfeldt A, Sahafi A, Asmussen E. Characterization of resin composites polymerized with plasma arc curing units. Dent Mater. 2000;16:330.

31. Powers JM, Hostetler RW, Dennison JB. Thermal expansion of composite resins and sealants. J Dent Res. 1979;58:584.

32. Puckett AD, Fitchie JG, Kirk PC, Gamblin J. Direct composite restorative materials. Dent Clin N Am. 2007;51:659-75.

33. Puckett AD, Holder R, O'Hara JW. Strength of posterior composite repairs using different composite/bonding agent combinations. Oper Dent. 1991;16:136-40.

34. Ramos RP, Chinelatti MA, Chimello DT, et al. Assessing microleakage in resin composite restorations rebounded with a surface sealant and three low-viscosity resin systems. Quintessence Int. 2002;33:450-6.

35. Rawls HR, Upshaw EJ. Restorative resins. In: Ansavice KJ (Ed). Phillip's Science of dental materials, 11th edition. Philadelphia: WB Saunders; 2003. pp. 399-441.

36. Roberson TM, Heymann HO, Ritter AV. Introduction to composite restorations. In: Roberson TM, Heymann HO, Swift EJ (Eds). Sturdevant's Art and Science of Operative Dentistry, 5th edition. Philadelphia: Mosby Inc; 2006. pp. 497-525.

37. Roeder LB, Tate WH, Powers JM. Effect of finishing and polishing procedures on the surface roughness of packable composites. Oper Dent. 2000;25:534-43.
38. Roulet J. The problems associated with substituting resin based composites for amalgam: a status report on posterior composites. J Dent. 1988;16:101.
39. Summitt JB, Robbins WJ, Hilton TJ, et al. Fundamentals of Operative Dentistry: A Contemporary Approach, 3rd edition. Chicago: Quintessence Publishing Co, Inc; 2008.
40. Swartz ML, Phillips RW, Rhodes B. Visible light activated resins: depth of cure. J Am Dent Assoc. 1983;106:634.
41. Tirtha R, Fan PL, Dennison JB, et al. In vitro depth of cure of photo-activated composites. J Dent Res. 1982;61:1184.
42. Wataha JC, Hanks CT, Strawn SE, Fat JC. Cytotoxicity of components of resin and other dental restorative materials. J Oral Rehabil. 1994;21:453.
43. Watts DC, Al Hindi A. Intrinsic 'soft start' polymerization shrinkage–kinetics in an acrylic based resin composites. Dent Mater. 1999;15:39.
44. Weinmann W, Thalacker C, Guggenberger R. Siloranes in dental composites. Dental Mater. 2005;21:68-74.

# Dental Cements

ADA Specification No. 96; ISO Specification No. 9917–1:2007

*'The men who try to do something and fail are infinitely better than those who try to do nothing and succeed.'*
—***Lloyd Jones***

## INTRODUCTION

Dental cements, through the years have been used as restorative material, luting agent and as a base. Although they exhibit limited strength, solubility and resistance to oral environment, they are one of the most important materials used in clinical dentistry. These materials are usually inorganic, nonmetallic substances which on hardening act as a liner, base, restorative material or a luting agent.

Mostly dental cements are supplied in the form of powder and liquid or automixing syringe or capsules. Except for resin cements, powders are basic in nature and liquid are acidic solutions. On mixing these components form a paste-like consistency which sets within a reasonable time. The reaction between powder and liquid is usually an *acid-base reaction.*

## DEFINITION

Dental cement is defined as *substance that hardens to act as a base, liner, filling material or adhesive to bind devices and prostheses to tooth structure or to each other.*
—Anusavice

## IDEAL REQUIREMENTS FOR DENTAL CEMENTS (FLOWCHART 18.1)

There is no single material developed so far which fulfills all the requirements.

- Should be nontoxic, nonirritant to pulp and other tissues
- Should have adequate working time to place the restoration
- Should have sufficient flow to permit complete seating of the restorations
- Should have low film thickness and low viscosity
- Should be insoluble in oral fluids
- Should possess sufficient strength to resist functional forces
- Should maintain a sealed intact restoration
- Cement should ideally be *adhesive* to enamel and dentine, and to gold alloys, porcelain and acrylics, but not to dental instruments
- Should be *bacteriostatic*, if inserted in cavity with residual caries
- Should have *obtundent* effect on pulp

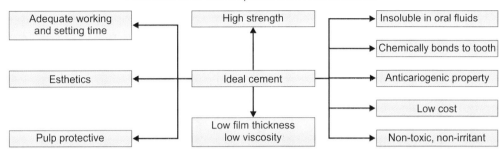

**Flowchart 18.1:** Ideal requirements for dental cement.

- *Optical properties*: For cementation of translucent restoration like porcelain crown, the optical property should be parallel to those of tooth substance
- Should develop strong bond through micromechanical bonding and adhesion
- Should be cost-effective
- Should protect pulp from effect of other restorative material
  - *Thermal insulation*: Cement used under metallic restoration should protect pulp from temperature changes
  - *Chemical protection*: Cement should be able to prevent penetration of harmful chemicals from material to pulp
  - Electric insulation under metallic restoration to minimize galvanic effects.

## GENERAL PROPERTIES

Dental cements are materials which are usually used in small amounts but can make a big difference in determining success of the treatment. Therefore, it is important to understand the general properties of the dental cements before discussion of the individual cements.

### Working Time

All dental cements should have adequate working time so that they can be correctly manipulated and used in the clinical situation. It is time elapsed from the start of mix till the time the material is to be placed or handled. It usually varies between 2 minutes and 5 minutes.

### Setting Time

Again for clinical success, dental cement should be adequate setting time so that it can be adapted to the tooth structure and carved before final setting. It is the time elapsed from the start of mixing till the material hardens. It usually varies between 2.5 minutes and 8 minutes. For light activated resin cement setting time is decided when the cement is exposed to light.

### Viscosity

It is the measure of flow. Viscosity of cement increases with increase in time and temperature. The cement should be used immediately after mixing well within the working time. Resin cements are available with different viscosities.

### Strength

Dental cement should possess minimum compressive strength of 70 MPa after 24 hours. Cements when used as base should be sufficiently strong to bear the functional load. Restorative cements require greater strength as compared to the luting cement. Resin cements exhibit better mechanical properties than conventional cements.

### Biocompatibility

All dental cements should be biocompatible. They should be nonirritating, nonreactive to the pulpal tissues. Cements based on acid-base reaction can show irritation to pulp at the time of placement due to low pH but as cement sets pH increases.

### Film Thickness and Consistency

This factor varies with the purpose of use of dental cement. If it is a luting cement then it should exhibit low viscosity when mixed and the film thickness should be less than 25 μm. This film thickness allows the cement to flow under pressure and into the irregularities of the tooth surface and the restoration. In case of restorative cement, the consistency should be thick and plastic so that it can be easily manipulated and placed into the prepared tooth cavity.

### Solubility

Cements exhibit varying degree of solubility. Water-based cements are more soluble than the oil-based cements. Low powder/liquid (P/L) ratio of cement show higher solubility and disintegration rate in the oral cavity. According to American Dental Association (ADA) specification maximum dissolution permitted after 24 hours for glass ionomer cement (GIC) is 0.1, for zinc phosphate is 0.2 and for zinc polycarboxylate, it is 0.3 mm. Dissolution of dental cement can be reduced by mixing in proper P/L ratio, correct manipulation and proper moisture control. Resin-based cements are virtually insoluble in oral fluids.

## CLASSIFICATION

### According to Craig (Table 18.1)

**Table 18.1:** Cements and its functions as well as special applications.

| Functions | Cements |
|---|---|
| Final cementation of completed restoration | $ZnPO_4$, Zn silico $PO_4$, reinforced ZnO-Eug, Zn polycarboxylate, glass ionomer cement (GIC) |
| Temporary cementation of completed restoration | ZnO-Eug, non-Eug-ZnO |
| High strength bases | $ZnPO_4$, reinforced ZnO-Eug., Zn poly F, GIC |
| Temporary fillings | ZnO-Eug, Zn poly-F |
| Low strength bases | ZnO-Eug, $Ca(OH)_2$ |
| Liners | $Ca(OH)_2$ in suspension |
| Varnishes | Resin in solvent |
| *Special applications* | |
| Root canal sealers | ZnO-Eug, Zn poly-F |
| Gingival tissue pack | ZnO-Eug |
| Surgical dressings | ZnO-Eug |
| Cementation of orthodontic bands | $ZnPO_4$, Zn poly-F |
| Orthodontic direct bonding | Acrylic resin and composite resin |

*Abbreviation*: Eug, eugenol.

### According to Phillips based on the Use of Cements (Table 18.2)

**Table 18.2:** Principal and secondary use of cement.

| Cement | Principal use | Secondary use |
|---|---|---|
| Zinc phosphate | Luting agent for restorations and orthodontic bands | Intermediate restoration, base |
| $ZnPO_4$ with Ag/Cu salts | Intermediate restorations | |
| ZnO-Eug | Intermediate restoration, luting agent, base and pulp capping agent | Root canal sealer, and periodontic bandage |
| $CuPO_4$ (red/black) | Intermediate restorations | |

*Contd...*

*Contd...*

| Cement | Principal use | Secondary use |
|---|---|---|
| Polycarboxylate | Luting agent and base | Intermediate restorations, and luting for orthodontic bands |
| Silicate | Anterior restorations | |
| Silicophosphate | Luting agent | Intermediate restoration |
| Glass ionomer | Coating for eroded/abraded areas and luting | Pit and fissure sealant, base and anterior restoration |
| Resin | Luting agent | Intermediate restoration |
| Calcium hydroxide | Pulp capping agent and base | |

*Abbreviation*: Eug, eugenol.

### According to EC Combe

- Acid-base reaction cements
- *Polymerizing materials*:
  - Cyanoacrylates
  - Dimethacrylate polymers
  - Polymer-ceramic composites
- *Other materials*:
  - Calcium hydroxide
  - Gutta-percha
  - Varnishes.

### According to American Dental Association Specification No. 8

- *Type I:* Fine grain for cementation-luting
- *Type II:* Medium grain for bases, orthodontic purpose.

### According to O'Brien based on the Bonding Mechanism (Table 18.3)

**Table 18.3:** Bonding mechanism as well as types of cement.

| Type of bonding mechanism | Type of cement |
|---|---|
| Phosphate bond | • *Zinc phosphate:*<br>  – Zinc phosphate fluoride<br>  – Zinc phosphate copper oxide<br>  – Zinc phosphate silver salts<br>• Zinc silicophosphate |
| Phenolate bond | • *Zinc oxide eugenol:*<br>  – Zinc oxide eugenol polymer<br>  – Zinc oxide eugenol EBA (orthoethoxy-benzoic acid)/alumina<br>• Calcium hydroxide salicylate |

*Contd...*

*Contd...*

| Type of bonding mechanism | Type of cement |
|---|---|
| Polycarboxylate bond | • *Zinc polycarboxylate:*<br>  – *Zinc polycarboxylate fluoride*<br>• Glass ionomer |
| Resin bond | • Acrylic-polymethyl methacrylate<br>• *Dimethacrylate:*<br>  – Dimethacrylate unfilled<br>  – Dimethacrylate filled<br>• Adhesive 4-methacryloyloxyethyl trimellitic anhydride (4-META) |
| Resin-modified glass ionomer bond | *Hybrid ionomers:*<br>• Self-cure<br>• Light cured |

## Donovan's Classification

- *Conventional cements:*
  - Zinc phosphate
  - Zinc oxide eugenol
  - Zinc polycarboxylate
  - Glass ionomer cement.
- *Contemporary cements:*
  - Resin cements
  - Resin-modified glass ionomer cement (RMGIC).

## SELECTION OF DENTAL CEMENTS BASED ON ITS USES (TABLE 18.4)

**Table 18.4:** Types of dental cement and its uses.

| Uses | Type of dental cement |
|---|---|
| Luting of inlays, crowns, fixed partial dentures and onlays | Glass ionomer cement, hybrid ionomer cements and resin cement |
| Vital teeth with average retention, thin dentin, average pulp recession, single crowns and small fixed partial denture | Zinc polycarboxylate |
| Nonvital teeth with advanced pulp recession and average retention | Zinc phosphate |
| Fixed partial dentures on vital teeth with above average retention, thin dentin and hypersensitive patient | Zinc oxide eugenol-polymer |
| Temporary cementation | Zinc oxide eugenol |
| Temporary cementation and stabilization of old restorations | Dimethacrylate resin |
| When remaining thickness of dentin is more than 0.5 mm, cavity base/liner used | Glass ionomer cement, zinc polycarboxylate and resin ionomer |
| As base/liner in cavity with remaining dentin thickness less than 0.5 mm | Calcium hydroxide salicylate and zinc oxide eugenol polymer |

## LUTING AGENTS

- *The term luting agent refers to a moldable substance which is used to seal a space or two components together*
- Luting agents are used to attach prosthesis or appliance to the tooth structure
- Commonly used cements for luting are resin-modified glass ionomer (RMGI), conventional glass ionomer, zinc phosphate, resin cement, zinc polycarboxylate or compomer
- Luting cements are of two types: (1) definitive cement and (2) provisional luting cement
- The type of luting agent is selected on the basis of planned longevity of the restoration.
- They should be fluid enough to flow into the continuous film of 25 μm thickness or less without cracking. The low viscosity of the luting agent should wet and flow into the interfaces between the tooth surfaces and the fixed prosthesis. Proper wetting of both the surfaces is important to retain the prosthesis in place.
- The procedure of luting consists of applying the luting agent on the inner surface of the prosthesis, seating the prosthesis on the prepared tooth and removing the excess cement once it is hardened (**Figs. 18.1A to C**).

**CLINICAL SIGNIFICANCE**

Water-based luting agents continue to mature over a period of time even after they have passed the defined setting time. For such cements coat of varnish or bonding agent is applied along the accessible marginal area.

## BONDING AND RETENTION

The principal means of *retention* of luting cements is by micromechanical interlocking with rough surfaces. Shillingburg has described this luting mechanism as nonadhesive, micromechanical and molecular adhesion.

### Nonadhesive Luting (Fig 18.3)

- Cement holds the restoration by engaging into small irregularities on the surface of the tooth and the restoration
- Hardened cement providing a void free seal is capable of resisting shear stress along the tooth restoration interface
- For example, zinc phosphate cement.

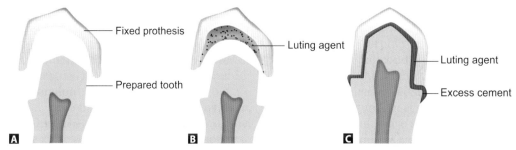

**Figs. 18.1A to C:** Diagram showing the process of luting fixed prosthesis; (A) Assembly of fixed prosthesis and prepared tooth; (B) Luting cement applied on the inner surface of prosthesis; (C) Fixed prosthesis seated in final position.

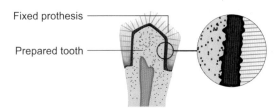

**Fig.18.2:** Nonadhesive luting.

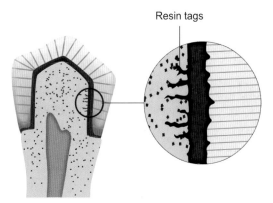

**Fig.18.3:** Micromechanical Bonding.

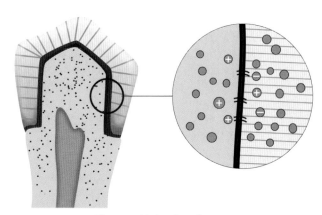

**Fig. 18.4:** Molecular adhesion.

## Micromechanical Bonding (Fig.18.3)

- This type of bonding is produced by creating deep irregularities by etching with phosphoric acid gel, hydrofluoric acid, air abrasion or electrolytic etching
- The cements have high tensile strength in the range of 30–40 MPa
- For example, resin cements and RMGI.

## Molecular Adhesion (Fig 18.4)

- It results from bipolar Van der Waals forces and weak chemical bond formation between the cement and the tooth structure
- For example, GIC zinc polycarboxylate cement

## SILICATE CEMENT

- Silicate cement [ADA specification no. 9 (New: 96)] is the oldest direct tooth colored material which was first introduced by *Fletcher* in 1873. This cement was marketed as anterior restorative material in 1903
- They have high esthetic value because of their translucency and resemblance to porcelain
- They have high solubility rate in the oral environment
- Fluoride based silicate cement were introduced in 1908 by Schoenbeck
- Average life of silicate cement is 4 years
- Silicate cement is obsolete with the advent of composites and GICs and because of its drawbacks **(Fig. 18.5)**.

### Composition

*Powder*

- *Silica ($SiO_2$)*: 40%
- *Alumina ($Al_2O_3$)*: 30%
- *NaF, CaF, cryolite $Na_3AlF_6$*: 19% (lowers the fusing temperature of glass)
- *Calcium salts such as $Ca(H_2PO_4)_2$*: Small amounts
- *Calcium oxide* (CaO).

*Liquid*

- *Phosphoric acid*: 52%
- *Aluminum phosphate*: 2%
- *Zinc phosphate*: 6%
- *Water*: 40%.

## Manufacture

- The powder ingredients are fused or sintered at around 1400°C to form glass. The fluoride content helps in lowering the fusing temperature of the glass. These fluoride salts are called as *ceramic fluxes*
- After sintering, the material is cooled rapidly causing the glass to crack. Thus, permitting the glass to be grinded to fine powder. This process is called as *fritting.*

## Setting Reaction (Fig. 18.6)

- When powder and liquid are mixed, typical acid-base reaction takes place
- Water is essential for the reaction

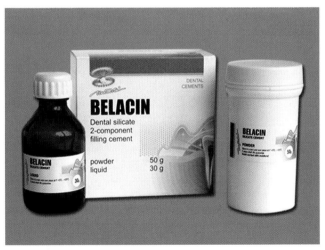

**Fig. 18.5:** Silicate cement.

- The hydrogen ions of the phosphoric acid attacks the surface of the glass particle displacing the aluminum ions and fluoride ions
- A hydrated gel of aluminosilicate is formed at the surface of the powder as the ions are liberated
- As the pH of the liquid phase rises, the metal ions precipitate as phosphates and fluorides
- The structure of set cement consists of core of unreacted glass particles which are covered by hydrated aluminum phosphate gel **(Fig. 18.7)**
- *Setting time:* 3–6 minutes.

## Properties

- *Mechanical properties:*
  - *Compressive strength*: 180 MPa—it is strongest of all the cements
  - *Tensile strength*: 3.5 MPa
  - *Hardness*: 70 KHN
- *Thermal properties*: Coefficient of thermal expansion is lower than other restorative material. It is close to that of tooth enamel and dentin
- *Biological properties*: It is classified as severe irritant to pulp. At the time of insertion, it has pH of less than 3 and even after a month it remains below 7. It serves as reference material to compare pulpal response to other material
- *Solubility and oral disintegration:* Silicate cement dissolves and disintegrates in oral fluids. The rate of solubility is 0.7% in the first 24–48 hours, but reduces after this. They are easily attacked by organic acids
- *Anticariogenic properties:* It is due to the presence of 15% fluorides. Fluoride release is slow and it occurs throughout the life of the restorations. This makes the adjacent tooth structure resistant to acid decalcification. Due to this the incidence of secondary caries around silicate restoration is markedly less
- *Esthetics*: It has excellent esthetics initially. The refractive index of silicate cement is similar to enamel and dentin. Although over a period of time the restoration gets stained

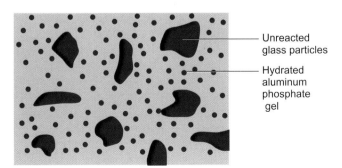

**Fig.18.6:** Schematic diagram showing setting reaction of silicate cement.

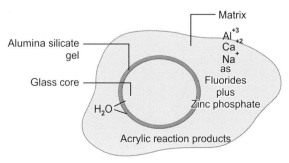

**Fig. 18.7:** Set cement consists of alumina silicate gel.

easily due to abrasion and erosion. Silicate restorations are contraindicated in *mouth breathers* as they tend to become powdery and opaque on drying. Also, it is difficult to finish and polish silicate restorations

- *Pulp protection:* Because silicate cement is severe irritant to pulp, in deep cavities it should be protected by a layer of ZnO
- *Adhesion:* Bonds mechanically with the tooth structure.

## Manipulation

- *Powder/liquid (P/L) ratio*: 1.6 g/4 mL
- Agate or plastic spatula is used to mix powder with liquid. Stainless steel spatula should not be used as it may get abraded by the silicate powder leading to discoloration of the mix
- Prescribed quantity of powder and liquid are dispensed on a cool, dry glass slab and is divided into two-three increments
- Liquid should be dispensed just prior to mixing as water can evaporate and alter the acid water balance
- The increments are rapidly folded into the liquid over the small area to form into putty-like consistency which has a shiny appearance
- Too thick a mix produces a crumbly mass whereas as too thin mix increases the setting time and solubility reducing the pH and its strength.

## Insertion

- Isolation is required during insertion of silicate cement
- If the cement is exposed to oral fluids during insertion it will result in higher solubility
- The mixed material should be inserted into the cavity in one part

- A cellulose acetate strip is held against the setting material in the cavity
- After setting the strip is removed and excess cement is removed from the margins
- The set cement is then protected with cavity varnish for the first 24 hours.

## Finishing and Polishing

Final finishing and polishing of the restoration should be delayed for several days. Early finishing of the restoration may disturb or fracture the margins.

## Advantages

- Highly esthetic anterior restorative material
- Anticariogenic properties
- High strength.

## Disadvantages

- High solubility
- Severe pulp irritant.

## ZINC PHOSPHATE CEMENT (FIGS. 18.8A AND B)

### Zinc Phosphate Cement or Crown and Bridge or Zinc Oxyphosphate Cement

It is the oldest luting cement [ADA specification no. 8 (New: 96)] which is a *gold standard* with which other newer cements are compared. It was first introduced in 1879 by *Dr Otto Hoffmann*. This cement is referred to as gold standard based on its long-term use and excellent clinical performance. However, it has certain drawbacks including irritation to

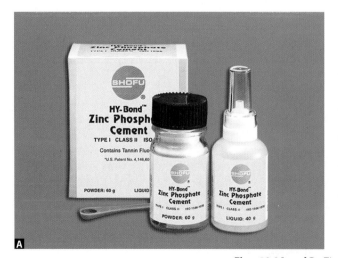 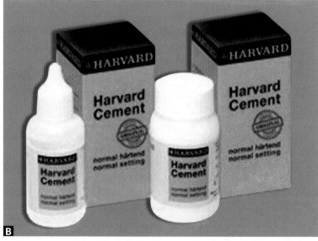

**Figs. 18.8A and B:** Zinc phosphate cement.

the pulp. Before application of zinc phosphate cement, it is highly recommended to apply coat of dental varnish in order to protect the pulp from chemical irritation.

## Supplied

- Powder liquid system
- Capsules of pre-weighed powder and liquid.
  For example, HY-Bond (Shofu), DeTrey Zinc (Dentsply), Harvard, etc.

## Applications

- For permanent luting of indirect restorations
- Can provide thermal insulation as high strength cavity base
- For cementing orthodontic bands
- Can be used as temporary restorative material.

### Classification of Zinc Phophate Cement

American Dental Association specification No 96 classified them as:
- *Type I:* Smaller particle cement used for luting or fine grained
  - Film thickness—25 micrometer or less.
- *Type II: Medium grained* or larger size particle cement used for luting and filling
- Film thickness—not more than 40 µm.

## Composition

*Powder*

- *Zinc oxide*: 90%—principal constituent
- *MgO*: 8.2%—aids in sintering by reducing the temperature of the calcination process at the time of manufacturing. It improves strength as well as imparts white color to the cement
- *Other oxides (CaO, BaO, and Ba$_2$SO$_4$)*: 0.1%—radiopacity
- *Silica*: 1.4%—inactive filler, aids in sintering
- *Bi$_2$O$_3$*: 0.1%—improves smoothness of the mix and prolongs the setting time
- *Fluorides:* Anticariogenic property.

*Liquid*

- *Phosphoric acid*: 38%—primarily reacts with ZnO
- *Water*: 36%—helps in controlling rate of reaction
- *Al$_3$PO$_4$ or ZnPO$_4$*: 16%—provides buffering action
- *Aluminum*: 2.5%—forms complex with phosphoric acid
- *Zinc*: 7.1%—increases zinc availability.

## Manufacture

- The powder ingredients are sintered between 1,000°C and 1,400°C to form a cake
- This cake is then grounded into fine powder (process called as *fritting*)
- Powder size influences the rate of setting of the cement. Smaller the particle size of the powder, faster the set of the cement
- Liquid is formed by adding aluminum and occasionally zinc, or their compounds to the solution of orthophosphoric acid
- Water controls the rate of reaction.

## Setting Reaction

- A chemical reaction takes place as soon as powder particles are mixed with the liquid. The phosphoric acid reacts with the surface of powder particles releasing zinc ions into the liquid
- Aluminum which is present in the liquid forms a complex with phosphoric acid and then reacts with the released zinc ions to form a *Zn aluminophosphate gel* on the surface of remaining powder particles
- Without Al, a noncohesive, crystalline structure matrix of *hopeite* Zn$_3$(PO$_4$)$_2$.4H$_2$O is formed in the presence of excess moisture
- It is an *exothermic reaction.* Therefore, mixing is done in increments and over large surface area of cooled glass slab to dissipate heat.

### CLINICAL SIGNIFICANCE

The glass slab should not be cooled below the dew point because water condensation will reduce the setting time. On the other hand if frozen glass slab is used, it will increase the setting time and provide more time for cementing restorations.

- The cored structure of set cement consists primarily of unreacted ZnO particles surrounded by cohesive amorphous matrix of Zinc aluminophosphate **(Fig. 18.9)**
- Water in the liquid is critical for reaction. Loss of water from the liquid can increase the setting reaction and addition during mixing can accelerate the setting reaction
- *Setting time:* 2.5–8 minutes.

### Factors Influencing Setting Time

- *Powder/liquid ratio*: Reducing the ratio results in thinner mix, which increases the setting time of zinc phosphate cement. It adversely affects the physical properties of the set cement

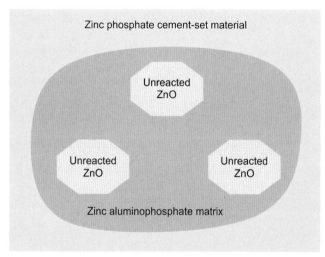

**Fig. 18.9:** Cored structure of set zinc phosphate cement.

- *Addition of powder to liquid*: In small increments, increases working and setting time as it permits more powder to be incorporated into the liquid
- *Rate of spatulation*: If it is prolonged, then matrix is effectively destroyed
- *Temperature of glass slab*: As the reaction is exothermic, cool glass slab should be used. Cooling the glass slab retards the reaction between the powder and the liquid and thus aiding in addition of adequate powder to liquid
- *Powder particle size*: Finer the size of the particles, faster the set of the cement
- *Water content*: More water accelerates the setting time whereas lesser water retards the setting reaction.

## Properties

- *Compressive strength:*
  - Strength of zinc phosphate cement is influenced by composition of powder and liquid, P/L ratio, method of mixing and handling during placement of cement
  - Properly mixed cement has compressive strength of 104–119 MPa. It achieves about 75% strength in 1 hour of mix and attains maximum strength in next 24 hours. It is due to this reason that zinc phosphate cement is the preferred base material before condensing amalgam into the prepared cavity
  - The mix cement has adequate strength to bear functional forces and is used as high strength base or luting agent
  - When exposed to oral environment, it disintegrates and there is loss of strength
  - *Factors affecting strength are:*
    - *Powder/liquid ratio:* Greater the amount of powder, greater the strength

- *Water content:* Either gain or loss of water will reduce the strength of the cement.
- *Tensile strength:* Brittle in nature has low diametral tensile strength of 5.5 MPa
- *Modulus of elasticity:* Comparatively high making it stiff, resistant to elastic deformation—13.7 GPa
- *Solubility:*
  - It has low solubility (0.06% wt), but it shows greater dissolution over a period of time as other factors come into play such as abrasion, presence of acid especially citric acid, lactic acid and acetic acid
  - *Effect of P/L ratio*: Thicker mix shows less solubility.
  - *Effect of water content in liquid*: Any change, increases solubility
  - *Effect of moisture*: Premature contact with moisture results in dissolution and leaching of surface
  - Varnish should be applied over the exposed cement.
- *Film thickness:* Thinner film more beneficial for luting (cementation) because they provide:
  - Better flow
  - Aids in complete seating of casting over the prepared tooth
  - Minimizes air spaces and structural defects present in bulk of cement. Smaller the size of the particles lesser is the film thickness
  - Film thickness can be reduced by applying pressure on casting during seating
- *Thermal properties*: Good insulator, effective in reducing galvanic effects
- *Adhesion property*: Bonding occurs by mechanical interlocking of the interfaces
- *Biologic properties*:
  - Acidity high due to phosphoric acid at the time of insertion
  - Two minutes after mixing the cement the pH is 2.14. As the setting takes place of the cement, the acid is neutralized
  - After 24 hours the pH is around 5.50
  - When thin mix is used the pH is lower and remains lower for a longer time. Thus, thin mix should be avoided.

### CLINICAL SIGNIFICANCE

Thickness of dentine as great as 1.5 mm can be penetrated by acid and therefore pulp should be protected using zinc oxide eugenol (ZnOE), $Ca(OH)_2$ or cavity varnish. Younger patient as compared to older patients are more susceptible to pulp response because greater number of dentinal tubules are open which can be penetrated by the acid. In older adults more sclerotic dentin is present which resists the penetration of the acid due to its tortuous pathway.

- In general pulp response is moderate.
- *Optical property*: Set cement—radiopaque.

## Manipulation

- *Powder/liquid ratio*: 1.4 g/0.5 mL
- A cool dry glass slab is taken so that it can help in dissipating the heat released during exothermic reaction
- Powder is dispensed on the glass slab and is divided into four to six increments
- Liquid is dispensed just before mixing **(Fig. 18.10)**. The cap of the liquid bottle should be replaced as soon as the liquid is dispensed because any loss or gain of water depending on the ambient humidity of the environment can alter the setting time and properties of the cement. In hot and dry conditions, phosphates can crystallize on the sides of the bottle as the water evaporates. In such case the liquid bottle should be replaced with a new one
- Powder is added to liquid in small portions to attain desired consistency using a long, narrow bladed stainless steel spatula. Mixing is initiated by adding smallest increment of powder to the liquid with brisk spatulation
- Each increment is mixed using brisk circular motion for 10–15 seconds before adding another increment **(Fig 18.11).** Cement is mixed in circular motion over large surface area
- Mixing is done slowly over larger area of cool glass slab to *dissipate heat* (exothermic reaction) and permit greater incorporation of powder to liquid. More the powder incorporated into the liquid, stronger and less acidic the cement. Mixing over wider area aids in neutralizing the acid and retarding the setting time.

- Correct consistency of the mix will string out 12–19 mm between the spatula and the slab before it runs back onto the slab **(Fig. 18.12)**. If the string is more than 19 mm then the mix is too thick to allow proper seating of the prosthesis. Such mix should be discarded and fresh mix should be made
- *Mixing time*: 1 minute 30 seconds
- *Frozen slab method*: Frozen thick glass slab reduces the initial reaction and permits incorporation of more powder resulting in superior properties of cement. With this method, there is substantial increase in working time (4–11 minutes). This method is also recommended for cementation of orthodontic bands and cementation of fixed bridges with multiple pins
- The temperature of the glass slab should not be below the dew point because moisture condensation will reduce the setting time
- Cement liquid should always be kept sealed in order to prevent alteration in water content
- Cloudy liquid should be discarded.

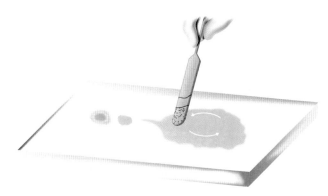

**Fig. 18.11:** Cement is mixed in circular motion over large surface area.

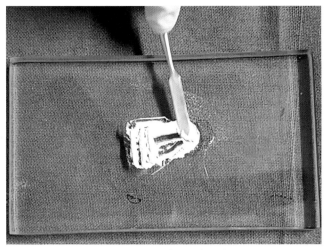

**Fig. 18.10:** Manipulation of zinc phosphate cement.

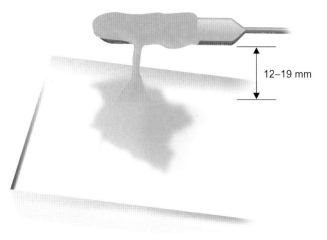

12–19 mm

**Fig. 18.12:** Correct mix should string out from the spatula.

## Insertion

- Isolation is must during cementation with zinc phosphate cement
- The mixed cement is applied to the internal surface of the crown before matrix formation occurs **(Fig.18.13)**
- Crown is firmly seated onto the prepared tooth under pressure to minimize air incorporation
- Once the cement is set, excess cement is removed and the margins are coated with varnish. Any excess cement should be immediately removed from the interproximal area using dental floss
- Varnish is applied to allow greater time for the cement to mature and to provide increased resistance to dissolution of the oral fluids.

## Mode of Retention

Zinc phosphate cement does not bond chemically with the tooth structure rather it bonds mechanically. If cavity liner is applied for pulp protection before cementing the restoration then the bond is somewhat weakened because of less interlocking caused by the surface of liner.

## Techniques to Increase Working Time

There are several techniques which can be employed to increase the working time of the zinc phosphate cement. Increasing working time is especially useful when cementing multiple crowns.

### By Reducing Powder/Liquid Ratio

This will cause the mix to be less viscous, i.e. thin in consistency resulting in reduced pH of the cement. The drawback of this method is that it will cause greater postoperative sensitivity to the patient and alter the mechanical properties of the cement.

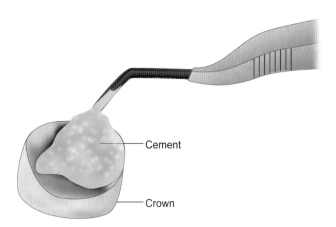

**Fig.18.13:** Internal layer of crown is coated with thin layer of cement.

### By Mixing Smaller Portions of Powder Particles for First Few Increment

The benefit of initially mixing smaller portions of powder particles into the liquid is to reduce the acidity and retard the rate of reaction. Also, heat generated during the reaction will be dissipated during spatulation. Instead of smaller portions if large portions are initially mixed the heat generated during the reaction will not be dissipated at faster rate rather it will prevent acceleration of the reaction.

### By Prolonging the Spatulation of the Last Increment of Powder

The working time of the cement can be increased by prolonging the spatulation of the last increment of the powder. Spatulation actually destroys the matrix formed and therefore extending time of spatulation will result in weak mix. This method for increasing working time is not preferred.

### By Reducing the Mixing Temperature

If powder and liquid are mixed at lower temperature, the chemical reaction is retarded resulting in delayed formation of the matrix. This is possible if cool glass slab is taken. But care should be taken that the temperature of the slab should not be cooled below the dew point as condensed water will dilute the liquid and lead to alteration of properties of the set cement. Among all the method, this is the most preferred and viable method for increasing the working time of the cement. Whenever multiple unit restoration is to be cemented, cool glass slab should be taken.

## Advantages

- Reduced film thickness
- Greater clinical record
- Inexpensive
- Good thermal and electric insulation
- Has good compressive strength.

## Disadvantages

- Bonds micromechanically only
- Technique sensitive
- Initial mix irritates the pulp
- Relatively high solubility
- Brittle in nature has low tensile strength.

## ZINC SILICOPHOSPHATE CEMENT

- This cement [ADA specification no. 21 (New: 96)] is a combination of zinc phosphate cement and silicate cement

- Presence of silicate glass improves strength, esthetics and fluoride release.

## Uses

- For cementation of fixed restorations
- As intermediate restorative material (IRM)
- For cementing orthodontics band
- As a die material.

### Classification of Zinc Silicophosphate Cement

American Dental Association specification No. 21 classified as:
- *Class I:* Luting agent
- *Class II:* Provisional posterior restorative material
- *Class III:* Dual purpose material.

## Composition

### Powder

- Zinc oxide
- Silicate glass
- Fluoride.

### Liquid

- *Orthophosphoric acid*: 55–60%
- *Water*: 40%
- *Zinc and aluminum salts*: 2–5%.

## Properties

- *Compressive strength:* 140–170 MPa
- *Tensile strength:* 7 MPa
- *Toughness and abrasion resistance:* Higher than zinc phosphate cement
- *Anticariogenic property:* Due to fluoride release
- *Esthetics:* Greater due to translucency of silicate glass
- *Solubility:* 1% by weight after 7 days
- *Pulp protection:* Needed in all vital teeth as pH is low.

# ZINC OXIDE EUGENOL CEMENT (FIG. 18.14)

- Zinc oxide eugenol cement (ADA specification no. 30, ISO specification no. 3107:2011) has been in use since 1890s. It was introduced as cement which was easy to manipulate even in presence of moisture and was well tolerated by the pulp
- It is less irritating than other cements but has reduced strength. Although modified cement have much

improved strength. It has *obtundent* effect on exposed dentin because of neutral pH
- Noneugenol cements used for patient sensitive to eugenol.

## Uses

- For temporary cementation of provisional crowns and bridges
- For temporary restorations
- Modified ZnOE cements used for permanent cementation of fixed prosthesis
- As cavity liners and bases
- As IRM
- As root canal sealers, e.g. Grossman's or Ricket's sealer
- For periodontal dressings and for giving surgical packs
- To cement implant superstructure which require less retentive properties for easy retrievability.

### Classification of Zinc Oxide Eugenol Cement

- American National Standards Institute (ANSI)/ADA specification No 30 classifies ZnOE cement as:
  - *Type I:* For temporary cementation
  - *Type II:* Permanent cementation of fixed prosthesis
  - *Type III:* Temporary filling material and thermal insulating base
  - *Type IV:* Intermediate restorations, cavity liners.
- According to O' Brien, ZnOE are of three types:
  1. Unmodified ZnOE
  2. Reinforced ZnOE
  3. Orthoethoxybenzoic acid (EBA) cement.

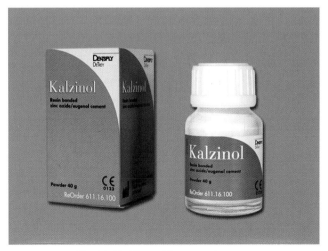

**Fig. 18.14:** Zinc oxide eugenol cement

## Mode of Supply

Dispensed in two forms:
1. Powder and liquid
2. Two paste system.
   For example, TempoSIL (Coltene/Whaledent) and Tempbond (Kerr).

## Composition

### Powder

- *ZnO:* 69.0%; principal ingredient
- *White rosin:* 29.3%; to reduce brittleness of set cement
- *Zn stearate:* 1.0%; acts as accelerator and plasticizer
- *Zn acetate:* 0.7%; acts as accelerator and improves strength
- *MgO:* Acts with eugenol similar to ZnO.

### Liquid

- *Eugenol:* 85.0%; reacts with ZnO or MgO
- *Olive oil:* 15%; plasticizer.

## Two-Paste System

- *Base paste:* Zinc oxide powder
- *Catalyst or accelerator paste:* Eugenol.

## Setting Reaction

- The setting of ZnOE cement is a *chelation* reaction. In first reaction hydrolysis of ZnO to its hydroxide takes place
- Water is essential to initiate the reaction and is also the by-product of the final reaction

$$ZnO + H_2O \rightarrow Zn(OH)_2$$

- Zinc hydroxide form chelates with eugenol and then solidifies. It proceeds as acid-base reaction while forming chelate.

$$\underset{\text{base}}{Zn(OH)_2} + \underset{\text{acid}}{2HE} \rightarrow \underset{\text{salt}}{ZnE_2} + 2H_2O$$

- Chelate formed is an amorphous gel that crystallizes and imparts strength to the set cement
- The reaction takes place more rapidly in the presence of hot humid environment (water acts as accelerator). The above reaction is also referred as *autocatalytic reaction*
- Setting reaction can be accelerated by the addition of zinc acetate dihydrate, as it is more soluble than $Zn(OH)_2$

- Set cement consists of residual particles of ZnO embedded in matrix of Zn eugenolate
- *Setting time:* About 4–10 minutes
- Setting time is controlled by moisture content, accelerators and P/L ratio.

Eugenol · · · zinc eugenolate

## Manipulation

- *Powder/liquid ratio:* 4:1–6:1 by weight. The P/L ratio varies depending on the desired consistency to be used either for luting or restorative purpose. For luting consistency the P/L ratio is 4:1 and for restorative consistency it is 6:1
- Both powder and liquid bottles are shaken gently
- Measured quantity of powder and liquid dispensed onto cool glass slab or paper mixing pad. Powder is measured and dispensed with a scoop whereas liquid is dispensed as drops. Powder is divided into uneven increments, i.e. larger increments are added first then smaller increments are incorporated to get the desired consistency
- Glass slab is recommended for mixing EBA-alumina modified cement. Mixing on cool glass slab slows down setting and enables formation of thick consistency. However, glass slab should not be cooled below the dew point because water condensed will accelerate the reaction
- Bulk of powder is incorporated in liquid and spatulated thoroughly in circular motion with stainless steel spatula
- Mixture is thoroughly kneaded with a stiff spatula. First large increments are added followed by smaller increments till desired consistency of the mixture is achieved
- In general, more the powder added, stronger the cement and more viscous the mixed cement. For restorative consistency thick dough is achieved which can be rolled into a rope. This thick dough can be packed and condensed into the cavity. Care should be taken not to add too much of powder as the mix will become crumbly. Likewise if less powder is added then the mix becomes sticky and is thin in consistency which is difficult to pack into the cavity

**CLINICAL SIGNIFICANCE**

- Oil of orange can be used to remove eugenol cements from instruments. As ZnOE is difficult to remove from the tissues it is advisable to apply petrolatum jelly on patient's lips and adjacent teeth before using this material
- Surgical pack is manipulated by mixing ZnOE in thin consistency
- Small cotton fibers are added to increase strength and durability. Tannic acid and chlorhexidine are added to the mixture. Tannic acid acts as hemostatic agent whereas chlorhexidine has antibacterial properties. The mixed pack is placed at the surgical site to alleviate postoperative pain and provide comfort to the patient.

- Equal length of each paste dispensed and mixed until uniform color is observed
  *Setting time:* 4–10 minutes
- Zinc oxide eugenol cements set quickly in mouth due to presence of moisture and heat.

## Properties

### Mechanical Properties

- *Compressive strength*:
  - Relatively weaker cement
  - Strength depends on the type of its use. Type I and type IV have lower strength
  - Type II and intermediate restoration are stronger
  - Compressive strength ranges from 3 MPa to up to 55 MPa
  - Size of particle size influences strength, smaller the size stronger the cement
  - Strength can be increased by reinforcing with alumina EBA or polymers
  - Maximum strength required for temporary cementation is 35 MPa
  - Minimum strength required for permanent cementation is 35 MPa, for bases is 25 MPa and for cavity lining is 5 MPa
  - Strength can be increased by adding alumina—EBA or polymers to the cement.
- *Tensile strength:* Ranges from 0.32 MPa to 5.8 MPa.
- Modulus of elasticity:
  - Important if used as base
  - Ranges from 0.22 GPa to 5.4 GPa.

### Thermal Properties

- *Thermal conductivity*:
  - Are excellent thermal insulators, same as dentin
  - $3.98$ (Cal. $sec^{-1}$ $cm^{-2}$ $(°C/cm)^{-1}$) $\times 10^{-4}$

- *Coefficient of thermal expansion* is close to that of tooth dentin $35 \times 10^{-6}/°C$ (dentin: $8.3 \times 10^{-6}/°C$). For this reason, it has good sealing ability and has minimal microleakage.

### Solubility and Disintegration

- Solubility of set cement highest among the cement
- Disintegrates rapidly in oral fluids due to hydrolysis of Zn eugenolate matrix to form $Zn(OH)_2$ + Eugenol
- Solubility is decreased by increasing P/L ratio.

### Film Thickness

Film thickness is higher than other cements. It is 40 µm when used for temporary cementation and 25 µm when used for permanent cementation.

### Adhesion

- Do not adhere well to enamel or dentin
- Shows good sealing characteristics despite volumetric shrinkage of 0.9%. Lower the P/L ratio better the sealing at the tooth-restoration interface.

### Biologic Properties

- *pH and effect on pulp*:
  - Least irritating of all the cements
  - Pulpal response is mild
  - pH: 6.6–8.0. Its neutral pH has mild response on the pulp. Eugenol should never be used directly on the pulp as it can be toxic.
- *Bacteriostatic and has obtundent effect on the pulp*:
  - Reparative dentin formation on the exposed pulp is variable
  - Eugenol is found to be potential allergen and some patient can be sensitive to it. Noneugenol cement is recommended for patients who are sensitive to eugenol.

### Optical Properties

Opaque.

## Advantages

- Zinc oxide eugenol cement has obtundent effect on the pulp. It also has soothing or anodyne effect on the inflamed pulp
- Provides excellent thermal insulation
- Has good sealing characteristics
- Bacteriostatic.

### Disadvantages

- Low strength
- High solubility
- Do not adhere well to tooth structure
- Should not be used directly over the pulp.

# MODIFIED ZINC OXIDE EUGENOL CEMENT

Modified ZnOE cements are of two types:
1. Orthoethoxybenzoic acid—alumina modified cement
2. Polymer reinforced cement.

## Orthoethoxybenzoic Acid—Alumina Modified Cements

Introduced to improve mechanical properties of basic ZnOE cement formulation by adding EBA as chelating agent **(Fig. 18.15)**.

### Composition

*Powder*

- *ZnO*: 70%
- *Alumina*: 30%.

*Liquid*

- *Orthoethoxybenzoic acid*: 62.5%
- *Eugenol*: 37.5%.

### Uses

- For permanent cementation of indirect restorations
- For temporary and intermediate restorations
- As base or liner.

### Manipulation

- *Powder/liquid ratio*: 3.5 g/mL for cementation and 5–6 g/mL for liners and bases
- Manipulation similar to conventional ZnOE cement
- A glass slab is used for mixing EBA cements. It need not be cooled as the reaction is not exothermic
- A bulk of powder is dispensed on the glass slab and it mixed thoroughly using a steel stiff blade spatula
- The mix is well kneaded with the spatula for 30 seconds and then strobbed for another 60 seconds to produce a creamy consistency
- Properly mixed cement flows under pressure on account of longer working time
- For achieving optimal properties, greater P/L ratio is desired
- The setting reaction in EBA cement occurs by forming a chelate with zinc oxide resulting in formation of crystalline zinc eugenolate which provides increased strength
- Moisture is essential for the setting of the cement
- Setting time: 7–13 minutes.

### Properties

- *Compressive strength increased:* 55–70 MPa
- *Tensile strength:* 3–6 MPa
- *Modulus of elasticity:* 5 GPa
- *Film thickness:* 40–70 μm
- *Solubility and disintegration in water:* 0.05% weight.
- Biologic properties similar to ZnOE cements
- Effect on pulp—mild
- *Adhesion:* Good with the tooth structure.

### Advantages

- Easy to manipulate
- Working time is long
- Good flow
- Minimum pulp irritation
- Strength and film thickness comparable to zinc phosphate cement.

### Disadvantages

- Proportioning of powder and liquid is critical
- Disintegration in saliva and blood
- Chances of plastic deformation
- Retention is less than zinc phosphate cement.

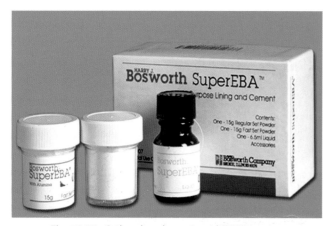

**Fig. 18.15:** Orthoethoxybenzoic acid (EBA) cement.

## Polymer Reinforced Zinc Oxide Eugenol Cement

### Uses

- For luting crowns and fixed partial dentures
- Base
- Temporary filling material
- Cavity liner **(Fig. 18.16)**.

### Composition

*Powder*

- *ZnO*: 70%
- *Finely divided natural or synthetic resins, polystyrene*: 10–40%.

*Liquid*

- Eugenol
- *Acetic acid*: Accelerator
- *Thymol or 8 hydroxyquinoline*: Antimicrobial agent.
  ZnO powder is surface treated. The combination of surface treatment and polymer reinforcement results in good strength, improved abrasion resistance and toughness.

### Manipulation

- A dry glass slab or mixing pad is used for mixing cement
- To achieve desire properties P/L ratio is critical
- Powder is mixed with liquid vigorously in small portions till uniform creamy mix is achieved
- *Setting time*: 6–10 minutes.

### Properties

- *Compressive strength*: 35–55 MPa
- *Tensile strength*: 5–8 MPa

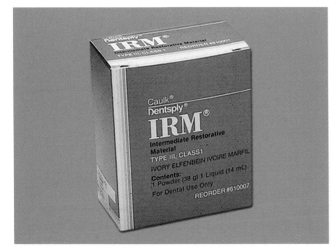

**Fig. 18.16:** Modified zinc oxide eugenol cement.

- *Modulus of elasticity*: 2–3 GPa
- *Film thickness*: 35–70 μm
- *Solubility and disintegration*: 0.03% wt
- *Biologic properties*: Similar to unmodified ZnOE.

### Advantages

- Good initial sealing property
- Adequate strength
- Minimum biologic effect.

### Disadvantages

- Greater solubility and disintegration
- Tends to discolor and soften composite resin as they interfere with its polymerization.

## ZINC OXIDE/ZINC SULFATE TEMPORARY RESTORATION

These are temporary restorative materials (ADA specification no. 96) which are supplied as single component in paste form.

### Uses

- Temporary restoration after caries excavation
- Temporary restoration during endodontic therapy
- Temporary restoration when required for short duration.

### Composition

- Zinc oxide
- Zinc sulfate 1-hydrate
- Calcium sulfate hemihydrate
- Dibutyl phthalate (plasticizer)
- Diatomaceous earth.

### Manipulation

- Paste-like material is inserted into the cavity with the help of cement carrier after caries removal
- The filling material is condensed into the cavity using a condenser
- The cavity walls should not be completely dried as the material sets by hydration.

### Setting Reaction

- The material sets chemically by reacting with water
- Setting reaction takes place slowly and the material expands on setting
- *Setting time:* 20–30 minutes.

## Properties

- Poor strength with short life span
- Good initial marginal seal. The seal improves as the material expands on setting
- It slowly disintegrates with time and therefore should not be used for long-term temporary restoration
- Radiopaque material.

# ZINC POLYCARBOXYLATE CEMENT (FIG. 18.17)

- Also called as polyacrylate cement [ADA specification no. 61 (New: 96)] It was introduced by D Smith in 1968 as first luting agent that chemically bonds with the tooth surface
- It was developed to combine the strength of phosphate cement and biological properties of ZnOE
- This cement is not used for restorations because it is opaque.

## Uses

- For permanent cementation of cast restorations and porcelain restorations
- For cementation of orthodontic bands
- As provisional restorative material
- As cavity liner and base.

## Composition

### Powder

- Zinc oxide: 55–60%—principal constituent
- Magnesium oxide: 1–5%—principal modifier, aids in sintering

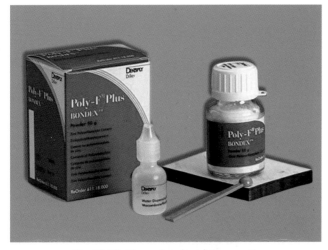

**Fig. 18.17:** Zinc polycarboxylate cement.

- Aluminum oxide: 10–40%—as filler
- *Stannous fluoride:* Small amount—improves mechanical properties, modifies setting time and has anticariogenic property. Fluoride release from this cement is only 15–20% of that released from GICs.

### Liquid

- Aqueous solution of polyacrylic acid—40%. The molecular weight of the polyacids ranges from 30,000 to 50,000
- Liquid is usually a copolymer of acrylic acid such as itaconic acid or maleic acid which is added for stabilization of the liquid, i.e. it prevents gelling of the liquid on storage. The viscosity of the liquid is controlled by altering the molecular weight or by adjusting the pH using sodium hydroxide during the manufacturing process.

## Supplied As

- Powder and liquid
- Capsules—which is mixed in amalgamator.

## Manipulation

### Conditioning

- The tooth surface should be properly isolated for better bonding
- The surface of the tooth is conditioned using 10% polyacrylic or maleic acid solution for 10–15 seconds followed by irrigation and drying
- Drying can be done by blotting or by air syringe
- The internal surface of the casting should be air abraded or sandblasted using alumina abrasive to remove contamination. Care should be taken that sandblasting for longer duration or applying excessive air pressure can damage the internal surface of the casting
- After sandblasting the surface is thoroughly rinsed to remove the debris and then surface is dried. The polished surface of the crown should be coated with petroleum jelly to prevent excess polycarboxylate cement to adhere to it.

### Procedure

- *Powder/liquid ratio is 1.5/1 by weight*
- *Working time: 2.5–3.5 minutes*
- In order to prolong working time powder should be cooled but the liquid should not be stored in a refrigerator as it tends to become more viscous due to gelation because of hydrogen bonding.

- Powder bottle is gently shaken and dispensed using a scoop. Powder is dispensed on a cool and dry glass slab **(Fig. 18.18)**. Mixing of the cement is done on a nonabsorbent surface such as glass slab
- Accurate proportioning of powder and liquid is critical for manipulation
- Liquid is dispensed just before mixing as it tends to lose water rapidly to the atmosphere resulting in a viscous liquid
- Powder is rapidly mixed into the liquid using a stainless steel spatula in one large increment over a small area. Spatulation should be completed within 30 seconds **(Fig. 18.19)**
- For good bonding, the cement is adapted to the tooth surface when it is *glossy* in appearance. Glossy appearance of the mix indicates that there are sufficient free carboxylic acid group present for good bonding to the tooth surface
- If the mixing time is prolonged, it results in *dull appearance* of the mix which is too thick to allow proper seating of the restoration. Such mix should be discarded
- The mixed cement is slightly viscous in nature and is classified as *pseudoplastic*, i.e. it flows under pressure to a film thickness of 25 µm **(Fig. 18.20)**
- Spatulation and seating of the casting reduce the viscosity of the cement
- *Mixing time*: 30 seconds.

### Removal of Excess Cement

- After the insertion of the mixed cement, excess cement should not be removed immediately as it passes through a *rubbery stage*. Removing cement at this stage tends to pull out cement from the margins resulting in voids
- Excess cement should be removed once the cement is hardened.

### Setting Reaction

- When powder is mixed with liquid, the polyacid in liquid attacks the surface of the powder particles resulting in release of zinc, magnesium and tin ions
- These ions bind to the polymer chains via the carboxyl groups
- They also react with the carboxyl group of adjacent polyacid chains resulting in crosslinked salts. This results in the formation of crosslinked polycarboxylate matrix phase encapsulating unreacted powder particles.

### Structure of Set Cement

- The set cement consists of unreacted powder particles dispersed in an amorphous gel matrix of zinc polycarboxylate

- *Setting time*: 6–9 minutes
- The pH of the mix is initially less acidic than the zinc phosphate cement around 3. As the setting reaction proceeds the pH changes from 3 to 6
- The setting reaction is increased by increasing the temperature of the glass slab and decreased by using cool slab.

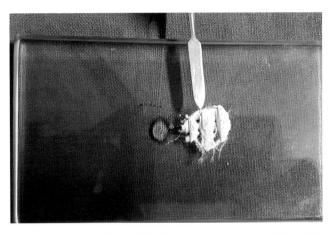

**Fig. 18.18:** Mixing of zinc polycarboxylate cement on cool glass slab.

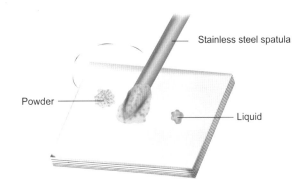

**Fig.18.19:** Powder of polycarboxylate cement should be added rapidly in large quantities.

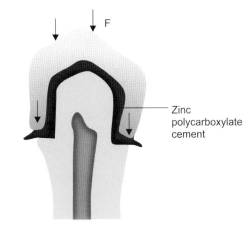

**Fig.18.20:** Polycarboxylate cement exhibits pseudoplastic behavior.

- Other factors which influence setting reaction are P/L ratio, size of powder particles, the presence of accelerators and retarders and concentration of the polyacrylic acid.

## Properties

### Mechanical Properties

- *Compressive strength*: 55–67 MPa; lower than zinc phosphate cement
- *Tensile strength*: 6.2 MPa; it is more than that of zinc phosphate cement
- *Modulus of elasticity*: 2.4–4.4 GPa; it is much less than zinc phosphate cement. It is not recommended for luting long span fixed partial dentures. Also since the elasticity of zinc polycarboxylate cement is more than that of zinc phosphate cement it makes removal of excess cement more difficult than zinc phosphate cement
- Strength increases with increased P/L ratio
- Set cement rapidly gains strength after initial setting period. Strength after 1 hour is 80% of 24 hours value.

### Solubility

- Solubility is low in water ranging between 0.1% and 0.6%
- It markedly increases when exposed to organic acid such as lactic acid or citric acid
- It also increases, if P/L ratio is decreased
- Solubility is comparable to zinc phosphate cement.

### Bonding to Tooth Structure

- Zinc polycarboxylate cement *chemically* bonds to the tooth structure
- Bonding occurs when polyacrylic acid react with calcium ions via the carboxyl group on the surface of enamel or dentin
- Bond strength to enamel is much stronger than with dentin because enamel contains higher concentration of calcium ions than dentin
- Bond strength to enamel is 3.4–13.1 MPa and to dentin 2.07 MPa
- It requires a clean, uncontaminated surface for better bonding
- Bonding to dentin is limited by presence of debris and contamination
- Bonding to stainless steel, amalgam, cobalt chromium and other alloys is excellent
- The bond strength of zinc polycarboxylate cement with tooth enamel or dentin on thermal cycling does not become zero as with zinc phosphate cement.

### Factors Influencing Bonding

- Shows better bonding to clean dry surface of the tooth
- Presence of saliva reduces bonding
- The internal surface of the casting should be sand-blasted or air abraded for better bonding.

### Biological Properties

- Has *mild* pulp response
- Has excellent biocompatibility comparable to ZnOE cement
- pH of the cement liquid is 1.7 which is rapidly neutralized by the powder
- As the setting reaction proceeds the pH of the cement rises rapidly
- Presence of fluoride exert *anticariogenic* effect
- Formation of reparative dentin in exposed pulp is *variable*

---

**CLINICAL SIGNIFICANCE**

Good biocompatibility of the cement is because of:
- *Rapid neutralization* of the liquid by powder
- Limitation of penetration of the polyacrylic acid into the dentinal tubules because of its *larger molecular weight and larger size*
- *Minimal* movement of fluids in the dentinal tubules.

---

### Advantages

- Chemically bonds with tooth structure and alloys
- Low irritation
- Ease of manipulation
- Film thickness and solubility comparable to zinc phosphate cement.

### Disadvantages

- Requires accurate proportioning of powder and liquid
- Lower strength and greater viscoelasticity than zinc phosphate cement
- Requires clean surface for better bonding
- Shorter working time.

## GLASS IONOMER CEMENT OR POLYALKENOATE CEMENT OR ALUMINOSILICATE POLYACRYLIC ACID

- First introduced by *Wilson and Kent in 1972 and originally called it as aluminosilicate polyacrylic acid (ASPA)* (ADA specification no. 96, ISO specification no. 9917-2:20170)

- This cement is based on chemical reaction between the silica glass powder and liquid containing polyacrylic acid
- These cements are adhesive tooth colored restorative materials which forms ionic bonds with the tooth structure
- It was originally used to restore anterior teeth with class III and class IV cavities but because of its anticariogenic properties and ionic bond to tooth structure its use was widely expanded
- It was developed to combine properties of *silicate cement* and *polycarboxylate* cements
- Since they bond chemically to the tooth structure, they require minimal tooth preparation. It is considered superior to other cements because it bonds chemically and is translucent. Newer formulations have been made in conventional GIC to improve mechanical properties. Also they are capable of being chemically cured, light cured or dual cured
- International Organization for Standardization (ISO) officially calls it as *glass polyalkenoate cement.*

## Applications

- As luting agent
- As restorative material for class III and class IV cavities
- For restoring class V cavities and eroded areas
- As high strength bases
- As cavity liner
- As core buildup material
- As pit and fissure sealant
- As IRM
- For atraumatic restorative treatment (ART)
- For cementation of orthodontic bands
- In geriatric dentistry.

## Classification of Glass Ionomer Cement

### According to Phillips

- *Type I:* Luting
- *Type II:* Restorative
- *Type III:* Liner and base.

### According to Davidson and Major

- Conventional/traditional:
  - Glass ionomer for direct restorations
  - Metal reinforced—GIC
  - High viscosity GIC
  - Low viscosity GIC
  - Base/liner
  - Luting.

- *Resin-modified glass ionomer cement*:
  - Restorative
  - Base/liner
  - Pit and fissure sealant
  - Luting
  - Orthodontic cementation material.
- Polyacid-modified resin composites/compomers.

### According to Sturdvent

- Traditional or conventional
- *Metal-modified GIC*:
  - Cermets
  - Miracle mix
- Light-cured GIC
- Hybrid (RMGIC)
- Polyacid-modified resin composites or compomer.

### According to Intended Applications

- *Type I:* Luting agent
- *Type II:* Restorative material
- *Type III:* Fast setting cavity lining
- *Type IV:* Pit and fissure sealants
- *Type V:* As orthodontic cements
- *Type VI:* For core buildup
- *Type VII:* As high fluoride releasing material
- *Type VIII:* For ART (Atraumatic Restorative Treatment)
- *Type IX:* In geriatric and pediatric dentistry.

### According to McLean, Nicholson and Wilson (1994)

- *Glass ionomer cement*:
  - Glass polyalkenoates
  - Glass polyphosphonates.
- Resin-modified GIC
- Polyacid-modified GIC.

### According to Anusavice (2013)

- *Type I*: Luting crowns, bridges and orthodontic brackets
- *Type IIa*: Esthetic restorative cements
- *Type IIb*: Reinforced restorative cements
- *Type III*: Lining cements and base.

## Mode of Supply

- Powder/liquid system **(Figs. 18.21A and B)**
- Pre-weighed powder/liquid capsules
- Light cure system
- Water settable type.

## Composition

Conventional GIC is composed of:

### Powder

The atomic ratio **(Table 18.5)** of alumina to silica is critical to their reactivity to the liquid component. The powder component is therefore called as "ion leachable glass". Adding more alumina can result in separate phase which will make the glass content more opaque. Other components added to adjust the setting reaction and improve the properties of the glass ionomer. Sodium fluoride and calcium fluoride acts as ceramic fluxes do not completely dissolve during the manufacturing process of glass ionomer powder. A large part of it is present in the final glass powder composition and is responsible for translucency and giving opal-like appearance.

### Liquid

Initially, the liquid of GIC cement used to contain 40–50% of aqueous solutions of polyacrylic acid but they were found to be very viscous and gel-like. Liquid of GIC should not be refrigerated because it has tendency to gel with time. Gelation occurs because of crosslinking occurring between polyacid chains by formation of hydrogen bonds.

Currently the liquid formulation of this cement is as:
- *Polyacrylic acid:* This is a copolymer of itaconic acid, maleic acid and tricarboxylic acid. These acids:
  - Increases reactivity of liquid
  - Decreases viscosity
  - Decreases gelation.
- *Tartaric acid:* This is rate controlling additive which help in improving properties of the GIC. When powder is mixed with liquid, tartrate ions first chelate with the initially released metal ions preventing direct

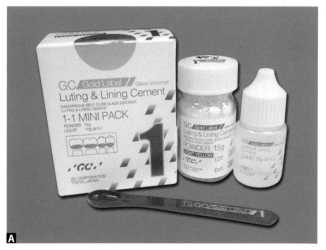
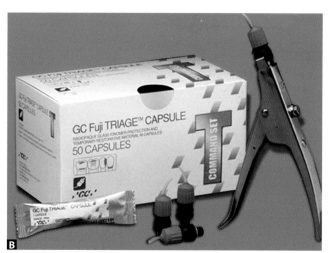

**Figs. 18.21A and B:** Glass ionomer cement supplied as powder and liquid system and in form of capsules.

| Component | Percentage | Function |
|---|---|---|
| Silica ($SiO_2$) | 41.9% | Increases translucency, skeletal structure |
| Alumina ($Al_2O_3$) | 28.6% | Increases opacity, skeletal structure, increases reactivity of the liquid |
| Aluminum fluoride ($AlF_3$) | 1.6% | Decreases fusion temperature, anticariogenicity, increases translucency, increases working time and increases strength |
| Calcium fluoride ($CaF_2$) | 15.7% | Acts as flux, increases opacity |
| Sodium fluoride (NaF) | 9.3% | Anticariogenic property. Both the fluorides acts as *ceramic flux* |
| Aluminum phosphate ($AlPO_4$) | 3.8% | Reduces melting temperature, acts as glass modifier and improves properties |
| Lanthanum, strontium, barium or ZnO | Small amounts | To impart radiopacity |
| Zirconium oxide | Traces | To improved strength |

**Table 18.5:** Percentage and functions of various components.

crosslinking with polyacid chains. Tartaric acid is a difunctional acid which forms complexes with calcium ions and the polyacids by coordinating with one or two COO⁻ groups. Titration of tartrate from ions coming into the solution delays the formation of calcium tartrate complex. This delay increases the working time without reducing the viscosity of the liquid. As soon as titration of tartaric acid is completed, released metal ions form crosslinked bridges and this causes rapid increase in the viscosity of the liquid

- Reduces setting time by increasing the formation of calcium polyacrylate chains. This helps in contributing to the early strength of the cement
- Improves working time by preventing premature formation of calcium polyacrylate chains.
- Eases handling.

- *Water:*
  - Acts as reaction medium
  - Forms a stable gel structure by hydrating the crosslinked matrix
  - Content of water is critical as more results in weak cement and less impair the setting reaction.

## Manufacture

The components of powder are fused (sintered) together at 1,100–1,500°C to form a fused or sintered uniform glass. The glass is then ground to particle size ranging between 15 μm and 50 μm.

### Setting Reaction

- Setting reaction of GIC is an acid-base reaction

- As powder is mixed with liquid, acids contained in the liquid etches the surface of glass particles releasing calcium, aluminum, sodium and fluoride ions into the aqueous medium **(Fig. 18.22)**
- Initially, *calcium ions* crosslink with the polyacrylic acid chains to form a solid mass
- In the next 24 hours, the calcium ions are replaced by the *aluminum ions* to crosslink with the polyacrylic acid.
- The sodium and fluoride ions do not participate in crosslinking of the cement
- However, certain sodium ions replace hydrogen ions of the carboxylic group and the remaining sodium ions along with the fluoride ions are evenly dispersed in the crosslinked matrix of the set cement
- Greater strength of the polyacrylate bond is indicated by charge on the aluminum complexes which has stronger affinity to bind with water than calcium. Thereby, increasing the gel strength
- Presence of water is critical for setting of the GIC. Initially, it serves as reaction medium but later on it slowly hydrates the crosslinked matrix to form a *stable gel structure*. This process is called as *maturation*
- The unreacted glass particles are surrounded by the hydrated silica gel.

### Structure of Set Cement

The set cement contains unreacted glass particles surrounded by silica gel in a matrix of polyanions crosslinked with ionic bridges. In between, the matrix are small crystallites of fluorides. Schematic diagram of set GIC cement is shown in **Figure 18.23**.

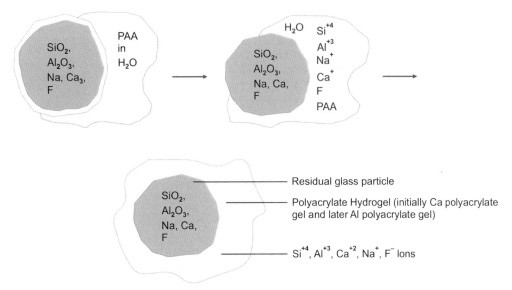

**Fig. 18.22:** Setting reaction of glass ionomer cement.

*Setting Reaction*

$$Fluoroaluminosilicate + Polyacrylic\ acid \rightarrow$$
$$\underset{(Base)}{} \qquad \underset{(Acid)}{}$$
$$Polyacid\ matrix\ (salt)$$

*Post-hardening Precipitation*
- Even after apparent set of cement, precipitation of polysalts occurs
- If the cement is exposed to water before complete hardening, it weakens because of the loss of cations and anions from the matrix
- Set cement should be protected by coating with varnish immediately after placing the restoration in order to prevent loss or uptake of unbound water.

### Factors Influencing Setting of Glass Ionomer Cement

- *Chemical constituents (Alumina: Silica) ratio:* Higher the ratio, faster the set
- *Particle size*: Finer the powder, faster the set and shorter the working time
- *Powder/liquid (P/L)* = more the P:L ratio, faster the set.
- *Temperature of mixing*: More temperature, faster the set.

### Setting Time

- *Type I:* 4–5 minutes
- *Type II:* 7 minutes.

### Properties

*Mechanical:*
- *Compressive strength:* Glass ionomer cement has compressive strength comparable to zinc phosphate cement. Type II GIC has compressive strength as 150 MPa and type I GIC has lower strength about 75 MPa (due to lower P/L ratio)
- *Tensile strength:* Diametral tensile strength of GIC is more than that of zinc phosphate cement
- *Hardness:* Wear resistance less than composite (48 KHN)

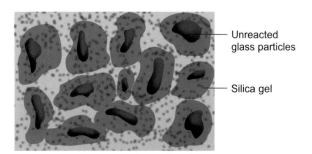

**Fig. 18.23:** Schematic diagram of set glass ionomer cement.

- *Modulus of elasticity:* 7 GPa. The modulus of elasticity of GIC is one-half that of zinc phosphate cement. Therefore, GIC is more susceptible to deformation.

*Solubility*
- The initial solubility of GIC is high because of leaching of intermediate products
- Resistant to attack by organic acid as compared to zinc phosphate cement. They are much less soluble in acidic environment in comparison to zinc phosphate and zinc polycarboxylate cements
- *Solubility:* 0.4–1.0% (for type II GIC solubility is 0.4% wt and for type I, it is 1.0% wt)
- Resistance to disintegration is improved by applying varnish over the conventional cements.

*Adhesion*
- Exhibit bonding to enamel, dentin and alloy similar to zinc polycarboxylate cement
- *Mechanism of adhesion*: There are two theories regarding mechanism of adhesion in GIC
  - *Theory 1:*
    - Glass ionomer bonds chemically with the tooth structure because of chelation reaction between the carboxyl groups of polyacids and the calcium ions of the hydroxyapatite crystals of tooth enamel and dentin **(Fig. 18.24)**
    - Bond to enamel is higher than that of dentin because of greater inorganic content of enamel and greater homogeneity
    - The bond strength to dentin is increased by treating with acid conditioner followed by application of dilute aqueous solution of $FeCl_3$.
  - *Theory 2:*
    - When freshly mixed GIC is applied to the tooth structure, it etches the tooth (hydroxyapatite crystals) to release calcium and phosphate ions.

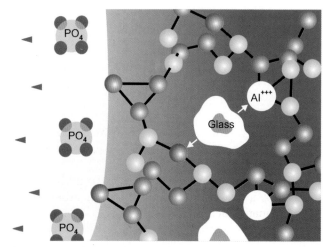

**Fig. 18.24:** Bonding mechanism of glass ionomer cement with tooth structure.

- Hydrogen ions present in the mixture rapidly buffers with the phosphate ions and raise the pH
- To maintain electrolytic balance calcium ions chelate with the carboxylic groups to form an ion rich calcium-phosphate-polyalkenoate complex with strongly bonds with the tooth enamel and dentin.

*Esthetics*
- The esthetic value of glass ionomer restorations is inferior to silicates and composites
- The restorations lack translucency and is opaque
- Surface topography is rough.

*Biocompatibility*
- Glass ionomers are relatively biocompatible. They elicit greater pulpal response than ZnOE cement but less than zinc phosphate cement
- Pulpal response to lining and restorative material is favorable
- Since luting GIC has lower P/L ratio they have lower pH for longer period of time resulting in postoperative sensitivity and is therefore having greater pulpal hazard than restorative GIC.

---

**CLINICAL SIGNIFICANCE**
- In deep preparation closer to pulp chamber, thin layer of protective Ca(OH)2 liner is recommended before placing GIC
- If adequate thickness of dentin is present then no liner or base is required to be placed below glass ionomer restorations. Remaining dentin thickness (RDT) of 1 mm or more is in itself an efficient buffer.

---

- Light-cured material have shown to exhibit greater cytotoxicity.

*Anticariogenic Properties*
- Glass ionomer release fluoride ions comparable to silicate cement and has action of sustained release
- Initially, large amount of fluoride are released into the matrix during the setting reaction, thereafter fluoride release is slow over longer period of time. **(Fig. 18.25)**: Release of fluoride ions from glass ionomer cement
- Because of chemical bonding with the tooth structure, there is reduced infiltration of oral fluids at the cement tooth interface. This helps in reducing incidence of secondary caries
- Anticariogenic activity is attributed to initial low pH, leaching of fluoride ions, release of other ions or combination of these
- There are three mechanism of anticariogenic property due to release of fluoride ions which are:

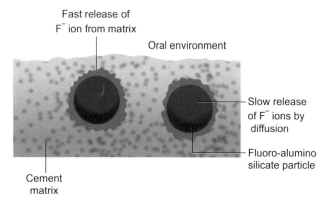

**Fig. 18.25:** Release of fluoride ions from glass ionomer cement.

- Inhibition of demineralization and promoting remineralization
- Formation of acid resistant fluorapatite
- Prevention of glycolysis and lactic acid production by inhibition of enzyme enolase.

*Coefficient of Thermal Expansion*
Glass ionomer cement has coefficient of thermal expansion closer to that of the tooth structure. It is $10 \times 10^{-6}/°C$ (tooth enamel: $11.4 \times 10^{-6}/°C$ and tooth dentin: $8.4 \times 10^{-6}/°C$).

## Manipulation

For long-term restoration and retentive fixed partial dentures, following conditions should be fulfilled:
- Tooth surface should be clean and dried but not desiccated
- The mix should seat completely into the prepared cavity
- Excess cement should be removed
- Proper finishing of the surface
- Protection of the restoration to prevent cracking or dissolution of the restoration.

## Tooth Surface Preparation

- The tooth surface is cleaned and smear layer formed during cavity preparation is removed by pumice slurry or by etching with 37% phosphoric acid or organic acid like polyacrylic acid (10–20%) for 10–20 seconds
- Once the tooth surface is conditioned, it is rinsed and thereafter dried but not desiccated.

## Proportioning and Mixing

- Powder/liquid ratio 3:1 by weight
- *Working time*: 2–3.5 minutes
- Reduced P/L ratio significantly compromise physical properties

- Increased P/L ratio reduces the working time and increases the viscosity of the mix
- Powder and liquid are dispensed on cool glass slab or paper pad just before mixing. Powder should be fluffed before dispensing by tumbling the powder bottle downward so that there is uniform distribution of the particles. One scoop of powder is dispensed onto the pad. Scoop provided by the manufacturer should be only used to ensure proper P/L ratio
- Cool glass slab can also be used to prolong the working time and retard the rate of reaction
- Care is taken that the glass slab should not be cooled below the dew point because moisture due to condensation changes the acid water balance of the reaction
- Powder is divided into two equal increments. Liquid is dispensed just prior to mixing because prolonged exposure can alter the ratio of water content in the liquid. First liquid bottle is tilted horizontally till the liquid comes to the tip of nozzle then the bottle is inverted vertically so that one full drop is dispensed on the paper pad **(Fig. 18.26)**
- The first increment is mixed rapidly using *agate or plastic* spatula over a smaller area. Stainless steel spatula should not be used because of the powder particles of GIC tends to abrade the spatula surface thereby incorporating impurities in the mix. First increment should be mixed within 5–10 seconds without spreading the mix
- Then second increment is taken and mixing is done using a *folding method* **(Fig. 18.27)**. Mixing of glass ionomer cement through folding method. Mixing is done within the small area unlike in zinc phosphate cement where mixing was done over large surface area. Second increment should be mixed within 15–25 seconds.

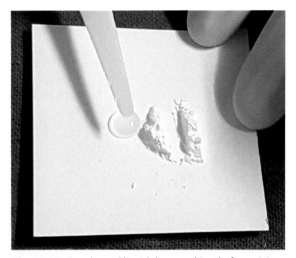

**Fig. 18.26:** Powder and liquid dispensed just before mixing.

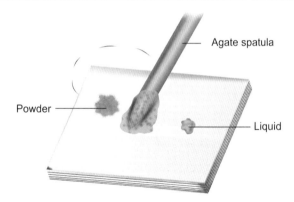

**Fig. 18.27:** Mixing of glass ionomer cement through folding method.

- *Mixing time*: 45–60 seconds
- The mixture should appear glossy. This glossiness is due to the unreacted polyacid ions on the surface of the mixture. These unreacted ions present on the surface are critical for bonding with the tooth surface
- *Dull appearance* of the mixture indicates insufficient free acid for bonding
- The mixed cement with restorative consistency is carried into the prepared cavity with help of plastic instrument whereas with luting consistency should flow easily to allow complete seating of the restoration onto the prepared tooth.

### Mechanical Mixing

The preweighed capsules of GIC are placed in an amalgamator or triturator to accomplish mixing. The thin septa between the powder and liquid are broken during trituration. The mixing time is 10 seconds at 3,000 cycles/min. Too short or long mixing time significantly affects the working time and physical properties of the cement.

### Advantages

- Powder and liquid mixed in accurate ratio
- Reduced mixing time
- Convenient delivery system as the mixture can be directly injected into the cavity.

### Disadvantages

- Selection of shade is limited
- As preweighed, the quantity of cement is limited by the manufacturer.

### Protection of Cement during Setting

- It is advised to slightly overfill the cavity with the cement
- Just after placement, the surface should be protected using a preshaped matrix in order to minimize the

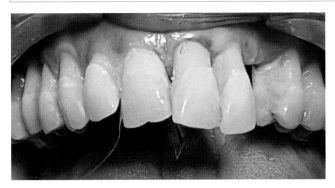

**Fig. 18.28:** Preformed transparent matrix used to protect the glass ionomer cement restorations.

chances of loss or gain of moisture during initial set **(Fig. 18.28)**
- This matrix is removed after 5 minutes and again the surface should be immediately protected after removing excess cement.

---

**CLINICAL SIGNIFICANCE**
- Surface protection after completion of the restoration is done by:
  - Varnish
  - Bonding agent
  - Petroleum jelly or cocoa butter.
- Unprotected surface results in chalky or crazed surface which is prone to dehydration and microcracking.

---

- Surface protection after completion of the restoration is done by:
  - Varnish
  - Bonding agent
  - Petroleum jelly or cocoa butter.
- Unprotected surface results in chalky or crazed surface which is prone to dehydration and microcracking.

*Finishing*

- Excess cement is removed from the margins
- Patient is further recalled for finishing after 24 hours
- It is not required if fast setting cement was used
- The finished restoration should be coated with protective agent before dismissing the patient.

## Advantages

- Easy to mix
- Good strength
- Chemically bonds with tooth structure
- Anticariogenic property due to sustained release of fluorides
- Translucency.

## Disadvantages

- Postoperative sensitivity
- Sensitive to moisture contamination during setting.

---

# METAL REINFORCED GLASS IONOMER CEMENT

Since conventional GIC lacked toughness, metal reinforced GIC were introduced to improve upon their physical and mechanical properties so that they could be used in the posterior teeth. The metallic fillers used in this cement are particles of silver which are sintered with glass or are silver alloy powder. They impart grayish color to the cement and make it more radiopaque.

*Metal reinforced GIC are of two types:*
1. *Silver alloy admixed:* Spherical amalgam alloy powder is mixed with glass powder *(Miracle mix)* **(Fig. 18.29)**. Miracle mix was first introduced by Simmons in 1980s as silver alloy admixed. Spherical silver alloy particles are added to cement in the ratio of 8:1 where 8 parts are of cement and 1 part is the silver alloy. The powder particles in above ratio are mixed with liquid in the ratio of 3:2 by weight. As silver alloy particles did not require mercury for mixing, this was referred to as "Miracle Mix"
2. *Cermet cement:* Glass powders are fused with silver particles through sintering at high temperature **(Fig. 18.30)**. Microfine silver alloy particles which are less than 3.5 μm in diameter are sintered with glass particles at 800°C under pressure. Small amounts of titanium oxide can be added to alter the color. Cermet cement was introduced by McLean in 1985.

## Uses

- Restorations of small class I cavities as alternative to amalgam in younger patients prone to caries

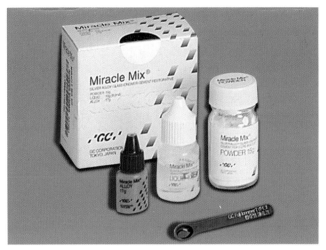

**Fig. 18.29:** Miracle mix cement.

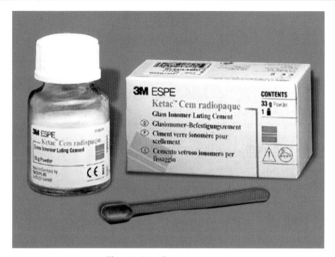

**Fig. 18.30:** Cermet cement.

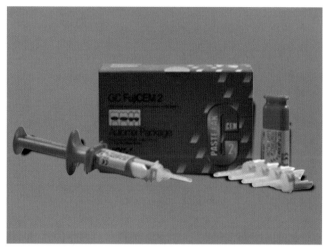

**Fig. 18.31:** Resin-modified glass ionomer cement.

- More prone for fracture when used for class II restorations
- For core buildup with caution as they have low fracture toughness and are brittle.

## Properties

### Mechanical

- Strength not greatly improved over the conventional GIC (150 MPa)
- Tensile strength higher (6.7 MPa)
- Fracture toughness low as compared to composite or amalgam
- Exhibit similar wear in solution pH between 6 and 7 but has greater wear at pH 5
- Metal reinforced cements are useful for core buildup teeth restored with cast crowns and occlusal surfaces of primary
- Since these restorations harden rapidly, they can be finished and polished in short duration as compared to amalgam or conventional GIC.

### Anticariogenic

- Anticariogenic property due to leaching of fluoride ions
- Less fluoride release is there with cermet cement as the glass particles are metal coated
- Admixed cement release more fluoride ions than conventional GIC, as metal filler do not bond to the cement matrix. Therefore, the interface of cement and matrix provide pathway for fluoride leaching.

### Esthetics

Gray in color due to metallic phase, therefore, not recommended in anterior teeth.

## RESIN MODIFIED GLASS IONOMER CEMENT (HYBRID IONOMER OR RESIN IONOMER) (FIG. 18.31)

- In 1980s, RMGICs were introduced with the desire to improve the fracture toughness and resistance to dissolution over the conventional GIC
- Water soluble polymer or polymerizable resins were added to conventional GIC to form RMGIC or hybrid ionomer
- In this, the water component of glass polyalkenoate cement is replaced by hydroxyethyl methacrylate (HEMA) along with a initiator/activator. The monomers can be polymerized either by chemical curing or light curing or both.

### Uses

- Permanent cementation of crowns, bridges, inlays, onlays and post
- As liners and bases
- For core buildup
- For cementation of orthodontic brackets and bands
- As pit and fissure sealants
- Repair material for damaged amalgam core or cusps
- Retrograde root filling material
- Restoration in low stress bearing areas such as class V cavities
- Restoration of deciduous teeth
- Restoration in high caries risk patient.

### Setting Reaction

- Resin-modified glass ionomer is a dual cured hybrid cement, as setting occurs by combination of long-term, complex acid-base reaction and chemical or light cure polymerization of the resin

- Initial hardening of such material results from polymerization of the resin as the acid-base reaction is slow in comparison to conventional GIC because of reduced water content. It is also possible to initiate the setting reaction with light activation which causes polymerization of resin to occur immediately. This polymerized resin provides the umbrella effect and protects the ongoing acid-base reaction within the resin cement. The protection provided by cured resin makes the uncured resin less sensitive to moisture and contributes to high early strength
- Although acid-base reaction continues to develop polyacid hydrogel matrix which hardens and strengthens the existing polymer matrix
- If resin percentage is high or the water content is low, then only polymerization reaction occurs and material behaves as filled, reinforced resin and is called as "compomer"
- These hybrid ionomer are designed for restorative purpose and contain nonreactive fillers which are similar to that in composite resin
- Some RMGIC can also be *tri-cured*, i.e. polymerization takes place due to chemical cure, light cure and acid base reaction of the glass ionomer.

## Composition

### Powder

- Fluoroaluminosilicate—ion leachable glass particles
- Initiator for light curing such as camphorquinone
- Initiator for chemical curing
- Polymerizable resin.

### Liquid

- Water
- Polyacrylic acid
- Polyacrylic acid with carboxylic group modified with methacrylate and HEMA monomer.

## Properties

### Strength

- Compressive strength is slightly lower compared to conventional GIC (105 MPa)
- Tensile strength is slightly higher (20 MPa) than conventional GIC because of their lower elastic modulus and sustenance of greater plastic deformation before fracture.

### Hardness

It has hardness of 40 KHN which is comparable to conventional GIC.

### Fracture Toughness

It is higher than the conventional GIC.

*Modulus of elasticity:* Resin-modified glass ionomer cement has lower modulus of elasticity than conventional GICs. They can sustain greater plastic deformation before fracture on load application.

### Adhesion to Tooth

- Bonding to the tooth structure is similar to conventional GIC
- Bond strength of RMGI is higher than the conventional GIC. This can be due to greater bonding between the resin component and the tooth structure.

### Adhesion to Restorative Materials

Exhibit higher bond strength to composite in comparison to conventional GIC.

### Marginal Adaptation

- Degree of shrinkage is higher because of polymerization of hybrid ionomer
- Reduced water and carboxylic acid content decreases the ability to wet tooth structure, thereby greatly increasing the chances of microleakage.

### Biocompatibility

- Similar to conventional GIC; although initial pH is less acidic than conventional GIC
- For deep cavities, protection with calcium hydroxide is required as with the conventional GIC
- Hybrid ionomer should not be used in direct pulp capping procedure

### Anticariogenicity

- Has significant anticariogenic effect due to fluoride release
- Fluoride release is similar to that of the conventional GIC
- Low viscosity hybrid ionomer or conventional GIC can be used as pit and fissure sealants.

### Esthetics

They are less translucent due to difference in the refractive index between the resin matrix and powder particles.

*Pulp response:* Mild.

## Manipulation

- Powder/liquid ratio: 1.6/1
- Powder is fluffed before dispensing
- Liquid and powder are dispensed on a mixing pad and should be mixed within 30 seconds. There are chances of porosity due to air incorporation during mixing of powder and liquid. Hand mixing showed formation of larger pores than when capsules are triturated mechanically. Viscosity of cement greatly influences the amount of porosity
- The mixture should yield a *mousse-like* consistency
- *Working time:* 2.5 minutes
- Most RMGI cements are supplied as preproportioned capsules for ease of mixing.

## Advantages

- Has shorter setting time and is less susceptible to water loss or gain
- Improved physical and mechanical properties
- More esthetic due to improved translucency
- Rapid setting improves color stability.

# CALCIUM ALUMINATE GLASS IONOMER CEMENT

This hybrid GIC recently introduced for luting fixed partial dentures have composition similar to other GIC. The powder particles are formed after sintering a mixture of CaO and $Al_2O_3$ in the ratio of 1:1 to form monocalcium aluminate. Sintered mass is milled to desired particle size. This component is mixed with conventional GIC to form hybrid calcium aluminate GIC.

## Composition

### Powder

- Calcium aluminate
- Strontium-fluoroalumino glass
- Strontium fluoride.

### Liquid

- Polyacrylic acid
- Tartaric acid
- Water
- Additives.

## Setting Reaction

When powder particles are mixed with liquid, the calcium aluminate component starts to dissolve calcium ions, $Al(OH)_4^-$ and $OH^-$ ions leading to a weak acid-base reaction.

The powder acts as base and the liquid as weak acid and form immediate precipitation of hydrates which sets with time. This cement is also called as *hydraulic cement* which can be used as restorative material.

## Supplied As

Capsules which are mixed mechanically.

## Properties

Calcium aluminate provides basic pH during polymerization and contributes toward long-term stability and improving strength. It provides excellent biocompatibility and helps in reducing microleakage.

The components of GIC control viscosity, setting time and strength. The polyacrylic acid have dual function, i.e. it not only crosslinks with calcium ions leached with soluble glass and calcium aluminate but also acts as dispersing agent for calcium aluminate. This material is a composite of hydrated ceramic material and a crosslinked polyacrylate polymer.

### Strength

- Has excellent compressive strength
- *Working time:* 2 minutes
- *Setting time:* 5 minutes
- *Film thickness:* 15+ 4 µm
- *Setting expansion:* 0.4%.

# COMPOMERS (FIGS. 18.32A AND B)

- Also known as *polyacid-modified composite resin*
- Compomers were introduced in late 1990s and were described as combination of composite and glass ionomers
- They are anhydrous resin that contains ion leachable glass as filler material and dehydrated polyalkenoic acid
- These materials possess properties which are different from both glass ionomers and composite resins.

## Rationale

To integrate fluoride-releasing capacity of GIC and superior properties of composite resin.

## Supplied As

- *Powder and liquid:* For luting purpose
- Single paste system which is light activated—for restorative purpose
- Two single-component system.

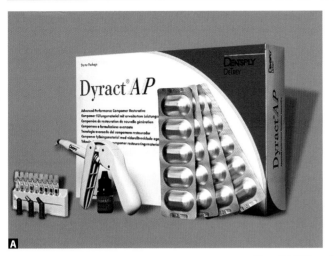 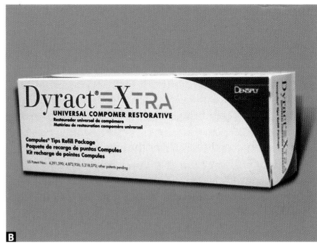

**Figs. 18.32A and B:** Compomers.

## Composition

For *restorative* purpose supplied as single paste, light curable material which is composed of:
- Silicate glass particles
- Inorganic filler particles
- Sodium fluoride
- Polyacid-modified monomer without water such as diester of 2-hydroxyl methacrylate with butane carboxylic acid
- Photoactivators.

For *luting* purpose supplied as two pastes or in form of powder and liquid.

### Powder
- Strontium aluminum fluorosilicate glass
- Metallic oxides
- Sodium fluoride
- Self- and light-cured initiators.

### Liquid
- Polymerizable methacrylate/carboxylic acid monomer
- Multifunctional acrylate/phosphate monomer
- Diacrylate monomer
- Water.

## Uses
- For restoration of low stress bearing areas limited to class III and class V cavities
- Can also be used as alternative to restorative GIC or resin-based composites
- Cementing cast alloy, porcelain fused to metal and gold restorations. Compomers are useful in luting restoration with metallic substrate.

### Contraindications

Cementing all ceramic crowns, inlays, onlays and veneers.

## Setting Reaction
- For single paste system, setting reaction is initiated by photopolymerization of the acidic monomer which results in a hardened material
- Over the period of time when the set material begins to absorb oral fluids, then acid-base reaction is initiated. This acid-base reaction is responsible for sustained release of fluoride. The slow acid-base reaction takes place between the acidic functional group and silicate glass particles
- As *single paste* system does not contain water, they are *not self-adhesive* and thus require a separate dentin bonding agent. After application of bonding agent, the bond strength of compomer is similar or higher than the hybrid ionomers
- For *two paste system* since water is present in the liquid, these materials are *self-adhesive* and *acid-base reaction* begins at the time of mixing as in hybrid ionomers.
- *Setting time: 3* minutes.

## Manipulation
- For *single paste system*, similar process as for composite is followed as first etching is done, followed by dentin bonding agent and then cement application. Finishing of the restoration is done similar to that for composites
- For *two paste system*, the powder and liquid is mixed and is applied over the internal surface of the prosthesis. Prosthesis is seated over the tooth with finger pressure for 90 seconds to reach the gel state. Excess cement is then removed and the margins are light-cured

immediately to stabilize the prosthesis. Chemical cure completes the setting reaction in about 3 minutes.

*Properties*

- Have higher compressive and flexural strength than RMGI, but have inferior properties to composites. It is observed that compressive strength and flexural strength of compomers reduce if they are stored in saline water. However, this is not noticed in composite resins. Another different property observed is during manufacturing when the reactive glass is treated with silane, its water uptake capacity is reduced and strength is improved
- Elastic modulus is 3.6 GPa
- Has good bond strength of 18–24 MPa with dentin
- Has limited sustained fluoride release and is less than the conventional GIC
- Has low solubility
- Little adhesion occurs without the resin bonding agent
- Water absorption—compomers have high water absorption which is as high as 3.5% by weight. This water uptake is desirable as it contributes to acid-base reaction and aids in subsequent fluoride release. Since restorative compomers do not have water, they have less fluoride release than the conventional GIC and hybrid ionomers.

## GIOMERS

These are fluoride releasing, light activated hybrid restorative materials which have properties of both GIC and composite resin. The benefits of using this material are better esthetics, easy handling and superior properties. Giomers are based on pre-reacted glass ionomer (PRG) technology in which as stable phase of pre-reacted GIC is used as filler material **(Fig. 18.33)**.

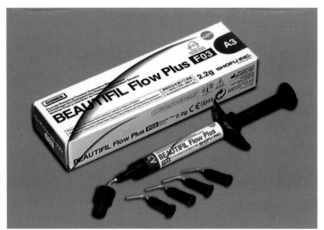

**Fig. 18.33:** Giomer.

### Classification of Giomers

Giomers are of two types depending on the type of PRG filler created:
1. *S-PRG:* Surface prereacted type of glass ionomer
2. *F-PRG:* Fully prereacted type of glass ionomer.

Recent improvement in the S-PRG technology has resulted in the development of modified S-PRG filler which consists of a glass core and two surface layers called the trilaminar structure. This special layer has a glass core made of multifunctional fluoro-boroaluminosilicate glass which is PRG phase. This layer greatly improves the properties of the hybrid material. They are second-generation giomers which are commercially available as FL Bond II (Shofu), Beautiful II (Shofu).

## RESIN CEMENTS (FIGS. 18.34A AND B)

- Resin cements (ADA specification no. 27) are flowable composites of low viscosity
- Resin cements based on methyl methacrylate has been in market since 1952 for cementation of indirect restorations
- With the increasing demand for all ceramic and bonded restorations, there has been drastic increase in the popularity of resin cements
- They can be methyl methacrylate, Bis-GMA dimethacrylate, or urethane dimethacrylate based, with fillers of colloidal silica or barium glass 20–80% by weight
- These materials are virtually insoluble in oral fluids. Organosilanes are used with the fillers to ensure that they form a wear resistant material
- Bonding agent is required to promote bonding between the cement and the tooth structure. Bonding takes place because of the adhesive monomer in the bonding agent which include HEMA, 4-META, carboxylic acids and an organophosphate such as 10-methacryloxy decamethylene phosphoric acid MDP)
- Once the surface of the tooth is demineralized by acid-etching a bonding agent is applied. The resin primer partially infiltrates the collagen fibrils which are demineralized by etching process
- All the resin cements do not require application of bonding agent for adhesion. If a resin cement contain component such as 4-META, it does not require a separate bonding agent
- Newer resin cements which are supplied as single paste system do not require etching, priming and bonding but are directly applied on the surface to the bonded.

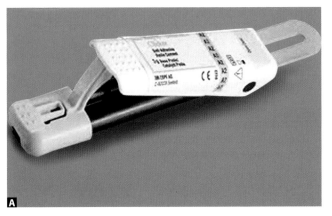
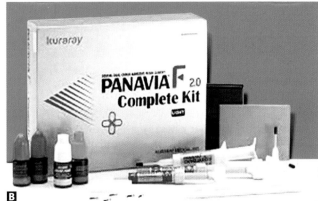

**Figs. 18.34A and B:** Resin cements.

## Uses

- For cementation of all ceramic crowns and fixed partial dentures
- For cementation of porcelain veneers, inlays and onlays
- For bonding of orthodontic brackets
- For cementation of resin bonded bridges
- For cementation of prefabricated and cast metal dowels in endodontically treated teeth.

### Classification of Resin Cement

*Based on the Method of Polymerization*

- *Class I:* Self-cured
- *Class II:* Light-cured
- *Class III:* Dual-cured.

*Based on Adhesive Technique*

- *Class I*: Etch and rinse resin cement
- *Class II*: Self-etch resin cement
- *Class III*: Self-adhesive resin cement.

## Composition

*Powder*

- Resin matrix
- Silane-treated inorganic fillers
- Coupling agent
- Photo or chemical initiators
- Activators.

*Liquid*

- Adhesive monomer (HEMA and 4-META)
- Organophosphate such as MDP
- Tertiary amines.

## Methods of Polymerization

- Self-cure or chemical cure
- Light-cure
- Dual-cure, i.e. both chemical and light-cure.

## Supplied

- *Chemical cure*: Supplied as powder or liquid of two paste system
- *Light-cure*: Supplied as single component system
- *Dual-cure*: Supplied as two component system.

## Bonding Mechanism

- Resin bonding to tooth enamel is by micromechanical interlocking into an acid-etched surface
- Resin bonding to dentin is more complex, requiring removal of smear layer, surface demineralization and application of dentin bonding agent.

The bonding mechanism in three types of resin cements based on different adhesive technique is given below:

1. *Etch-and-rinse resin cement*: It is a methacrylate-based resin cement which uses etch and rinse adhesive technique for bonding. Phosphoric acid is commonly used for etching the tooth surface followed by the application of primer and bonding agent. The surface of the tooth should not be completely dried before application of bonding agent in order to avoid collapse of collagen fibrils. Then resin composite is applied and polymerized. Bonding here is achieved by micromechanical interlocking. Dual-cure method of polymerization is recommended to achieve adequate bond strength.

2. *Self-etch resin cement*: In this system, self-etching primer is applied on the tooth surface before applying the resin cement. Self-etch resin cement can be a two-step or one-step system. Two-step system consists of self-etching primer and a hydrophobic adhesive resin

whereas one-step system consists of etchant, primer and bonding agent in a single bottle. In this method, the tooth surface is demineralized and infiltrated at the same time. Although the smear layer is not removed but is impregnated with acidic monomer. Bonding in this method also depends on micromechanical interlocking.

3. *Self-adhesive resin cement*: This type of cement does not require etching or bonding step. The bonding in this type of cement is mainly chemically and not by micromechanical means. The phosphoric acid present in the resin reacts with the filler particles and the tooth surface in presence of water to form a bond. The resin polymerizes into crosslinked polymer. Prior to using this cement the tooth surface is recommended to be etched separately. The bond strength achieved by self-adhesive resin cement is usually inferior to that achieved from etch-and-rinse resin cement.

## Manipulation

- Powder and liquid are dispensed on the mixing pad in accurate proportions as directed by the manufacturer
- Paste materials are normally proportioned 1:1 (equal lengths)
- The two components are mixed rapidly to minimize air inclusion and attain uniform mix.

- On mixing, polymerization of the monomers occurs resulting in the formation of highly crosslinked composite structure
- Conditioning of the tooth surface remains same for all types of resin cement, but treatment of the prosthesis varies with the composition
- Noneugenol provisional cement is recommended when resin cement is to be used as definitive cement
- Eugenol is found to interfere with polymerization of the resin cement.

### Bonding of Ceramic Prosthesis

Resin cements are material of choice to cement all ceramic prosthesis **(Fig. 18.35)**.

Surface treatment of some of the commonly used all ceramic prosthesis is given here.

- All ceramic prostheses are highly translucent and require specific shade to provide optimal esthetics
- Desired shade of resin cement is selected to cement the ceramic prosthesis
- The inner surface of the ceramic prosthesis with a glassy phase is etched and silane coupling agent is applied before cementation to achieve better retention.
  - *Glass-based ceramic prosthesis*:
    - The surface treatment of glass-based ceramic prosthesis is done using 5–9.5% hydrofluoric acid

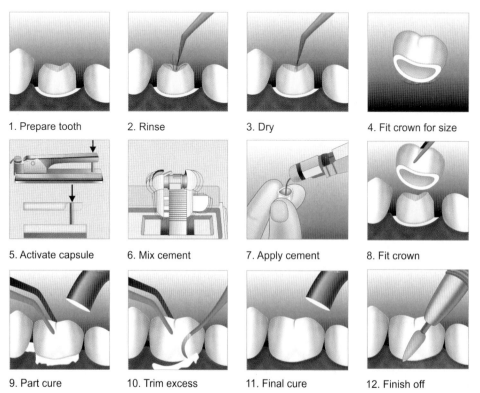

1. Prepare tooth    2. Rinse    3. Dry    4. Fit crown for size

5. Activate capsule    6. Mix cement    7. Apply cement    8. Fit crown

9. Part cure    10. Trim excess    11. Final cure    12. Finish off

**Fig. 18.35:** Cementation of all ceramic restorations with resin cement.

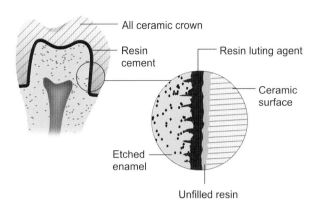

**Fig.18.36:** Bonding of All ceramic restoration with resin cement.

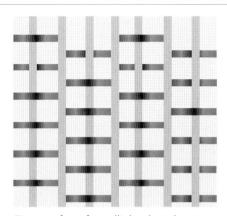

**Fig. 18.37:** Tissue surface of metallic brackets showing meshwork to aid in retention.

- Hydrofluoric acid selectively dissolves the glass matrix creating microporosities around the leucite crystals **(Fig. 18.36)**
- The surface is then conditioned with silane coupling agent
- Sandblasting for such prosthesis is contraindicated.
  – *Glass-infiltrated alumina-based ceramics*:
    - The surface of such prosthesis is treated with tribochemical silica coating process
    - Then the surface is cleaned with 110 μm high purity $Al_2O_3$. Later the surface is conditioned with silane coupling agent.
  – *Zirconia-based ceramics*:
    - Surface treatment of zirconia-based ceramics is done by either air particle abrasion or by tribochemical silica coating.

### Bonding of Metal Prosthesis

- The inner surface of the metal prosthesis is grit blasted or sand blasted with 30–50 μm alumina particles at an air pressure of 0.4–0.7 MPa
- Roughening can also be done by electrochemical etching
- Some resin cements use metal primer containing adhesive promoter for bonding
- Naturally forming oxide on the surface of base metal alloys can also aid in bonding when MDP or 4-META-based resin cements are used
- However, noble metal alloys used in metal ceramic prosthesis do not form stable oxide
- In order to enhance bonding thin layer of tin can be electrochemically deposited on the metals surface.

### Bonding of Orthodontic Brackets

- Proper isolation and etching of the tooth surface is essential for proper bonding of orthodontic brackets

- The tissue surface of the bracket requires some kind of mechanical retention such as metal mesh available in metallic brackets **(Fig. 18.37)**
- The resin cement flows into these mesh and locks to provide adequate retention
- Bonding of resin to the ceramic bracket is achieved by etching it and applying organosilanes on the surface
- Plastic bracket is primed with a solvent containing methyl methacrylate monomer to attain good bonding
- Debonding of the metal brackets usually occurs at the cement/bracket interface whereas debonding of ceramic/plastic brackets occurs at the wing of the brackets.

## Cementation of Restorations

### Chemical Cure Resin Cement

- Supplied as two-component system
- Two components mixed on the paper pad
- Mixing time 20–30 seconds
- Removal of excess cement becomes difficult if it is delayed until the cement is polymerized
- This type of cement is suitable to bond all types of prostheses.

### Light Cure Resin Cement

- Supplied as single-component system
- Composed of methacrylate monomers, photoinitiators
- Indicated to cement thin ceramic restorations, resin-based prosthesis and ceramic/plastic orthodontic brackets
- Time of exposure of light for polymerization should never be less than 40 seconds
- Time of exposure depends on intensity of light transmitted and the thickness of resin cement
- Excess of cement should be removed as the prosthesis is completely seated

- Alternately, brief exposure of 10 seconds aids in removal of excess cement.

### Dual-cure Resin Cement

- Supplied as two-component system
- *Base paste* consists of methacrylate monomers, fillers, chemical or light activated initiators
- *Catalyst paste* consists of methacrylate monomers, fillers and activators
- Mixing done similar to chemically cure system
- Chemical activation is very slow and provides extended working time until light activation starts
- With light activation cement hardens rapidly
- It continues to gain strength over an extended period of time due to chemically activated polymerization process
- Dual-cure cement should not be used, if the thickness of light transmitting prosthesis is more than 2.5 mm.

### Properties

- *Strength:*
  - *Compressive strength*: 180–265 MPa
  - *Tensile strength*: 34–37 MPa
  - *Elastic modulus*: 2.1–3.1 GPa
- *Film thickness*: Less than or equal to 25 µm
- *Solubility:* Insoluble in oral fluids
- *Bond strength to dentin:* 18–25 MPa
- *Pulp response:* Moderate
  - Pulp protection with calcium hydroxide or glass ionomer liner is essential if the remaining dentin thickness is less than or equal to 0.5 mm to prevent penetration of chemical irritants.
- *Esthetics:* Excellent with availability of different shades.
- *Polymerization shrinkage:* High enough to generate stresses that can result in gaps at the cement/tooth interface **(Fig. 18.38)**
- *Adhesion:* Micromechanical bonding with enamel and dentin (possible chemical bonding).

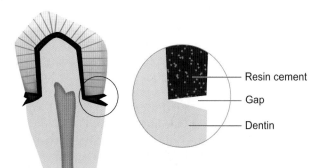

**Fig.18.38:** Gap formation at cement tooth interface due to polymerization shrinkage.

### Advantages

- High strength
- Low oral solubility
- Excellent esthetics
- Good bonding with tooth enamel, dentin, alloys and ceramic surfaces.

### Disadvantages

- Technique sensitive
- No fluoride release
- Film thickness relatively high
- Polymerization shrinkage
- Pulpal sensitivity
- Difficulty in removing excess cement
- Costly.

## Adhesive Resin

- In early 1980s, conventional Bis-GMA resin cement was modified to achieve chemical bonding and micromechanical bonding with tooth structure and base metal alloys by adding phosphate ester to the monomer component
- Panavia and C&B Metabond represent adhesive resin luting agent
- Currently, Panavia F is a popular adhesive resin which is *dual-cured, self-etching, self-adhesive and with fluoride-releasing* capability. They exhibit good bonding with base metal alloys after it is air abraded with alumina oxide and silane treatment. Bonding to noble metal is fair after tin plating and application of metal primer
- *C&B Metabond* has physical properties similar to resin cements but have *good tensile strength*. They are indicated for prosthesis which has compromised retention.

---

# SANDWICH TECHNIQUE (FIG. 18.39)

- Also called as *bilayered technique* or *laminated restoration technique* or *replacement dentin technique*
- This technique was first developed by *McLean* et al. in 1985.

## Rationale

- To place GIC between the tooth and the composite resin. The purpose is to take advantage of adhesive property of GIC and esthetic and durability of resin based composites
- Resin-modified glass ionomer cement reduces gap between the gingival margins located in the dentin or cementum caused by the polymerization shrinkage of the resin due to its adhesion to the tooth structure

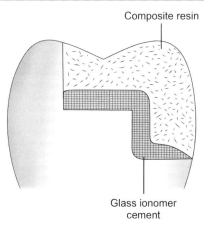

**Fig. 18.39:** Sandwich technique.

- Composite resin micromechanically bonds to the set glass ionomer and chemically to HEMA in RMGI
- Resin-modified glass ionomer cement has better properties than conventional GIC and also have good bonding with the composite resins.

## Indications

- For class II and class V restorations in patient with moderate to high caries risk
- For small class I and II defects.

## Advantages

- This technique shows improved resistance to caries and reduced microleakage as compared to the composite resin
- Anticariogenic property due to release of fluoride
- Reduced bulk of composite resin reduces chances of polymerization shrinkage
- Good pulpal response as GIC is in direct contact of the tooth
- Reduced chances of postoperative sensitivity.

## Disadvantages

- Time consuming
- Technique sensitive.

## Procedure

- Prepared tooth is isolated
- Pulp is protected with calcium hydroxide paste if required. Although it reduces the area for adhesion with GIC
- The prepared tooth is conditioned with polyacrylic acid for optimal adhesion

- Freshly mixed fast setting GIC is placed over the conditioned tooth surface
- Acid etching is done only GIC is fully matured
- After etching the surface is washed and dried
- The dried surface is coated with dentin bonding agent and cured for 20 seconds
- Then composite resin is filled into the cavity in increments and cured in conventional manner
- The completely filled cavity is finished and polished in conventional manner.

## ATRAUMATIC RESTORATIVE TREATMENT

- Atraumatic restorative treatment technique was first introduced by *Jo Frencken* in 1996 in South Africa
- Although this technique was first evaluated in Tanzania in 1980
- This technique is useful in countries which lack modern auxiliary equipment and basic infrastructure such as water, electricity and equipment
- In such places, ART technique is used to preserve as many teeth as possible
- Only hand instruments are used to remove carious lesions **(Fig. 18.40)**
- Material that bonds chemically such as GIC, with the tooth structure is desired for cavity restoration
- After removal of caries, the tooth is restored with *highly viscous GIC*
- Highly viscous glass ionomer is used because of its adhesiveness and fluoride release property
- Also viscous GIC is pressed into the excavated cavities and pits and fissures similar to amalgam restoration

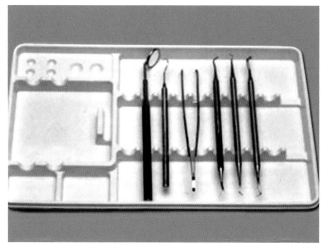

**Fig. 18.40:** Hand instruments used in atraumatic restorative treatment.

## Goals

- To preserve as many teeth as possible
- Minimize tooth preparation
- To provide maximum prevention
- To minimize surgical intervention.

## Indications

- Restoration of primary teeth
- Intermediate restoration of permanent posterior teeth
- Mentally retarded, physically disabled and elderly patient
- Small to moderate pit and fissure caries.

## Atraumatic Restorative Technique (**Fig. 18.41**)

- Isolation of the carious tooth with cotton rolls
- Hand instruments are used to remove the carious lesion
- Better access is gained by removing the undermined enamel with hand instruments
- Carious tissue is removed with spoon excavators
- Soft demineralized dentin is excavated before restoration
- Highly viscous GIC is material of choice to restore such lesions

- They pressed into the cavity
- Excess of GIC after restoration is removed
- To improve chemical bonding, the tooth surface can be treated with weak acid prior to filling with GIC.

## Advantages

- Only hand instruments used
- Modern equipment not required
- Reduced discomfort and pain to patient
- High survival rate of partially or fully retained single surface restorations.
- Low cost of treatment
- Minimal tooth preparation
- Minimal intervention
- Less technique sensitive.

## Disadvantages

- Operator fatigue during instrumentation
- Accessibility is poor especially in posterior teeth.

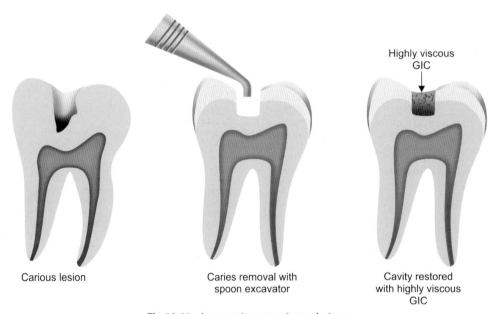

Carious lesion  •  Caries removal with spoon excavator  •  Cavity restored with highly viscous GIC

Highly viscous GIC

**Fig.18.41:** Atraumatic restorative technique.

---

# TEST YOURSELF

## Essay Questions

1. Classify dental cements. Write in detail about zinc phosphate cement.
2. Classify dental cement. Discuss in detail glass ionomer cement.
3. Enumerate various cements based on uses in dentistry. Describe composition, setting reaction and properties of zinc oxide eugenol cement.
4. Discuss in detail zinc polycarboxylate cement.

5. Compare the properties and setting reaction of zinc phosphate, zinc oxide eugenol and glass ionomer cement.
6. Discuss various resin cements.
7. Describe composition, setting reaction, bonding mechanism and fluoride release mechanism of glass ionomer cement.

## Short Notes

1. Aluminosilicate polyacrylic acid (ASPA).
2. Hybrid ionomer.
3. Atraumatic restorative treatment (ART).
4. Giomer.
5. Miracle mix.
6. Sandwich technique.
7. Resin modified glass ionomer cement (GIC).
8. Water settable cement.
9. Hydraulic cement.
10. Calcium aluminate cement.
11. Resin cement.
12. Compomer.
13. Orthoethoxybenzoic acid (EBA) cement.
14. Cermet cement.

## Multiple Choice Questions

1. Truly adhesive restoration is:
   A. Unfilled resins
   B. Composites
   C. Polycarboxylate
   D. Bis-GMA.
2. Primary drawback of zinc polycarboxylate cement is:
   A. Irritation to pulp
   B. Lacks adhesion
   C. Short working time
   D. All of the above
3. Composition of polycarboxylate cement is:
   A. Zinc oxide powder and phosphoric acid
   B. Zinc oxide powder and polyacrylic acid
   C. Aluminum silicate powder and polyacrylic acid
   D. Aluminum silicate powder and phosphoric acid
4. Which cement has maximum solubility?
   A. Silicate
   B. Zinc phosphate
   C. Poly carboxylate
   D. Glass ionomer
5. Manipulation of silicate cement is:
   A. Mixed with agate spatula
   B. Mixed on cool glass slab not below dew point
   C. As quickly as possible in short area
   D. All of the above

6. Material of choice for geriatric patient with some teeth remaining:
   A. Glass ionomer
   B. Porcelain
   C. Composites
   D. Pit and fissure sealants
7. If small drop of eugenol is mixed with the cement base:
   A. Setting time is reduced
   B. Sensitivity of tooth is reduced
   C. Setting time is increased
   D. Strength is reduced
8. Minimum film thickness is important property for which luting cement:
   A. Zinc phosphate cement
   B. Zinc oxide eugenol
   C. Silicate
   D. Polycarboxylate
9. Resin modified GIC have all of the following except:
   A. Controlled fluoride release
   B. Both acid base and polymerization reaction
   C. Improved strength compared to conventional GIC
   D. Improved esthetics
10. Ionic bonding in glass ionomer cement is due to:
    A. Polyacrylic acid
    B. Phosphate ion
    C. Fluoride ion
    D. Silicate ion
11. As compared to zinc phosphate cement, modified zinc oxide eugenol cement is:
    A. Practically insoluble in saliva
    B. Has minimum film thickness
    C. Does not require varnish for pulp protection
    D. Has high initial strength
12. Which of the following is not present in GIC?
    A. Tartaric acid
    B. Polyacrylic acid
    C. Eugenol
    D. Silicate glass
13. What would be the rationale for placing a liner of glass ionomer under a large and deep composite restoration in a premolar tooth?
    A. Provide thermal insulation for the tooth
    B. Reduce postoperative sensitivity
    C. Seal the dentinal surfaces under the composite restorations
    D. Improve the strength of the restoration
14. Which of these factor will have least effect on the setting rate of zinc phosphate cement?
    A. Powder/liquid ratio
    B. Size of powder particles
    C. Size of mixing area
    D. Stiffness of mixing spatula

15. The test for properly mixed luting cement is:
    A. Putty consistency
    B. Granular consistency
    C. Cement will hold a thin string, breaking when the spatula is raised an inch
    D. Cement will break and form a drop at the end of the spatula

16. Which cement shows exothermic reaction during mixing?
    A. Glass ionomer cement
    B. Resin cement
    C. Zinc phosphate
    D. Calcium hydroxide

17. Zinc phosphate cement is mixed over large surface area of the glass slab to
    A. Help lengthen the working time
    B. Help dissipate the exothermic reaction
    C. Help neutralize the chemicals
    D. All of the above

18. Luting cement should:
    A. Have a film thickness allowing for complete seating
    B. Have a film thickness for proper insulation
    C. Have a film thickness for complete filling of the crown
    D. None of the above

19. Which cement bonds to dentin, mild to pulp and resists recurrent caries?
    A. Zinc oxide eugenol
    B. Polycarboxylate
    C. Calcium hydroxide
    D. Glass ionomer

20. Many cement should only be dispensed at the time of mixing and not before because:
    A. Chances of dehydration from exposure of air
    B. Contamination from moisture in the air
    C. To avoid materials coming in contact with each other
    D. All of the above

---

## ANSWERS

| 1. C | 2. C | 3. B | 4. A |
|------|------|------|------|
| 5. D | 6. A | 7. B | 8. A |
| 9. A | 10. A | 11. C | 12. C |
| 13. B and C | 14. D | 15. C | 16. C |
| 17. D | 18. A | 19. D | 20. D |

---

## BIBLIOGRAPHY

1. Behr M, Rosentritt M, Wimmer J, Lang R, Kolbeck C, Bürgers R, et al. Self-adhesive resin cement versus zinc phosphate lining material: A prospective clinical trial begun 2003. Dent Mater. 2009;25:601-4.

2. Blackman R, Barghi N, Duke E. Influence of ceramic thickness on the polymerization of light cured resin cement. J Prosthet Dent. 1990;63:295-300.

3. Chaar MS, Att W, Strub JR. Prosthetic outcome of cement-retained implant-supported fixed dental restorations: a systematic review. J Oral Rehab. 2011;38:697-711.

4. Chan KC, Boyer DB. Curing light-activated composite cement through porcelain. J Dent Res. 1989;68:476-80.

5. Craig RG, Powers JM. Restorative Dental Materials, 11th edition. St. Louis: Mosby; 2002. pp. 594-634.

6. Crisp CAS, Kent BE, Lewis BG, et al. Glass-ionomer cement formulations. II. The synthesis of novel polycarboxylic acids. J Dent Res. 1980;59:1055-63.

7. Davidson CL, Mjor IA. Advances in Glass Ionomer Cements. Chicago; Qunitessence; 1999.

8. Donovan TE, Cho GC. Contemporary evaluation of dental cements. Compend Contin Edu Dent. 1999;20:197-219.

9. Duarte S Jr, Sartori N, Neimar A. Adhesive resin cements for bonding esthetic restorations: a review. Quintessence Dent Technol. 2011;34:40-66.

10. Farah JW, Powers JM. Esthetic resin cements. Dent Advis. 2000;17:1.

11. Francken JE, Taifour D, van't Hof MA. Survival of ART and amalgam restorations in permanent teeth of children after 6.3 years. J Dent Res. 2006;85:622-6.

12. Gandolfi MG, Chersoni S, Acquaviva GL, Piana G, Prati C, Mongiorgi R. Fluoride release and adsorption at different pH from glass-ionomer cements. Dent Mater. 2006;22:441-9.

13. Goldman M. Fracture properties of composite and glass ionomer dental restorative materials. J Biomed Mater Res. 1985;19;771-83.

14. Jefferies SR, Pameijer CH, Appleby DC, Boston D, Galbraith C, Lööf J, et al. Prospective observation of a new bioactive luting cement: 2-year follow-up. J Prosthodont. 2012;21:33-41.

15. McComb D. Adhesive luting cements—classes, criteria and usage. Compend Contin Educ Dent. 1996;17:759-73.

16. McKinney JE, Antonucci JM, Rupp NW. Wear and microhardness of a silver-sintered glass-ionomer cement. J Dent Res. 1988;67:831-5.

17. Mount GJ. An Atlas of Glass Ionomer Cements: a Clinicians Guide, 3rd edition. New York: Martin Duntiz; 2002. pp. 1-73.

18. Nicolson JW. Polyacid-modified composite resins ("compomers") and their use in clinical dentistry. Dent Mater. 2007;23:615-22.

19. Platt JA. Resin cements: into the 21st century. Compend Contin Educ Dent. 1999;20:1173-6.

20. Rosenstiel SF, Land MF, Crispin BJ. Dental luting agents: a review of the current literature. J Prosthet Dent. 1998;80:280-301.

21. Shillingburg HT, Hobo S, Whitsett LD, et al. Fundamentals of Fixed Prosthodontics, 3rd edition. Chicago: Quintessence; 1997. pp. 400-12.

22. Sidhu SK, Watson TF. Resin modified glass ionomer material: A status report for the American Journal of Dentistry. Am J Dent. 1995;8:59-67.

23. Smith DC. Dental cements current status and future prospects. Dent Clin North Am. 1983;6:763-93.

24. Swartz ML, Phillips RW, Clark HE. Long-term F release from glass ionomer cements. J Dent Res. 1984;63:158-60.

25. Tyas MJ. Milestones in adhesion: glass ionomer cements. J Adhes Dent. 2003;5:259-66.

26. Wang L, Sakai VT, Kawai ES, et al. Effects of adhesive systems associated with resin-modified glass ionomer cements. J Oral Rehabil. 2006;33:110-6.

27. Weigand A, Buchalla W, Attin T. Review on fluoride releasing restorative materials—fluoride release and uptake characteristics, antibacterial activity and influence on caries formation. Dent Mater. 2007;23:343-62.

28. Welbury RR, McCabe JF, Murray JJ, et al. Factors affecting the bond strength of composite resin to etched glass-ionomer cement. J Dent. 1988;16:188–193.

29. Wilson AD, McLean JW. Glass Ionomer Cements. Chicago: Quintessence; 1988.

30. Zhen CL, White S. Mechanical properties of dental luting cements. J Prosthet Dent. 1999;81:597-609.

# Pulp Protective Agents

*'Success is not final, failure is not fatal: it is the courage to continue that counts.'*

—*Winston Churchill*

## INTRODUCTION

Most of the restorative procedures can cause pulpal injury especially those involving extensive preparations. It is important to recognize hazards associated with different restorative procedures and minimize injury to the pulp. Protection of the pulp from different restorative material, trauma and chemical irritant or bacterial invasion is important to preserve the vitality of the pulp. There are number of causes for pulpal inflammation or dystrophy, which are identified below.

## ETIOLOGY OF VARIOUS PULPAL IRRITANTS (FLOWCHART 19.1)

- *Bacterial irritant*: This is one of the most common irritants to the pulp.
  - Caries
  - Accidental pulp exposure
  - *Fracture*: Complete or incomplete
  - Extension of infection from the gingival sulcus
  - Anomalous tract infection such as dens invaginatus and dens evaginatus
  - Periodontal pocket and abscess
  - *Anachoresis*: It is a process in which microorganisms carried by the bloodstream from another source localize on inflamed tissue of the pulp.
- *Traumatic*:
  - *Acute trauma*: Fracture of tooth, luxation and avulsion
  - *Chronic trauma*: Parafunctional habits such as bruxism
  - Attrition, erosion and abrasion.
- *Iatrogenic*:
  - Thermal changes during tooth preparation
  - Trauma during restoration
  - Orthodontic movement
  - Periodontal curettage
  - Periapical curettage
  - Electrosurgery
  - Laser burn.
- *Idiopathic*:
  - Aging
  - Internal or external resorption
  - Hereditary hypophosphatemia
  - Sickle cell anemia.
- *Chemical*:
  - *Restorative materials*: Cements, plastics, etchants, liners and bonding agent
  - *Disinfectants*: Sodium fluoride, silver nitrate and phenol
  - *Desiccants*: Alcohol and ether.

## PULP PROTECTING AGENTS

Pulp protecting agents are following:
- Cavity varnish
- Cavity liner
- Cement bases.

Flowchart 19.1: Showing etiology of various pulpal irritants.

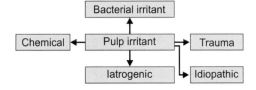

# CEMENT BASES

- Cement base is a layer of cement, which is placed under the restoration to protect the pulp against thermal injury, galvanic shock or chemical irritation **(Fig. 19.1)**
- It should be thick enough to resist the masticatory stresses and withstand condensation pressure during restoration placement
- Thickness of cement base should be more than 0.75 mm.

## Indications of Cavity Base

- To provide pulp protection against thermal injury, galvanic/electric shock and chemical irritation
- To act as shock absorber
- To withstand the forces of condensation

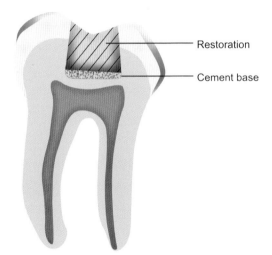

**Fig. 19.1:** Cement base applied to protect the pulp.

- To substitute dentin in deep cavities
- To serve as an intermediate bonding material between the tooth and the composite restoration
- To prevent ingress of bacteria and their toxins into the dentinal tubules through microleakage.

## Types of Cement Bases

- High-strength bases
- Low-strength bases.

### High-strength Bases

- For example, *glass ionomer, resin-modified glass ionomer (RMGI), zinc phosphate, zinc polycarboxylate, polymer reinforced zinc oxide eugenol (ZnOE)* and *compomer*
- Used to provide thermal protection of the pulp and mechanical support for the restorations
- Used under direct and indirect metallic restorations
- Commonly used high-strength bases are given in **Table 19.1**
- Low-strength bases flow more easily and are less rigid than the high-strength bases.

### Properties

- Greater compressive strength, tensile strength and modulus of elasticity as compared to the low-strength bases
- Zinc phosphate bases are the most rigid bases whereas polymer-based ZnOE are least rigid
- Thickness and elastic modulus of the cement base affect the deflection of the base and the restorations
- Mismatch between the elastic modulus of the cement base and the restoration results in tensile stresses, which

| Type of material | Indication | Advantages | Disadvantages |
|---|---|---|---|
| GIC<br>For example, Vitrebond, Ketac-Bond, Fuji Lining LC | RDT = 1–2 mm<br>Placed below composite restoration | • Chemical bonding to tooth structure<br>• Anticariogenic<br>• Highly biocompatible | • Increased solubility<br>• Technique and moisture sensitivity |
| Reinforced zinc oxide eugenol<br>For example, IRM | RDT = 1–2 mm below amalgam restoration | • Good sealing<br>• Obtundent effect on pulp | • Excess base removal is difficult |
| Zinc phosphate<br>For example, Harvard cement, Hy-Bond | RDT = 1–2 mm below amalgam restorations, inlay, onlays | • High-compressive strength to withstand forces of condensation<br>• Good thermal and electrical insulator | • Retention by mechanical means<br>• Pulpal irritation due to high initial pH |
| Zinc polycarboxylate | RDT = 1–2 mm below composite and amalgam restoration | • Chemical bonding<br>• Biocompatible<br>• Anticariogenic | • Short-working time<br>• Difficult to manipulate |

**Table 19.1:** Commonly used in high-strength bases.

*Abbreviations:* RDT, remaining dentin thickness; IRM, intermediate restorative material; GIC, glass ionomer cement.

lead to failure of either the cement base or restorative material
- Zinc phosphate cement is recommended under the amalgam restoration, whereas glass ionomer, RMGI or zinc polycarboxylate are recommended under composite restoration
- Glass ionomer cement (GIC), when used as base, provides benefits of chemical bond with tooth structure, additional retention, as it can be etched and ability to release fluoride **(Fig. 19.2)**
- Thermal conductivity and thermal diffusivity of most cements are similar to those of tooth enamel and dentin.

## Low-strength Bases

- For example, *calcium hydroxide [Ca(OH)₂], ZnOE cement* and *light-cured Ca(OH)₂*
- These bases have minimum strength and low rigidity
- They serve as a barrier to the irritating chemicals and provide therapeutic benefits to the pulp
- Commonly used low-strength bases are given in **Table 19.2**.

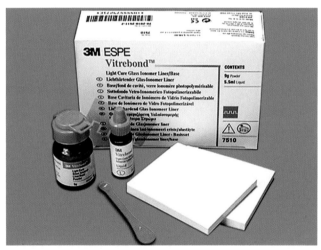

**Fig. 19.2:** Glass ionomer cavity base and liner.

### Properties

- *Thermal protection*: Base should provide thermal protection to the pulp
  - The thermal conductivity of the cement bases is similar to the tooth structure.
- *Therapeutic value*: $Ca(OH)_2$ acts as pulp capping agent; ZnOE has obtundent effect on the pulp
- *Strength*: Should have sufficient strength to withstand masticatory stresses and condensation pressure
- *Protection against chemical insults*: It should act as barrier against the penetration of the irritating constituents.

---

**CLINICAL SIGNIFICANCE**

- Base is selected on the basis of the design of the cavity, type of restorative material and proximity to the pulp
- Thickness of the cavity base should not be more than 0.5–0.75 mm thickness. Thick base compromises the bulk of the restoration and increases susceptibility to fracture
- Sound tooth structure should never be reduced to create space for the base. Tooth structure should always be conserved to increase support and provide the protection to pulp
- Cavity base should only be applied on the internal wall of the prepared cavity to prevent dissolution by saliva
- The modulus of elasticity of the base and the restorative material should match each other. Any mismatch between the two can result in generation of tensile stresses at the base restoration interface resulting in failure
- Calcium hydroxide is used in direct pulp capping and indirect pulp capping
- Zinc oxide eugenol is used in deep cavities to protect pulp from penetration of chemical irritants
- For amalgam restorations, $Ca(OH)_2$ or ZnOE bases are used.

---

**Table 19.2:** Commonly used low-strength bases/suspension liner.

| Type of material | Indications | Advantages | Disadvantages |
|---|---|---|---|
| Calcium hydroxide For example, Dycal, Calcimol, Pre-Line | RDT <1 mm Used below GIC and composite restorations | • Capable of inducing reparative dentin formation • Forms a stable adherent layer | • High solubility • Very-short working time • Placement is difficult, as it sticks to the instrument |
| Light-cured calcium hydroxide For example, Calcimol LC, Septocal LC | RDT <1 mm used below GIC and composite restorations | • Adequate working time as sets on command • Available in single tube, so no mixing required | • Does not provide thermal and electrical insulation |
| Zinc oxide eugenol For example, Kalzinol | RDT = 1–2 mm used under interim restorations | • Adequate working time | • Difficulty to maintain consistency of the mixture |

*Abbreviations:* RDT, remaining dentin thickness; GIC, glass ionomer cement; LC, light-cured.

- For direct-filling gold stronger base such as zinc phosphate, zinc polycarboxylate or glass ionomer are recommended
- For resin-based composites, $Ca(OH)_2$ and GIC are used as cement bases
- Cavity varnish or dentin bonding agents are usually required to prevent microleakage and acid penetration
- Type of cement base used to determine the order in which cavity varnish and base are applied
- When zinc phosphate cement is used as a base then cavity varnish is applied before the base
- When $Ca(OH)_2$, zinc polycarboxylate or GIC is used then cement base should be placed first, followed by varnish or bonding agent once the base has hardened.

## SUB-BASES

Sub-bases are very low-strength cement, which are placed below the high-strength bases to reduce pulpal inflammation and initiate formation of reparative dentin. $Ca(OH)_2$ is the most commonly used sub-base because of its beneficial effect on the pulp.

### Calcium Hydroxide

- Calcium hydroxide gained prominence after the pioneering work of Dr Hermann in 1930s. After World War II, the use of $Ca(OH)_2$ expanded and was widely used for dental use. This type of cement was introduced in early 1960s. It is relatively weak cement, which is based on phenolate type reaction between $Ca(OH)_2$ and salicylate esters **(Fig. 19.3)**

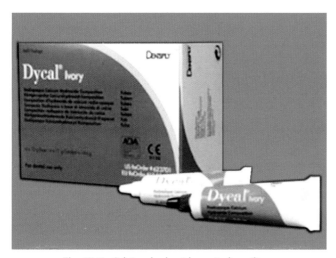

**Fig. 19.3:** Calcium hydroxide cavity base/liner.

- It is primarily used as direct or indirect pulp capping agent because of its alkaline nature and remineralization effect, which helps in forming reparative dentin
- It serves as protective barrier against irritants from restorations **(Fig. 19.4)**.

### Applications

- Used as direct or indirect pulp capping agent
- As low-strength base below restoration to protect the pulp
- As cavity liner **(Fig. 19.5)**
- In apexification procedure in young permanent dentition where the root formation is incomplete.
- As endodontic sealer
- For management of traumatized teeth
- For management of resorption
- As intracanal medicament.

### Modes of Supply (Figs. 19.6A and B)

- Supplied as two-paste systems, i.e. base and catalyst paste in tubes
- Light-cured syringe
- Single paste in a syringe form.

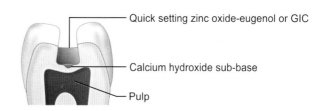

Very deep cavity-calcium hydroxide sub-base beneath ZOE or GIC lining

**Fig. 19.4:** Calcium hydroxide used as sub-base in deep cavity restorations.
*Abbreviations:* ZOE, zinc oxide eugenol; GIC, glass ionomer cement.

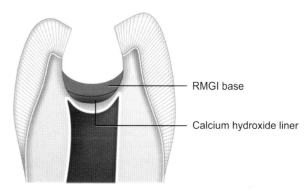

**Fig. 19.5:** Calcium hydroxide used as cavity liner.
*Abbreviation:* RMGI, resin-modified glass ionomer.

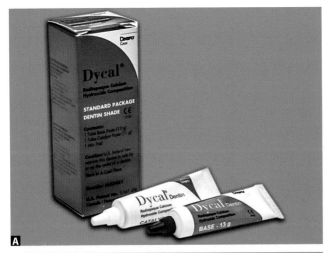

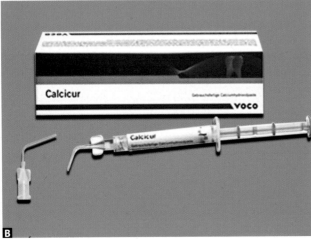

**Figs. 19.6A and B:** Calcium hydroxide supplied as two-paste systems and syringe form.

## Composition

*Base paste:*
- *Disalicylate ester of 1,3 butylene glycol*—40%
- Calcium phosphate
- Zinc oxide and iron oxide
- *Titanium dioxide*: Inert fillers and pigments
- *Calcium tungstate* or *barium sulfate*: Provides radiopacity.

*Catalyst paste:*
- *Calcium hydroxide*: 50%—principal reactor
- *Zinc oxide* and *iron oxide*: 10%
- *Zinc stearate*: 0.5%—accelerator
- *Ethylene toluene sulfonamide*: 39.5%—oily compound act as carrier
- *Titanium dioxide*: Inert filler.

## Classification of Calcium Hydroxide Base

*Based on availability:*
- Single-paste system, e.g. Endocal, VLC Dycal
- Two-paste system. e.g. Dycal
- Powder mixed with different vehicles.

*Based on the setting time:*
- *Fast setting*—this is chemically activated $Ca(OH)_2$ paste, which is used as sub-base or liner. The normal setting time is 2.5–3.5 minutes. Although, it sets fast in presence of moisture. It is a low-strength base, For example, Dycal
- *Controlled setting*—this is light-activated $Ca(OH)_2$ paste, which is indicated in direct pulp capping procedure. It contains photoinitiator such as camphorquinone. E.g. light cure $Ca(OH)_2$, VLC Dycal, Calcimol LC
- *Slow setting*—it is used as temporary sealing material, which sets slowly in presence of moisture. For example, Proviplast
- *Nonsetting*—this type of $Ca(OH)_2$ powder needs to be mixed with various vehicles and is used as intracanal medicament.

### Setting Reaction

$Ca(OH)_2$ and salicylate ester to form a chelate called amorphous calcium disalicylate:

$$Ca(OH)_2 + Salicylate\ ester \rightarrow Ca\text{-}disalicylate$$
$$(amorphous\ chelate)$$

### Manipulation

- Both the base paste and catalyst paste are mixed in equal volume. Mixing should be complete in 10 seconds
- The mixture should be homogeneous and streak free, which is carried to the cavity with the help of cement carrier
- Increased humidity and temperature reduce the working time and the setting time. Likewise, reduced humidity and temperature will increase the working time and the setting time
- Setting time is 2.5–3.5 minutes, but clinically it sets much faster.

### Properties

- *Mechanical*: Has poor mechanical properties:
  - *Compressive strength*: Low but increases with time after setting. After 24 hours, it is 10–27 MPa
  - *Tensile strength*: Low (1.5–2.0 MPa)
  - *Modulus of elasticity*: 0.37 $GPa/m^2$ is low (cannot be used in load-bearing areas). It is not recommended to be used as sole base or luting agent

- *Thermal properties*: If used in thick layer then provides some thermal insulation (minimum 0.5 mm thickness). However, it should not be used with thickness greater than 0.5 mm because it has low strength
- *Solubility and disintegration*:
  - Solubility is highest among cements ranging between 0.4% and 7.8% by weight in distilled water in 24 hours
  - These cements subjected to hydrolytic breakdown
  - It there is continued marginal leakage then complete dissolution of the lining material occurs
  - Slight solubility is desirable for therapeutic benefits. Although, it is higher in contact with ether or phosphoric acid. Therefore, it is important to take precautions when this cement is used in presence of varnish or after acid etching
- *Biologic properties*:
  - This cement has strong antibacterial effect and also aids in remineralization of carius dentin
  - Has alkaline pH and has therefore, soothing or obtundent effect on the pulp. Its pH varies between 9.2 and 11.7
  - Assist in formation of secondary dentin when used as pulp capping agent
  - *Calcific barrier formation*: $Ca(OH)_2$ produces organic matrix, which mineralizes within 4–6 weeks. $Ca(OH)_2$ stimulates the dentin matrix formation through adenosine triphosphate (ATP) activation and diffusion of growth factors. It activates alkaline phosphatase activity and induces odontoblast like cell differentiation. This process is followed by formation of reparative dentin. The newly formed calcific barrier consists of two layers—(1) the outer layer is dense acellular cementum and (2) the inner layer is the dense fibrocollagenous-connective tissue
  - Calcium hydroxide can also act in presence of blood and other tissue exudate. It produces calcium ions resulting in less leakage at the capillary junction and reducing the plasma flow. It is considered as material of choice for the "*Weeping canal*". Increase in concentration of calcium ions accelerates bone formation
  - *Antibacterial effects*—because of its high-alkaline pH most of the pathogens are destroyed. The antibacterial effect of $Ca(OH)_2$ is due to:
    - Protein denaturation
    - Damage to DNA
    - Damage to bacterial cytoplasmic membrane
    - Acts as barrier and exerts pulp protective action by neutralizing and preventing passage of chemical irritants
    *Factors limiting the antibacterial action of Ca(OH)₂ are:*
    - Permeability and buffering capacity of dentin
    - Inaccessible area
    - Low-water solubility and diffusibility of $Ca(OH)_2$
    - Resistant strains
- *Adhesion*:
  - The cement is sensitive to saliva, moisture, blood, etc. and does not bond properly to tooth structure in their presence.

*Advantages*

- Ease of manipulation
- Rapid hardening in thin layers
- Forms stable adherent layer
- Has good sealing property
- Antibacterial property
- Formation of reparative dentin.

*Disadvantages*

- Has low strength
- Very short-working time
- High solubility
- Tends to stick with the instrument
- Shows plastic deformation
- Shows greater dissolution in acidic conditions.

## Light-activated Calcium Hydroxide (Figs. 19.7A and B)

- It is composed of $Ca(OH)_2$ and barium sulfate, which are dispersed in urethane dimethacrylate resin. It has hydroxyethyl methacrylate (HEMA), some polymerizing activators, photoinitiators and fluoride
- Has longer working time because polymerizes on light exposure
- Indicated when remaining dentin thickness (RDT) is less than 1 mm
- Used under the glass ionomer and composite resin restoration
- Is less brittle
- Has high-compressive strength (96 MPa) and tensile strength (38 MPa).
- Shows low solubility ($\leq 1.0\%$)
- Shows low dissolution in acid ($\leq 0.5\%$)
- Do not show antibacterial property
- For example, Calcimol LC, Septocal LC and Cal LC.

*Advantages*

- Long-working time as sets on command
- Available in single tube where mixing is not required

*Disadvantage*

Does not provide adequate thermal and electrical insulation.

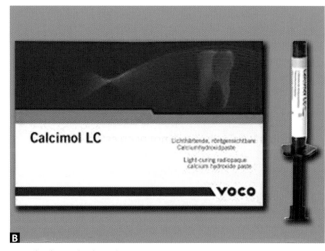

**Light-cured calcium hydroxide cavity liner**
Indirect pulp capping
Lining under all filling materials
Protection when applying the total etch technique

**Figs. 19.7A and B:** Light-activated calcium hydroxide.

## Calcium Hydroxide as Root Canal Sealer (Fig. 19.8)

- These root canal sealers contain $Ca(OH)_2$
- Calcium hydroxide as root canal sealer is effective when it dissociates into $Ca^{2+}$ and $OH^-$ ions. This will happen when it dissolves. This can lead to formation of obturation voids
- They are radiopaque and contain greater amount of retarders to increase the working time
- They have antibacterial property because of high-alkaline pH and also due to absorption of carbon dioxide
- Supplied as base and catalyst paste
- Not commonly used.

*Advantages*
- Have antibacterial property
- They have ability to promote the formation of calcific barrier.

*Disadvantage*
Forms obturation voids.

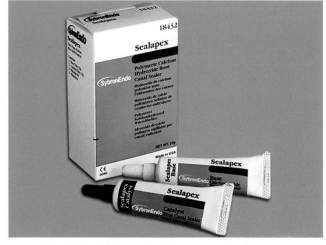

**Fig. 19.8:** Calcium hydroxide root canal sealer paste.

## CAVITY VARNISH

- Cavity varnish consists of mixture of resins, which are dissolved in a solvent such as chloroform, alcohol, ether, etc.
- When they are applied on the surface of the cavity, they form a coating by evaporation of the solvent preventing ingress of oral fluids at the restoration tooth interface into the underlying dentin **(Fig. 19.9)**
- They reduce postoperative sensitivity when applied to the dentinal surface under newly placed restorations
- They are rapidly been replaced by bonding agents.

### Applications

- Minimizes penetration of acid from cement into the dentinal tubules

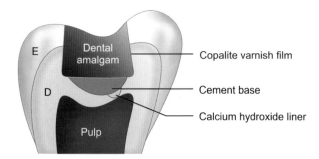

**Fig. 19.9:** Cavity varnish is applied on the surface of the cavity.

- Prevents penetration of oral fluids around the metallic restorations into the dentinal tubules
- Reduces microleakage around margins of newly placed amalgam and reducing postoperative sensitivity
- Reduces passage of irritants into tubules from overlying restorations or base. For example, silicate and zinc phosphate cement.

- Prevents penetration of corrosion products from amalgam into tubules, thus minimizing discoloration
- Used as surface coating over restorations such as silicate cement or glass ionomer to protect from dehydration or contact with oral fluid
- Applied on surface of metallic restorations as temporary protection against galvanic shock
- Fluoride-containing varnish has anticariogenic property although effectiveness is not been established.

## Composition

Cavity varnish is a solution containing:
- Principally natural gum such as copal rosin or synthetic resins dissolved in organic solvent such as alcohol, chloroform, benzene, ethyl acetate, toluene, acetone or ether
- Medicinal agents like chlorobutanol, thymol and eugenol may be added.

## Supplied As

Liquid in dark-colored bottles **(Fig. 19.10)**.

## Manipulation

- Applied in thin layers by means of small cotton pledget or disposable applicator brush
- Disposable applicator brush is discarded after every use to prevent contamination of the varnish
- In order to achieve uniform coating on the surface of the cavity, at least two layers of varnish are applied
- When first layer dries, small voids are formed on the surface

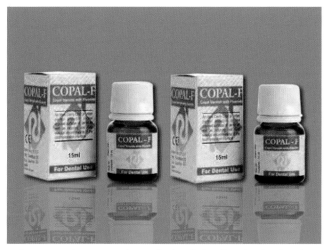

**Fig. 19.10:** Cavity varnish supplied in dark-colored amber bottles.

- Second or third coat fills up these voids
- Two layers are found to be more effective than single heavy layer.

## Properties

- Cavity varnish reduces but not prevents the passage of acid content into underlying dentin
- Because of thin film thickness, it does not possess mechanical strength and does not provide thermal insulation
- Film thickness of varnish varies between 2 μm and 40 μm
- Contact angles of varnish on dentin ranges between 53° and 106°
- Solubility low and insoluble in distilled water.

## Precautions

- Solution should be tightly capped after every use to prevent evaporation of the solvent
- Should be applied in thin multiple layers
- Excess varnish should not be left on margins of the restorations, as it prevents proper finishing of the restoration at the margins.

### CLINICAL SIGNIFICANCE

- Cavity varnish is contraindicated with adhesive materials like glass ionomers and composite resins because solvent in varnish softens the resin
- Also, it eliminates potential for adhesion and biocompatibility of GIC.

### Fluoride Varnish

This type of varnish contains fluoride and helps in preventing smooth surface caries in deciduous and young permanent teeth. This varnish when applied onto the tooth hardens in contact with saliva. The child is instructed to brush after 1 day. It is advised to apply fluoride varnish two times in a year. For example, Duraphat and Fluor Protector **(Fig. 19.11)**.

## CAVITY LINER

Cavity liners are suspensions of $Ca(OH)_2$ in an organic liquid, which provides barrier against passage of irritants from restorative materials to the dentin.

They are used similar to cavity varnish, but unlike varnish they provide therapeutic benefits to the tooth **(Fig. 19.12)**.

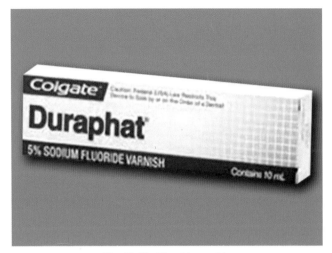

**Fig. 19.11:** Fluoride varnish.

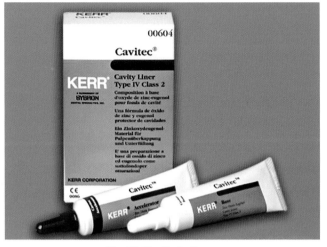

**Fig. 19.12:** Cavity liners.

## Composition

- Suspensions of Ca(OH)$_2$ in an organic liquid such as methyl ethyl ketone or ethyl alcohol or in aqueous solution of methyl cellulose
- Methyl cellulose acts as thickening agent
- May also contain acrylic polymer beads or barium sulfate
- Fluoride compounds such as calcium monofluorophosphate are also added in some liners
- On evaporation of the volatile substance, liner forms a thin film on the prepared tooth.

## Manipulation

- Cavity liners are fluid in consistency and are easily applied over the dentin surface
- Solvents evaporate to leave behind thin layer of Ca(OH)$_2$ that protects the underlying pulp
- Thin film of Ca(OH)$_2$ with alkaline pH can also neutralize or react with acid released form phosphate-based cements.

## Properties

- They do not possess mechanical strength or provide thermal insulation. It neutralizes acids, which move toward and pulp
- As Ca(OH)$_2$ is soluble in oral fluids, it should not be applied at the margins of the restorations. Ca(OH)$_2$ also induces formation of secondary dentin
- Fluorides are added to prevent secondary caries below the restorations
- Cavity liners have shown to improve sealing at the tooth restoration interface preventing influx of chemical irritants from the restoration into the dentin.

## Types of Cavity Liners

- Calcium hydroxide
- Zinc oxide eugenol liner
- Flowable composites
- Glass ionomers.

## DIRECT PULP CAPPING

- It is a technique of treating a pulp exposure site by material that promotes reparative dentin formation
- This procedure is done following a *mechanical pulpal exposure* in an area of normal dentin where bacterial contamination has not occurred
- If there is *carious pulpal exposure* then endodontic therapy is indicated.

### Indications

- When small mechanical pulpal exposure (≤0.5 mm in diameter) in area of normal dentin has occurred
- Bleeding from the exposure site is easily controlled
- Tooth is asymptomatic before operative procedure, i.e. vital without any pain
- Exposure site is in clean uncontaminated area
- When mechanical exposure was atraumatic with minimal desiccation of the tooth.

### Contraindications

- When pulpal exposure site is more than 0.5 mm in diameter
- Exposure is due to carious lesion extending into the pulp
- When there is radiographic evidence of periapical pathology

- When there is excessive bleeding at the exposure site
- When there is spontaneous pain at the exposure site.

*Factors influencing success of direct pulp capping:*
- Age of the patient
- Size of the exposure
- Type of the exposure
- History of pain.

## Procedure

- Tooth is isolated after administering local anesthesia
- All undesirable and undermined enamel is removed
- The cavity floor and the exposure site are gently washed and irrigated with distilled water **(Fig. 19.13)**
- The site is dried with the help of cotton pellets but never desiccated
- Calcium hydroxide paste is mixed into thin creamy consistency and gently applied at the exposure site
- Light-activated $Ca(OH)_2$ paste can also be used as direct pulp capping material
- If unmodified ZnOE is used then some dentinal shavings are cut from the surrounding dentin and deposited at the exposure site
- After capping, interim restoration is done with ZnOE for 6–8 weeks
- After 6–8 weeks, the exposure site is inspected carefully for dentin bridge formation (reparative dentin)
- If reparative dentin has formed then permanent restoration is done after using appropriate base
- If the pulp is degenerated then endodontic therapy should be started immediately.

## INDIRECT PULP CAPPING

- This technique involves deliberate retention of softened dentin near the pulp and medicating the remaining dentin with $Ca(OH)_2$ **(Fig. 19.14)**

- It aims at preventing pulp exposure and recovery of pulp through medication
- Calcium hydroxide helps in the formation of reparative dentin bridges over the area of frank pulpal exposure.

## Indications

- Deep carious lesion approximating the pulp
- When there is no history of pain or any radiographic evidence of periapical pathology
- When the tooth does not show any sign of root resorption or radicular disease
- When tooth is nontender on percussion.

## Contraindications

- There is radiographic evidence of periapical pathology
- When there is frank pulpal exposure
- Patient gives history of pain and shows sign of tooth mobility
- When there is evidence of root resorption.

## Procedure

- Tooth is isolated after administering local anesthesia
- All *infected dentin* is removed using a spoon excavator leaving behind *softened affected dentin*
- Any undermined or softened tooth structure is removed.
- The portion of the remaining softened affected dentin is covered with thin creamy mixture of $Ca(OH)_2$
- Calcium hydroxide promotes formation of reparative dentin over the affected area
- Resin-modified glass ionomer liner is placed over $Ca(OH)_2$ for better result
- Temporary restoration of ZnOE is done.

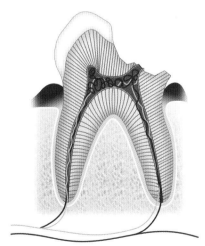

**Fig. 19.13:** Mechanical exposure of pulp is indicated for direct pulp capping.

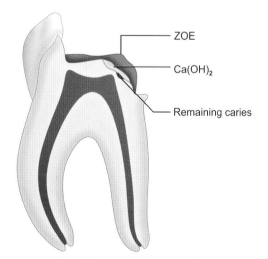

**Fig. 19.14:** Indirect pulp capping.
*Abbreviation:* ZOE, zinc oxide eugenol.

- The tooth is evaluated after 6–8 weeks, which is the time required for reparative dentin formation
- To evaluate dentin formation radiographically 10–12 weeks' time is required
- If there is no evidence of pulpal degeneration, then permanent restoration is done otherwise endodontic therapy should be started.

# METHODS OF PULP PROTECTION UNDER DIFFERENT RESTORATIONS

- *Amalgam:*
  - Since amalgam is a metallic restoration, it shows high-thermal conductivity and therefore, a bases or liner should be placed under the restoration
  - Amalgam is one of the least irritating permanent restorative material to the pulp
  - Corrosion must be considered when amalgam restorations are inserted
  - If the RDT is more than 2 mm then cavity varnish or dentin bonding agent is applied at the margins
  - If the RDT is 0.5–2.0 mm then cavity liner or an appropriate base is used
  - If the RDT is less than 0.5 mm then Ca(OH)$_2$ is used as sub-base below the cavity base as a pulp protective measure.
- *Gold foil:*
  - The use of gold foil should be avoided in the teeth of young patients because pulp horns are large and higher and the remaining dentin thickness is less
  - Also, pressure applied during insertion of gold foil can result in inflammatory reaction to the pulp
  - If remaining dentin thickness is between 0.5 mm and 2.0 mm then cavity base is used
  - And if it is less than 0.5 mm then calcium hydroxide is used as sub-base to protect the pulp.
- *Composite resins:*
  - Acid-etching procedure and unbound components of resins may induce inflammation of the pulp
  - Although adequately cured composites are relatively biocompatible

- Inadequately cured resins can results in leaching out of components capable of long-term pulpal inflammation
- Pulp protection is required under deep preparation
- Cavity liners are usually recommended with calcium hydroxide sub-base for deep preparations
- Eugenol-based cavity liners should be avoided as they interfere with the polymerization of the resin.
- *Silicate cements:*
  - Acid content in silicate cement results in severe inflammation of pulp especially if cavity liner is not used below the restoration
  - Reparative dentin formation is inhibited initially, owing to the death of the underlying odontoblasts and other pulp cells
  - Depth of cavity determines the effect of silicate cement on the pulp
  - The closer the silicate restoration to the pulp, the more severe the inflammatory reaction
  - In deep cavities, where less than 0.5 mm of dentin remains between the base of the cavity and the pulp, chronic inflammation may persist for 6 months to a year, resulting in total pulp necrosis
  - It is necessary to protect the pulp under silicate restoration with cavity liner and base.
- *Glass ionomer cement:*
  - Glass ionomer cement shows mild pulp response
  - More the amount of liquid in the mixture, greater the reaction to the pulp especially with luting consistency
  - Freshly mixed glass ionomer cements causes more damage than set cement because of the presence of unbound acid
  - Good adhesion accounts for its good biocompatibility, less leakage and thus reduced invasion of bacteria at tooth restoration interface
  - To reduce postoperative sensitivity, the vital tooth should be protected with dentin bonding agent before cementing the prosthesis
  - Deeper cavity preparation requires cavity liner and or base before restoring with glass ionomer.

---

# TEST YOURSELF

### Essay Questions

1. Discuss pulp protecting agents under metallic restorations.
2. Describe pulp protection under composite resin restorations.
3. Describe the role of Ca(OH)$_2$ in direct and indirect pulp capping.
4. Describe in detail direct pulp capping and indirect pulp capping procedures.
5. Discuss various cavity bases used in general dentistry.

## Short Notes

1. High-strength bases.
2. Calcium hydroxide.
3. Cavity liners.
4. Cavity varnish.
5. Light cure $Ca(OH)_2$.
6. Root canal sealers.
7. Low-strength bases.
8. Pulp irritants.

## Multiple Choice Questions

1. A cavity base is placed on the floor of a deep cavity under a gold restoration to:
   A. Prevent gold atoms from penetrating into the tooth
   B. Improve the stiffness of the restoration
   C. Seal the dentin from toxic gold particles
   D. Provide thermal protection for the pulp

2. If a patient requires an amalgam restoration in maxillary molar, which of the following will be the best base material:
   A. Glass ionomer
   B. Zinc phosphate
   C. Zinc oxide eugenol
   D. Light-cured $Ca(OH)_2$

3. What will explain the rationale of placing a liner of glass ionomer under a large and deep composite restoration in a molar tooth?
   A. Provide thermal insulation for the tooth
   B. Seal the dentinal surfaces under the composite
   C. Improve the strength of the restoration
   D. Minimize the chances for postoperative sensitivity

4. Which material is often placed into the deep cavity for promoting secondary dentin formation?
   A. Zinc oxide eugenol
   B. Calcium hydroxide
   C. Glass ionomer
   D. Zinc phosphate

5. Insulating base is placed under the restoration to:
   A. Encourage secondary dentin formation
   B. Reduce acidity
   C. Seal the dentinal tubules
   D. Protect the pulp from sudden temperature changes

6. Cements mixed with primary consistency are used for:
   A. Luting and high-strength bases
   B. Luting and low-strength bases
   C. Core buildup
   D. Surgical dressing

7. Cavity varnish when painted on the tooth:
   A. Forms an impermeable resin film
   B. Forms a semipermeable resin film
   C. Acts as medicament
   D. Prevents thermal changes from reaching the pulp

8. Cavity varnish should not be used below all these restorations, *except*:
   A. Amalgam
   B. Composite
   C. Glass ionomer
   D. Silicate

## ANSWERS

| | | | |
|---|---|---|---|
| 1. D | 2. B | 3. B and D | 4. B |
| 5. B | 6. B | 7. B | 8. A |

## BIBLIOGRAPHY

1. Anusavice KJ. Dental amalgam. Phillip's Science of Dental Materials, 11th edition. St. Louis: Saunders; 2003.
2. Costa CAS, Mesas AN, Hebling J. Pulp response to direct capping with an adhesive system. Am J Dent. 2000;13:81.
3. Craig RG, Powers JM. Amalgam. Restorative Dental Materials, 11th edition. St. Louis: Mosby; 2002.
4. Hilton TJ. Cavity sealers, liners and bases: Current philosophies and indications for use. Oper Dent. 1996;21:134.
5. Leinfelder KF. Changing restorative traditions: the use of bases and liners. J Am Dent Assoc. 1994;125:65.
6. Phillips RW, Crim G, Swartz ML, et al. Resistance of calcium hydroxide preparations to solubility in phosphoric acid. J Prosthet Dent. 1984;52:358-60.
7. Swartz ML, Phillips RW, Norman RD, et al. Role of cavity varnishes and bases in the penetration of cement constituents through tooth structure. J Prosthet Dent. 1966;16:963.
8. Tam LE, McComb D, Pulver F. Physical properties of proprietary light cured lining materials. Oper Dent. 1991;16:210-7.
9. Weiner R. Liners and bases in general dentistry. Aus Dent J. 2011;56:11-22.

*'More gold has been mined from thoughts of men than has been taken from the earth.'*

—*Napoleon Hill*

## INTRODUCTION

Direct gold restorations have long been considered standard by which clinical performance of other restorative materials have been compared. A properly done direct gold restoration has excellent clinical longevity and durability. However, direct gold restorations are rarely used in clinical practice because of its demand for high technical excellence; time involved, cost, metallic appearance and increased patient demand for esthetic restorations. It is important for the clinician to have thorough knowledge about these materials so that correct clinical decisions can be made relative to oral rehabilitation.

*Factors influencing high-quality direct gold restorations are:*
- Isolation—dry and clean field required
- Proper manipulation of direct gold with proper instruments.
- Appropriate type of gold used in specific clinical situation.
- Material used only where indicated.

## DEFINITION

*Direct gold restorations are gold restorative materials that are manufactured for compaction directly into the prepared cavity.*

## HISTORICAL EVENTS

- *3000 BC:* Evidence of gold jewelry in Roman and Greek culture
- *3000–2000 BC:* Gold jewelry found in Sumerian, Babylonian and Assyrian tomb
- *1570–1293 BC:* Use of gold in Egyptian mummies and tomb
- *1483 AD: Giovanni d'Arcoli* first recommended use of gold foil for filling diseased teeth
- *1510–1590: Ambroise Pare* used lead of cork to fill teeth
- *1678–1761: Pierre Fauchard*, Father of modern dentistry used tin foil or lead cylinder for filling tooth cavities
- *1715–1767: Philip Pfaff*, dentist to Frederick the Great of Prussia, used gold foil for pulp capping
- *1795: Robert Woofendale* introduced gold foil for restoration purposes in America
- *1812: Marcus Bull* of Hartford, Connecticut started manufacturing beaten gold for dental use
- *1838: E. Merrit* introduced principles of condensation of gold foil
- *1853:* Sponge Gold was introduced in the United States and England
- *1855: Robert A Arthur* first introduced the cohesive gold
- *1871:* Corrugated gold made by burning gold foil sheets between papers in the absence of air.

## GENERAL PROPERTIES

- *Noble metal*: Pure gold is the most noble metal among all the metals
- *Corrosion resistant*: It has excellent resistance to tarnish and corrosion
- *Inertness*: It is chemically inactive and is not affected by heat, moisture, air or solvents
- *Ductility*: It is the most ductile metal amongst all the metal as it can be drawn into thin wire
- *Malleability*: It is the most malleable metal amongst all the metal as it can be rolled into thin sheets which are almost transparent. Manufacturing for dental use the thickness starts from 25 μm
- *Hardness*: After cold working, hardness of pure gold is 52–75 VHN. This hardness is equivalent to the hardness of type I gold alloy. After work hardening, hardness is increased to 90 VHN which approaches hardness value of type II gold alloy
- *Elongation*: Percent elongation after cold working is 12.8% which allows lateral displacement and wedging desired to enhance retention during condensation process
- *Color*: It has rich yellow metallic appearance
- *Density*: Density of pure gold is highest among all metals, i.e. 19.3 g/cm$^3$. Because of high density greater mass of gold is required to restore given volume of the prepared tooth
- *Condensation*: Excellent malleability and lack of surface oxide after degassing permit condensation of gold pellets directly into the cavity. Pieces of gold are cold welded at room temperature using a condensing instrument
- *Weldability*: Gold pellets can be cold welded, i.e. welding of gold increments together at mouth temperature under pressure
- *Cohesiveness*: Cohesion of gold during condensation occurs due to metallic bonding between the overlapping increments of gold under pressure
- *Coefficient of thermal expansion*: Coefficient of thermal expansion is 14.4 × 10$^{-6}$/°C. It is similar to the tooth dentine.
- *Thermal conductivity*: It has high thermal conductivity.
- *Biocompatibility and marginal adaptation*: It has excellent biocompatibility and marginal integrity.

## USES

- Class I restorations of pits and fissures of most posterior teeth and lingual surfaces of anterior teeth
- Class V restoration of posterior teeth where access and esthetics permits

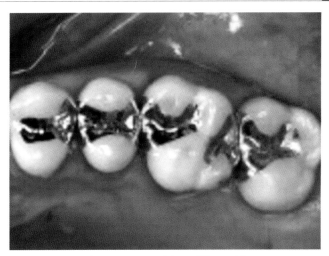

**Fig. 20.1:** Uses of direct filling gold.

- Restorations of abraded, eroded or abfraction areas
- Class III incipient interproximal lesion of anterior teeth
- Class II restorations of small proximal lesions on mesial or distal surfaces of mandibular first premolar and maxillary premolars **(Fig. 20.1)**
- Class VI direct gold restorations on the incisal or cusp tips
- Repair of defective margin of otherwise acceptable gold casting
- Repair cement vent holes in gold crowns.

## CONTRAINDICATIONS

- Inaccessible areas with large lesions
- Young patients with large pulp chamber
- Periodontally weakened teeth with poor prognosis
- Uncooperative patient, lacking patience
- Handicapped or elderly patient
- In high esthetic zone
- Where large amount of tooth structure is destroyed
- Areas where large occlusal stress is expected
- Root canal treated teeth as they are brittle
- Cost.

## ADVANTAGES

- Excellent biocompatibility
- Least tarnish and corrosion of all the metals
- Excellent malleability provides self-sealing margins
- Good adaptation to the cavity wall and does not require any cementing media
- Cohesive gold allows cold welding to occur at mouth temperature on applying pressure
- Can be polished to high luster, permit lesser plaque accumulation

- Density and hardness of compacted gold enable the restoration to withstand the compressive forces of occlusion
- Thermal expansion similar to dentin
- Chemically inactive and insoluble in most of the solvents
- High wear resistance
- Less chances of molecular change.

## DISADVANTAGES

- It cannot be used in esthetic areas because of metallic appearance
- Technical difficulty to form dense restorations
- Requires great skill and patience
- Use limited to low stress bearing areas and small lesions
- Costly
- Because of its high density it requires greater mass of gold in a given volume of prepared tooth compared to other metals with lower densities
- Improper compaction can damage the pulp
- Gold restoration opposing the amalgam restoration can cause "galvanic shock".

### Classification of Direct Filling Gold

*1. On the basis of its availability, direct gold can be classified as (Phillips')* **(Flowchart 20.1)**.
- Gold foil
  - Sheet
    - Cohesive
    - Noncohesive.
  - Ropes
  - Cylinders
  - Laminated foil
  - Platinized foil.
- Electrolytic precipitate (crystalline gold)
  - Mat gold
  - Mat foils (mat gold plus gold foil)
  - Gold calcium alloy.
- Granulated gold (encapsulated gold powder)

*2. According to WJO Brien*
- Foil
  - Platinized gold foil
  - Gold foil
  - Mat foil.
- Electrolytic
  - Mat gold
  - Calcium alloy (e.g. Electralloy).
- Powdered gold (e.g. Goldent)
  - E-Z gold.

## GOLD FOIL

- It is also called as *fibrous gold*
- It is one of the oldest and most durable form of direct gold
- It is available in the form of sheets, pellets, cylinders, ropes and partially precondensed laminates of various thickness **(Fig. 20.2)**
- It is manufactured by beating cast ingot into sheets of thickness of 15–25 µm foils by alternately subjecting to cold working and strain hardening process
- These thin sheets are separated by 4 inch square of parchment and rolled into a bundle
- Bundle is beaten into desired thickness
- Weight of gold in each 4 inch square sheet is designated by a number
- Standard No. 4 gold foil indicates—4 × 4 inch sheet which weighs 4 grains (0.259 g) and which is about 0.51 µm thick
- Similarly standard No. 3 gold foil indicates—4 × 4 inch sheet which weighs 3 grains (0.194 g) and which is 0.38 µm thick
- Other foils which are available are No. 20 (20 grains), No. 40 (40 grains). No. 60 (60 grains) and No. 90 (90 grains)
- Cross-section of properly condensed cohesive gold foil shows 400–600 µ of superficial and 200 µ of deepest layer of restoration to composed of solid gold
- Serrated solid gold exists in bulk of the restorations with scattered voids in between them **(Fig. 20.3)**.

### Cohesive and Noncohesive

Sheets of gold foils can be supplied by the manufacturer into either cohesive or noncohesive form.

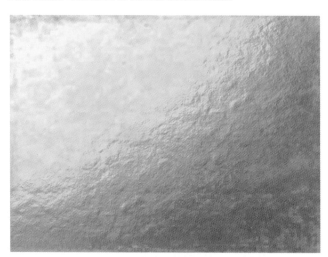

**Fig. 20.2:** Gold foil supplied in form of sheets.

**Flowchart 20.1:** Types of direct filling gold.

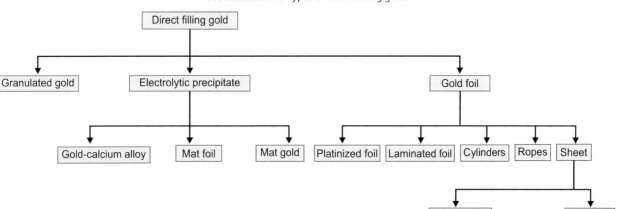

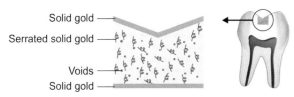

Solid gold
Serrated solid gold
Voids
Solid gold

**Fig. 20.3:** Cross-section of cohesive gold foil.

*Cohesive Foil*

- Type of gold foil which is free of surface contaminants is called as *cohesive gold foil*
- For a gold foil to cold weld at mouth temperature, it should have absolutely clean surface
- The gold supplied by the manufacturer should be in cohesive state
- Gold like other metals adsorbs gases on its surface which prevents cohesiveness of individual increments of gold during condensation
- Manufacturer supplies the gold foil essentially free of surface contaminants, but they can be contaminated during storage.

*Noncohesive Foil*

- The manufacturer usually supplies the gold foils with an adsorbed protective gas film such as ammonia
- Ammonia reduces the adsorption of the less volatile substances and prevents the premature cohesion of the sheets
- The ammonia treated foil is called as *noncohesive foil*
- Noncohesive gold can also have adsorbed agents like iron salt or an acidic gas on its surface
- To restore the cohesive property of foil, it is heated or degassed to remove the volatile film
- E-Z Gold pellets are supplied with a wax coating which must be burned off before condensing

- Sometimes only noncohesive direct gold are required for certain procedures. This noncohesive gold is manufactured by permanently contaminating the surface with phosphorus and sulfur gases
- Noncohesive gold are used to build-up the bulk of a direct gold restoration.

**Gold Foil Cylinders**

- Type of gold foil formed by rolling cut segments of No. 4 foils into a desired width of 3.2 mm, 4.8 mm and 6.4 mm
- The desired width foil is rolled around No. 22 tapestry needle
- Alternately, No. 60 or No. 90 gold foils can also be used to form gold foil cylinders.

**Gold Foil Pellets**

- As 4 × 4 inch sheet of gold foil is too large to use it in restorative procedure. It is rolled into pellets of desired size before inserting into the prepared cavity
- Pellets of gold foil are generally rolled from 1/32, 1/64 or 1/128 sections cut from No. 4 sheet foil **(Fig. 20.4)**
- The book of foil is marked and cut into squares or rectangles
- Each piece of desired width is lightly rolled into pellet form
- Gold pellets are then stored in *gold foil boxes* which is divided into sections of various sizes.

**Preformed Gold Foils**

- Preformed gold foils are marketed in from of cylinders or ropes
- Both these preformed shaped foils are made from No. 4 foil that is *carbonized or corrugated*
- This form of gold was incidentally discovered during the *Great Chicago Fire* in 1871

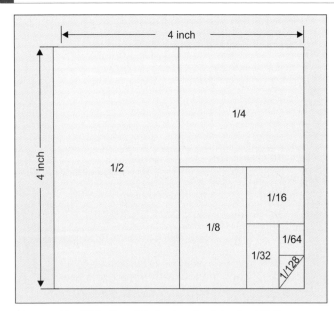

**Fig. 20.4:** Template for size of pellets of gold foil.

- Corrugated gold foil is obtained by burning gold foil between the sheets of paper in an airtight container
- This occurs because of shriveling of the paper in air tight safe
- After removing carbon, gold exhibit superior welding properties
- The preformed ropes and cylinders are cut into various lengths and sizes to restore the prepared cavity
- Preformed laminates are formed by placing number of sheets one over another and cutting them into desired size.

## Platinized Gold Foil

- This type of gold foil is a laminated structure
- It can be produced in either of the two ways:
  - Firstly, by sandwiching a layer of pure platinum foil between two No. 4 pure gold foils **(Fig. 20.5)**
  - Second, by bonding layers of platinum and gold together by *cladding process* during rolling operations before the hammering process
- This type of foil is available only in No. 4 sheet form
- Platinum increases hardness and wear resistance of the gold restorations
- It is recommended in stress bearing areas to provide improved mechanical properties to the gold foil restorations.

## Electrolytic Precipitates or Crystalline or Sponge Gold

- This type of direct filling gold (DFG) is available in the form of microcrystalline powder which is formed by electrolytic precipitation or atomization

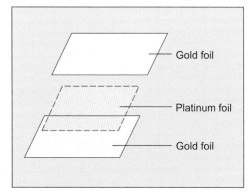

**Fig. 20.5:** Platinized gold foil.

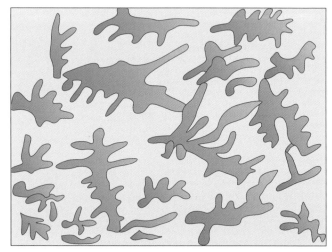

**Fig. 20.6:** Dendritic crystals of mat gold.

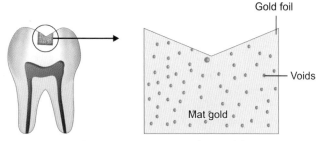

**Fig. 20.7:** Cross-section of mat gold.

- The gold powder is in the form of dendritic crystals of approximately 0.1 mm length formed into shapes by sintering at a raised temperature below the melting point of gold which is 1,063°C **(Fig. 20.6)**
- The process of sintering causes interdiffusion between particles which help to Coalesce or grow together
- Cross-section of mat gold restoration shows spread throughout the restoration without any areas of solid gold, i.e. mat gold restoration are veneered by gold foil to avoid porosities at the surface **(Fig. 20.7)**.

## Mat Gold

- It is a crystalline form of electrolytically precipitated gold which is sandwiched between sheets of gold foil
- They are supplied in the form of strips of desired sizes.

### Advantages

- It is used to build-up the internal bulk of the restoration
- It can be easily condensed and adapted to the retentive portions of the prepared cavity.

### Disadvantages

- Since, it is loosely packed it is friable and contain numerous void spaces between particles
- Inorder to avoid this, foil gold is recommended to be veneered on the external surface of the restorations
- This type of gold is not recommended on the external surface of the restorations because of its loosely packed crystalline form which does not cold weld into the solid mass as gold foil.

## Mat Foil

- Marketed since early 1960s
- It is sandwich of electrolytic precipitated gold powder between sheets of No. 3 gold foils
- Sandwich is sintered and cut into strips of different widths
- This was done to eliminate the need to veneer the restoration with a layer of foil
- This type of gold is not used nowadays.

### Advantage

The combined adaptability of mat gold with surface density of gold foil that was effective throughout the restoration.

### Disadvantage

Greater chances of voids which are observed as pits on the outer surface of the restoration.

## Alloyed Electrolytic Precipitate

- This form of direct filling fold is alloyed with calcium
- Calcium content in the finished product is 0.1%
- The alloy form is converted into mat form by sintering at raised temperature
- The process of sintering produces the product of greater initial density which can be more rapidly condensed into the prepared cavity

- It is capable of producing hardest surface of all DFG by *dispersion strengthening*
- Further hardness can be increased by adding elements such as palladium, platinum, indium and silver
- Electrolytic gold alloyed with calcium is referred to as *electralloy RV*.

### Advantages

- Easy to manipulate
- Higher density and can be rapidly condensed
- Greater hardness and superior mechanical properties.

### Disadvantages

- Can cause bridging if improperly stepped.
- May create over contouring during condensation.

## Powdered or Granular Gold

- This type of direct gold is available in the form of irregularly shaped, precondensed pellets or clumps of particles formed by comminution, chemical precipitation or atomization of the molten gold
- The average size of gold powder is 15 µm and the maximum size is 74 µm
- The gold powder particles are enclosed in No. 3 gold foil
- The atomized and chemically precipitated powders are mixed with soft wax to form pellets
- These wax gold pellets are then wrapped with No. 3 gold foil
- The pellets are cylindrical in shape and are available in several diameters and lengths
- Cross-section of the granular gold shows voids which are spread throughout the restorations with thin strips of solid gold corresponding to gold foil found in between the restoration. Therefore, as with mat gold, powdered gold restorations should also be veneered with gold foil at the surface and at the margins **(Fig. 20.8)**

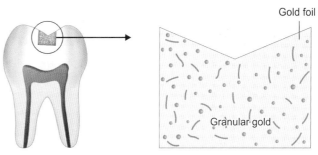

**Fig. 20.8:** Cross-section of granular gold.

### Advantages

- Upon condensation spreads laterally from its point of impact; important for early stages of condensation
- Overlaying with gold foil is recommended.

### Goldent

- Type of granular gold introduced in early 1960s
- The individual granules averaging 15 μm are produced into the masses of irregular shapes of 1–3 mm
- They are lightly precondensed to improve its handling
- The masses are enclosed in envelope of foil for better handling during condensation
- It consists of 95% powder and 5% foil
- It does not require veneering
- Compacting property can be further improved by mixing granules with spherical atomized particles.

### Stopfgold

- Produced from chemically precipitated gold powder, which is subjected to milling process after precipitation
- The individual particles are loosely sintered together and cut into strips
- Thickness available 0.7 mm, 1–1.5 mm
- High luster due to reflection by the flat particles
- It has lesser porosity and thus gives better cold welding ability
- It has much improved shear strength.

### E-Z Gold

- Marketed as Williams E-Z Gold (Ivoclar—Williams, Amherst, NY)
- Formed by combination of chemical precipitation and atomization
- Average particle size is 15 mm
- The atomized particles are mixed with wax and wrapped in No. 3 and No. 4 foil and cut into desired sizes
- Has property of inertness and permanence
- Has improved softness and working characteristics.

## STORAGE OF DIRECT FILLING GOLD

Direct filling gold (DFG) are stored in gold foil boxes which are having compartments of various sizes **(Fig. 20.9)**. To prevent contamination from other sources, damp cotton dipped in 18% ammonia is placed in each compartment of the box. This makes the gold foil noncohesive and prevents oxides forming on the surface of gold. Ammonia treated gold is readily used after degassing it.

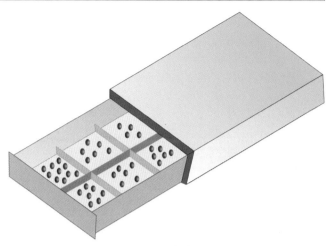

**Fig. 20.9:** Gold foil box.

## DESORPTION OR DEGASSING

It is a process of heating the foil or pellet immediately before carrying into the prepared cavity in order to remove volatile protective coating is called *degassing*. The process is also called as *desorption, annealing or heat treatment*. The term annealing should be avoided as it is a misnomer.

### Objectives of Degassing

- To remove adsorbed ammonia gas and other surface impurities from the surface to make it cohesive
- To prevent the surface from getting contaminated until complete cohesion occurs.

### Methods of Degassing

#### Piece Method

- A single piece is degassed at a time
- It is usually accomplished by using a simple alcohol lamp and a gold foil carrier
- It is most practical method of degassing regardless of the type of DFG used
- Acetone free alcohol should be used for this purpose.

##### Advantages
- Wastage of foil is avoided as only required amount is used
- Desired size pellet can be selected for use
- Chances of contamination between degassing and its use is eliminated.

*Disadvantage:* Technique sensitive.

*Bulk Method*

- It is degassing of several gold pellets at the same time
- It is accomplished by using electric or gas source of heat.

*Advantage:* Convenient and requires lesser time for the restoration.

*Disadvantages*
- Accidental movement during heating can cause sticking of the pellets to each other
- Chances of overheating
- Greater wastage of unused gold
- Inability to select desired piece of gold that fits into the prepared cavity.

## METHODS OF DEGASSING OR DESORPTION

*Degassing or desorption can be done in either of the three ways*:
1. By an open alcohol flame
2. Mica over a flame
3. Electrical degassing.

### By an Open Alcohol Flame

- Each individual pellet is picked up and is heated directly over the open flame before compacting into the prepared cavity
- The pellet is held over the flame for *3–5 seconds over the middle zone* of the flame or the high energy reducing zone [blue zone **(Fig. 20.10)**]
- Desorption is said to be complete when gold pellet shows *dull red glow*
- Fuel which is used for the flame can be alcohol or gas, but acetone free *alcohol* is usually preferred, as there is less chance of contamination.

- Alcohol should be pure methanol/ethanol without any additives or colorants
- Denatured alcohol may be used if the other denaturant available is methanol
- Only E-Z gold pellet is heated ½ to 1 inch *above* the ethanol flame until a bright flame occurs and the pellet turns *dull red* for 2–3 seconds.

### Precautions

- Lamp should be free of waxes and other surface contaminants
- Wick should be trimmed to produce—teardrop shaped clear light blue flame of ¾ inch in height
- Overheating or underheating should be avoided
- Overheating leads to direct gold becoming more stiff, less ductile and difficult to condense
- Underheating leads to partial cohesiveness and peeling away of the adjacent layers.

### Advantages

- Desired size gold to be condensed are only selected for desorption
- Chances of contamination is less
- Wastage of gold is avoided.

### Mica over a Flame

- Sheet of mica is held over any type of flame **(Fig. 20.11)**
- The surface of the mica sheet is divided into several areas
- These areas indicate the time the piece of gold is held over the mica sheet
- Maximum time of 5 minutes is allowed for gold to be heated over mica.

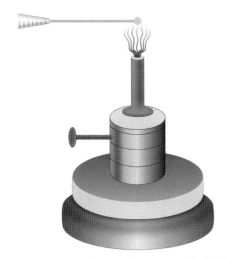

**Fig. 20.10:** Gold pellet degassed using open alcohol flame.

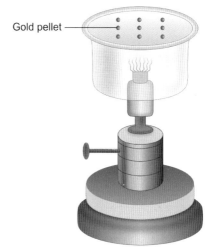

Gold pellet

**Fig. 20.11:** Mica tray mounted over alcohol lamp for degassing.

- Care should be taken to hold the gold pieces with stainless steel wire points or similar instruments that will not contaminate it
- Incomplete tray desorption can occur because of nonuniform air current, heating excessive amount of gold, excessive sintering, adhesion of pellets and exposure to contamination.

### Electrical Degassing

- It is the most controlled and standardized way of degassing **(Fig. 20.12)**
- It consists of a heating compartment area which is made of aluminum
- An electric heater controls the time and temperature of heating
- Surface of heater is divided into small compartments, each of which accommodates a gold piece
- This eliminates the chances of cohesion before placement into the prepared cavity
- Maximum of 5 minutes are allowed for heating in the electric decontaminator.

#### *Advantages*

- Electric heater controls the time and the temperature
- Allows the operator to work alone.

#### *Disadvantage*

800°F may not be high enough for powdered gold which require a temperature of 900–1200°F.

## HAZARDS OF OVERHEATING OF DIRECT FILLING GOLD MATERIALS AND THEIR REMEDY

- Overheating causes the gold to become stiffer, less ductile and more difficult to compact
- Overheating can cause recrystallization and grain growth time which can severely hamper the mechanical properties of the material. Therefore, minimum time and temperature should be used for degassing
- It can cause incorporation of impurities from the surrounding atmosphere. This can be avoided by degassing in polluted atmosphere and by controlling time and temperature of degassing
- Overheating can cause over sintered situation resulting in the adherence of the entire mass of the particles. It can be avoided by using controlled time and temperature of heating sintered gold

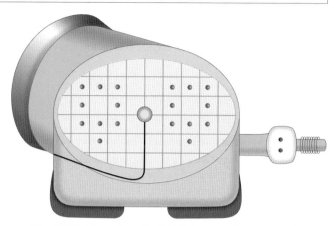

**Fig. 20.12:** Degassing of gold foil done on electric annealer.

- Overheating can cause complete melting of the gold surface making the gold completely noncohesive
- During bulk degassing, pieces of gold may adhere to each other before inserting them into the prepared cavity. This can be prevented if gold pellets are heated in separate compartments on the mica sheet.

## UNDERHEATING OF DIRECT FILLING GOLD

- Incomplete removal of protective gases—causing it to be partially cohesive
- Can cause pitting and porosity in the final restoration.

## CONDENSATION OR COMPACTION OF DIRECT FILLING GOLD

*Compaction is defined as* "the process of increasing the density of the metal foils, pellets or powder through compressive pressure".

*Cold welding:* It is a process of forming atomic bonds between pellets, segments or layers as a result of condensation.

*Wedging:* It "refers to the pressurized adaptation of the gold form within the space between the tooth structure walls or corners that have been slightly deformed elastically".

#### *Objectives of Compaction of DFG*

- To wedge initial pieces of gold into the retention points created in the prepared cavity
- To cold weld the pieces of gold together by complete cohesion

- To closely adapt the gold to the margins and walls of the prepared cavity. It improves retention, reduces microleakage and secondary caries
- To minimize voids in general and to eliminate them from critical areas like margins and surfaces so that uniform compactness is achieved
- Strain hardening of gold material by cold working during condensation. This enhances the mechanical properties of the material
- To develop strength within the restoration.

## PRINCIPLES OF CONDENSATION

- *Line of force:* It is that direction through which the force is exerted by the condenser. The line of force should be directed at an angle of 45° to cavity walls and floors, i.e. the condenser point should bisect line angles and trisect point angles formed by the cavity walls. This ensures maximum adaptation of gold against the walls, floors and minimum irritation to the pulp-dentin complex **(Fig. 20.13)**
- *Forces of condensation* should be directed at an angle of 90° to previously condensed material. This prevents any shear forces to develop which may displace already condensed gold pieces **(Fig. 20.14)**
- Minimal thickness of gold pellet should be condensed as it easier to achieve the objectives of condensation. At the same time, the pellet should be thick enough so that condenser tip does not penetrate it
- Condensation should always start at a point on one side and proceed in a straight line to another point on the opposite side then back to the original side on a different straight line. This ensures that the condenser has covered the entire surface of that piece of gold. It should overlap at least ¼ of the previously condensed area. This

process is called as *"stepping"*. Stepping ensures dense restoration, minimal voids and maximal adaptation of gold into the prepared cavity **(Fig. 20.15)**
- *Energy of condensation* should be dissipated. Condensation energy can be increased by increasing the frequency or the amplitude of the condensing instrument or by reducing the size of the face of the condenser
- Pieces of direct gold should be condensed from the *center of the increment to the periphery* or from one periphery of the increment to the other. The former method of condensation minimizes entrapment of air bubbles on the surface of the final restoration
- Precipitated type of direct gold should be hand condensed.

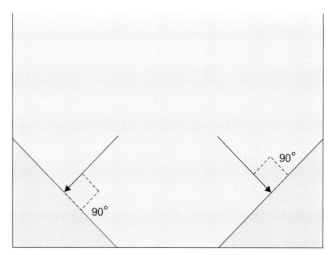

**Fig. 20.14:** Forces of condensation should be directed at an angle of 90° to previously condensed gold.

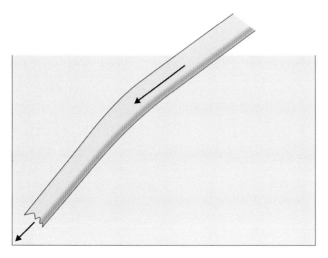

**Fig. 20.13:** Line of force.

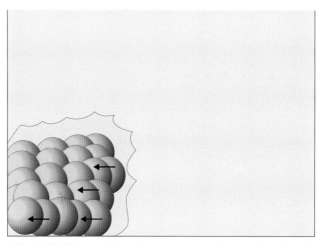

**Fig. 20.15:** Process of stepping to ensure maximum adaptation of gold to the cavity walls.

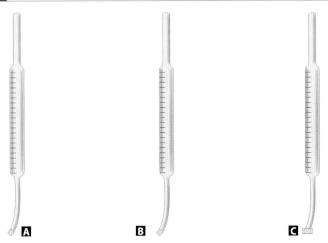

**Figs. 20.16A to C:** Types of condensers: (A) Round condenser; (B) Parallelogram condenser; (C) Foot condenser.

## TYPES OF GOLD CONDENSERS

### Classification of Gold Condensers

- *Based on the shape of the condensers (**Figs. 20.16A to C**):*
  - Round condensers
  - Parallelogram and hatchet condensers
  - Foot condensers.
- *Based on the surface of the tip of the condenser:*
  - Smooth surface
  - Serrated surface.
- *Based on the type of tip of the condenser:*
  - Flat faced
  - Convex faced.
- *Based on the type of shank of the condenser:*
  - Straight
  - Monoangled
  - Offset.
- *Based on different shapes, gold condensers are of following types:*
  - *Round condensers (Bayonet condenser):* This type of condenser is mainly used to begin direct gold restorations and to establish *ties* in the inner parts of restorations. They are 0.4–0.55 mm in diameter
  - *Parallelogram and hatchet condensers:* They are used for initial condensation and to form bulk of the restorations. They are useful only for hand pressure compaction and have nib faces that measure 0.5–1 mm in diameter
  - *Varnley foot condensors:* These condensers are mainly used for cavosurface condensation and surface hardening of the restoration. They are also employed for bulk built up of the gold restorations. The nib face is rectangular in shape and has diameter of 1–1.3 mm.

### Common Features of Gold Condensers

All gold condensers have pyramidal serrations on the nib faces. *This type of configuration serves following functions:*
- They prevent slipping on the gold
- They increase the surface area of the condenser face
- Creates lateral force to properly condense the pieces of gold by acting as swaggers
- They make triangular indentations on the condensed piece of gold, such that succeeding increment interlocks into these indentations.

*Condenser for mechanical condensation are provided in Condensers different shapes for contra-angle or straight handpiece:*
- They can be monoangled, binangled or bayonet shanked or no angled.
- The smaller the nib face size—the greater the pounds/sq inch.

## GENERAL STEPS FOR INSERTION OF DIRECT FILLING GOLD RESTORATION IN A PREPARED CAVITY

### Buildup for the Restoration

#### Tie-formation (Fig. 20.17)

First step involves connecting two opposing point angles or starting points filled with gold with a transverse bar of gold. It forms the foundation for any restoration of direct gold.

#### Banking of Walls (Fig. 20.18)

It is covering each wall from its floor or axial wall to the cavosurface margin with direct gold foil or material.

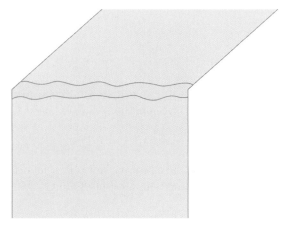

**Fig. 20.17:** Tie-formation.

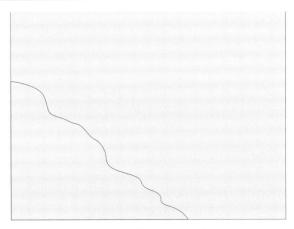

**Fig. 20.18:** Banking of walls.

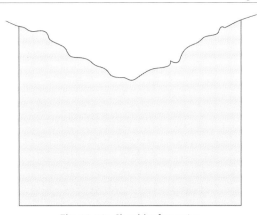

**Fig. 20.19:** Shoulder formation.

### *Shoulder Formation (Fig. 20.19)*

To complete the buildup, it is important to connect two opposing walls with DFG material. The buildup should continue until the preparation is overfilled.

### Paving of the Restoration

Cohesive gold foil should be used to cover the entire surface of restoration. Foot condenser is useful for this procedure.

### Surface Hardening of the Restoration

The surface gold should be strain hardened by utilizing highest condensation energy in all directions.

### Burnishing

Burnishing is accomplished by moving the burnisher from gold to the tooth surface. It helps in providing better adaptation of the material at the margins by eliminating the surface and marginal voids and improves the surface hardening.

### Margination

Excess gold is removed in small increments from the margins using a sharp instrument. This procedure is done to visualize the original outline of the prepared cavity. It follows margination to close any marginal discrepancies and to strain harden the surface of the restoration.

### Contouring

Contouring is accomplished by using knifes, files or finishing burs to create proper anatomy of the restoration to coincide with that of the tooth.

### Finishing and Polishing

Finishing is done using tin oxide powder on soft bristle brushes or rubber cups. Satin finish is preferred over high gloss finish as it gives better esthetics because reflection of light is reduced.

### Final Burnishing

It is done to close any marginal voids and other surface discrepancies.

## TECHNIQUE FOR COMPACTING DIRECT FILLING GOLD

- Compaction of DFG is done by using hand pressure alone, by hand pressure with mallet or by using mechanical condenser activated by spring, pneumatic pressure or electromallet
- Factors which influence the quality of gold restorations are amount of condensation pressure applied, direction of force and pattern of compaction
- Condensers are basically designed to direct the forces of compaction to DFG
- The process of compaction starts when a piece of gold is placed in a prepared cavity and is initially pressed by hand
- Then an appropriate size condenser is used to begin malleting in the center of mass
- Each succeeding step of the condenser overlaps (by half) the previous one as the condenser is moved toward the periphery of the cavity
- Gold is compacted as it moves under the nib face of the condenser. Most effective compaction occurs directly under nib face
- Compaction can also occur by lateral movement of the piece of gold against the surrounding walls

- The process of compaction helps in condensing gold at the point angles and line angles, in removing voids within each increment and in retaining succeeding increment in already condensed direct gold
- Porosity or voids are likely to occur in all types of direct gold restorations
- Each type of gold requires modification in technique to minimize porosities in the restoration
- Gold foil and electrolytic gold are compacted by using direct thrust from hand followed by use of mallet
- Powdered gold is best compacted by using heavy hand pressure with slight rocking movement along with direct thrusts
- Mechanical condensers can also be used as they provide consistent force
- Electromallet is an acceptable condenser if manufacturer's instructions are followed properly.

## MECHANICAL CONSIDERATIONS IN DIRECT FILLING GOLD

- Pure cohesive gold foils when used alone provide the strongest and hardest of all the other forms of direct gold. This is because they have fewer voids, fewer foreign bodies and lesser number of component ingredients.
- The smaller the size of the increments during condensation, the stronger will be the final restoration.
- The greater the resistance to condensation, the harder and stronger will be the restoration
- The smaller the size of condenser, the better will be the resulting mechanical properties of the restoration—due to the high energy dissipated by smaller condensers
- Combination of different materials is used to produce stronger and denser restoration. Like the bulk of the restoration is done using precipitated gold and the remainder is veneered using cohesive gold foil
- In general DFG's do not possess high strength and hardness as compared to cast restorations
- They cannot be used in large stress bearing areas such as cast crown
- They are primarily used to restore small class I restorations, pits, for repair of casting margins and small class III and class V restorations.

## BIOLOGICAL CONSIDERATIONS OF DIRECT FILLING GOLD

The direct gold restorations can sometimes irritate the pulp—dentin organ. The causes are:
- If the condensation forces are not directed at 45° angle to the axial walls and pulpal floor. They will be dissipated to the vital dental tissues and may lead to irritation of the pulp
- If the gold pellets are subjected to greater amount of heat required for degassing, this heat will be transmitted to the dentin pulp organ
- The frictional heat builtup during finishing and polishing procedure can irritate dentin pulp organ.

## PROPERTIES OF COMPACTED GOLD (TABLE 20.1)

### Strength

Greatest strength of DFG is achieved when the resulting compacted gold is dense and homogeneous. If it is porous, having voids it has least strength as gold is not closely compacted. In DFG, failure occurs from tensile stress because of incomplete cohesion. Thus, transverse strength is an indirect measure of cohesion.

### Hardness

Hardness indicates overall quality of compacted gold. Presence of voids or porosity indicates low hardness of the compacted gold.

### Density

Density of pure gold is 19.3 g/cm$^3$. Although DFG restorations are characterized by nonuniform density as porosities are likely to occur in all direct gold restorations. Pure density of gold in never achieved in the direct gold restorations regardless of the form of gold or technique used.

### Voids

Presence of voids in the restorations increases its susceptibility to corrosion and plaque accumulation. It may further lead to gross leakage and secondary caries. Factors

| Table 20.1: Physical properties of direct filling golds. | | | |
|---|---|---|---|
| Type of material | Strength | Hardness | Density |
| Gold foil | 265–296 MPa | 69 KHN | 15.8–15.9 g/cm$^3$ |
| Mat gold | 161–169 MPa | 52–62 KHN | 14.3–14.7 g/cm$^3$ |
| Powdered gold | 155–190 MPa | 55–64 KHN | 14.4–14.9 g/cm$^3$ |
| Mat/gold foil | 196–227 MPa | 70–79 KHN | 15.0–15.1 g/cm$^3$ |

which influence voids in direct gold restorations are—skill of the dentist, size and shape of the condenser tip and the compacting technique.

The physical properties of direct gold restorations is greatly influenced by the skill of the clinician in manipulating and compacting gold in prepared cavity.

## DECLINE IN DIRECT GOLD RESTORATIONS

- In spite of many favorable properties, the placement of gold foil restorations is at decline, both in the university-based practice and in private practice globally
- Gerald D Stibbs (1987), critically evaluated the reasons for this decline

– Lack of emphasis of direct gold restoration in dental curriculum
– Lack of trained staff in direct gold restorations
– Change in overall attitude to settle for less than the best restoration.

Tooth colored restorative material with both optical and physical properties similar to that of tooth structure is the current emphasis of research. The metallic restorations including DFG definitely cannot satisfy the esthetic demands of the patients. However, there is no cost-effective esthetic material that can last functionally and durably as DFG for small lesions. Hence, when indicated for selected posterior teeth where the esthetic demand is not critical, DFG is an ideal material.

## TEST YOURSELF

### Essay Questions

1. Classify direct filling gold (DFG). Discuss in detail gold foil.
2. What are direct filling gold? Write indication and contraindications of DFG. Describe the compaction of DFG in detail.
3. Write properties of DFG which makes it unique. Discuss the method of degassing procedure of DFG.

### Short Notes

1. Cohesive gold.
2. Noncohesive gold.
3. Sponge gold.
4. Mat gold.
5. Mat foil.
6. Annealing of gold.
7. Crystalline gold.
8. Compaction of gold.
9. Powdered gold.

### Multiple Choice Questions

1. Which of the following is not a part of direct filling gold procedure?
   A. Condensing each piece of foil with 10–15 pounds of force
   B. Using cement to weld each increment to the next one
   C. Isolating the tooth with rubber dam
   D. Dipping each piece of gold in alcohol to improve cohesion
2. It is common to use more than one type of direct filling gold to restore a cavity because:
   A. Some are manufactured with less density as bulk filling materials only

B. Smoothness is increased when dense foils are used on the surface
C. Only alloys with calcium can be used in the final layer for optimal hardness
D. It is not possible to actually condense certain materials in the base of the cavities

### ANSWERS

1. B and D        2. A and B

### BIBLIOGRAPHY

1. Anusavice KJ. Direct-filling gold. Phillip's Science of Dental Materials, 11th edition. St. Louis, Missouri: Saunders; 2003.
2. Birkett GH. Is there a future for gold foil? Oper Dent. 1995;20:41.
3. Charbeneau GT. The direct filling gold restorations. Principles and Practice of Operative Dentistry, 3rd edition. Philadelphia: Lea and Febiger; 1975.
4. Hodson JT. Structure and properties of gold foil and mat gold. J Dent Res. 1963;101:78-83.
5. Johansson G, Bergman M, Anneroth G, et al. Human pulpal response to direct filling gold restorations. Scand J Dent Res. 1993;101:78-83.
6. Lambert RL. Stopfgold: a new direct filling gold. Oper Dent. 1994;19:16-9.
7. Ritcher WA, Cantwell KR. A study of cohesive gold. J Prosthet Dent. 1965;15:722-731.
8. Roberson TM, Heymann HO, Swift ED. Sturdevant's Art and science of operative dentistry. A contemporary approach, 5th edition. St. Louis: Mosby, 2006.
9. Thomas JJ, Stanley HR, Gilmore HW. Effects of gold foil condensation on human dental pulp. J Am Dent Assoc. 1969;78:788-94.
10. Waikakul A, Punwutikorn J. Clinical study of retrograde filling with gold leaf: comparison with amalgam. Oral Surg Oral Med Oral Pathol. 1991;71:228-31.

# Section 6

## Indirect Restorative Materials

# Dental Ceramics

ADA Specification No. 69; ISO Specification No. 6872:2015

*'Take up one idea. Make that one idea your life, think of it, dream of it, live on that idea.'*
*—Swami Vivekanand*

## INTRODUCTION

Dental ceramics are currently the most sought after restorative and prosthetic materials because they are best able to mimic the appearance of the natural teeth, have long-term color stability, wear resistance and excellent biocompatibility. However, despite having excellent esthetics, they are susceptible to fracture under tensile or flexural loading as they are brittle in nature. Several desirable properties of dental ceramics such as low-fusing temperature, high viscosity and resistance to devitrification are obtained by adding oxides to the basic structure. Broadly ceramics can be classified as:

- *Silicate ceramics*: Comprise of amorphous glass phase with porous structure, e.g. dental porcelain
- *Oxide ceramics*: Consist of principal crystalline phase with either no or small glass phase. Partially stabilized zirconia ($ZrO_2$) used widely because of its high-fracture toughness
- *Nonoxide ceramics*: Not used in dentistry
- *Glass ceramics*: Used in high-esthetic areas but has low-fracture toughness.

Different types of ceramics are made suitable to be used in dentistry by precisely controlling the amount and type of components used in its manufacturing.

## DEFINITION

Dental ceramics are inorganic compound with nonmetallic properties typically consisting of oxygen and one or more metallic or semimetallic elements that are formulated to produce whole or part of a ceramic-based dental prosthesis.

The term ceramic is derived from the Greek term "*Keramos*", which means "*A Potter or Pottery*".

## EVOLUTION

Right from the Stone Age, some 10,000 years ago, ceramics have been important material to mankind. Around 700 BC, Etruscans used ivory and bone to make teeth, which were held by gold framework **(Fig. 21.1)**. Even human teeth were used to replace missing teeth for many years.

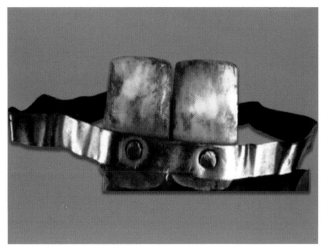

**Fig. 21.1:** Etruscans used ivory teeth held by gold framework.

- *400–900 AD:* Mayan civilization—first evidence of milled plugs (inlays) of jade for esthetic purposes
- *1728: Pierre Fauchard,* known as father of modern dentistry suggested the use of porcelain in dentistry
- *1789: Duchateau* (French pharmacist) and *De Chemant* (French dentist)—patented the first porcelain tooth material
- *1808: Fonzi* an Italian dentist—introduced the *terrometallic porcelain tooth* that was held in place by platinum pin or frame
- *1817: Planteau*, a French dentist—first introduced porcelain teeth in United States
- *1822: Peale,* an artist *developed* baking process for porcelain teeth in Philadelphia
- *1837: Ash* developed improved version of porcelain tooth material
- *1844: SS White Company* was established, which manufactured porcelain denture teeth on large scale
- *1851: John Allen* patented "Continuous Gum Teeth" prosthesis, which consisted of two to three porcelain teeth fused to small block of gum-colored porcelain
- *1885: Logan* fused porcelain to platinum post and called it as Richmond crown
- *1900–1905:* Introduction of first electric porcelain furnace
- *1903: Dr Charles Land* fabricated first ceramic crown using platinum foil matrix and high-fusing feldspathic porcelain
- *1933: Brodsky* reported first manufactured refractory material for dental use (German-Brillat)
- *1955: Buonocore* reported method of chemically etching enamel
- *1959: Morrison and Warnick* reported findings of ethyl silicate refractory material for dental use
- *1962: Weinstein and Weinstein*—introduced porcelain fused to metal restorations
- *1963: Vita Zahnfabrik*—first development of commercial porcelain
- *1965: McLean and Hughes*—improved the fracture resistance by introducing aluminous porcelain
- *1968: MacCulloch* first proposed the application of glass ceramics
- *1971: Francois Duret* first to consider the automatic production for dental restorations [computer-aided design and computer-aided manufacturing (CAD-CAM) technique]
- *1980: Mormann* and *Brandestini* developed chairside CAD-CAM system for machining dental porcelain (CEREC)
- *1983: Sozio* and *Riley* developed the Cerestore injection-molded core

- *1984: Adair and Grossman*—first introduced the castable glass ceramic (Dicor)
- *1989:* Alceram a replacement for Cerestore was introduced
- *1990:* Wohlwend and Scharer reported on a technique for pressed glass restorations (Empress)
- *1992:* Duceram LFC (low-fusing ceramic) was marketed
- *1996:* Techceram commercial introduction of thermal spray technique into dentistry
- *2005:* CEREC 3 system was first introduced in the market **(Fig. 21.2)**.

## GENERAL PROPERTIES

- Dental ceramics are nonmetallic, inorganic structures containing oxides of one or more metallic or semimetallic elements
- They are brittle in nature and can fracture on flexion
- Exhibit excellent biocompatibility
- Ceramics are highly resistant to corrosion
- Exhibit high-temperature stability in oxygen-free environment
- Has high modulus of elasticity
- Do not react with most liquids, acids, alkalis and gases. Ceramics are usually chemically inert
- Exhibit high-fracture toughness and hardness. $ZrO_2$-based ceramics have flexural strength similar to that of steel but their fracture toughness is much lower than that of steel
- Has high-wear resistance
- Exhibit excellent long-term color stability
- Have ability to form into precise shape

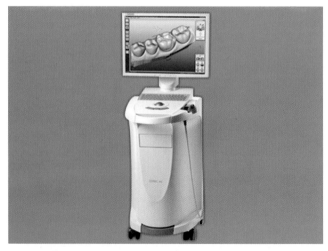

**Fig. 21.2:** CEREC 3 system first introduced in 1980.

- Has high potential for matching natural tooth
- Exhibit low-thermal conductivity, thermal diffusivity and electrical conductivity
- Low-fusing feldspathic porcelain has firing shrinkage of 14% and high-fusing porcelain has shrinkage of 11.5%.

## BASIC STRUCTURE

Most of the dental ceramics contain a crystal phase and silicate glass matrix phase. Basic structure of all silicate structures is silicon-oxygen tetrahedron $(SiO_4)^{4-}$ chains, which consists of two oxygen atoms for each silicon atom. It has central silicon cation $(Si^{4+})$, which is covalently bonded by four oxygen anions located at the corners of the regular tetrahedron **(Fig. 21.3)**. In cases of feldspathic porcelain alkali ions such potassium or sodium ions are positioned so that they can bond to electrons from unbalanced oxygen ions. In this situation, these ions tend to disrupt silicate chains and increase the thermal expansion of the glass. The coefficient of thermal expansion can be further increased by adding crystalline particles such as tetragonal leucite $(K_2O. Al_2O_3.4SiO_2)$. Only dental ceramic in which the crystal phase is made of sanidine is the VITABLOCS MarkII. *Sanidine* is a potassium aluminosilicate phase $(KAlSi_3O_8)$, which mostly exists at high temperature but can also be retained on cooling as monoclinic crystals. The glass matrix in these ceramic can be either potash or soda feldspar $(KAlSi_3O_8$ or $NaAlSi_3O_8)$.

### Classification of Dental Ceramics

*According to type:*
- Feldspathic porcelain
- Aluminous porcelain
- Leucite-reinforced ceramic

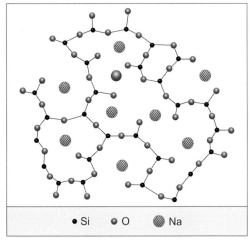

**Fig. 21.3:** Diagram representing structure of silicate glass.

- Lithia-based glass ceramic
- Glass-infiltrated alumina
- Glass-infiltrated spinel
- Glass-infiltrated $ZrO_2$
- Glass ceramic.

*According to use:*
- Anterior crowns
- Posterior crowns
- Veneers
- Porcelain denture teeth
- Ceramic inlays or onlays
- Metal ceramic
- Stain and glaze ceramic
- Fixed partial dentures (FPDs).

*According to processing methods:*
- Sintered porcelain
- Partial sintering and glass infiltration
- Castable porcelain
- Machined porcelain
- Infiltrated porcelain
- Pressed porcelain
- CAD-CAM
- Copy milling.

*According to firing technique:*
- Air fired (at atmospheric pressure)
- Vacuum fired (at reduced pressure)
- Diffusible gas firing.

*According to firing temperature:*
- High fusing—1,300°C
- Medium fusing—1,101–1,300°C
- Low fusing—850–1,100°C
- Ultra-low fusing—less than 850°C.

*According to substrate material:*
- Cast metal
- Sintered metal
- Swaged metal
- Glass ceramic
- CAD/CAM.

*According to microstructure:*
- Glass
- Crystalline
- Crystal-containing glass.

*According to translucency:*
- Opaque
- Translucent
- Transparent.

# MANUFACTURE OF PORCELAIN

Dental porcelain is manufactured by heating ingredients (quartz, feldspar and other oxides) at high temperature to form a glassy mass, which is then rapidly quenched in water to fracture this glassy mass. This process is called as *Fritting* and the resulting product is called as *Frit*. The frit products are ball milled into desired particle size and pigments are added to provide desired shade to porcelain. As fritting takes place at much higher temperature than that used during fabrication of the restoration, much of the chemical reaction (pyrochemical reaction) already occurs between the ingredients before they are used in the laboratory. Dental porcelain is usually supplied by manufacturer in the form of powder of different shades.

## Composition

Basic composition of porcelain varies with its different types:

### High-fusing Porcelain

- Feldspar (60–80%)—basic glass former
- Kaolin (4–5%)—binder
- Quartz (15–25%)—filler
- Alumina (8–20%)—glass former and flux
- Oxides of Na, K, Ca (9–15%)—fluxes (glass modifier)
- Metallic pigments—1%—color matching.

### Feldspar

- Potassium and sodium feldspar are naturally occurring mineral consisting mainly of potash ($K_2O$) and soda ($Na_2O$)
- They also contain alumina ($Al_2O_3$) and silica ($SiO_2$) particles
- Potassium feldspar when mixed with metal oxides and fired at high temperature, it undergoes incongruent melting and forms crystals of leucite in a glass phase, which softens and has tendency to flow slightly
- Softening of glass phase during firing results in coalesce of powder particles to form a dense mass
- This process of coalesce of powder particles is called as *Liquid Phase Sintering*
- Feldspar when melted at high temperature forms crystalline mineral leucite
- Leucite is a potassium-aluminum-silicate mineral, which has high coefficient of thermal expansion (20–25 ppm/°C) as compared to that of feldspar glasses (10 ppm/°C)
- Crystals of leucite are formed when feldspar is heated between 1,150°C and 1,530°C by process called as *Incongruent Melting*.

### Kaolin/Clay ($Al_2O_3.2SiO_2.2H_2O$)

- It is hydrated aluminum silicate, which acts as binder
- It is present in the concentration of 4–5%
- Helps in forming a sticky mass with water, which allows unfired porcelain to be easily molded
- It provides opacity and rigidity to the mass
- It is primarily used for formulations of high-fusing porcelain and ceramic denture teeth.

### Pure quartz

- Pure quartz crystals are ground to finest grain size
- Silica is mixed to give stability to the mass during heating
- It also provides a framework for other ingredients
- It is present in concentration of 13–14% and provides strength, translucency and firmness
- Silica forms the matrix phase of feldspathic porcelain
- It exists in four forms—(1) crystalline quartz, (2) crystalline cristobalite, (3) crystalline tridymite and (4) noncrystalline fused form
- Fused silica has high-melting temperature because of three-dimensional network of covalent bonds between silica tetrahedral.

### Alumina

- Dental ceramics form binary compounds of metallic and nonmetallic elements such as alumina or $ZrO_2$ by bonding of metals
- They release valence electrons and share with the nonmetals to enhance bonding
- The free-surface energy of positive metal ions should be lower than that of negative nonmetal ions in order to attract other nonmetallic ions
- These are used as stabilizers and can also be added as crack blockers or toughening crystals
- $ZrO_2$ possesses high-fracture toughness. Although, they are not used in pure form because cracks appear during sintering as a result of transformation from tetragonal to monoclinic phase
- This transformation is disrupted by adding certain oxides of magnesium oxide (MgO), yttria ($Y_2O_3$), calcium oxide (CaO) or CeO
- Current $ZrO_2$-based ceramic is based on tetragonal $ZrO_2$ particles (TZP), which are completely stabilized by $Y_2O_3$
- Sometimes to prevent leaching of $Y_2O_3$, 0.25% of $Al_2O_3$ can be added

- Commonly used crystal phase in ceramics include—leucite, lithia disilicate, alumina, alumina and $ZrO_2$ combination, $ZrO_2$ and apatite.

### Medium- and Low-fusing Porcelain

The low- and medium-fusing porcelain powders are essentially glasses, which have been ground from blocks of matured porcelain. They are manufactured by the process called as *Fritting* and the resultant products are called as *Frits*. The basic ingredients are same as high-fusing porcelains, but certain balancing oxides are additionally added.

*Glass modifiers*
- Act as fluxes and help in reducing the softening temperature of glass and increase flow of porcelain during firing
- The most commonly used glass modifiers are potassium, sodium and calcium oxides
- Other oxides added may be lithium oxide, MgO, phosphorous pentoxide, etc.

*Intermediate oxides*
- For example, $Al_2O_3$
- It increases viscosity at low-firing temperatures.

### CLINICAL SIGNIFICANCE
Glass modifiers not only lower the softening temperature but also reduce the viscosity of the glass, which causes slumping or pyroclastic flow during firing.

*Boric oxide*
- It reduces the softening temperature and increases flow
- It is a glass modifier and a glass former.

*Coloring agents*
- They are metallic oxides, which are added to give various shades
- These coloring agents are manufactured by fusing metallic oxides with feldspar and fine glass and then subjecting to fritting process
- They are added to unpigmented porcelain powder to obtain the desired shade and color
- Some examples of coloring agents are given below **(Table 21.1)**.

*Opacifying agents*
- Translucency of porcelain is reduced by adding opacifying agents
- Zirconium oxide is the most commonly used opacifier
- Other opacifying agents are cerium oxide ($Ce_2O_3$), titanium oxide, tin oxide.

### Indications of Porcelain (Table 21.2)

- Single crowns made of all ceramic, porcelain jacket crowns, porcelain fused to metal or castable glass ceramics
- Anterior and posterior FPDs
- Porcelain laminates veneers
- Porcelain denture teeth
- Ceramic inlays and onlays
- Ceramic brackets used in orthodontics
- Prefabricated labial veneers for natural teeth.

### Contraindications

- Long-span FPDs in posterior region
- Patient with parafunctional habits such as bruxism
- When esthetics is not critical
- When patient cannot afford.

### Advantages

- Excellent esthetics
- High strength when bonded to tooth structure
- Does not stain
- Has high-compressive strength
- Low-thermal conductivity and thermal expansion
- Biocompatible
- Higher abrasive resistance than tooth enamel.

### Disadvantages

- Brittle and fragile
- Technique sensitive
- Costlier
- Need special and costly laboratory equipment
- Can abrade opposing natural tooth.

## METAL CERAMIC PROSTHESIS

Also called as porcelain fused to metal, porcelain bonded to metal, porcelain to metal and ceramometal restorations.

Metal ceramic prosthesis combines the esthetic property of ceramic with the strength and accuracy of cast metal. It consists of a metal coping, which fits over the prepared tooth

**Table 21.1:** Coloring agents.

| Metallic oxide | Color |
|---|---|
| Cobalt oxide | Bluish color |
| Copper oxide | Green |
| Titanium oxide | Yellowish-brown |
| Manganese oxide | Lavender |
| Iron oxide | Brown shade |

**Table 21.2:** Indications and contraindications of various dental ceramics.

| Type of ceramic | Indications | Contraindications |
|---|---|---|
| Feldspathic porcelain | • Anterior laminate veneer<br>• Metal ceramic veneers | • Patient with parafunctional habits such as bruxism<br>• Inlays, onlays, crowns and bridges |
| Aluminous porcelain | • Core ceramic for anterior crowns | • Patient with parafunctional habits<br>• Fixed partial dentures<br>• Crowns on molar tooth |
| Leucite glass ceramic | • Anterior single unit crown<br>• Anterior laminate veneers | • Fixed partial dentures<br>• Patient with parafunctional habits such as bruxism<br>• Areas under high-functional load |
| Lithium disilicate glass ceramic | • Anterior three unit fixed partial denture<br>• Anterior and posterior crowns<br>• Premolar crowns | • Patient with parafunctional habits such as bruxism<br>• Fixed partial dentures in posterior region involving molar tooth<br>• Areas under high-functional load |
| Alumina | • Anterior Fixed partial dentures<br>• Core ceramic for crowns | • Patient with parafunctional habits such as bruxism<br>• Areas under high functional load<br>• Anterior laminate veneers |
| Glass-infiltrated alumina | • Anterior and posterior crowns | • Anterior laminate veneers<br>• Posterior fixed partial dentures<br>• Patient with parafunctional habits such as bruxism |
| Glass-infiltrated spinel | • Anterior crowns | • Anterior fixed partial denture<br>• Posterior fixed partial denture<br>• Patient with parafunctional habits such as bruxism |
| Glass-infiltrated alumina/zirconia | • Posterior crowns<br>• Posterior fixed partial denture up to three units | • Anterior laminate veneers<br>• Anterior crowns<br>• Patient with parafunctional habits such as bruxism<br>• In cases, where high translucency is required |
| Zirconia (Y-TZP) with veneering ceramic | • Posterior crowns<br>• Posterior fixed partial denture up to five units | • Anterior laminate veneers<br>• Anterior crowns and fixed partial denture<br>• In cases where high translucency is required<br>• Patient with parafunctional habits such as bruxism |
| Zirconia (Y-TZP) without veneering ceramic | • Posterior crowns<br>• Posterior fixed partial denture | • Anterior laminate veneers<br>• Anterior crowns and fixed partial denture<br>• In cases, where high translucency is required<br>• Patient with parafunctional habits such as bruxism |

and ceramic is fused over the coping. The metal coping is covered with three layers of porcelain namely opaque porcelain, dentin and enamel porcelain **(Fig. 21.4)**.

## Opaque Porcelain

It masks the metal underneath and helps in the development of shade. It plays a vital role in developing bond between the ceramic and the metal. It is about 0.3 mm thick layer.

## Dentin or Body Porcelain

It provides the bulk of the restorations and gives most of the color or shade. Thickness of body porcelain is 1 mm.

## Enamel or Incisal Porcelain

It provides translucency to the restorations.

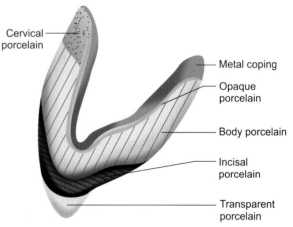

**Fig. 21.4:** Parts of metal ceramic crown.

*Definition*
*A tooth or/implant retained fixed dental prosthesis that uses a metal substructure upon which a ceramic veneer is fused.*
                                        —*GPT 8th edition*

Metal ceramic prosthesis has high-clinical durability as suggested by clinical data of over 50 years. There are number of advantages of using metal ceramic prosthesis as compared to all ceramic prosthesis.

- High resistance to fracture
- Less tooth preparation is required
- Less abrasion or wear of opposing enamel.

However, there are few disadvantages of using metal ceramic prosthesis as compared to all ceramic prosthesis:

- Sensitivity to nickel alloy
- Allergic reaction
- Less esthetic due to presence of metal especially in anterior region
- Visibility of metal collar in the labial margin of metal ceramic crown.

## METAL-CERAMIC BOND (FIG. 21.5)

For proper bonding between metal and ceramic, both alloys and ceramic should have the following properties:

- Both porcelain and alloy should form a strong bond, as common cause of failure is debonding of porcelain from metal
- Both porcelain and alloy should have almost similar coefficient of thermal expansion
- Porcelain should fuse at a much lower temperature than the melting temperature of the metal
- The metal alloy should have high modulus of elasticity and should not deform at firing temperature
- The metal should not interact with ceramic, as this will visibly discolor it and affects the esthetics

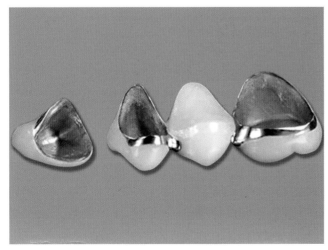

**Fig. 21.5:** Porcelain-metal bond.

- Metal-porcelain bond must be durable and stable at interface to withstand masticatory stresses
- Metal alloy having slight higher coefficient of thermal expansion causes the porcelain to be in state of residual compression at the alloy interface. Porcelain is much stronger in compression than tension.

### Bonding Mechanisms

There are generally four types of bonding mechanisms present between metal substructure and ceramic:

1. Mechanical interlocking
2. Compressive forces
3. Van der Waals forces
4. Chemical bonding.

#### Mechanical Interlocking

- Mechanical interlocking of the ceramic occurs with microabrasions on the surface of the metal coping
- Microabrasions on the surface of the metal are produced by finishing the metal with uncontaminated stone and by air abrasion
- Air abrasion increases wettability, provides mechanical interlocking and also increases surface area for chemical bonding
- In some systems such as palladium silver alloys, there is no external oxide formation for bonding with porcelain. In such alloys, oxidation occurs internally to bond mechanically with porcelain
- This type of bonding mechanism is needed where oxide layer is not present such as in noble metal alloys. These alloys depend on mechanical interlocking for bonding with ceramic
- Alternately, addition of small amount of tin to the noble metal alloys can result in the formation of surface oxides, which can help in bonding. This process of formation of oxides is done by *electrodeposition*.

**CLINICAL SIGNIFICANCE**

Electrodeposition has shown to achieve adequate bonding with ceramic. The benefits of this technique are—improved wettability of surface of metal with ceramic, acts as barrier-preventing diffusion of metal ions into ceramic and reduces porosity at the metal-ceramic interface.

#### Compressive Forces

- These are developed within the metal ceramic prosthesis by having coefficient of thermal expansion for metal coping slightly higher than the ceramic veneer and by properly designing the metal coping

- The difference in coefficient of thermal expansion causes the ceramic to be drawn toward the metal coping when the restoration cools after firing.

### Van der Waals Forces

- Developed by mutual attraction of the charged molecules
- Plays minor role in bonding.

### Chemical Bonding

- This is the most accepted mechanism of bonding between porcelain and alloys
- Oxidation behavior of metal ceramic alloys determines the potential for bonding with porcelain
- During the degassing cycle, adherent oxides are formed which are responsible for chemical bonding between the porcelain and alloys
- Chemical bonding occurs between the ceramic and the surface oxide layer present on the base metals such as iron, indium and tin of gold alloys
- Bond strength is further increased by firing in an oxidizing atmosphere
- Base metal alloys readily forms chromium oxide that bonds ceramic without the addition of any trace elements.

## Failures of Metal-Ceramic Bond

- Fractures can occur due to excessive stress development, deficiency in material and discrepancy during processing
- Clinical fractures of metal-ceramic restorations can occur primarily at three sites:
  1. Between opaque porcelain and interaction zone
  2. Within the interaction zone
  3. Between the metal and interaction zone.

### Classification of Bond Failures in Metal-Ceramic Restorations (O'Brien 1977) **(Fig. 21.6)**

*Type 1: Metal-porcelain*: In this type, fracture occurs at the metal porcelain interface where the fracture shows a clean surface of metal. The cause for this failure is contamination or porous metal surface, which may result in metal surface which is devoid of oxide layer needed for bonding.

*Type II: Metal oxide-porcelain*: This type of fracture occurs at the metal oxide and porcelain interface where porcelain fractures at the metal oxide surface leaving oxide firmly attached to the metal. Common in base metal alloys.

*Type III: Cohesive within the porcelain:* This type of fracture occurs cohesively entirely within the porcelain, which is due to tensile failure within the porcelain. Bond strength exceeds the strength of porcelain. Seen in high-gold content

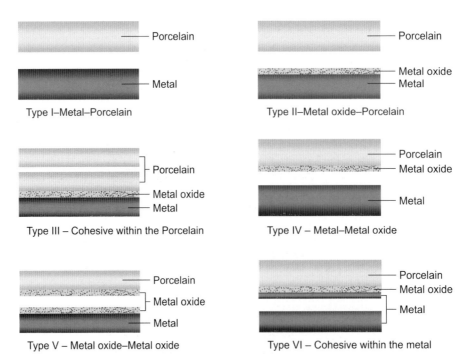

**Fig. 21.6:** Failures of metal-ceramic bond.

alloys. This type of fracture can occur because of error in design of crown or due to excessive occlusal load. It is commonly observed in high gold content alloys.

*Type IV: Metal-metal oxide*: This type of fracture occurs at the metal-metal oxide interface where the metal oxide breaks away from the metal and is left attached to porcelain. The common cause of failure is due to error in processing of the metal. Seen in base metal alloys due to excess of chromium and nickel oxide.

*Type V: Metal oxide-metal oxide*: In this type, fracture occurs through the metal oxide. Caused due to overproduction of oxides.

*Type VI: Cohesive within the metal*: This type of fracture occurs cohesively within the metal and is more common in FPDs where the joint area breaks.

## Technical Considerations

### Fabrication and Design of Metal Coping or Framework

- The metal coping should be designed such that it should allow porcelain to remain in compression by supporting the incisal edges, the occlusal surfaces and the marginal ridges
- Wax pattern is fabricated over the die, which is then casted to get the metal coping
- Wax is cut back by 1 mm in the esthetic areas to ensure sufficient space for porcelain **(Fig. 21.7)**
- All sharp angles are rounded in order to prevent stress concentration
- Methods of fabricating metal coping for metal-ceramic restorations are:
  - Electrodeposition of gold or other metal on a duplicate die
  - Burnishing and heat treating metal foils on die
  - Casting of alloy through lost wax technique
  - CAD-CAM processing of metal ingot

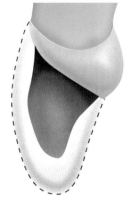

**Fig. 21.7:** Wax pattern cut back.

- Metal coping or framework is fabricated by using either of the above mentioned technique.

### Metal Preparation

- Investment material is removed ultrasonically with airborne particle abrasion or with steam
- Metal surface is smoothened using ceramic-bound stones or carbide burs and then is air abraded with aluminum oxide
- Air abrasion creates satin finish on the veneering surface, which is easily wetted by porcelain slurry **(Fig. 21.8)**
- Metal thickness should not be less than 0.3 mm, as it can lead to distortion during porcelain firing
- Metal coping or framework is immersed in ultrasonic cleanser for 5 minutes to remove grinding debris, small particles or oil
- Steam cleaning can also be used as an alternative to ultrasonic cleaning. Clean surface is absolutely necessary for good metal to porcelain bonding.

### Degassing or Oxidizing

- For proper chemical bonding between the metal and porcelain, a controlled oxide layer should be created on the metal surface
- The oxide layer is formed by placing the coping or framework in the porcelain furnace at a specified temperature that should sufficiently exceed the firing temperature of porcelain.

### Porcelain Application

- Dental porcelain is supplied in the form of powder and water-based glycerin liquid
- Appropriate amount of opaque powder is dispensed on a glass slab and then modeling liquid is added. Both powder and liquid are mixed with the help of spatula to form a paste of workable consistency

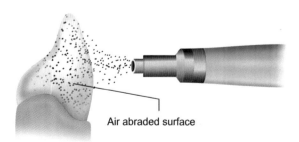

Air abraded surface

**Fig. 21.8:** Air abrasion creates surface which is readily wet by porcelain slurry.

- Metal spatula should not be used for mixing as metal particles can rub off and act as contaminants
- Mixed paste is picked with the help of brush or spatula and applied over the metal substructure **(Fig. 21.9)**
- First opaque porcelain is applied in thin layer with a brush. The thickness of opaque layer of porcelain should not be less than 0.3 mm **(Fig. 21.10)**
- Porcelain is then condensed to spread the material evenly.

### Porcelain Condensation

- Proper condensation of the powder particles is important, as it produces lower firing shrinkage and reduced porosity in the fired porcelain
- Condensation of porcelain can be achieved by using either method such as vibration, spatulation and brush techniques

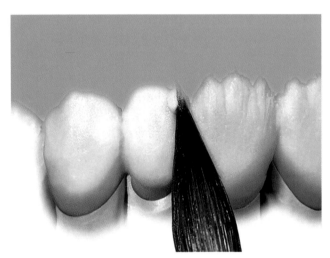

**Fig. 21.9:** Application of paste porcelain with the help of brush.

- *Vibration method:* Mild vibration is used to pack the wet powder particles densely on the underlying framework. Excess water, which comes on the surface, is blotted off using a clean tissue. In this method, condensation occurs toward the blotted area **(Fig. 21.11)**
- *Spatulation method:* A small spatula is used to apply and smoothen the wet porcelain. The smoothening action brings excess moisture on the surface, which is blotted out with tissue
- *Brush method:* In this method, dry powder particles are applied with the brush to the surface to absorb water. Dry powder is applied on the side opposite from the increment of wet porcelain
- When the entire veneering surface is covered, any excess material is removed with the help of stiff, dry, short bristle brush.

### Porcelain Sintering

- *Sintering—It is a process of heating mass of loosely packed particles held by a binder to a specified temperature to densify and strengthen it as a result of bonding, diffusion and flow phenomenon to form a fused coherent solid*
- As these particles fuse to form coherent solid, the formed ceramic undergoes considerable amount of shrinkage.

*Rationale:*
To sinter the powder particles for specific time and temperature to result in a coherent solid.

*Medium used for sintering process:*
- Three different media are used for sintering—*air, vacuum and diffusible gas* **(Table 21.3)**
- Firing in vacuum furnace helps in greatly reducing the porosity. For metal-ceramic restorations vacuum firing

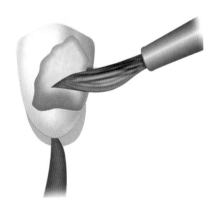

**Fig. 21.10:** Opaque porcelain applied with the help of a brush.

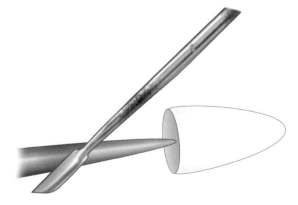

**Fig. 21.11:** Mild vibration used for condensation of porcelain.

is preferred. However, complete sintering of a structure is not possible even if fired in vacuum.

*Stages in sintering or firing:*
There are number of stages of dental porcelain, which have been identified when it is "sintered" or "fired". The commonly used terminology for referring the surface appearance of unglazed porcelain is "bisque".

*Drying or green stage:*
- The condensed mass of low-fusing porcelain is placed in front of the preheated furnace at approximately 650°C for 5 minutes
- The preheating procedure helps in dissipating of the remaining water vapor. If the condensed mass is directly placed into the furnace without preheating, it results in fracture of large areas of ceramic or formation of voids
- The sintered glass particles when heated, flows resulting in wetting and bridging between such particles (**Fig. 21.12**)
- Pores are formed by air trapped during the sintering process
- In this stage, slight contraction occurs.

**Table 21.3:** Sintering process by different media.

| Air firing | Vacuum firing |
|---|---|
| Tendency to trap air within porcelain | Results in dense pore free porcelain |
| Results in pits and roughness on grinding | Shows reduced surface roughness |
| Results in reduced strength and translucency | Greater strength and translucency |
| Voids of larger size | Voids of extremely small size |

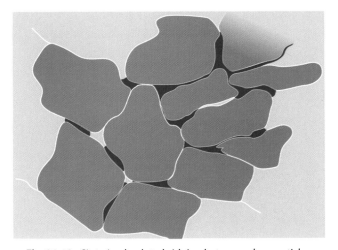

**Fig. 21.12:** Sintering leads to bridging between glass particles.

*Low bisque:*
- As the temperature increases, the furnace is closed and the particles start to fuse together
    - The surface of porcelain is highly porous having grains, which soften at the contact points
    - Coalescence occurs at the point of contact between the powder particles. The material is still porous at this stage
- Has minimal shrinkage and the fired body is highly friable or weak
- Particles lack cohesion as well as translucency or glaze.

*Medium bisque:*
- As the temperature continues to increase at this stage, there is complete cohesion of powder particles
- Although, pores still exists on the surface of porcelain, but the flow of glass grains is increased
- Since it is porous, it lacks translucency and high glaze
- There is an evidence of definite shrinkage during this stage, approximately 20%.

*High bisque:*
- At this stage, there is further increase in the flow of glass grains, which completely seals the surface and provides smoothness to the porcelain
- The sintered body at this stage is strong and corrections, if any, can be made by grinding before final glaze
- There may be evidence of slight porosity at this stage
- In the case of nonfeldspathic porcelains, a slight shine appears at this stage.

*Cooling stage:*
- Very slow rate of cooling is required to avoid cracks or crazing in the sintered ceramic
- Rapid cooling can lead to thermal shock resulting in catastrophic fracture of glass.

## Dentin and Enamel Porcelain Application

- After the opaque porcelain application is fired, dentin and enamel porcelain is added
- Initially, shoulder porcelain is added on the coping, it is condensed and then fired at appropriate temperature (**Fig. 21.13**)
- Body dentin is mixed to creamy consistency and applied over the opaque layer with a brush or spatula (**Fig. 21.14**)
- Complete contour of the crown is developed with dentin porcelain with the brush or spatula
- Porcelain is then condensed and dried using a tissue paper
- Dentin porcelain is slightly overbuilt beyond the intended final contour of the crown to compensate for shrinkage (**Fig. 21.15**)

- At this stage, dentin is carved back to allow the placement of the enamel porcelain
- Enamel porcelain is then applied to restore the complete contour of the restoration **(Fig. 21.16)**
- When complete, the restoration should be slightly larger incisally to compensate for firing shrinkage
- The restoration is carefully removed from the die and small amount of porcelain is added to the interproximal areas
- Finally, the restoration is condensed and blotted with tissue
- The initial buildup is dried in front of the furnace for several minutes and is then sintered under vacuum at the temperature specified by the manufacturer
- After firing, the restoration is placed back on the die and is inspected for any corrections
- Insufficient contours are corrected by buildup and are then fired
- Firing or sintering is done at 10–20°C lower than the initial firing.

## Characterization and Staining

- Characterization and internal staining is done to provide a lifelike appearance to the final restoration
- Different stains are available, which help in characterization of the restoration
- Stain powders are mixed with special liquid and are layered within the buildup powders to create special effects
- One disadvantage of internal staining is that if desired result is not achieved then the entire porcelain needs to be stripped from the substructure.

## Glazing and Surface Characterization (**Fig. 21.17**)

- Glazing is defined as the final firing of porcelain in which the surface is vitrified and a high gloss is imparted to the material
- Objectives of glazing are—to improve strength, esthetics and hygiene; to reduce crack propagation
- Before glazing, the restoration is tried in the patient mouth and any necessary changes or corrections are made
- After satisfactory bisque trial, the restoration is smoothened and surface is treated by either methods:
  - Natural or autoglaze
  - Applied overglaze
  - Polishing.

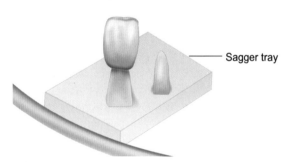

**Fig. 21.13:** Condensed procelain is placed in front of furnace.

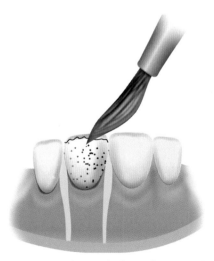

**Fig. 21.14:** Dentin porcelain applied over the opaque layer with the help of a brush.

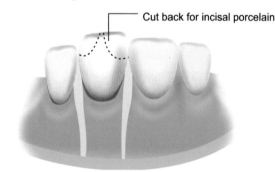

**Fig. 21.15:** Overbuilt dentin porcelain.

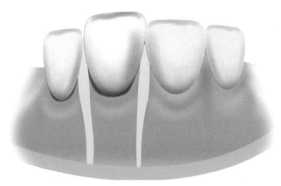

**Fig. 21.16:** Complete porcelain build up on the cast.

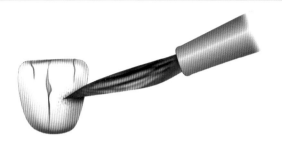

**Fig. 21.17:** Surface characterisation and glazing of final restoration.

- *Natural or autoglaze or self-glaze*—porcelain has ability to glaze naturally when held at its fusing temperature in air for 1–4 minutes. A pyroclastic surface flow occurs and surface glaze is formed. This ability of natural glaze is lost with multiple firing of porcelain
- *Applied overglaze or add-on glaze*—low fusing clear porcelain in painted over the smoothened restoration and is fired at much lower fusing temperature of dentin and enamel porcelain. Add on glaze is highly recommended for large restoration requiring multiple corrections
- *Polishing*—is accomplished using commercially available polishing systems. It is useful on relatively small areas of adjustments such as proximal or small occlusal contact. Jacobi et al. has shown that polished porcelain is less destructive to opposing natural tooth than glazed porcelain.

## Cooling of the Restoration

- Cooling of the metal-ceramic restoration from its firing temperature to room temperature is very critical (**Fig. 21.18**)

- Sudden cooling of the restoration can cause fracture of the porcelain

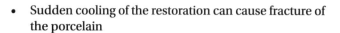

**CLINICAL SIGNIFICANCE**

Cooling slowly is very important process especially in metal-ceramic restorations. Multiple firing of metal-ceramic restoration can cause increase of coefficient of thermal contraction of leucite present in ceramic. This increase can result in tensile stress development forming cracks.

## Other Metal Reinforced Systems

### Captek System (Fig. 21.19)

- This system based on capillary attraction to produce a gold composite metal. Captek (Precious Chemicals Co. Inc) is an acronym for *"Capillary assisted technology"*. This technique is based on fabricating metal coping without using conventional melting and casting process. These are available as laminated gold alloy metal strips of Captek P (Au-Pt-Pd) and Captek G (Au-Ag) variety
- Captek P and G metals produce thin metal copings for single crowns or frameworks for FPDs with maximum span length of 18 mm
- In this system, metal coping is fabricated from two metal impregnated wax sheets, which are adapted and burnished to the die using swaging instrument. Then bonder layer is applied over it and veneering ceramic is then sintered at firing temperature
- The first sheet develops a porous three-dimensional capillary network of gold-platinum-palladium layer (Captek P), which is impregnated with 97% gold (Captek G) when second sheet is fired

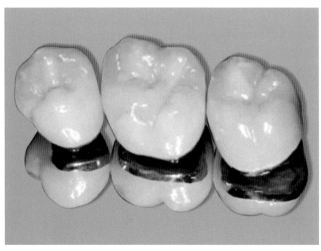

**Fig. 21.18:** Finished metal-ceramic restoration.

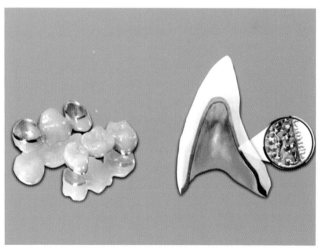

**Fig. 21.19:** Captek crowns.

- The Captek G sheet contains 97.5% gold and 2.5% by weight silver. Captek P acts like a metal sponge, which draws molten gold completely onto it. Once this composite material is burnished on the die, the margins are trimmed and finished. The thickness of metal coping is about 0.25 mm, which is much smaller than produced by cast metal technique (0.50 mm). The metal coping is then fired in porcelain furnace with two thin coats of opaque porcelain and then subsequent layers of body and enamel porcelain.
    - Captek P and G metal alloys are capable of producing thin metal copings for crowns or making frameworks for metal-ceramic bridges
- This system provides excellent esthetics and marginal adaptation.

*Drawbacks*
- Highly technique sensitive
- Difficulty of bonding dissimilar metals
- Atomic bonding of veneering ceramic dependent on bonded layer rather than the oxides as in cast metal process
- Use in high-stress area is doubtful
- Clinical data is limited.

### Helioform HF 600 System *(Fig. 21.20)*

- This system uses electroforming technique to produce thin pure gold copings
- Gold is deposited onto the polyurethane die that is coated with silver spacer using computer-controlled plating equipment to control its thickness
- Before porcelain firing, the coping is coated with noble metal paste primer
- This primer helps to improve metal porcelain bonding and improves esthetics by blocking color of the dark metal oxide
- Electroforming enables good marginal adaptation.

### Advantages

- High strength and resistance to fracture
- Improved marginal fit
- Permanent esthetic quality of properly designed restorations
- Less tooth reduction in comparison to all ceramic preparation.

### Disadvantages

- Increased opacity
- Difficult to create depth of translucency because of the mirror effect of the dense opaque masking porcelain

- Porcelain used in metal-ceramic restorations can result in cloudiness due to devitrification
- The fit of long-span bridges or splints may be affected by the creep of the metal during successive bakes of porcelain
- More difficult to obtain good esthetics than regular or aluminous porcelain.

### Indications

- In cases of parafunctional mandibular activity where an esthetic restoration is essential
- Teeth requiring fixed splinting or being used as bridge abutments
- In all posterior teeth, where full coverage is necessary for esthetic reasons.

### Contraindications

- Adolescent teeth where minimal tooth preparation is essential
- Teeth, where enamel wear is high and there is insufficient bulk of tooth structure to allow room for metal and porcelain
- Anterior teeth where esthetic is of prime importance, e.g. high shades of very translucent teeth.

### Troubleshooting in Metal-Ceramic Restorations **(Table 21.4)**

Some of the commonly occurring troubleshooting in fabrication of metal ceramic restorations and their causes are given below.

### Methods of Strengthening Ceramics

The structure of ceramic is inherently weak because they are brittle material and have low-tensile strength.

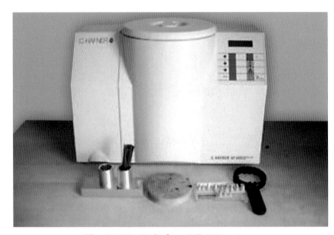

**Fig. 21.20:** Helioform HF 600 system.

Ceramics can be strengthened by following methods:
- Minimize the effects of stress raisers
- Minimize the number of firing cycles
- Minimize tensile stress through optimal design of prosthesis
- Development of residual compressive stresses:
  - Ion exchange
  - Thermal tempering
  - Coefficient of thermal expansion mismatch
- Interruption of crack propagation:
  - Dispersion of crystalline phase
  - Transformation toughening.

### Minimize the Effects of Stress Raisers

- Stress raisers are discontinuities in brittle materials such as ceramic and metal-ceramic restorations, which cause stress concentration in these areas
- Sudden changes in shape and thickness of porcelain contour should be avoided as they behave as stress raisers
- Any sharp line angles in the preparation should be rounded.

#### CLINICAL SIGNIFICANCE
- Creases or folds in the platinum foil become embedded in porcelain-producing notches, which behave as stress raisers
- Large changes in porcelain thickness, which are essentially determined by the tooth preparation have tendency to create areas of stress concentration.

### Minimize the Number of Firing Cycles

- Leucite is a high-expansion and high-contraction crystal phase, which greatly influences the thermal contraction coefficient of porcelain
- Multiple firings can change the leucite content which can alter the coefficient of thermal contraction of porcelain
- If this coefficient of expansion increases above the value for metal then the mismatch between the porcelain and metal produces stresses during cooling that can cause formation of crack in porcelain.

### Minimize Tensile Stress through Optimal Design of Prosthesis *(Fig. 21.21)*

- Stronger and tougher ceramic should be selected as they can sustain higher tensile stresses
- Conventional feldspathic porcelain should be avoided, as the core especially in the posterior teeth as occlusal forces can induce tensile stresses
- Aluminous porcelain crowns are contraindicated for restoring posterior teeth as occlusal forces can induce tensile stresses
- Porcelain is much stronger in compression rather than in tension. Therefore, tensile stresses should be avoided in porcelain to prevent fracture of the restoration
- The ceramic prosthesis should be designed such that exposure to high-tensile strength is avoided

#### CLINICAL SIGNIFICANCE
- Tensile stresses in all ceramic FPD can be reduced by greater connector height (≥4 mm) and by widening the radius of curvature of the gingival embrasure
- However, the connector height should not be more than 4 mm as this makes the prosthesis too bulky and unesthetic.

| Table 21.4: Troubleshooting in metal-ceramic restoration. | |
|---|---|
| *Troubleshooting* | *Causes* |
| Cracks or fracture during bisque stage | • Poor design of framework<br>• Improper condensation<br>• Incompatible metal alloy porcelain combination<br>• Incomplete moisture control |
| Voids | • Multiple firing<br>• Air incorporation during buildup<br>• Incomplete moisture control<br>• Poor casting technique<br>• Poor metal preparation |
| Clinical failure | • Poor framework design<br>• Improper metal preparation<br>• Centric stops too close to ceramic-metal junction |
| Esthetic failure | • Inadequate tooth preparation<br>• Poor shade selection<br>• Too thick opaque layer<br>• Multiple firing<br>• Poor communication with the technician |

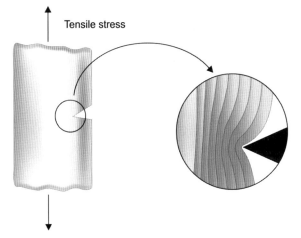

Tensile stress

**Fig. 21.21:** Tensile stresses in porcelain can lead to failure of the restoration.

- Premature contact on ceramic restoration can produce large localized stresses. If these premature contacts are not eliminated then it can lead to formation of *Hertzian Cone cracks* resulting in chipping of occlusal surface. Therefore, it is important to ensure elimination of any interfering contact before cementation of the ceramic restoration.

### Development of Residual Compressive Stresses

#### Ion exchange
- Also called as *Chemical Tempering* (Anusavice et al. 1992)
- This is one of the most effective ways of introducing compressive stresses onto the surface of ceramics
- In this method, ceramic article-containing sodium is placed in a bath-containing molten potassium nitrate. The larger potassium ions exchange with the smaller sodium ions on the surface **(Fig. 21.22)**
- Potassium ions are 35% larger than the sodium ions and have to squeeze through to replace sodium ions from the glass surface
- This squeezing of the potassium ions creates a very large residual compressive stresses
- According to Anusavice et al. (1994) the depth of compression zone achieved by this method is less than 100 μm and its strengthening effect will be lost, if the ceramic is grinded, worn or eroded more than this thickness.

#### Thermal tempering
- This is the most common method of strengthening glass **(Fig. 21.23)**
- In this method, compressive stresses are created on the surface by rapid cooling of an object when it is in molten state

- This sudden cooling results in the formation of outer rigid skin of glass, which surrounds the molten core of an object
- When this molten core hardens, it contracts and creates a residual tensile stress in the core whereas there is residual compressive stress on the outer surface
- This method is commonly employed in strengthening glass used as automobile windows, windshields, sliding glass door, etc.
- For dental use, hot glass phase ceramic is suddenly cooled in silicone oil or other special liquid.

#### Thermal compatibility
- Metal and porcelain when selected for porcelain fused to metal restorations should have slight mismatch in the coefficient of thermal contraction
- The value of coefficient of thermal contraction of metal should be slightly higher than the porcelain on cooling from the firing temperature to the room temperature
- The difference in coefficient of thermal contraction between the metal and porcelain provide additional strength to the restoration by placing it in the state of residual compression

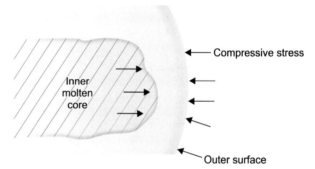

**Fig. 21.23:** Strengthening of glass by thermal tempering

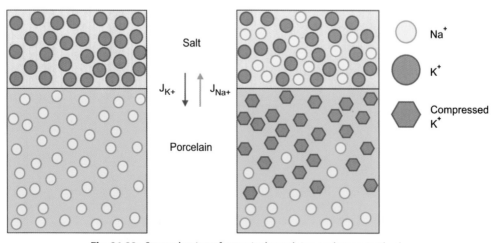

**Fig. 21.22:** Strengthening of ceramic through ion exchange method.

- Likewise, residual compressive stresses can be introduced in ceramic by selecting veneering ceramic with different coefficient of thermal expansion than the core ceramic. When veneering ceramic, which is fired over the core ceramic is allowed to cool to room temperature. The core ceramic with higher coefficient of thermal expansion tends to produce compressive stress in the veneering ceramic. This increases the fracture resistance of the ceramic structure.

### *Disruption of Crack Propagation*

*Dispersion of a crystalline phase*
- It is a method of reinforcing ceramic with a foreign material capable of blocking crack propagation in the material
- Ceramic, which is primarily composed of glass can be strengthened by adding stronger foreign material such as leucite, $ZrO_2$, alumina or lithium disilicate
- Strengthening of ceramic is influenced by size and volume of the crystal, its coefficient of thermal expansion relative to glass matrix.

#### CLINICAL SIGNIFICANCE
Glass is strengthened by adding stronger crystal particle such as alumina to the glass as crack cannot propagate through these tough particles, e.g. aluminous porcelain developed for porcelain jacket crowns.

*Transformation toughening:*
- Dental ceramics is toughened and strengthened by homogenously distributing small tough crystals in a glass matrix
- These tough crystals include alumina, leucite, tetrasilicic fluormica, lithia disilicate or magnesia-alumina-spinel
- $ZrO_2$-based ceramics undergo transformation toughening by transforming $ZrO_2$ from tetragonal phase to a monoclinic phase at the crack tips, which are in areas of tensile stress
- This transformation from tetragonal phase to monoclinic phase is prevented by adding 3 % mol of $Y_2O_3$
- The resulting structure is extremely strong and tough with flexural strength of 900 MPa
- $Y_2O_3$ stabilized $ZrO_2$ ceramic is sometimes referred to as *ceramic steel.*

## ALL CERAMIC RESTORATIONS

All ceramic restorations are those restorations which do not have any metallic core or in other words are made solely of ceramics. These restorative materials have become very popular nowadays because of high esthetics, improved fracture resistance and improved CAD-CAM technology. Although all ceramic crowns have been in use for more than five decades but had limitation because of inferior strength. They were not indicated in high-stress areas such as posterior teeth. This has led to development of high strength all ceramic restorations, which can be used both in anterior and posterior region. Also, advancement in ceramic processing methods have allowed greater quality control and increased mechanical reliability. The ceramics can be glass ceramic, feldspathic or alumina- or $ZrO_2$-based ceramic. Currently available all ceramic restorations claim to have adequate strength to be used as anterior and posterior FPDs.

### Classification of All Ceramic Restorations

*Based on composition—according to Anusavice (2003):*
- *Predominantly alumina:* In-Ceram alumina, Procera
- *Predominantly $ZrO_2$:* Lava, cercon
- *Silica glass:* VITABLOCS Mark II
- *Leucite-based glass ceramics:* IPS Empress
- *Lithia-based glass ceramic:* IPS Empress 2.

*Based on microstructure—according to Kelly (2004):*
- *Predominantly glassy materials:* Alpha VMK
- *Particle-filled glasses:* Dicor, In-Ceram, IPS Empress
- *Polycrystalline ceramics:* Procera, lava, cercon.

*Based on processing method—according to McLaren (2009):*
- *Conventional powder slurry*—Optec HSP, Duceram LFC
- *Castable ceramics*—Dicor
- *Machinable ceramics:*
  - *Copy milling*—Celay
  - *CAD-CAM*—Cerec 1 and 2, Cicero, automill
- *Pressable ceramics*—IPS Empress
- *Infiltrated ceramics*—In-Ceram (Vita Zahnfabrik)

*Based on composition—according to O'Brien:*
- *Feldspar:*
  - High leucite
  - Low leucite (porcelain jacket crown)
- *Glass ceramic:*
  - Lithium disilicate
  - Mica
- *Core reinforced:*
  - Alumina
- Magnesia.

### Criteria for Selection of Dental Ceramics

- All ceramic crowns should be used when the adjacent anterior teeth show high degree of translucency

- All ceramic restorations not indicated for patient with evidence of parafunctional habits such as bruxism and clenching
- When patient demands for high-esthetic restorations
- Adequate interarch space should be available and adequate tooth reduction should be possible
- Dentist should be skilled to provide perfect impressions from preparations, which are free of undercuts and have well-defined finish lines with adequate tooth reduction
- Informed consent should be obtained from patients after informing about the potential benefits, risks, cost and alternative of the treatment
- Laboratory technician should be experienced to provide excellent restorations
- Distance of the edentulous span should not be more than 42 mm for the fabrication of $ZrO_2$-based restorations.

## Methods of All Ceramic Fabrication

All ceramic restorations can be fabricated by using the following methods **(Table 21.5)**:

1. Powder condensation
2. Slip casting
3. Hot pressing
4. CAD-CAM sintered
5. Densely sintered
6. Glass infiltrated.

## Aluminous Core Ceramics

- In 1965, McLean and Hughes introduced the high-strength aluminous ceramic core to overcome the low strength of high-fusing feldspathic porcelain
- The porcelain jacket crown developed by them had inner core made of 40–50% alumina porcelain dispersed in a glass matrix **(Figs. 21.24A and B)**
- The reinforcing inner core was layered by feldspathic porcelain resulting in restoration twice as strong as conventional porcelain
- Flexural strength of aluminous porcelain core was approximately 131 MPa
- Although the strength improved, but it was not enough to be used in posterior region
- Fracture resistance in aluminous porcelain jacket crown was further improved by using platinum matrix
- In this method, aluminous porcelain is bonded to thin platinum foil coping
- Porcelain bonding to the foil is facilitated by electroplating the platinum foil with thin layer of tin and then oxidizing in the furnace to provide a layer of tin oxide for porcelain bonding
- Clinical longevity of anterior crowns is excellent but McLean has reported a failure of 15% after 5 years when used in molar region

**Table 21.5:** Methods of all ceramic fabrication.

| Method of fabrication | Composition | Commercial brands |
|---|---|---|
| Powder condensation | Glass<br>Leucite-glass<br>Fluorapatite-glass<br>Leucite-glass<br>Alumina-glass | • Duceram LFC (Dentsply)<br>• Finesse low fusing (Dentsply)<br>• IPS e.max Ceram (Ivoclar Vivadent), IPS Eris (Ivoclar Vivadent)<br>• LAVA Ceram (3M ESPE), Vitamin D (Vita Zahnfabrik), Vitadur Alpha (Vita Zahnfabrik)<br>• Vitadur N (Vita Zahnfabrik) |
| Hot pressing | Leucite-glass<br>Lithium disilicate-glass<br>Fluorapatite-glass | • Finesse All ceramic (Dentsply), IPS Empress (Ivoclar Vivadent)<br>• IPS Empress 2 (Ivoclar Vivadent), IPS e.max Press (Ivoclar Vivadent),<br>• IPS e.max ZirPress (Ivoclar Vivadent) |
| Slip casting | Glass-Alumina<br>Glass-Alumina-Spinel<br>Glass-Alumina-PS Zirconia | • In-Ceram Alumina (Vita Zahnfabrik)<br>• In-Ceram Spinel (Vita Zahnfabrik)<br>• In-Ceram Zirconia (Vita Zahnfabrik) |
| CAD-CAM presintered | Partially stabilized zirconia<br>Alumina | • Cercon (Dentsply), DC-Zirkon (DCS), Everest ZS-Blanks (Kavo), IPS e.max ZirCAD (Ivoclar Vivadent), LAVA Frame (3M ESPE), Procera All Zirkon (Nobel Biocare)<br>• Procera All Ceram (Nobel Biocare) |
| Densely sintered | Partially stabilized zirconia<br>Leucite-glass<br>Lithium disilicate glass | • Digizon (Digident), Everest ZH-Blanks (Kavo), ZirKon (Cynovad)<br>• Everest G-Blanks (Kavo), ProCAD (Ivoclar Vivadent), Vitablocks Marck II (Vita Zahnfabrik)<br>• IPS e.max CAD (Ivoclar Vivadent) |
| Glass infiltrated | Glass-Alumina<br>Glass-Alumina-Spinel<br>Glass-Alumina-PS Zirconia | • In-Ceram Alumina (Vita Zahnfabrik)<br>• In-Ceram Spinel (Vita Zahnfabrik)<br>• In-Ceram Zirconia (Vita Zahnfabrik) |

*Abbreviations:* PS, partially stabilized; CAD-CAM, computer-aided design/computer-aided manufacturing

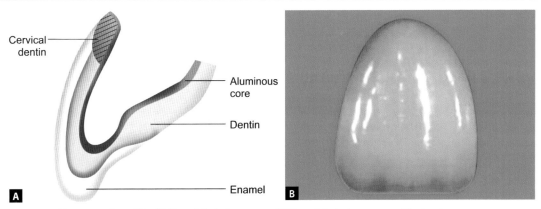

**Figs. 21.24A and B:** (A) Porcelain jacket crown; (B) Porcelain jacket crown with aluminous core.

- Aluminous crowns provide slightly better esthetics for anterior teeth as compared to metal ceramic crowns.

## Glass Ceramics

These are those materials, which can be shaped in the desired form just like glass and are then subjected to firing in the porcelain furnace. Glass ceramic was introduced to dentistry by McCulloch in 1968. He produced denture teeth using glass-molding process. Glass ceramics are mostly available in powder form, which are mixed with liquid to form slurry and are applied on the die with a brush in desired shape. Excess moisture is removed by blotting to compact the powder particles. Further compaction of these particles occurs once they are placed for firing in the porcelain furnace. The glass component flows under vacuum during firing leading to crystallization of the glass. Crystalline particles formed during firing interrupts the propagation of cracks thereby increasing strength and toughness of ceramic. Recently, glass ceramics-containing leucite, lithium disilicate and hydroxyapatite are in use. These materials are available in powder form or as solid blocks, which can be heat pressed or machined using CAD-CAM process.

### Castable Glass Ceramic

*Dicor* (**Figs. 21.25**):
- Dicor was the first commercially available castable ceramics by Corning Glass Works in 1984
- This castable glass ceramic was composed of $SiO_2$, $K_2O$, MgO, fluoride from $MgF_2$ and small amounts of $Al_2O_3$ and $ZrO_2$, added for durability and esthetics
- Fluoride acts as nucleating agent and improves fluidity of the molten glass
- It is formed into inlay, labial veneer or complete crown by lost wax casting technique

- Dicor restorations were fabricated by waxing the crown to complete anatomic contour with precise control of occlusion and axial contours
- The wax pattern is invested in phosphate-bonded investment material and after casting, it is divested. The casting is sandblasted and sprues are removed
- The casting is then embedded in investment and reheated to allow nucleation and growth of crystalline phase. This process of crystal nucleation and crystal growth is called as "*ceramming*". The cerammed casting is checked for fit on the die and is veneered and stained according to the requirement
- The Dicor glass ceramics consist of 55% of tetrasilicic fluormica crystals
- The ceramming process results in increased toughness and strength, and increased abrasion resistance
- *Cerapearl*, another type of castable glass ceramic having microstructure similar to tooth enamel. Not available currently
- *CAD-CAM ceramic Dicor machinable glass ceramic (MGC)* consists of 70% volume of tetrasilicic fluromica crystals, which are 2 µm in diameter. Their mechanical properties are similar to Dicor glass ceramic except they exhibit lesser translucency. Dicor and Dicor MGC

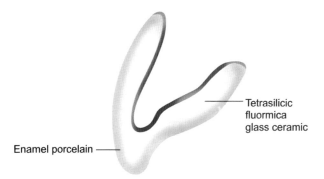

**Fig. 21.25:** Castable ceramic crowns.

is no more used in dentistry because of availability of materials with superior properties

- Tooth preparation of the glass ceramic is similar to that of metal ceramic restorations
- Minimum occlusal and incisal reduction of 1.5 mm and axial reduction of 1 mm is recommended
- Heavy chamfer or shoulder with rounded gingivoaxial line angle finish line is recommended for glass ceramic restorations.

*Properties:*
The physical properties of Dicor are given in the **Table 21.6.**

*Advantages:*
- Excellent marginal fit
- Moderately high-flexural strength
- Ease of fabrication
- Improved esthetics
- Increased chemical durability and thermal shock resistance
- Minimal abrasiveness to natural tooth
- Low-thermal expansion similar to the tooth structure
- Minimal processing shrinkage.

*Disadvantages:*
- Susceptible to fracture when used in posterior region
- Inability to be colored internally
- Low-tensile strength.

*Indications:*
- Inlays
- Onlays
- Complete crowns
- Partial veneer restorations.

*Contraindications:*
- Fixed partial dentures
- Removable partial dentures with internal rests.

## Pressable Ceramics

### Definition

*A ceramic that can be heated to a specified temperature and forced under pressure to fill a cavity in a refractory mold.*
                                                                    *—Anusavice*

| Table 21.6: Physical properties of Dicor. | |
|---|---|
| *Property* | *Dicor* |
| Density | 2.7 g/cm$^3$ |
| Translucency | 0.56 |
| Flexural strength | 152 MPa |
| Modulus of elasticity | 70.3 GPa |
| Microhardness | 362 kg/mm$^2$ |

- Pressable ceramics are available as prefabricated ingots, which are made of crystalline particles distributed throughout the glass material
- These ceramics contain leucite crystals and lithium disilicate crystals, which are well known to be used clinically for making anterior veneers, crowns, inlays and onlays. Recently, this technique is used for heat pressing on veneer ceramics on metal and ZrO$_2$ core ceramics
- Leucite-based ceramic contains about 35% by volume of these crystals (K$_2$O.Al$_2$O$_3$4SiO$_2$). These ceramics have relatively less flexural strength and fracture toughness as compared to lithium disilicate crystals, e.g. IPS Empress (Ivoclar Vivadent), Finesse All Ceramic system (Dentsply Ceramco)
- Lithia disilicate ceramics contain about 65–70% by volume of these crystals. They have narrow-sintering range, which makes them highly technique sensitive. They are much stronger ceramics than the leucite-based ceramic, e.g. IPS Empress 2 (Ivoclar Vivadent), Optec OPC 3G (Pentron Laboratory Technologies).

### Technique

- Heat pressing method is based on Lost-wax technique to obtain empty mold. In this method, heated ceramic ingot is pressed into the mold **(Fig. 21.26)**
- The ceramic ingot consists of higher concentration of leucite crystals, which increase its resistance to crack propagation
- The heat-pressing process takes 45 minutes to produce the ceramic substructure
- The heated ceramic cools and hardens into the shape of the mold
- Then investment material is broken to retrieve the ceramic substructure
- This ceramic substructure can be either stained or glazed or built up using conventional-layering method

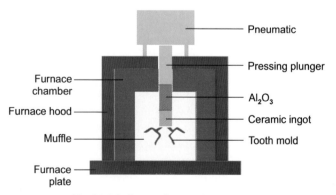

**Fig. 21.26:** Process for pressing ceramics.

- Wide ranges of shades and translucency help in providing lifelike appearance of the restorations **(Figs. 21.27A and B)**
- Unlike other glass ceramic, pressable ceramics do not require another heating cycle for crystallization of the leucite crystals
- Heat pressing is also called as *"high temperature injection molding"*.
- IPS Empress and IPS Empress 2 are examples of pressable ceramics **(Fig. 21.28 and Table 21.7)**
- IPS e.max press was introduced in 2005 as improved version of IPS empress 2.

| **Table 21.7:** IPS Empress and IPS Empress 2 specifications. | |
|---|---|
| *IPS Empress* | *IPS Empress 2* |
| Core consists of 35% leucite crystals | Contains 70% elongated lithia disilicate crystals |
| Flexural strength—112 MPa | Flexural strength—400 MPa |
| Coefficient of thermal expansion—15 ppm/°C | Coefficient of thermal expansion—10.6 ppm/°C |
| Pressing temperature—1,180°C | Pressing temperature—920°C |
| Indications—veneers, anterior crown, inlays and onlays | Inlays, onlays, veneers, anterior and posterior crowns, anterior FPD |

*Abbreviation:* FPD, fixed partial dentures

## Advantages

- Moderately high-flexural strength
- Lack of metal
- Translucent ceramic core
- Excellent marginal fit
- Excellent esthetics.

## Disadvantages

- Potential to fracture in posterior teeth
- Low-to-moderate fracture toughness

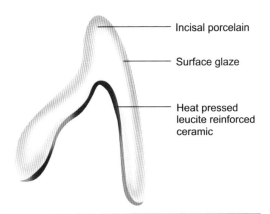

Incisal porcelain

Surface glaze

Heat pressed leucite reinforced ceramic

**A**

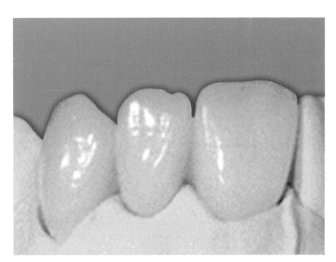

**Fig. 21.28:** IPS Empress crowns.

- Require resin cement to bond the crown micromechanically to the tooth structure.

## Indications

- Porcelain veneers
- Inlays and onlays
- Anterior and posterior crowns
- Anterior FPDs.

## Contraindications

- Moderate-to-high stress areas
- Patient with parafunctional habits
- Young patient with high-pulp horns
- Posterior FPDs
- Cantilever bridges
- Patient with worn-out dentition.

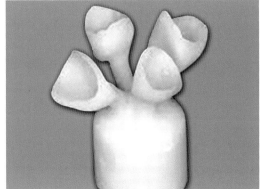

**B**

**Figs. 21.27A and B:** Heat pressed ceramic crowns.

## In-Ceram

- In-Ceram was first developed by Sadoun in 1985, using alumina as the core
- Slurry of finely ground material, which is mixed to thin and creamy, consistency is applied onto the porous refractory die. This process is called as *slip-casting* **(Fig. 21.29)**
- The die is then heating in a furnace to produce partially sintered coping or framework
- Then glass is applied to the surface of porous core and is subjected to second firing process. During this process, glass is infused or absorbed into the porous core material by capillary action **(Fig. 21.30)**
- The densely packed alumina crystal improves the strength by inhibiting crack propagation and eliminating residual porosity.

Based on the type of core ceramic, In-Ceram is of three types:
1. In-Ceram spinel
2. In-Ceram alumina
3. In-Ceram $ZrO_2$

- The final core of In-Ceram spinel consists of glass-infiltrated magnesium spinel, In-Ceram alumina consists of 70% weight of alumina infiltrated with 30% sodium lanthanum glass and In-Ceram $ZrO_2$ consists of 20% weight $ZrO_2$ and 62% weight alumina and 18% infiltrated glass

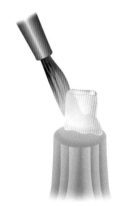

**Fig. 21.29:** Slip applied on the porous refractory die.

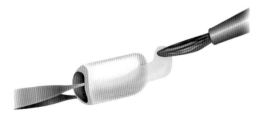

**Fig. 21.30:** Glass infiltrate applied on the alumina coping.

- Each of these In-Ceram ceramics can be infiltrated with lanthanum glass without any significant dimensional change
- In-Ceram alumina core possesses 2.5 times greater strength than conventional feldspathic porcelain and glass ceramics
- Flexural strength of glass-infiltrated core material is 350 MPa for In-Ceram spinel, 500 MPa for In-Ceram alumina and 700 MPa for In-Ceram $ZrO_2$
- In-Ceram cores are highly abrasive
- It is difficult to cut or remove In-Ceram prosthesis.

### Procedure

- Tooth preparation is done with occlusal reduction of 1.5–2.0 mm and with heavy chamfer finish line
- Impression is made and two dies are poured
- Alumina is applied on the porous duplicate die
- Die is heated in furnace for 2 hours at 120°C to dry alumina
- Then coping is sintered for 10 hours at 1,120°C
- Sodium lanthanum glass slurry mixture is applied on the coping and is fired for 4 hours at 1,120°C to allow infiltration of glass
- After trimming the excess, dentin and enamel porcelain is applied on the core
- Sintering done in furnace and the prosthesis is finished and glazed.

### Advantages

- Relatively high-flexural strength and toughness
- Lack of metal
- Can be luted by conventional-luting agents.

### Disadvantages

- Greater marginal discrepancies (161 μm)
- Greater chances of fracture
- Higher opacity (In-Ceram spinel has less)
- Technique sensitive
- Cannot be etched
- Require greater clinical skills.

### Indications

- In-Ceram spinel is indicated for inlays, onlays, veneers and anterior crowns
- In-Ceram alumina is indicated for anterior and posterior crowns and anterior three unit FPDs
- In-Ceram $ZrO_2$ is indicated for posterior crowns and anterior and posterior FPD.

## Yttria-stabilized Zirconia (**Figs 21.31A and B**)

Zirconia is being used in medical field as reliable biomaterial for hip replacement since 1970s. This material was introduced to dentistry in 2004 and since then has been widely used for crowns and fixed prosthesis. $ZrO_2$ is a white crystalline oxide of zirconium. Pure $ZrO_2$ is present as three different crystalline forms namely (**Fig. 21.32**):

- $ZrO_2$ with cubic structure obtained at temperature above 2,367°C
- $ZrO_2$ with tetrahedral structure obtained between 1,167–2,367°C
- $ZrO_2$ with monoclinic structure obtained below 1,167°C.

The tetragonal phase of $ZrO_2$ can be stabilized at room temperature by addition of elements like Mg, Ca, Sc, Y or Nd. It can also be done by reducing the crystal size to less than 10 nm.

### Properties

- $ZrO_2$ is a chemically inert and nonmetal
- It has very-low thermal conductivity about 20% as high as that of alumina. Its thermal conductivity 2.5–2.8 Wm.K and coefficient of thermal expansion is 10.3 $(10^{-6}K)$

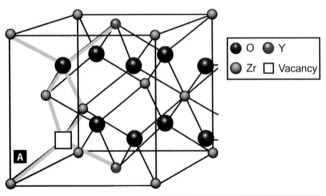

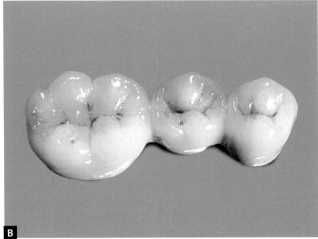

**Figs 21.31A and B:** Yttria-stabilized Zirconia

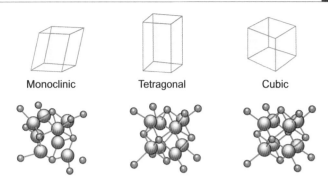

Monoclinic    Tetragonal    Cubic

**Fig. 21.32:** Crystalline forms of $ZrO_2$.

- It is highly corrosion resistant
- At room temperature, pure $ZrO_2$ has monoclinic crystalline structure and as the temperature is raised, it converts into tetragonal and cubic structure. During transformation, $ZrO_2$ can crack at the time of cooling from the processing temperature. To avoid cracking, $ZrO_2$ structure is stabilized by adding stabilizing oxides such as MgO, $Y_2O_3$, CaO and $Ce_2O_3$. The most commonly used stabilizer used in dentistry is $Y_2O_3$, as it is highly soluble trivalent stabilizer
- Addition of $Y_2O_3$ (3–5% mol) results in stabilized tetragonal $ZrO_2$ ceramic core and is called as $Y_2O_3$-stabilized $ZrO_2$ or $Y_2O_3$-stabilized tetragonal $ZrO_2$ polycrystals (Y-TZP)
- Stabilization of $ZrO_2$ using $Y_2O_3$ produces metastable tetragonal structure at room temperature. This transformation toughening considerably increases flexural strength and fracture toughness. Apart from transformation, toughening other methods of crack shielding are ductile zone formation, transformation zone formation and microcracking.

### CLINICAL SIGNIFICANCE

When the tetragonal phase is cooled to room temperature, it can transform into monoclinic phase with increase in volume. This change can lead to generation of stress, which may lead to crack formation, prompting metastable tetragonal crystals to migrate next to the crack tip and transform it to stable monoclinic form. In this event, there is 3% volume expansion of the $ZrO_2$ crystals, which inhibit propagation of crack by placing it in state of compressive stress. This mechanism helps in gaining strength and toughness to the ceramic structure. Due to this reason $Y_2O_3$-stabilized $ZrO_2$ ceramic is called as *"ceramic steel"*.

Density of $ZrO_2$ can be increased during sintering by controlling the composition, particle size and temperature time cycle. It is 6.07 g/cm³.

- It has high compressive and tensile strength. Its flexural strength is more than 900 MPa
- The fracture resistance of all $ZrO_2$ crown is exceptionally high. This is major challenge in using these materials because they can wear the opposing tooth enamel and also it will be difficult to adjust occlusion in such crowns
- The fracture toughness of $Y_2O_3$-stabilized $ZrO_2$ is 9–13 $MPa.m^{1/2}$
- Modulus of elasticity is 200 GPa
- Poisson's ratio—0.30

Yttria-stabilized tetragonal $ZrO_2$ polycrystals are usually used for CAD-CAM milling and are of three types:
1. Those that are milled in Green state (compacted), e.g. Cercon (Dentsply), Lava (3M ESPE), ZirkonZahn (USA).
2. Those that are milled in partially sintered state, e.g. IPS e.max ZirCAD (Ivoclar Vivadent), VITA In-Ceram YZ Cubes (VITA Zahnfabrik), Everest (Kavo Dental), Precident DCS (DCS).
3. Those that are milled in fully sintered state, e.g. Zirkon Pro 50 (Cynovad), Everest ZH Blanks (Kavo Dental).

## Machinable Ceramics

Machinable ceramics can be milled to form inlays, onlays and veneers using special equipment.

### Classification of Machinable Ceramics

- *Digital systems (CAD-CAM):*
  - *Direct*: Multidimensional surface scanning directly of the tooth, e.g. Cerec 1 and 2
  - *Indirect*: Surface scanning via impression making and model fabrication, e.g. Automill, DCS president, Cicero, denti CAD, Sopha bioconcept
- *Analogous system (copying methods):* Copy milling/copy grinding or pantography systems
  - Manual copy milling, e.g. Celay
  - Automatic copy milling, e.g. Ceramatic II DCP.

### *Computer-aided Design and Computer-aided Manufacturing Ceramics*

Acronym for CAD-CAM is *computer aided design–computer aided manufacturer*. It was introduced to dental profession in 1970's by Duret in France, Altschuler in USA and Mormann and Brandestini in Switzerland. CAD-CAM technology in dentistry is used to replace time-consuming Lost-wax technology for fabricating prosthesis. This technique allows the clinician to create complex-shaped prosthesis using ceramic ingots. These ingots are machined to reproduce the planned restoration accurately. Although densely sintered ceramic ingot is available, which is nonporous but is difficult to mill. Therefore, they are wet milled and do not require further sintering. These restorations are produced within an hour thus, reducing the need for temporary restorations. It is possible to make highly esthetic, precise and quality restoration using this method.

*Historical background:*
- *1957: Dr Patrick J Hanratty*—Father of CAD-CAM technology—developed CAM software program called pronto
- *1971: Dr Francois Duret (France)*—First dental CAD-CAM device
- *1983: Dr Matts Anderson (Sweden)*—developed Procera
- *1980's: Dr Dianne Rekow (USA)*—developed CAD-CAM system using photographs and high-resolution scanner—mill restorations using 5 axis machine
- *1983:* First CAD-CAM restoration by *Dr Duret*—the Ganaciene Conference (France)
- *1985: Dr Werner Mormann* and *Dr Marco Brandestini (Switzerland)*—first commercial CAD-CAM system (CEREC).

*Component of computer-aided design and computer-aided manufacturing system:*
All CAD-CAM systems are complex and involve three steps:
1. *Step 1: Data acquisition:* The first step is collection of information to record the intraoral condition to the computer. This can be done by using an intraoral camera or by using a scanner. The scanning process can take place by using either **(Figs. 21.33A and B):**
   - *Optical scanner:* This scanner is used intraorally using either a white light or laser beam to scan the object of interest. In this method, information is obtained directly from the patient's mouth, e.g. Omnicam in CEREC system
   - *Mechanical scanner:* In this technique, the master cast, which is made after pouring the final impression, is scanned mechanically. It consists of a ruby ball and the master cast is read line-by-line. In this method, information is obtained indirectly by reading the master cast, e.g. Procera scanner from Nobel Biocare
2. *Step 2: Data processing:* The data obtained is transferred to the CAD software in the computer and the restoration is designed. This step is one of the important elements for successfully fabricating restoration **(Fig. 21.34)**
3. *Step 3: Digital fabrication process:* In this final step, the CAD model is transformed into the physical part by fabricating or manufacturing digitally. The restoration can be produced either chairside or in the laboratory **(Fig. 21.35).**

This digital manufacturing can take place in two ways:
1. Additive manufacturing
2. Subtractive manufacturing.

*Advantages:*
- Negligible porosity
- Impression is not required
- Single patient appointment
- Excellent patient acceptance
- Acceptable esthetics
- Good fracture resistance and strength.

*Disadvantages:*
- Expensive equipment
- Lack of computer-controlled processing support for occlusal equilibration

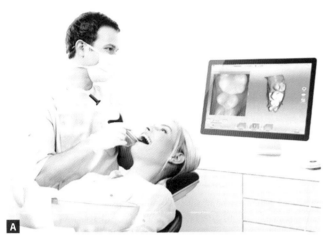

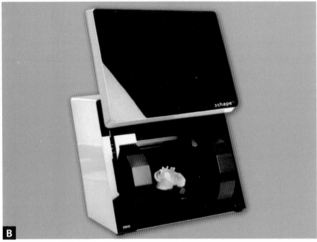

**Figs. 21.33 A and B:** Collection of digital data: (A) intraoral scanning; (B) Mechanical scanning.

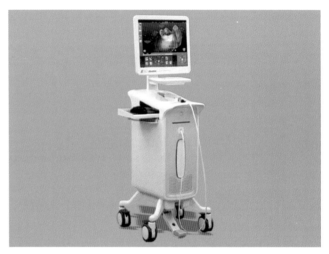

**Fig. 21.35:** Fabrication of the restoration either chairside or in the laboratory.

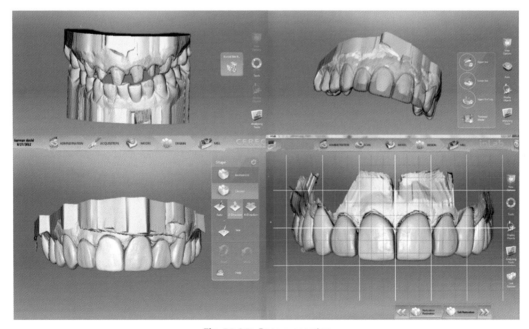

**Fig. 21.34:** Data processing.

- Highly technique sensitive.

Current CAD-CAM systems are:
- CEREC system **(Fig. 21.36)**
- DCS Precedent system
- Procera system
- Lava system
- Everest system
- Cercon system.

### Subtractive Manufacturing

In this technology, the material is removed from a block to form an object of desired geometry. This technique is used in conventional machining process such as milling process. This method is most commonly used in CAD-CAM dentistry currently because power-driven machines such as lathes, saw, milling machines, etc. are used to create the desired geometry of the object, which is digitally controlled.

*Milling procedure of CAD-CAM prosthesis:*
- Milling of $ZrO_2$ ceramics can be done in three forms:
  1. Green state milling
  2. Partially sintered milling
  3. Fully sintered milling.

*Procedure of CAD-CAM milling:* Any one of the above mentioned form of $ZrO_2$ blank is set in the milling machine holder. The machine is programmed as to compensate for the expected sintering shrinkage. The milling tool is inserted and set according to the manufacturer's instructions. Ceramic blank is milled and machined as desired. Then the milled restoration along with the residual blank is removed from the mount. The milled restoration is separated from the residual blank using a diamond disk. The restoration is cleaned and dried. It is then placed in the hot zone of the sintering furnace for sintering. This process aids in achieving adequate density of the restoration. After sintering process, allow it to cool and then inspect for any surface or subsurface flaws. Any adjustment needed is done using water-cooled diamond disk. The final restoration may require ceramic veneering or can be used in the monolith form.

### Copy Milling Method

This method of milling ceramic blanks is based on a mechanical scanner, which traces the surface of the prefabricated pattern of the restoration made of composite resin. The resin pattern can be made directly on the tooth in the patient mouth or can be prepared on the die after making impression. A copy milling machine has two areas one in which resin pattern is mounted and another area where a ceramic blank is mounted. As the mechanical scanning tool passes over the resin pattern **(Fig. 21.37)**, the milling tool simultaneously cuts through the ceramic blank duplicating the movement. Milled restoration is then veneered with porcelain **(Fig. 21.38)** and characterized using appropriate shades. Currently, In-Ceram spinel or In-Ceram alumina is used to fabricate inlays, onlays and crowns. This technique is commonly used in Celay system (Mikrona Technologies, Spreintenbach, Switzerland). Since this technique is dependent on the profile tracing ability of the technician, the restoration formed is inferior to that formed through other method such as heat pressing.
- *Advantages*:
  - Create fine details such undercuts and voids
  - Create precise internal geometry.
- *Disadvantages*:
  - Wastage of material by milling
  - Cannot be effectively used for mass production.

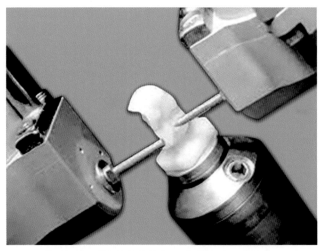

**Fig. 21.36:** CEREC CAD/CAM milled by diamond disc.

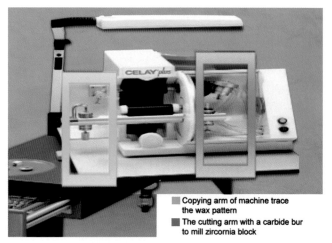

■ Copying arm of machine trace the wax pattern
■ The cutting arm with a carbide bur to mill zircornia block

**Fig. 21.37:** Copy milling method

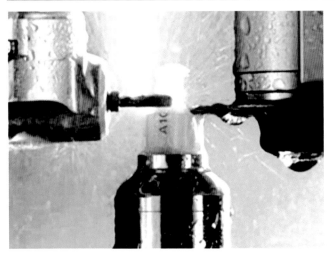

**Fig. 21.38:** Milling of ceramic blank.

## Additive Manufacturing

Also called as *3D printing, desktop manufacturing, rapid manufacturing, rapid prototyping and additive layer manufacturing* (**Figs. 21.39A and B**).

### Definition
*It is a process of joining materials to make objects from three-dimensional (3D) model data, usually layer upon layer, as opposed to subtractive manufacturing methodologies.*
                    *—ASTM International (ASTM 2792-12)*

*Uses of additive manufacturing in dentistry*
- Fabrication of surgical guides
- Fabrication of study models
- Veneers and laminates for try-in
- Aligners used in orthodontics
- Wax patterns for fabricating inlays, onlays, crowns and bridges
- For fabrication of maxillofacial prosthesis
- Has potential to create human clones, bioengineer living organs, tissues, etc.

*Types of additive manufacturing*
- Stereolithography (SLA)
- Laminated object manufacturing
- Laser powder-forming techniques
- Solid ground curing
- Fused deposition modeling
- Selective electron beam melting
- 3D ink-jet printing
- Robocasting.

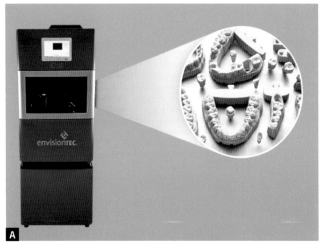

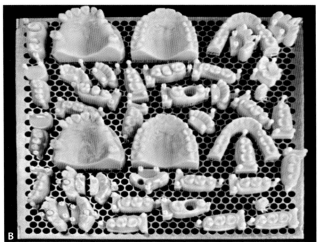

**Figs. 21.39A and B:** Additive manufacturing.

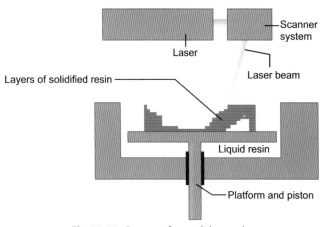

**Fig. 21.40:** Process of stereolithography.

1.  *Stereolithography (Fig. 21.40):*
    – First introduced by *Charles W Hull* in 1986
    – It is method of making solid object by successfully printing thin layers of an ultraviolet (UV) curable material one on top of the other
    – First 3D model is created in CAD model up into thin layers
    – Laser scans the liquid resin in vat and creates the first layer
    – Successive layers are printed until the object is complete
    – Final object is rinsed with solvent to remove uncured resin.

    *Uses:*
    – Builds model by laser fusing a photopolymer layer-by-layer
    – Used for making surgical guides for implant placement
    – Also used to fabricate temporary crowns and bridges **(Fig. 21.41)**
    – Used for fabricating customized implants such as cranioplasties, orbital floors and onlays.
2.  *Fused deposition modeling:*
    – It is an additive manufacturing technology, which is used to model, prototype and produce appliances **(Figs. 21.42A and B)**
    – First developed by *Scott Crump* in late 1980s
    – Principle—laying down materials in layers
    – Material used are polycarbonates, polycaprolactone, polyphenylsulfones and waxes.
3.  *3D Bioplotter from Envisiontec:*
    – Bioplotter is capable of printing multiple materials to build 3D structure **(Fig. 21.43)**

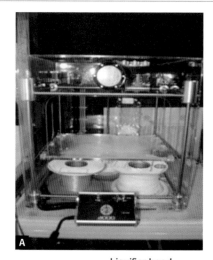

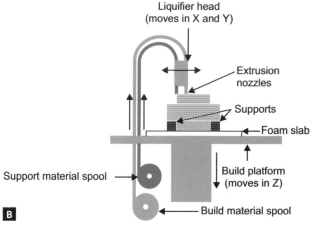

**Figs. 21.42A and B:** Fused deposition modeling.

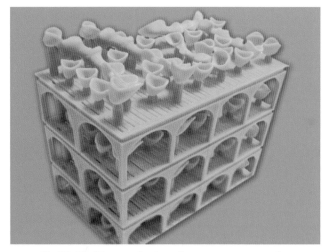

**Fig. 21.41:** Mass production of temporary crowns using stereolithography method.

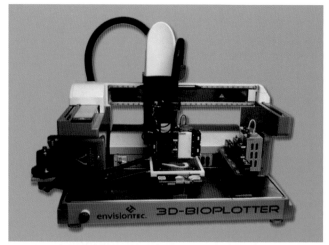

**Fig. 21.43:** 3D Bioplotter by Envisiontec.

- Used for modeling scaffolds for tissue engineering and organ printing
- Ceramic pastes used for creating bone, bioresorbable polymers
- Human body parts can be created through this technique.

4. *Selective electron beam melting*:
   - This technology manufactures parts by melting metal powders layer-by-layer with an electron beam in a high vacuum
   - Stream of electrons is created by heating tungsten filament
   - Powder particles fuse together giving shape to desired object
   - Powder particles can be polyethylene, polyamide, metal powders of titanium or cobalt-chromium (Co-Cr) alloys
   - Has wide application in orthopedics, maxillofacial surgery, implant dentistry, maxillofacial reconstruction **(Fig. 21.44)**.

5. *Laser powder forming technique*:
   - Selective laser melting (SLM) or selective laser sintering **(Fig. 21.45)**
   - It directs high power laser using mirrors at a substrate consisting of fine layers of powder
   - Creates melt pool and the particle fuse together
   - After each cross-section is scanned, the powder bed is lowered by one layer thickness, new layer of material is applied and the process is continued
   - Range of metal powders such as steel, titanium, titanium alloys, Co-Cr alloys
   - Range of polymers such as polyamides, ultra-high molecular weight polyethylene, polycaprolactone, composite resins

- Widely used in prosthodontics to create complex geometries
- For ceramic industry, it is called as *direct metal laser sintering (DMLS)*
- Used for making facial prosthesis, drug delivery devices and in tissue engineering.

6. *3D ink-jet printing*:
   - Ink-jet printing is accomplished using ink-jet printer, which have a capacity to print at a high resolution by ejecting small ink drops. This ink drops can be aqueous solution of ceramic suspension, cell solution to form tissue extracts, polymers, etc.
   - Its mechanism of action is by selectively depositing binding material through a print head in order to fuse a thin layer of powder to a previously fused layer. The fusing of previous layer can be by UV light, heat, drying or chemical reaction
   - Used in fabrication of ceramic inlays, onlays, crowns, maxillofacial prosthesis **(Fig. 21.46)**.

7. *Robocasting*:
   - Also called as *Direct Ink Writing (DIW)*
   - It is a rapid prototyping technique, which helps in fabricating objects based on layering method
   - It uses aqueous solution of colloidal paste, which is controlled by computers to extrude on a flat substrate without using molds
   - This method does not require drying or solidification as in fused deposition modeling. It maintains its shape as soon as it contacts the substrate
   - It creates 3D-printed structure by the conversion of SLA file
   - Used in orthopedics for bone and tissue engineering
   - It is used in *Bioprinting* of biocompatible tissue implants.

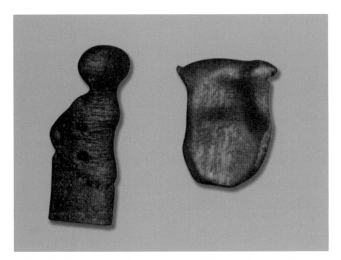

**Fig. 21.44:** Selective electron beam melting used to reconstruct temporomandibular joint.

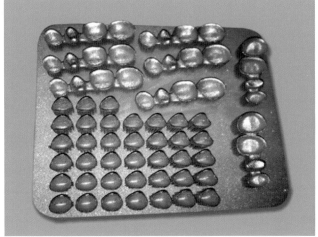

**Fig. 21.45:** Metal crowns formed using laser powder forming technique.

8. *Bioink:*
   - It is a colloidal paste or hydrogel, which is used to 3D print tissue models in a Bioprinter **(Fig. 21.47)**
   - It is capable of promoting cell adhesion, migration and cell differentiation
   - It can simulate natural extracellular matrix and is biodegradable
   - It is used in skin grafting.

*Advantages of additive manufacturing:*
- Ability to create any geometry
- Capability to spatially grade composition and microstructure
- Does not require previous mold
- Precise control of internal morphology, shape distribution and connectivity
- With advancements and broader acceptance cost of materials and laboratory can be lower in long run

- Dental care can improve drastically for medically compromised, old patients
- Has potential to improve quality of life, better patient satisfaction in terms of function, esthetics and comfort.

*Disadvantages of additive manufacturing:*
- Limitation in relation to speed
- Costly
- Choice of materials is limited
- Need both hard and soft skills to operate
- Patient input is minimal
- Current material and laboratory cost is much higher
- Greater research needed
- Evidence-based research (real world proofing)
- Maintenance and safety issues
- Environmental aspects
- Legal aspects especially printing of living tissues.

## Procera System

- *Dr Matts Anderson* developed the Procera system in Sweden
- This system uses CAD-CAM to fabricate a framework in alumina, $ZrO_2$ or titanium and then uses specialized ceramic with compatible coefficient of thermal expansion
- It is one of the hardest ceramic used in dentistry. Procera zirconia has flexural resistance of 1,100–1,200 MPa and compression resistance of 900 ncm
- Indicated for veneers, inlays, onlays, anterior and posterior crowns
- The Procera system consists of Procera scanner, which scans the surface of the die which obtained from the impression using mechanical profiling device and transfers the data to the milling unit **(Fig. 21.48)**

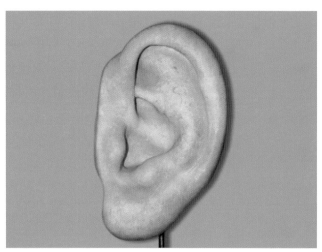

**Fig. 21.46:** Fabrication of maxillofacial prosthesis using 3D printing technique.

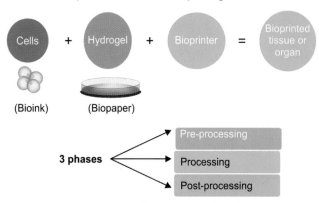

**Fig. 21.47:** Essential components of bioprinting.

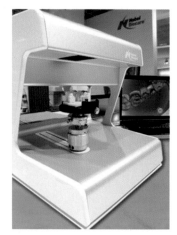

**Fig. 21.48:** Procera scanner.

- Milling unit produces an enlarged die with the help of CAD-CAM process
- Core ceramic is dry pressed on the die and is then sintered and veneered
- 15–20% of the core shrinkage is compensated by fabricating oversized ceramic pattern, which will shrink to the desired size during sintering to fit the prepared tooth
- Procera All Ceram core is more translucent than the In-Ceram $ZrO_2$.

## CLINICAL SIGNIFICANCE

Internal surface of alumina core is sandblasted using silica-coated alumina particles to ensure adequate bonding. Acid etching of this surface does not provide micromechanical retention and should be avoided.

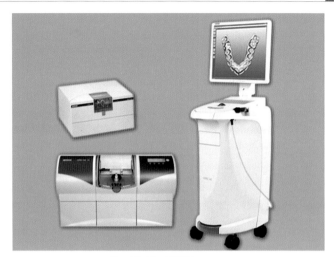

**Fig. 21.49:** CEREC system.

- CEREC system consists of a 3D video camera, an electronic image processor, digital processor and miniature milling machine **(Fig. 21.49)**.

*Procedure:*
- Tooth is prepared for all ceramic restorations
- Preparation is coated with opaque powder
- Preparation is imaged with an optical scanner and the best view image is stored in the computer
- The finish lines and contours are identified and marked on the screen with the help of the software
- Appropriated shade of ceramic block is inserted into the milling machine and the grinding procedure is initiated
- The ceramic block is grinded by a diamond-coated disk, which is controlled by the computer
- The fabrication time for single crown is 20 minutes. The crown is characterized by adding appropriate shades
- Restoration is then acid-etched and silane-coupling agent is applied in preparation to bond onto the tooth preparation.

*Types*
- Procera All Ceram—consists of 99.9% alumina core
- Procera All Titan—contains titanium used for making framework
- Procera All Zirkon—consists of densely sintered zircon oxide stabilized by $Y_2O_3$
- Procera custom abutments—can be made of alumina, titanium or $ZrO_2$.

*Advantages*
- Excellent esthetics
- Good shade stability
- Reduced laboratory time
- Excellent adaptation
- Less-technique sensitive
- Better flexural resistance when compared to other ceramic systems.

*Disadvantages*
- Costly equipment
- Need special laboratory with a scanner
- Require special training for technician
- Limited clinical use confined to single crowns and selected cases of three unit FPDs.

*Indications*
- Anterior and posterior crowns
- Veneers
- Inlays and onlays
- Crowns for implants
- Three unit FPDs with distal abutment being the first molar.

### CEREC System

- The CEREC system was originally developed by *Brains AG*, Switzerland 1986

## PORCELAIN REPAIR

- As porcelain is brittle in nature, occasionally it can fracture
- Porcelain repair can be done rather than replacing the restoration
- Number of porcelain repair systems are available for this purpose.

### Procedure

- The fractured restoration is isolated
- The porcelain surrounding the fractured area is trimmed using a diamond abrasive bur
- The fractured area is etched using an etching gel

- After etching the area is washed and dried
- Then silane-coupling agent is applied over the porcelain surface and metal-bonding agent is applied over the exposed metal portion
- Bonding resin is applied over the entire surface
- Then appropriate shade composite is applied and cured following manufacturer's instructions **(Figs. 21.50A and B)**
- Shear bond strength of repair systems usually varies between 10 MPa and 15 MPa.

## CEMENTATION

### Cementation of Metal Ceramic Restorations

- The internal surface of the restoration is sandblasted with alumina particles
- Any conventional luting agent can be used to lute metal ceramic restoration with tooth structure
- Commonly used luting agents are zinc phosphate cement, glass ionomer cement, zinc polycarboxylate cement, etc.

### Cementation for Conventional Glass Ceramics

- Glass ceramic restoration is surface treated by etching with 5–9.5% hydrofluoric acid and the prepared tooth structure is etched by using 37% phosphoric acid gel

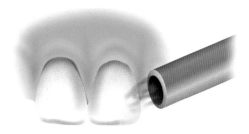

**Fig. 21. 50A:** Repair composite is applied and cured.

- Then silane coupling agent is applied on the internal surface of ceramic restorations to facilitate bonding between the tooth and the restorations
- Appropriate shade of the resin luting agent is selected
- Resin is used to lute the glass ceramic restorations
- Chemical cure, light cure or dual cure resin cement can be used to lute ceramic restorations.

### Cementation for Glass-infiltrated and Alumina-based Ceramic

- Glass-infiltrated and alumina-based ceramics are effectively roughened by tribochemical silica-coating process
- Surface of the restoration is coated with 110 µm of high-purity aluminum oxide for 14 seconds to create uniform pattern of roughness
- The surface is then conditioned with silicone coupler to facilitate bonding with composite resin
- Appropriate shade of resin cement is selected **(Fig. 21.51)**
- The restoration is luted with the selected resin cement.

### Cementation with Zirconia-based Restorations

- Since $ZrO_2$-based restorations have high-fracture resistance, they do not require an adhesive interface for retention
- $ZrO_2$-based restorations can be luted with conventional glass ionomer cement, resin-modified glass ionomer and resin cement.

## PORCELAIN DENTURE TEETH

- Porcelain denture teeth have composition and properties, which vary from the ceramics used for fixed prosthodontics
- Usually porcelain teeth are composed of feldspar, 15% quartz and 4% kaolin

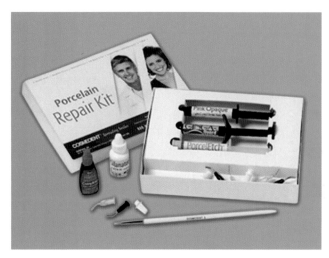

**Fig. 21.50B:** Porcelain repair kit.

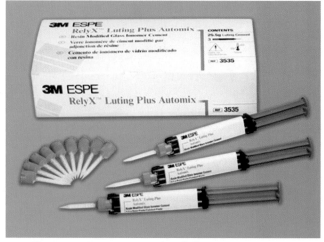

**Fig. 21. 51:** Resin cement to bond all ceramic restorations.

- They are retained on the denture base by mechanical interlocking
- Anterior porcelain teeth are retained by metal pins and posterior teeth are retained by creating diatoric holes through which resin flows **(Figs. 21.52A and B)**
- Either acrylic teeth or porcelain teeth can be used to fabricate complete or partial dentures.

## Advantages

- Excellent esthetics
- Excellent biocompatibility
- High resistance to wear and distortion
- Allows the denture to be rebased.

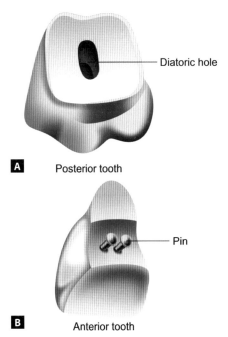

**A**  Posterior tooth

**B**  Anterior tooth

**Figs. 21. 52A and B:** Porcelain teeth attached by mechanical means.

## Disadvantages

- Require mechanical attachments for retention
- Brittle in nature
- Produce clicking sound on contact with opposing teeth
- Require greater inter-ridge distance
- Cannot be polished easily after grinding
- Greater density increases weight of the denture
- Mismatch in thermal expansion coefficient produces stresses in acrylic denture base.

## ABRASIVENESS OF PORCELAIN

Dental porcelain is known to cause catastrophic wear of the opposing tooth enamel. Wear is extremely high when rough unglazed surface of ceramic restoration opposes the natural tooth in patient with parafunctional habits.

Abrasiveness of porcelain against the tooth enamel is affected by number of factors such as:

- Hardness, fatigue resistance, tensile strength, fracture toughness, particle glass bonding, amount and frequency of force, chewing patterns, lubrication with saliva and abrasiveness of food particles. More the difference of hardness between two sliding surfaces greater will be degree of wear.

*Steps to minimize wear of tooth enamel by dental ceramics are*:

- Eliminate occlusal prematurities
- Provide canine-guided occlusion
- To use metal restorations in functional bruxing patients
- If occlusion is ceramic, then ultra-low fusing ceramics should be used
- Polish the functional ceramic contacts
- Readjustment of occlusion periodically
- Repolishing of ceramic surfaces periodically.

## TEST YOURSELF

### Essay Questions

1. Classify dental ceramics. Describe in detail composition of feldspathic porcelain.
2. Discuss in detail metal-ceramic restorations.
3. Discuss the metal alloys used in metal ceramic restorations.
4. Classify all-ceramic materials. Discuss zirconia-based ceramics.
5. Discuss composition and properties of dental ceramics.
6. Discuss methods to strengthen ceramics.
7. Discuss CAD-CAM ceramics.
8. Discuss bonding of ceramic with metals and its failures.
9. Describe the steps in fabrication of metal-ceramic prosthesis.

### Short Notes

1. In-Ceram alumina.
2. Hot-pressed ceramics.
3. Zirconia ceramics.
4. Dicor ceramics.
5. Transformation toughening.
6. Partially stabilized zirconia.
7. Additive manufacturing in CAD-CAM ceramics.
8. Copy milling.

9. Glazing in ceramics.
10. Glass ceramics.

## Multiple Choice Questions

1. Most of shrinkage during firing occurs in which stage?
   A. Fusion
   B. Low-bisque stage
   C. Medium-bisque stage
   D. High-bisque stage
2. Shrinkage during firing can be reduced to great extent, if:
   A. Particle size is increased
   B. Fusion temperature is increased
   C. By thorough condensation before firing
   D. All of the above
3. "Pop-off" of ceramic veneer from the underlying gold crown is due to:
   A. Too thick an application of a pure gold surface conditioner
   B. Contamination at the metal-ceramic interface
   C. Underfiring of the opaque layer
   D. All of the above
4. Porcelain bonded to metal is strongest when it is fired:
   A. Slowly
   B. Under tension
   C. Under compression
   D. Fired number of times before completion
5. First commercially castable ceramic material for dental use was:
   A. Dicor
   B. Cerestore
   C. Magnesium aluminate spinel
   D. None of the above
6. To prevent porosity in dental porcelain it should be baked:
   A. In an atmosphere of nitrogen
   B. In presence of air
   C. In vacuum
   D. Under pressure
7. Yttria-stabilized zirconia is added in porcelain to:
   A. Provide opacity
   B. Undergoes crystalline change when placed under stress
   C. Interferes with crack propagation
   D. All of the above
8. When sintering porcelain on metal between which two stage it is critical to prevent contamination for better bonding?
   A. Heat treatment and opaque firing
   B. Opaque firing and bisque firing
   C. Heat treatment and presoldering
   D. Bisque and glazing
9. Indium is added to metal alloy for porcelain fused to metal for:
   A. Improve bonding
   B. To increase strength
   C. To reduce porosity
   D. To match thermal expansion of metal and porcelain
10. Constituent used in porcelain preparation that fuses at high temperature and forms a matrix is:
    A. Soda ash
    B. Quartz
    C. Feldspar
    D. Kaolin
11. Stains in porcelain restoration result in all of the following, *except*:
    A. Reduced value
    B. Increased metamerism
    C. Difficulty in glazing
    D. None of the above
12. Part of the CAD restoration, which is more vulnerable to wear during polishing is:
    A. Occlusal surface
    B. Cemental margin
    C. Proximal surface
    D. Labial surface

## ANSWERS

| | | | |
|---|---|---|---|
| 1. D | 2. C | 3. D | 4. C |
| 5. A | 6. C | 7. D | 8. A |
| 9. A | 10. C | 11. C | 12. B |

## BIBLIOGRAPHY

1. Albakry M, Guazzato M, Swain MV. Influence of hot pressing on the microstructure and fracture toughness of two pressable dental glass-ceramics. J Biomed Mater Res B Appl Biomater. 2004;71:99-107.
2. Albakry M, Guazzato M, Swain MVA. Fracture toughness and hardness evaluation of three pressable all-ceramic dental materials. J Dent. 2003;31:181-8.
3. Anusavice KJ. Phillip's Science of Dental Materials, 11th edition. St. Louis: Elsevier, 2003. pp. 655-719.
4. Anusavice KJ. Recent developments in restorative dentistry. J Am Dent Assoc. 1993;124:72-4.
5. Barnes A, Gingell JC, George D, Adachi E, Jefferies S, Sundar V. Clinical evaluation of an all ceramic restorative system: 24 month report. Am J Dent. 2006;19:206-10.
6. Beuer F, Edelhoff D, Gernet W, Sorensen JA. Three year clinical prospective evaluation of zirconia-based posterior fixed dental prosthesis (FDPs). Clin Oral Invest. 2009;13:445-51.
7. Cesar PF, Soki FN, Yoshimura HN, Gonzaga CC, Styopkin V. Influence of leucite content on slow crack growth of dental porcelains. Dent Mater. 2008;24:1114-22.
8. Conrad JH, Seong JW, Pesun JI. Current ceramic materials and systems with clinical recommendations: A systematic review. J Prosthet Dent. 2007;98:389-404.

9. DeHoff PH, Anusavice KJ. Viscoelastic finite element stress analysis of the thermal compatibility of dental bilayer ceramic systems. Int J Prosthodont. 2009;22:56-61.

10. Della Bona A, Kelly JR. The clinical success of all ceramic restorations. J Am Dent Assoc. 2008;34:841-7.

11. Denry IL, Kelly J, Donovan TE. State of the art of zirconia for dental applications. Dent Mater. 2008;24:299-307.

12. Denry IL. Recent advances in ceramics for dentistry. Crit Rev Oral Biol Med. 1996;7:134-43.

13. El Attaoui H, Saadaoui M, Chevalier J, Fantozzi G. Static and cyclic crack propagation in Ce-TZP ceramics with different amounts of transformation toughening. J Eur Ceram Soc. 2007;27:483-6.

14. Griggs JA. Recent advances in materials for all ceramic restorations. Dent Clin N Am. 2007;51:713-27.

15. Grossman DG. Cast glass ceramics. Dent Clin North Am. 1985;29:719-23.

16. Guazzato M, Albakry M, Swain VM. Mechanical properties of In-Ceram Alumina and In-Ceram Zirconia. Int J Prosthodont. 2002;15:339-46.

17. Guazzato M, Walton TR, Franklin W, et al. Influence of thickness and cooling rate on development of spontaneous cracks in porcelain/zirconia structure. Aust Dent J. 2010;55:306-10.

18. Hummel M, Kern M. Durability of the resin bond strength to the alumina ceramic Procera. Dent Mater. 2004;20:498-508.

19. Karl M, Fischer H, Graef F, Wichmann MG, Taylor TD, Heckmann SM. Structural changes in ceramic veneered three-unit implant supported restorations as a consequence of static and dynamic loading. Dent Mater. 2008;24:464-70.

20. Kelly JR, Denry I. Stabilized zirconia as a structural ceramic: An overview. Dent Mater. 2008;24:289-98.

21. Kelly JR, Nishimura I, Campbell SD. Ceramics in dentistry: historical roots and current perspectives. J Prosthet Dent. 1996;75:18-32.

22. Kelly JR. Dental ceramics: What is this stuff anyway? J Am Dent Assoc. 2008;139:4S-7S.

23. Kelly JR. Dental ceramics: current thinking and trends. Dent Clin North Am. 2004;48:513-30.

24. Kohorst P, Herzog TJ, Borchers L, Stiesch-Scholz M. Load-bearing capacity of all-ceramic posterior four unit fixed partial dentures with different zirconia frameworks. Eur J Oral Sci. 2007;115:161-6.

25. Kosmac T, Oblak C, Marion L. The effects of dental grinding and sandblasting on ageing and fatigue behavior of dental zirconia Y-TZP ceramics. J Eur Ceram Soc. 2008;28:1085-90.

26. Layton DM, Clarke M. A systemic review and meta-analysis of the survival of feldspathic porcelain veneers over 5 and 10 years. Int J Prosthodont. 2012;25:590-603.

27. Layton DM, Clarke M. A systemic review and meta-analysis of the survival of non-feldspathic porcelain veneers over 5 and 10 years. Int J Prosthodont. 2013;26:111-24.

28. Lee JJ, Kwon JY, Bhowmick S, Lloyd IK, Rekow ED, Lawn BR. Veneer vs. core failure in adhesively bonded all-ceramic crown layers. J Dent Res. 2008;87:363-6.

29. Lohbauer U, Petschelt A, Greil P. Lifetime prediction of CAD/CAM dental ceramics. J Biomed Mater Res. 2002;63:780-5.

30. Luthardt R, Holzhuter M, Rudolph H, et al. CAD-CAM machining effects on Y-TZP zirconia. Dent Mater. 2004;20:655-62.

31. Mantri SS, Bhasin AS. CAD/CAM in dental restorations: An overview. Ann Ess Dent. 2010;11:123-8.

32. Mc Laren AE. Ceramics in dentistry—Part I: classes of material. Inside Dentistry. 2009: 94-103.

33. Mc Lean JW, Hughs TH. The reinforcement of dental porcelain with ceramic oxides. Br Dent J. 1965;119:251-67.

34. Mc Lean JW. Evolution of dental ceramics in the twentieth century. J Prosthet Dent. 2001;85:61-6.

35. Noort RV. The future of dental devices is digital. Dental Mater. 2012;28:3-12.

36. Oilo M, Gjerdet NR, Tvinnereim HM. The firing procedure influences properties of a zirconia core ceramic. Dent Mater. 2008;24:471-5.

37. Pjetursson BE, Sailer I, Zwahlen M, et al. A systematic review of the survival and complication rates of all ceramic and metal ceramic reconstructions after an observation period of at least 3 years. Part 1: Single crowns. Clin Oral Implants Res. 2007;18:73-85.

38. Raigrodski JA. Contemporary materials and technologies for all ceramic fixed partial dentures: A review of literature. J Prosthet Dent. 2004;92:557-62.

39. Rosenstiel SF, Gupta PK, Van der Sluys RA, Zimmerman MH. Strength of a dental glass ceramic after surface coating. Dent Mater. 1993;9:274-6.

40. Sailer I, Feher A, Filser F, et al. Five-year clinical results of zirconia frameworks for posterior fixed partial dentures. Int J Prosthodont. 2007;20:383-8.

41. Scherrer SS, Quinn GD, Quinn JB. Fractographic failure analysis of a Procera All Ceram crown using stereo and scanning electron microscopy. Dent Mater. 2008;24:1107-13.

42. Shillingburg TH, Hobo S, Whitett DL, Jacobi R. Fundamentals of Fixed Prosthodontics, 3rd edn. Quitessence Publication; 1997. pp. 433-54.

43. Spear F, Hollaway J. Which all—ceramic system is optimal for anterior esthetics? J Am Dent Assoc. 2008;139:19S-24S.

44. Teixeira EC, Piascik JR, Stoner BR, Thompson JY. Dynamic fatigue and strength characterization of three ceramic materials. J Mater Sci Master Med. 2007;18:1219-24.

45. Tinschert J, Natt G, Mautsch W, Spiekermann H, Anusavice KJ. Marginal fit of alumina and zirconia-based fixed partial dentures produced by a CAD-CAM system. Oper Dent. 2001;26:367-74.

46. Tinschert J, Zwez D, Marx R, Anusavice KJ. Structural reliability of alumina-, feldspar-, leucite-, mica- and zirconia based ceramics. J Dent. 2000;8:529-35.

47. Wang H, Aboushelib MN, Feilzae AJ. Strength influencing variables on CAD/CAM zirconia frameworks. Dent Mater. 2008;24:633-8.

48. Zandparsa R. Digital imaging and fabrication. Dent Clin N Am. 2014;58:135-58.

49. Zhang Y, Lawn B, Rekow E, Thompson VP. Effect of sandblasting on the long-term performance of dental ceramics. J Biomed Mater Res B Appl Biomater. 2004;71:381-6.

50. Zhu Q, deWith G, Dortmans LJ, Feenstra F. Subcritical crack growth behavior of Al2O3—glass dental composites. J Biomed Mater Res B Appl Biomater. 2003;65:233-8.

# Nature of Metals and Alloys

*'Too little confidence and you're unable to act, too much confidence and you're unable to hear.'*

*—John Maeda*

## INTRODUCTION

Mostly metals used in dentistry are in the form of alloys or mixtures of one or more metals. The use of metal has reduced over period of time and has been replaced by esthetic materials such as composite resin or ceramics. However, cast metal is widely used to fabricate copings or substructures for metal-ceramic restorations which are currently one of the most commonly used restorations. It is, therefore, important to understand the basics of metals and alloys used in dentistry.

## DEFINITIONS

### Metal

*Any strong and relatively ductile substance that provides electropositive ions to a corrosive environment and that can be polished to a high luster.*

*—GPT 8th Edition*

### Alloy

*A mixture of two or more metals or metalloids that are mutually soluble in the molten state.*

*—GPT 8th Edition*

## METALS AND ALLOYS

The study of metal and alloys is called as *metallurgy*. Metals are one of the important class of material which are widely used in dentistry to replace missing teeth and adjacent structures. They are composed of metallic elements which has characteristic feature of high strength, high thermal and electrical conductivity, ductility, opacity and high luster. Each metal is distinguished from others on the basis of strength, hardness, ductility, malleability, melting point, nobility, thermal and electrical conductivity and specific gravity. Out of 118 elements in the periodic table, about 88 (or 74.6%) are pure metals **(Fig. 22.1)**. When two or more metals or nonmetals are mixed, they form *alloys*. This combination of metals is called as *alloying*.

Metals which are used in dentistry are usually in the form of alloys except for pure gold foil, commercially pure titanium and endodontic silver points. Metal and alloys used in restorations are crystalline solids. All solid metals are good conductors of heat and electricity, exhibit high luster, has high fracture toughness, has ability to absorb energy and inhibit crack propagation under increasing tensile load. Pure metals have limited use in dentistry and therefore combinations of one or more metals or nonmetals are used. All alloys used in dentistry should be biocompatible and corrosion resistant.

Each metal alloys have unique characteristics and properties. The metal alloys vary in properties than those of pure metals. They vary among each other in hardness, brittleness, toughness, ductility, electrical and thermal conductivity, color, density, malleability, specific gravity, wear resistance, corrosion resistance and weldability. For example, when elemental iron is alloyed with small amount of carbon it forms steel which can be used in high stress areas. If another element chromium is added to iron and carbon alloy it form stainless steel. The corrosion resistance of stainless steel is greatly improved because of the formation of passivating layer of chromium oxide.

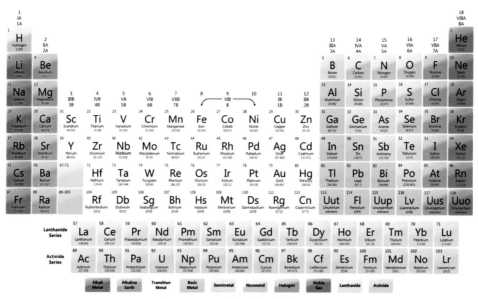

**Fig. 22.1:** Periodic table of elements.

Metals are grouped according to the electronic configuration of the outermost shell. They vary in their density, ductility, melting point and nobility in the periodic table. They are classified as alkali metal, alkaline earth metals, transition metals and rare earth metals. Properties of metals do not suddenly change from metallic to nonmetallic side of the table but the boundary is indistinct **(Fig. 22.1)**. The element close to the boundary have properties of both metal and nonmetal. As mentioned earlier mostly alloys are used in dentistry. Dental casting alloys are commonly made of metals such as cobalt, gold, chromium, iron, nickel, palladium, silver, copper and titanium.

Noble metals are highly corrosion resistant metals which do not require any other metal for protection against corrosion. However, they need to be alloyed with other elements to improve fracture toughness, strength and hardness. Noble metals are gold, iridium, osmium, palladium, platinum, rhodium and ruthenium. For use in metal ceramic restorations noble metals are alloyed with oxidizable elements such as iron, tin and indium to improve bonding of metal with ceramic.

## Uses of Metal or Alloys in Dentistry

- For direct intracoronal restorations such as using direct filling gold
- For fabrication of extracoronal restorations such as inlays, onlays, crowns and fixed partial dentures
- For fabricating superstructures, cast frameworks, cast partial dentures, etc.
- For surgical use such as making titanium plates, screws, etc.

- For orthodontic use in making wires, brackets, bands, etc.
- For making laboratory instruments and materials
- For making surgical instruments.

## Desirable Properties of Metal

- Should have high strength
- Should be malleable and ductile
- Should have good thermal and electrical conductivity
- Should have high fracture toughness
- Should have high luster
- Should have high corrosion resistance.

Complex dental alloys used in dentistry are: (1) Dental amalgam consisting of mercury, silver, tin and copper; (2) Noble metal alloys consisting primarily of gold, platinum, palladium, silver, etc.; (3) Base metal alloys majorly consist of nickel, cobalt, chromium, iron, titanium and number of secondary elements.

## Structure of Metal

All metals are crystalline in nature. It refers to regular arrangement of atoms. The crystallinity of each metal varies from one type of metal to another depending on the electronic configuration of each metal **(Fig. 22.2)**. For fabrication of a metallic structure, a metal or alloy is melted, molded and then cooled to the desired shape to again form a crystalline solid.

It is interesting to note that dental amalgam and gold are the only metallic dental materials which solidify at oral temperature as against the above discussion that solid is

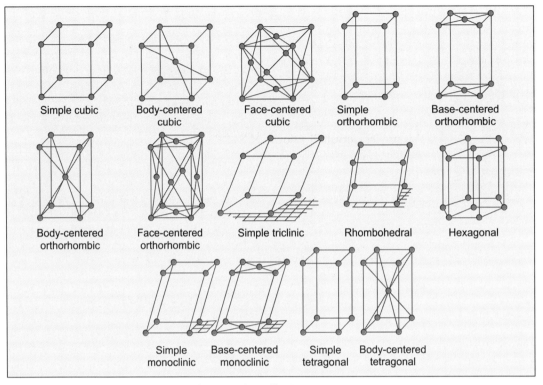

**Fig. 22.2:** Crystal lattice structure.

formed from high temperature (molten) to low temperature (cooling). In amalgam solidification takes place when silver and tin alloy powder is mixed with liquid mercury (metal) to form crystalline structure at oral temperature. The silver and mercury atoms organize to form a regular crystalline structure, i.e. $\gamma_1$ phase.

### Solidification of Metal

This process occurs during the freezing of a pure metal in a clean container. When the molten alloy is allowed to cool, alloy particles are first to solidify as the temperature lowers below the liquidus. The alloy particles acts as nuclei on which other alloy particles solidify. This process of formation of nuclei is called as nucleation. As the temperature lowers further to cool the molten alloy these nuclei forms crystals called as "grains". During the solidification phase the *crystals* or *grains* continue to grow as more atoms join them through metallic bonds. Ultimately each crystal grows to meet other growing crystal forming a boundary *(grain boundary)*. This grain boundary restricts further growth in that direction. Therefore, on solidification structure of solid consists of thousands of crystals haphazardly placed.

The solid structure is always more stable than the liquid phase. Also, in the liquid phase the atoms have higher energy than at the solid state. As the molten metal (liquid phase) is cooled to solid state, there is loss of energy. This

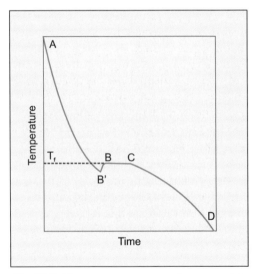

**Fig. 22.3:** Time-temperature curve for pure metal.

change of energy is called the latent heat of solidification and is equal to the heat of fusion.

If a pure metal is melted and allowed to cool to room temperature in a clean container, a time-temperature cooling curve as shown in **Figure 22.3.** As the molten metal cools, the temperature drops sharply from point A to point B'. Then temperature increases from point B' to point B. The temperature at this point remains constant till the point C.

Subsequently, the temperature reduces sharply to room temperature. The temperature $T_f$ indicated on the graph represents the *fusion temperature or the melting point* of the pure metal. During melting, temperature remains constant but at the time of freezing or solidification, latent heat of solidification is released as metal changes from high-energy liquid state to low-energy liquid state.

The initial cooling of the molten metal from $T_f$ to B' is called as *supercooling*. During this process, crystallization of the pure metal occurs. Once the crystals begin to form, release of latent heat of fusion causes the temperature to rise until the crystallization is completed at point C. Supercooling of pure metals only occurs in inert atmosphere and in clean containers.

## Nucleation

As the molten metal cools, solid structure forms rapidly. This solid structure forms atom clusters which are called as *nuclei of crystallization* or *embryos*. This process of nucleation can occur by two mechanisms:
1. Homogeneous nucleation
2. Heterogeneous nucleation.

### Homogeneous Nucleation

This process occurs when liquid phase is rapidly cooled to form solid structure. During this process, there is rapid loss of energy resulting in formation of irregular polycrystalline grains. In this process, there is no foreign particle added to promote uniform nucleation. The homogenously formed nuclei are randomly formed and are bonded together in a crystalline form. The nuclei act as seeds for the formation of embryos. The embryos are randomly formed small clusters of atoms which have same crystalline arrangement as the resultant atomic state found in the solidified alloy.

### Heterogeneous Nucleation

It is a process of seeding the nuclei with a foreign solid particle to reduce the grain size *(grain refiner)*. These are high melting elements such as Iridium added to the metal to promote uniform nucleation. They are called as grain refiners.

*Grain refiners* are metal of high melting point which are added to the alloy. As they remain solid when the rest of the alloy is molten, these small particles behave as seeds around which grain growth occurs. This helps in greatly improving the physical properties of the solid alloy. If grain refiner such as iridium is added in concentration of 0.005%, there is marked improvement in the ductility and tensile strength of the solid alloy. However, hardness and yield strength are not affected by its addition.

## Effect of Solidification on Properties

The crystallization of the solid metal occurs because of atomic diffusion from the molten metal to the nuclei. The crystals are formed in irregular position with structural discontinuities and imperfections and not in a single plane. Crystallization of pure metal characteristically resembles branch of tree, yielding elongated crystals called as *dendrites* (**Fig. 22.4**).

Three dimensionally they appear as frost crystals on window pane in winters. Dendrites grow during solidification by mechanism of *thermal supercooling*. *Protuberances* in the form of extensions or elevated areas form spontaneously on the front side of solidifying metal and advance into the regions of *negative temperature gradient*. Dendritic microstructure is not desirable for cast dental alloys because of increased chances of microcracks *(hot tears)* in the thin areas of the casting.

### CLINICAL SIGNIFICANCE
Dental base metal alloys solidifies with *dendritic microstructure* whereas noble metal alloys solidifies with an *equiaxed polycrystalline microstructure* because of incorporation of small quantities of indium, ruthenium or rhenium as grain refining elements.

## ALLOY SYSTEMS

Alloy system is referred to as all possible combinations of two or more elements, at least one of which is metal, e.g. Au-Ag system includes all possible alloys of gold and silver varying from 100% gold to 100% silver. Most of the pure metals are soluble in each other in molten state. Although alloys are combination of two or more metallic elements which are not necessarily pure. Alloys have superior properties than the pure metal and can be easily fabricated.

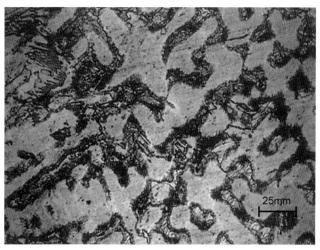

**Fig. 22.4:** Crystallization of pure metal form dendrites.

In dentistry alloys and not pure metal are most commonly used.

If the alloy system is made of two metals, it is called the *binary alloy*, if three or four metals form alloy then it is called as *ternary* or *quaternary* alloys.

## Classification of Alloys

- *On the basis of use*:
  - All metal inlays
  - All metal crown and bridges
  - Metal ceramic prosthesis
  - Posts and cores
  - Removable partial dentures
  - Dental implants.
- *On the basis of major elements*:
  - Gold-based
  - Palladium-based
  - Silver-based
  - Nickel-based
  - Cobalt-based
  - Titanium-based.
- *On the basis of nobility:*
  - High noble
  - Noble
  - Predominantly base metals.
- *On the basis of principal three elements*:
  - Au-Pd-Ag
  - Pd-Ag-Sn
  - Ni-Cr-Be
  - Co- Cr- Mo
  - Ti-Al-V
  - Fe-Ni-Cr.
- *On the basis of dominant phase system:*
  - Single phase or solid solutions (isomorphous phase)
  - Eutectic alloys
  - Peritectic alloys
  - Intermetallic compounds.

## PHASE DIAGRAMS AND ALLOYS

The concept of phases and phase diagrams help in understanding the nature of alloys and metal solubility. Alloys possess crystal structure as pure metal or can possess atomic structures such as eutectics or intermetallic compounds.

A phase is a homogeneous, physically distinct and mechanically separable region of a metal microstructure. For example, mixture of ice and water has two phases as ice has crystalline arrangement of atoms of a solid and water has random atomic arrangement of a liquid. Although ice and water are chemically the same.

A dental alloy can have a single phase if composition of the alloy is entirely *homogeneous* and can be *multiphase alloy* if the composition of the alloy is different. The distinction between single and multiple phase alloys is important to the strength, corrosion, biocompatibility and other properties.

A phase diagram or constitution diagram is a graph of the phase which field limits as a function of temperature and composition. These diagrams usually represent the equilibrium conditions and sometimes metastable conditions. In a binary alloy system, binary phase diagram is used. For ternary alloys, three phase diagram is used. Phase diagrams describing alloys greater than three are avoided because of greater complexity. Dental alloys which contain four or more metals, the binary phase of two most abundant metals in the alloy is usually described.

Each phase diagram of alloy system has three components such as: (1) liquid phase, (2) liquid + solid phase and (3) the solid phase. Let us take an example of theoretical binary alloy AB.

A phase diagram of this system has x-axis which shows the composition of the elements in either weight percent or atomic percent. The y-axis represents the temperature of the alloy system. The phase diagram shows the composition and types of the phases at a given temperature and at equilibrium. In the **Figure 22.5**, anything above the line ACB is liquid and anything below line ADB is solid. The area which lies between the two lines contains some liquid and some solid. Phase diagram can be used to study the composition of solid and liquid phases.

When metals are allowed to mix in a molten state and then cooled to solid state, there are several types of alloy system which can result depending on the solubility of the metals in each other. If metals are soluble in each other at all temperature and compositions then it is called the

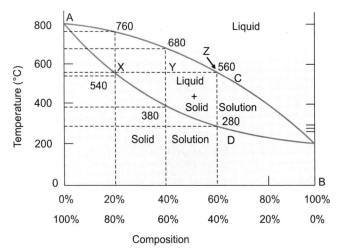

**Fig. 22.5:** Phase diagram of an alloy system.

*complete solid solutions*, if the metals are not soluble in each other *eutectic alloys* system results. Sometimes metals may react to form specific compounds called as the *intermetallic compounds*.

## SOLID SOLUTIONS

In this type of alloy system atoms of two metals are located in the same crystal structure. The structure of the alloy appears entirely homogeneous as only single phase is formed during solidification. For example, gold alloys, Ag-Pd alloys.

Most of the alloys belonging to this system are commonly used in dentistry. In such alloy system two metals are completely soluble in the solid state.

### Types of Solid Solutions

#### Substitutional Solid Solutions

In this type, atoms of the solute metal occupy the positions in the crystal structure that are usually occupied by the solvent atoms in the pure metal. These metals are completely soluble in each other at all temperature and compositions. They are also called as *complete solid solutions*. For example, Pd-Ag alloy in which palladium is a solvent is replaced by the silver atoms in the crystal which is structure.

#### Interstitial Solid Solutions

In this type of alloy system, the solute atoms are much smaller in diameter than the solvent atoms and are located between the atoms in the crystal structure of the solvent metal. For example, Cp-Ti (commercially pure titanium alloys), consists of highly pure titanium with oxygen, carbon, nitrogen and hydrogen atoms dissolved interstitially.

### PHYSICAL PROPERTIES OF SOLID SOLUTIONS

The strength, proportional limit, hardness is increased whereas the ductility is reduced. The strength of the solid solutions is increased with greater concentration of the solute atoms and with increasing dissimilar sizes of the solvent and the solute atoms. Since dislocation movement of the solid solution is limited and the ductility usually reduces as the strength and hardness is increased. Maximum hardness of the solid solution is reached at approximately 50% of each metal.

## EUTECTIC ALLOYS

Binary alloys which do not have complete solubility in both liquid and solid states are called as *eutectic alloys*. These alloys have limited solid solubility. However, all metal are at least partially soluble in each other if not completely. For example, silver-copper system.

The phase diagram of silver-copper system consists of: (1) Liquid phase; (2) A silver rich phase (α) which contains small quantity of copper atoms; (3) A copper rich phase (β) which contains small amount of silver atoms.

The α and β phases are called as *terminal solid solutions* as they are located at the left and right side of the phase diagram. The boundary of solidus is ABEGD since liquid phase is not found below this line and boundary of liquidus is identified as AED, as no solid phase occurs above this line. Both solidus and liquidus meet at E **(Fig. 22.6)**. This composition is called as the *eutectic composition* or *eutectic* (72% silver and 28% copper). On the left side of the phase diagram from A to B, the copper content of the silver rich α-phase varies between 0% and 9%. Similarly, on the right side from D to G, silver content of the copper rich phase varies between 0% and 8%.

### Characteristic of Eutectic Composition

• The melting temperature of eutectic alloy is lower than the melting points of either of the metal in the alloy
• No solidification occurs at E, i.e. the eutectic liquid composition freezes at a constant temperature which is similar to pure metal and the solid consist of both phases (α and β). The lower fusion temperature of the eutectic alloys is desirable for dental solders although, other properties are inferior to those of solid solutions alloys.

### Eutectic Reaction

When binary eutectic alloy solidifies it forms into a rod-shaped lamellar structure called as *eutectic constituent* which has areas of two nearly pure parent metals.

The eutectic reaction is written as:
Liquid → α solid solution + β solid solution

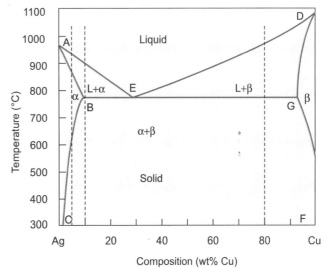

**Fig. 22.6:** Silver-copper system.

Since this reaction occurs at single temperature and composition, it is called as *invariant transformation*.

The phase diagram also contains lines CB and FG which are called as *solvus lines* as they are not present in phase diagrams of solid solutions systems. Under equilibrium conditions, the solvus line CB represents solid solubility of copper in the α phase increases from 1% at 300°C to almost 9% at B. Likewise solvus line FG that the equilibrium solid solubility of silver phase increases from very small value at 300°C to maximum of 8% at point G.

### Physical Properties of the Eutectic

*Hypoeutectic alloys* are those alloys which have compositions less than the eutectic whereas *hypereutectic alloys* have compositions greater than the eutectic. The majority of crystals in hypoeutectic alloys contains α solid solutions and in hypereutectic alloys contains β solid solutions. Hypo- or hypereutectic alloys are relatively brittle in comparison to the eutectic alloys which are ductile.

> **CLINICAL SIGNIFICANCE**
> Sometimes, the strength and hardness of eutectic alloys can be more than that of the pure metal because of composite structure of the alloy.

Silver copper eutectic is found in admixed high copper amalgam alloys. The α solid solution casting alloys of silver and copper is used in pediatric dentistry as they have greater tarnish resistance than the eutectic alloys.

## PERITECTIC ALLOYS

Like eutectic system, there is limited solid solubility of two metals in peritectic transformations. In this system, liquid and solid phase of fixed proportions react at a fixed temperature to yield as single solid phase. For example, the original dental amalgam alloy which consists of silver tin phase is the peritectic system, silver and platinum found in gold casting alloys, palladium and ruthenium has peritectic reaction at 16.5 wt% of Ru. Ruthenium being an important grain refining element for the palladium casting alloys.

As eutectic reaction, peritectic reaction also occurs at particular temperature and at particular composition. This reaction is also called as invariant reaction. The peritectic reaction is expressed as:

Liquid + β solid solution → α solid solution

In the phase diagram of silver-platinum alloy system, β phase is silver rich and the β phase is platinum rich and the (α + β) phase results from limited solid solubility of silver in platinum (less than approximately 56%) at 700°C. The peritectic transformation occurs at point P where liquid and the platinum rich β phase transforms to silver rich α

phase. For hypoperitectic composition, cooling through the peritectic temperatures results in following transformation:

Liquid + β → liquid + α

In both the reactions mentioned in **Figure 22.7**, α phase forms at the interface between the liquid and the β phase. There is substantial amount of diffusion between these phases for transformation and this makes the peritectic alloys more prone to coring during rapid cooling.

> **CLINICAL SIGNIFICANCE**
> Peritectic alloys are prone to coring during rapid cooling. Coring of these alloys results in inferior corrosion resistance and brittle alloys as compared to the homogeneous α solid solution phase.

## INTERMETALLIC COMPOUNDS

If two metals on mixing in the molten state results in a new compound on rapid cooling it forms an intermetallic compounds. For example, in Ag-Sn alloy system, an intermetallic compound of $Ag_3Sn$ is formed. Grains of these compounds are formed at definitive ratio.

### Coring

*It is defined as a microstructural condition in which a composition gradient exists between the center and the surface of a structural component such as a dendrite, grain or particle.*

It consists of core and matrix. The core consists of dendrites that are composed of compositions with higher solidus temperatures, and the matrix consists of portion of microstructure between the dendrites that contain compositions with lower solidus temperatures. For example,

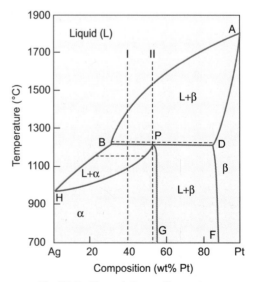

**Fig. 22.7:** Silver-platinum alloy system.

at the solidus temperature T, composition of dendrite is Pd 65% and Ag 35%. During coring, the last liquid to solidify is richer in silver and solidifies between the dendrites under rapid freezing conditions. In a photomicrograph, core is observed as light relatively broad dendrites with higher melting compositions and matrix are represented by dark narrow features with lower melting temperatures.

## Homogenization

Homogenization of the cast alloy occurs when it is held at a temperature near its solidus to achieve maximum amount of diffusion without melting. In this process, there is little or no grain growth as the grain boundary is mainly immobilized by secondary or impure elements and phases. After homogenization, ductility and tarnish and corrosion resistance increases of the cast alloys.

## ALLOY STRENGTHENING MECHANISMS

Dental casting alloys demand high strength and hardness to fulfill the restorative criteria. There are number of methods of increasing strength and hardness of the alloys.

## Solid Solutions

These alloys are usually stronger and harder than either of the component pure metal. Atoms of unequal sizes strengthen the alloy by making it more difficult for the atomic planes to slide by each other. Again ordered solutions further enhance the strength by providing pattern of dissimilar sizes throughout the alloy's crystal structure. Solid and ordered solution hardening is the most common method of strengthening of the casting alloys.

## Coherent Precipitation

In this method when the casting alloys are heated a new second phase is formed in the body of the alloy. This new phase blocks the movement of the dislocations, thereby increasing strength and hardness of the dental alloy. This process is more effective if the precipitate is still part of the normal crystal lattice.

## Grain Refining

Elements like Ir, Rh, and Ru are used as grain refiner to greatly increase the strength of the dental casting alloy. Using these elements, the ductility of the original composition is not altered.

## Cold Working

This process greatly improves the strength of the alloy. By this method, dislocations are worked out and further deformation becomes more difficult. However, cold working reduces the ductility and embrittles the alloy.

## TEST YOURSELF

### Essay Questions

1. Classify dental alloys. Write about eutectic and peritectic alloys.
2. What are solid solutions? Describe the palladium- silver alloy phase diagram.

### Short Notes

1. Solidification of alloys.
2. Eutectic alloys.
3. Peritectic alloys.
4. Classification of alloys.
5. Grain refiners.
6. Phase diagram.
7. Intermetallic compounds.

### Multiple Choice Questions

1. Which of the following has two different phases in solid state?
   A. Eutectic alloy
   B. Solid solution
   C. Intermetallic compound
   D. None of the above
2. A true eutectic alloy has:
   A. Melting point below the melting point of either metal
   B. Melting point above the melting point of component metals
   C. Melting point below that of the high fusing metal only
   D. Melting point above that of low fusing metal only
3. Eutectic components are characterized by:
   A. Brittleness and decreased ductility
   B. Elasticity and increased hardness
   C. Brittleness and increased malleability
   D. Decreased hardness and increased elasticity
4. If an intermetallic component is formed from two metals its properties:
   A. Are same that of constituent metals
   B. Is inferior to either of constituent metals

C. Is superior to both metals
D. Mechanical properties cannot be predicted
5. Compared to solid solution, eutectic alloy has:
   A. High melting range
   B. Low melting point
   C. Small grain size
   D. High malleability

## ANSWERS

1. A     2. A     3. A     4. D     5. B

## BIBLIOGRAPHY

1. Anusavice KJ. Phillips' science of dental materials, 11th edition. St. Louis, Missouri; Saunders; 2003.
2. Christensen GC. Longevity versus esthetics: the great restorative debate. J Am Dent Assoc. 2007;138:1013-5.
3. Craig RG, Powers JM, Wataha JC. Dental materials: properties and manipulations, 7th edition. St. Louis: Mosby; 2000.
4. Carr AB, Cai Z, Brantley WA, et al. New high-palladium casting alloys: Part 2. Effects of heat treatment and burnout temperature. Int J Prosthodont. 1993;6:233-41.
5. Flinn RA, Trojan PK. Engineering materials and their applications, 4th edition. New York: John Wiley and Sons; 1994.
6. Leinfelder KF. An evaluation of the casting alloys used for restorative procedures. J Am Dent Assoc. 1997;128:37-45.
7. Moffa J. Alternative dental casting alloys. Dent Clin North Am. 1983;27:733-46.
8. Morris HF, Manz M, Stoffer W, et al. Casting alloys: the material and the clinical effects. Adv Dent Res. 1992;6:28-31.
9. Neilsen JP, Tuccillo JJ. Grain size in cast gold alloys. J Dent Res. 1966;45:964-9.
10. O' Brien WJ. Dental materials and their election, 2nd edition. Carol stream IL: Quintessence Publishing; 1997.
11. Porter DA, Easterling KE. Phase transformations in metals and alloys, 2nd edition. London: Chapman and Hall; 1992.
12. Smith DL, Burnett AP, Brooks MS et al. Iron-platinum hardening in casting golds for use with porcelain. J Dent Res. 1970;49:283-8.
13. Vermilyea SG, Huget EF, Vilca JM. Observations on gold-palladium-silver and gold-palladium alloys. J Prosthet Dent. 1980;44:294-9.
14. Watanabe I, Atsuta M, Yasuda K, Hisatsune K. Dimensional changes related to ordering in an AuCu-3 wt% Ga alloy at the intraoral temperature. Dent Mater. 1994;10:369-74.
15. Wendt SL Jr. Nonprecious cast-metal alloys in dentistry. Curr Opin Dent. 1991;1:222-7.
16. Yasuda K, Ohta M. Difference in age-hardening mechanism in dental gold alloys. J Dent Res. 1982;61:473-9.
17. Yasuda K, Van Tendeloo G, Van Landuyt J et al. High-resolution electron microscopic study of age-hardening in a commercial dental gold alloy. J Dent Res. 1986;65:1179-85.

# Dental Casting Alloys

*' The only place where success comes before work is in the dictionary.'*

*—Vidal Sassoon*

## INTRODUCTION

Metals used in dentistry are mostly in the form of alloys or mixture of one or more metals. Alloys have distinct advantage over the pure metals in their improved mechanical and physical properties. Precious metal alloys were most popular form of restorative material prior to deregulation of gold prices in the open market in late 1960s. Due to this lower cost substitutes to gold alloys were introduced. Semiprecious alloys were chosen as they were semi-noble and at the same time economical. They included silver-palladium alloys and other alloys which have more than 10% and less than 75% of gold. Again steep rise in the cost of noble metals in 1973–74 brought widespread interest in base metal alloys which were called as nonprecious alloys. Currently nonmetallic tooth colored restorations have gained immense popularity because of greater esthetic value. The uses of metallic restorations have reduced tremendously in the last two decades. However, metal alloys continue to be used in metal-ceramic restorations to enhance strength, wear resistance and hardness. This chapter outlines different alloys used in dentistry.

## HISTORICAL BACKGROUND

- *1897: Philbrook* first introduced the cast restorations
- *1907:* Introduction of lost-wax technique by *William H Taggart.* He fabricated gold inlay using this method
- *1932:* National Bureau of Standards now called the National Institute of Standards and Technology, classified gold-based casting alloys on the basis of Vickers hardness number (VHN)

- *1933:* Replacement of Co-Cr for gold in fabricating removable partial dentures. Base metal alloys showed better strength, greater stiffness, lighter weight and less cost
- *1950:* Development of resin veneers for gold alloys
- *1959:* Development of porcelain fused to metal technique
- *1968:* Palladium-based alloys as alternatives to gold alloys
- *1971:* Nickel-based alloys introduced as alternatives to gold alloys. Gold was partially or completely replaced by nonprecious alloys because of high gold prices
- *1976:* Medical and Dental Devices Act in the United States placed dental industry under Food and Drug Administration (FDA)
- *1980s:* Introduction to all ceramic technologies
- *1996:* European Union directed that any import of dental equipment, devices will require seal of approval of CE (certification-expert)
- *1999:* Gold alloys as alternatives to palladium-based alloys.

## IDEAL REQUIREMENTS FOR CASTING ALLOYS

- *Biocompatibility*: Alloy used for dental casting should be biocompatible. The metal alloy should well tolerate oral fluids and should not release any harmful agent into the oral environment. However, an individual patient can be sensitive to particular component of the alloy. In such cases, clinician should take all necessary precautions and minimize the risk to the particular patient

- *Strength*: Alloys used should have high strength and sag resistance to ensure sufficient function and structural durability over long period of time
- *Modulus of elasticity*. Metal alloy used in thin sections should have enough rigidity to withstand masticatory forces without deformation. The alloy used in metal ceramic restoration should be thin in order to allow sufficient layer of ceramic to be sintered on it. Base metal alloys have greater modulus of elasticity as compared to gold alloys
- *Ductility and malleability*: Casting alloy should have adequate ductility and malleability so that it can be better adapted such as clasps in cast partial dentures
- *Hardness*: Casting metal should have good hardness value so that it can resist scratching and abrasion and can maintain smoothness of the restoration
- *Yield strength*: Casting alloys should have high yield strength in order to resist permanent deformation
- *Marginal fit*: Alloys used should have excellent fit without marginal gap. Good marginal fit improves the clinical longevity of the restoration
- *Economic reason*: Alloys used for casting should have reasonable cost
- *Corrosion resistance*: Should have excellent tarnish and corrosion resistance. Resistance to corrosion is achieved by either using noble metal alloys or by using alloy which has ability to form passivating layer
- *Castability*: Alloys used for casting should be easy to melt. The molten alloy should flow freely into the invested mold. The alloy should wet the surface of the mold without forming porosity within the surface of the alloy
- *Soldering and finishing* should allow easy carrying out of casting, brazing (soldering) and polishing. Hardness of the alloy is a good indicator to determine difficulty in grinding and finishing of the restoration
- *Porcelain bonding*: Alloy should have good chemical bonding with porcelain material. The alloy should be able to form thin adherent oxide layer over its surface to promote bonding
- *Thermal properties*: The melting range of casting alloy should be low in order to form smooth surface with the mold wall. It should compensate for solidification shrinkage by controlled mold expansion. The alloy should have closely matching coefficient of thermal expansion with porcelain in metal ceramic restorations
- *Chemical reactivity*: Alloy should show minimal or no reactivity with the mold material
- *Wear resistance*: Alloy should have good wear resistance
- *Ease of fabrication*: The alloy should be easy to manipulate and fabricate restorations and prosthesis

- *Color of the alloy*: Color of the metal alloy varies from white to yellow. The noble metals are usually yellow where gold is the primary constituent whereas base metal alloy is darker in color. The color of the metal especially in metal ceramic restorations should be masked by using opaque porcelain to improve esthetics.

## Classification of Casting Alloys

- *According to American Dental Association—based on total noble metal content (1984)* (*Table 23.1*)
- *Revised American Dental Association classification of prosthodontic alloys (2003)*
  - *High noble alloys:* Should contain ≥60% of noble content and ≥40% gold content
  - *Titanium and titanium alloys:* Should contain ≥85% of titanium
  - *Noble alloys:* Should contain ≥25% of noble content
  - Predominantly base metal: Should contain ≤25% of noble content.
- *Classification of casting alloys* [American National Standards Institute/American Dental Association (ANSI/ADA) specification No. 5 (1997)]
  - *Type I* (low strength or soft alloys): Casting can tolerate very less stress. For example, inlays, class III, class IV cavities. Least strength for these alloys is 80 MPa and least elongation after fracture is 18%
  - *Type II* (medium strength): Casting can tolerate moderate strength. For example, inlays, onlays, partial veneer crowns. Least strength for these alloys is 180 MPa and least elongation is 12%
  - *Type III* (high strength): Casting can tolerate high stresses. For example, onlays, pontics, full crowns, short span fixed partial dentures (FPDs). Least strength is 240 MPa and least elongation after fracture is 12%
  - *Type IV* (extra hard): These casting alloys can tolerate very high stresses and can be made in thin sections. For example, saddles, bar, thin veneer crowns, partial denture frameworks, long span FPDs. Least strength is 300 MPa and least elongation is 10%.
- *Classification of metallic material for dental application—ISO 22674 (2006)—based on the mechanical properties of the casting alloys* (*Table 23.2*).

- *Classification of casting alloys for all metal, metal-ceramic prosthesis and cast partial denture frameworks* (*Table 23.3*).

**Table 23.1:** Total noble metal content.

| Type of alloy | Total amount of noble content |
|---|---|
| High noble (HN) | Contains more than 40% gold and more than 60% noble metal alloys. Also called precious alloys |
| Noble (N) | Contains ≥25% of noble metal elements (Au, Pt, Pd, Rh, and Ir). Also called as semi-precious alloys |
| Predominantly base metal (PB) | Must contain ≤25% weight of noble metal. Also called as non-precious alloys |

**Table 23.2:** Mechanical properties of the casting alloys.

| Type | Yield strength | Elongation (%) | Uses |
|---|---|---|---|
| 0 | – | – | These alloys formed by electroforming or sintering. Commonly used for metal-ceramic crowns or small veneered one surface inlay |
| 1 | 80 | 18 | Single tooth restoration, veneered or non-veneered one surface inlay, veneered crowns |
| 2 | 180 | 10 | Single tooth fixed restoration, multiple surface inlay |
| 3 | 270 | 5 | Multiple unit fixed restoration—fixed partial dentures (FPDs) |
| 4 | 360 | 2 | Alloy used in thin sections which is subjected to high stress such as cast partial dentures, clasps, thin metal coping, long span fixed partial dentures or FPDs with small cross-sections, bars, attachments, implant supported superstructures |
| 5 | 500 | 2 | Alloys used in thin sections for fabricating thin cast partial dentures, clasps |

**Table 23.3:** Casting alloys for all metal, metal-ceramic prosthesis and cast partial denture frameworks..

| Type of casting alloy | All metal | Metal-ceramic prosthesis | Partial denture frameworks |
|---|---|---|---|
| High noble (HN) | Au-Ag-Pd<br>Au-Pd-Cu-Ag | Au-Pt-Pd<br>Au-Pd-Ag (5–12 weight % Ag)<br>Au-Pd-Ag (>12 weight % Ag)<br>Au-Pd | Au-Ag-Cu-Pd |
| Noble (N) | Ag-Pd-Au-Cu<br>Ag-Pd | Pd-Au<br>Pd-Au-Ag<br>Pd-Ag<br>Pd-Cu-Ga<br>Pd-Ga-Ag | |
| Predominantly base metal (PB) | $C_pTi$<br>Ti-Al-V<br>Ti-Al-Nb<br>Ni-Cr-Mo-Be<br>Ni-Cr-Mo<br>Co-Cr-W<br>Co-Cr-Mo<br>Cu-Al | $C_pTi$<br>Ti-Al-V<br>Ti-Al-Nb<br>Ni-Cr-Mo-Be<br>Ni-Cr-Mo<br>Co-Cr-Mo<br>Co-Cr-W | $C_pTi$<br>Ti-Al-V<br>Ti-Al-Nb<br>Ni-Cr-Mo-Be<br>Ni-Cr-Mo<br>Co-Cr-Mo<br>Co-Cr-W |

#All casting alloys which are used for metal-ceramic prosthesis can be used to fabricate all metal prosthesis but all metal alloys cannot be used for metal-ceramic prosthesis.

# PRECIOUS METAL ALLOYS

## Introduction

Precious metal alloys were traditionally used in dentistry in the form of castings. Taggart in 1907 introduced the casting method to cast metals using *lost-wax technique.* High gold containing alloys were used for inlays and are still used for this kind of restoration because they can be easily burnished as they are soft. Full veneer and partial veneer cast crowns can also be cast with gold alloys but are rapidly replaced by metal ceramic and all ceramic restorations especially in the anterior esthetic zone. Currently precious metal alloys use gold along with various alloying elements such as palladium, platinum, silver and copper in varying proportions **(Table 23.4).**

**Table 23.4:** Composition of precious metal alloys.

| Type of alloy | Classification | Au | Pd | Ag | Cu | Ga, In and Zn |
|---|---|---|---|---|---|---|
| Type I | High noble (Au based) | 83% | 0.5% | 10% | 6% | Traces |
| Type II | High noble (Au based) | 77 | 1 | 14 | 7 | Traces |
| Type III | High noble (Au based) | 75 | 3.5 | 11 | 9 | Traces |
| Type III | Noble (Au based) | 46 | 6 | 39 | 8 | Traces |
| Type III | Noble (Ag based) | — | 25 | 70 | — | Traces |
| Type IV | High noble (Au based) | 56 | 4 | 25 | 14 | Traces |
| Type IV | Noble (Ag based) | 15 | 25 | 45 | 14 | Traces |

## Karat and Fineness

- The amount of gold content in the dental alloy is specified on basis of Karat or Fineness
- Karat describes gold content of the alloy based on parts of gold per 24 parts of the alloy. For example, 24 karat gold means pure gold (100%), 22 karat gold means 91.67% gold, i.e. 22 parts of pure gold and 2 parts of other metal
- Fineness of gold alloy is percentage of gold multiplied by factor of 10. For example, 100% gold is 1,000 fine, 75% gold is 750 fine
- Fineness is used to identify dental gold solders but karat is rarely used to specify gold content in dental alloys. Currently carat or fineness is rarely used to describe gold content of the dental alloys **(Table 23.5)**.

## Classification of Casting Alloys

- *According to ISO Draft International Standard for casting gold alloys, they are classified on the basis of mechanical properties (2002):*
  - *Type I (low strength or soft alloy):* Casting can tolerate very less stress (for example, inlays). The minimum strength at 0.2% should be 80 MPa and minimum elongation after fracture is 18%
  - *Type II (medium strength):* Casting can tolerate moderate strength. For example, inlays, onlays and complete crowns. The minimum strength at 0.2% offset should not be less than 180 MPa and minimum percent elongation should not be more than 10%
  - *Type III (high strength or hard alloy):* These casting are capable of tolerating high stresses. For example, onlays, pontics, crowns and saddles. The minimum strength should not be less than 270 MPa and minimum percent elongation should not be more than 5% **(Fig. 23.1)**
  - *Type IV (extra high strength or extra hard alloy):* These castings are capable of tolerating very high stresses. For example, saddles, bar and partial denture frameworks. The minimum strength should not be less than 360 MPa and the minimum percent elongation should not be more than 3%.

**Table 23.5:** Gold content in carat and fineness.

| Gold content (%) | Carat | Fineness |
|---|---|---|
| 100 | 24 | 1000 |
| 75 | 18 | 750 |
| 58 | 14 | 583 |
| 42 | 10 | 420 |

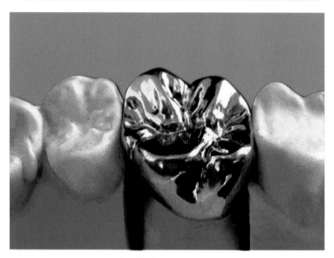

**Fig. 23.1:** Gold crown.

## FUNCTION OF ALLOYING ELEMENTS

### Gold

- It is the major constituents of most of the high noble and noble alloys
- Contributes to yellow color
- Excellent tarnish and corrosion resistance (should be at least 16 Karat)
- Most ductile and malleable among all metals
- To have noble properties, the alloy should have gold greater than 65–80%
- It has yellow color and is relatively insoluble in acids except aqua regia (mixture of hydrochloric and nitric acids)

- Has relatively low melting point of 1,063°C and has specific gravity of 19.32
- The space lattice structure is face-centered cubic (FCC)
- Along with copper contributes to heat hardening of the alloy
- It is used as direct filling material in the form of gold foil
- Gold is dense and provides excellent castability
- It is highly conductive and has modulus of elasticity and hardness similar to enamel

## Copper

- Acts as principal hardener
- Its melting point is 1,083°C and specific gravity is 8.96
- Aids in reducing melting point and fusion temperature of gold
- Its space lattice structure is FCC
- It is chemically very active
- It gives reddish color to the alloy
- In greater amounts it reduces resistance to tarnish and corrosion
- Maximum content should not be greater than 17%
- It is essential if the alloy is heat hardened
- Contributes to tarnish in flame or with sulfurous food items.

## Silver

- Silver is not considered as noble as it reacts with sulfides, halides and phosphates resulting in tarnished surface
- It is the principal whitener of the casting alloys
- It has low melting point of 961°C and specific gravity of 10.49
- Its approximate content is between 0% and 20%
- It whitens very slowly and counteracts the redness given by copper. It creates green gold
- Its space lattice structure is FCC
- Gives increased strength and hardness
- Decreases tarnish resistance in large amounts. It tarnishes in presence of sulfur
- Has high affinity for oxygen. This tendency makes the casting difficult as it readily produces porosity
- Increase heat hardening with copper
- Some silver alloys used for metal ceramic restorations especially those containing palladium shows greening of porcelain **(Fig. 23.2)**
- At raised temperature silver diffuses into porcelain and can lead to color change.

## Platinum

- It is bright white metal which has high hardness and density
- Strengthens the alloy

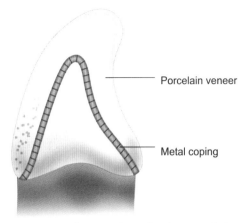

**Fig. 23.2:** Discoloration of porcelain because of silver.

- It has high melting point of 1,769°C and resists oxidation at raised temperatures
- Its specific gravity is 21.45
- When alloyed with gold, it becomes compatible with ceramometal bonding
- It is used as substrate in the form of platinum foil which is used for porcelain densification. Its coefficient of thermal expansion is close to porcelain and has melting temperature greater than porcelain sintering temperature
- Its high hardness gives excellent resistance to wear and is a common constituent in precision attachments
- Its space lattice structure is FCC
- Raises the melting point rapidly
- Has a whitening effect on the alloy
- Reduces the grain size
- It is the best hardener in the alloy superior to copper
- Its approximate content is between 0% and 20%
- Contributes to tarnish resistance
- Although it is highly biocompatible but when used with palladium it is can show hypersensitive reactions in some patients.

## Palladium

- Contributes to tarnish resistance. It is low cost substitute to gold
- It is white in color and its density is 60% that of gold
- Its melting point is 1,552°C and specific gravity is 12
- Its space lattice structure is FCC
- Helps in raising the fusion temperature
- Has great affinity for hydrogen gas. It can absorb almost 900 times its volume of hydrogen gas. It is used for industrial purpose to purify hydrogen
- Its approximate content is 0–12%
- It reduces the cost of the alloy as it is less expensive than platinum.

## Other Minor Additions

### Zinc

- It is a scavenger for oxygen. Without zinc, silver absorbs $O_2$ during melting, later during solidification; $O_2$ is rejected causing gas porosities
- Its meting point is 420°C and specific gravity is 7.31
- Its space lattice structure is close packed hexagonal
- Its approximate content in gold alloys is 0–2%
- Has tendency to tarnish but since use in low quantity its effect is less dominant
- It reduces surface tension and increases fluidity
- Used to form surface oxide formation needed for ceramometal bonding
- It helps to bind oxygen in the molten metal alloy but because of its low density, it has very low concentration in the final casting. Most of zinc is concentrated in the casting button
- It is common element in many dental solders.

### Gallium

- It is added to compensate for the decreased coefficient of thermal expansion that result when silver free alloy are used
- Elimination of silver is done to reduce the green stain at the porcelain metal interface.

### Iridium

- Its meting point is 2,443°C and specific gravity is 22.4
- Its space lattice structure is FCC
- Its approximate content in gold alloys is 0.005–0.1%
- It is white in color and added as grain refiner
- Help to harden metal ceramic gold-palladium alloys
- Small quantity of iridium and ruthenium acts as centers for nucleation and growth to reduce the grain size on cooling
- Used to increase surface oxide formation needed for ceramometal bonding.

## PROPERTIES

- *Melting range:* Since dental casting alloys are combinations of elements rather than pure elements, they have melting range and not melting points. The solidus-liquidus range should be narrow to avoid alloy in the molten state for longer period of time
- *Density:* Alloys with higher densities tends to form casting faster and easily
- *Strength:* Yield strength of the alloy should be adequate to tolerate the masticatory stresses
- *Hardness:* Greater the hardness, greater the difficulty in polishing the alloys

- *Elongation:* It is measure of ductility of the alloy. For FPDs, low elongation of the alloy is desirable. Alloys such as type I and II gold alloys, has high elongation which allows easy burnishing without fracture
- *Biocompatibility:* All casting alloys should be biocompatible. The issue of biocompatibility is related to elemental release of corrosion products from the alloy into the oral cavity.

### Heat Treatment of Precious Metal Alloys

Gold alloys significantly harden if it contains adequate amount of copper. Type I and type II gold alloys usually do not harden. However, type III and type IV gold alloys can be hardened or softened depending on the type of treatment given.

### Softening Heat Treatment or Solution Heat Treatment

The gold casting is placed in the furnace at the temperature of 700°C for 10 minutes and then it is quenched in water to room temperature. During this time, all the intermediate phases are changed to disordered solid solution and the rapid quenching do not allow ordering of the molecules to take place. With this treatment ductility is *increased* but tensile strength, proportional limit and hardness are *reduced*. Such treatment is indicated for alloys that are to be ground, shaped or cold worked in or outside the mouth.

### Hardening Heat Treatment or Age Hardening

This type of treatment is usually given after the alloy is given softening heat treatment in order to relieve all *strain hardening*. The gold casting is soaked or aged for 15–30 minutes at a temperature between 200°C and 450°C before it is quenched in water to room temperature. With this treatment, there is reduction in ductility and increase in strength, proportional limit and hardness. Modulus of resilience is considerably increased but the percent elongation in certain cases is significantly increased. This treatment is indicated for metallic partial dentures, saddles, FPDs, cast crowns and pontics in situations where rigidity is required. Age hardening is not indicated for small structures like inlays. This process reduces ductility of gold alloys.

## ALLOYS FOR METAL-CERAMIC RESTORATIONS

### Introduction

One of the primary limitation of dental ceramic as restorative material is its low strength to tensile and shear stresses although it possess sufficient compressive strength. If ceramic is directly bonded onto the cast alloy substructure then this limitation can be minimized to larger extent.

To achieve this, strong bond between the metal substructure and ceramic veneer is desirable.

## Uses

- For fabricating all metal restorations
- For fabricating porcelain fused to metal fixed restorations **(Fig. 23.3)**.

## Ideal Requirements of Metal-Ceramic Alloys for Bonding

- Fusing temperature of alloy should be higher than the porcelain firing temperature.
- Should have compatible coefficient of thermal expansion with ceramic.
- Should resist sag or creep resistance
- Should be able to bond with ceramic
- Should not stain or discolor ceramic
- Should have high modulus of elasticity in order to resist flexion of the metal or metal ceramic prosthesis.

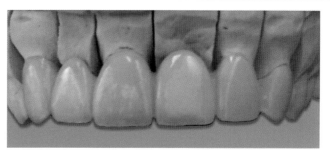

**Fig. 23.3:** Metal-ceramic fixed partial denture.

### Classification for Metal-ceramic Alloys

- *According to the composition, metal ceramic alloys are classified as:*
  - *High noble metal alloys:* Have noble metal content greater than 60% with at least 40% gold
    - Gold-platinum-palladium
    - Gold-palladium-silver
    - Gold-palladium
  - *Noble metal alloys:* Have noble metal content at least 25%
    - Palladium-silver
    - High palladium
  - *Base metal alloys:* Have less than 25% of noble metal content
    - Nickel-chromium
    - Cobalt-chromium
    - Nickel-chromium-beryllium
- *According to O'Brien metal ceramic alloys can be classified as:*
  - *Noble metal alloys:* Further divided into two types:
    1. *Gold based:*
       - Au-Pt-Pd
       - Au-Pd
       - Au-Pd-Ag
    2. *Palladium based:*
       - Pd-Ag
       - Pd-Cu
       - Pd-Co
  - *Base metal alloys:*
    - Ni-Cr-Be
    - Ni-Cr
    - Co-Cr
    - Ti and Ti alloys.

## Criteria for Selecting Metal-ceramic Alloys for Restorations

- *Physical properties:* Greater the noble metal content, greater the resistance to corrosion and inert properties of an alloy. Hardness of the alloy determines its load bearing ability, occlusal wear resistance, finishing and polishing properties. Yield strength determines the load bearing ability of the restoration. Elongation of the alloy determines its marginal adaptability
- *Porcelain-metal bond:* The alloy should have adequate porcelain bond with ceramic. Addition of small quantity of base metal to noble and high noble alloys promotes formation of oxides which greatly improves chemical bonding between the metal and the porcelain
- *Chemical properties:* The alloy should have high resistance to tarnish and corrosion and should have thermal stability
- *Thermal properties:* Metal ceramic alloys should have sufficiently high melting temperature to provide dimensional stability during porcelain firing. All metal ceramic alloys should have higher solidus temperature than the sintering temperature to minimize creep deformation. If the alloy is heated to its solidus temperature than the alloy flows under its own mass (creep). The amount of creep will also depend on the size of the prosthesis and the number of times the prosthesis framework is subjected to firing
- *Biocompatibility:* The metal alloy should be biocompatible. Nickel and beryllium containing base metal alloys are identified as potential biologic hazard
- *Porcelain metal compatibility:* Porcelain and metal used for restoration should have compatible coefficient of thermal expansion and melting temperatures. Differences between the coefficient of thermal contraction between the two induces high level of stress in porcelain which can lead to its cracking or delayed fracture **(Fig. 23.4)**
- *Casting accuracy:* It is required to provide clinically acceptable castings.

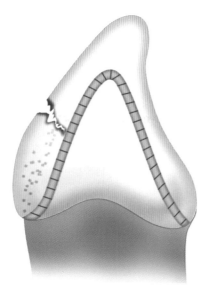

**Fig. 23.4:** Thermal expansion incompatibility between alloy and porcelain can result in formation of crack.

# HIGH NOBLE AND NOBLE ALLOYS

- Metal-ceramic restorations were first introduced to dentistry in 1958
- Ceramco No 1 alloy was the first to be used for this technology
- High noble alloys are composed of primarily gold and platinum. The percentage of gold varies from 78% to 87%. Other metals which are found in small amounts are tin, indium and iron which provide adequate strength
- Composition of high noble and noble metal alloys given in **Table 23.6**
  The physical and mechanical properties of commonly used precious alloys given in **Table 23.7**.

## Advantages

- As it contains greater quantity of high noble alloys, the restorations have excellent marginal adaptation and fit.
- Corrosion resistance is excellent
- No porcelain discoloration as silver content is very less.

**Table 23.6:** Composition of commonly used precious dental alloys.

| Composition | Au (%) | Pd (%) | Pt (%) | Ag (%) | Cu (%) | Others (%) |
|---|---|---|---|---|---|---|
| High noble | | | | | | |
| Au-Pt-Pd-Ag | 78 | 12 | 6 | 1.2 | | Fe-1, In-Sn, Ir <1 |
| Au-Pt-Pd | 86 | 1.95 | 10 | | | In-2, Ir <1 |
| Au–Pd-Ag-In | 40 | 37.4 | | 15 | | In-6, Ga-1.5, Ir <1 |
| Noble | | | | | | |
| Au-Cu-Ag-Pd | 46 | 6 | | 39.5 | 7.49 | Zn-1, Ir <1 |
| Pd-Cu-Ga | | 75.9 | | | 10 | Ga-6.5, In-7, Ru <1 |
| Ag-Pd | | 53.42 | | 38.9 | | Sn-7,Ga <1, Ru, Rh |
| Pd-Ga-Au | 2 | 85 | | | | Ga-10, In-1.1, Ag, Ru <1 |

**Table 23.7:** Physical and mechanical properties of commonly used precious metal alloys .

| Precious metal alloys | Melting range (°C) | Density (g/cc) | Vickers hardness (VHN) | Ultimate tensile strength (MPa) | Modulus of elasticity (GPa) | Percent elongation (%) |
|---|---|---|---|---|---|---|
| High noble | | | | | | |
| Au-Pd-Pt-Ag | 1,170–1,300 | 17.2 | 255 | 689 | 103.4 | 4 |
| Au-Pt-Pd | 1,060–1,230 | 18.7 | 190 | 586 | 82.7 | 6 |
| Au-Ag-Pd-In | 1,175–1,280 | 13 | 265 | 586 | 124 | 17 |
| Noble | | | | | | |
| Pd-Cu-Ga | 1,120–1,270 | 10.5 | 365 | 1,068 | 131 | 7 |
| Ag-Pd | 1,190–1,300 | 10.9 | 220 | 689 | 115.8 | 25 |
| Pd-Ga-Au | 1,105–1,330 | 10.9 | 285 | 717 | 131 | 25 |
| Pd-Ag-Au | 1,130–1,340 | 11 | 250 | 827 | 131 | 35 |

## Disadvantages

- High cost
- These alloys are less rigid and have poor sag resistance.

## Gold-Palladium-Silver Alloys

- This alloy was first marketed under the name of Will Ceram W in 1970
- Composed of Au, 42–68%; Pd, 25–40%; Ag, 5–16%; Sn, 0–4%; In, 0–6%; Ga, 0–2%; and Zn, 0–3%
- With the addition of high amount of silver and palladium, the cost of alloys is considerable reduced
- They have excellent tarnish and corrosion resistance
- The hardness value of alloy is 218 VHN and yield strength is 439 MPa
- Their elastic modulus is high and the alloy is less susceptible to dimensional change during porcelain firing
- Major drawback of this alloy is discoloration of porcelain (greening) due to presence of silver **(Fig. 23.5)**
- It is better to avoid the use of these alloys when lighter ceramic shade is to be used.

## Gold-Platinum-Palladium Alloys

This alloy was used to produce first successful metal ceramic restoration. Addition of platinum increased the melting temperature. Rhenium (Re) was added in some alloys as grain refiner to increase the hardness of the alloy. Iron is added for forming oxides which greatly improved bonding. Also, iron reacts with platinum to precipitate into FePt3 increasing its strength and proportional limit. These alloys have adequate strength, hardness, elastic modulus and

elongation but have low sag resistance. They are indicated for single crowns and small span FPDs. However, their use is very limited because of availability of more economical alloys with better properties.

## Gold-Palladium Alloys

- This type of silver-free alloy was first introduced in 1977 by Jelenko as Olympia
- This alloy was designed to overcome the discoloration effect of silver on porcelain
- The alloy is composed of Au, 45–68%; Pt, 0–1%; Pd, 22–45%; Sn, 0–5%; In, 2–10; Ga, 0–3%; and Zn ≤4
- It is white alloy which contains oxide formers such as indium and iridium and is commonly used for metal ceramic restorations **(Fig. 23.6)**
- The yield strength of the alloy is 572 MPa and hardness value is 220 VHN. Elastic modulus is 124 GPa. They have high strength, elastic modulus and hardness as compared to Au-Pt alloys
- Higher palladium content reduces density of the alloy and it affects the force of the alloy as it enters the investment during casting
- Although they have low density but are relatively easier to cast.
- They have excellent tarnish and corrosion resistance because of the high noble content
- Main drawback of this alloy is thermal expansion incompatibility with some higher expansion porcelains.

## Palladium-Silver Alloys

- This alloy was first introduced in 1974 as first gold-free alloy used for metal-ceramic restorations **(Fig. 23.7)**.

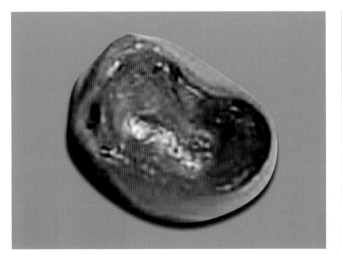

**Fig. 23.5:** Discoloration of porcelain due to presence of silver.

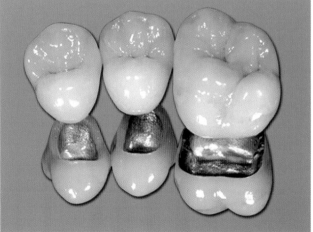

**Fig. 23.6:** Metal-ceramic restoration made with gold-palladium alloy.

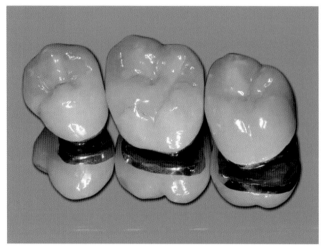

**Fig. 23.7:** Palladium-silver alloy used to fabricate metal-ceramic restorations.

- The alloy is composed of Au, 0–6%; Pt, 0–1%; Pd, 50–75%; Ag, 1–40%; Sn, 0–9%; In, 0–8%; Ga, 0–6%; Zn, 0–4%; and Mn, 0–4%
- Tin and indium are added to increase hardness of the alloy and to promote oxide formation and provide adequate bonding to porcelain
- The melting range of the alloy is high as gold is replaced by palladium
- Silver content increases the contraction coefficient and lowers the melting range. As the silver content is higher chances of porcelain discoloration is high. It causes greening of the porcelain
- The hardness of the alloy is 242 VHN, yield strength is 531 MPa and elastic modulus is 138 GPa
- The properties of these alloy resemble other noble metal alloys and are suited for fabricating metal ceramic restorations
- They have good tarnish and corrosion resistance
- The castings made with these alloy shows least flexion as compared to other precious alloys because of high modulus of elasticity. Only non-precious alloys have greater modulus of elasticity than these alloys
- They also show greater sag resistance during firing
- Their metal to porcelain bond is excellent
- Metal surface coupling agents are advised in order to avoid discoloration of ceramics **(Fig. 23.8)**
- The surface of palladium-silver alloys forms nodules to create an irregular surface to retain porcelain by mechanical rather than chemical means **(Fig. 23.9)**.

**CLINICAL SIGNIFICANCE**

High content of silver can produce discoloration and this alloy should be used with caution especially when using lighter shades.

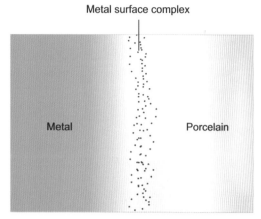

**Fig. 23.8:** Metal surface coupling agent is used to minimize discoloration of porcelain.

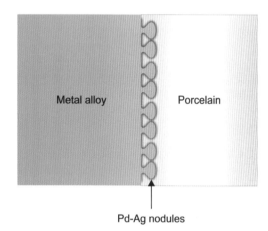

**Fig. 23.9:** Pd-Ag nodules aids in porcelain retention by mechanical means.

## Palladium-Copper-Gallium Alloys

- This type of alloy was first introduced in 1982 by Ney as option
- It is composed of Pd, 70–80%; Cu, 15% and Ga, 9% without any Au content
- They have excellent mechanical properties with yield strength as 520 MPa–1,200 MPa, percentage elongation at fracture ranging from approximately 7–30%
- There is difficulty in casting or melting these alloys as compared to the palladium-silver alloys
- Casting of these alloys tends to form dark brown or black oxide during oxidation and subsequent porcelain firing cycles **(Fig. 23.10)**
- This oxide layer should be completely masked during application of opaque porcelain
- Gallium reduces the liquidus temperature which is increased by palladium. It enhances porcelain bonding and also helps in increasing strength.

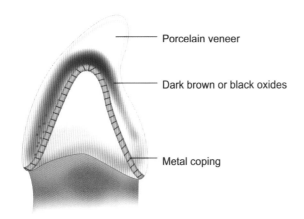

**Fig. 23.10:** Porcelain discoloration due to dark brown or black oxides formed on subsequent firing.

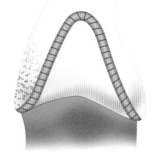

**Fig. 23.11:** Discoloration of porcelain is more severe in cervical area.

## Palladium-Gallium-Silver

- These types of alloys are compatible with low expansion porcelain
- They tend to produce slightly lighter colored oxide layer as compared to Pd-Cu alloys
- Silver content is low (5%) and is inadequate to cause greening of porcelain
- These alloy have lower hardness and can be adjusted chair side or in the laboratory.

## Palladium-Cobalt Alloys

- Such alloy contains Pd, 88% and Co, 4–5%
- The coefficient of thermal expansion of these alloys is higher and this property is advantageous with some porcelains
- Major drawback of this alloy is formation of dark oxide which is difficult to mask at thin margins **(Fig. 23.10)**
- These alloys are prone to hot tearing and embrittlement due to carbon if silver is not present. Their use in metal-ceramic restorations is limited.

## Silver-Palladium Alloys

- These alloys are white in color which contains pre-dominantly silver but at least 25% of palladium which provides nobility and promotes tarnish resistance
- They may or may not contain copper and small quantity of gold
- Copper free Ag-Pd alloy contains Ag, 70–72% and Pd, 25%. Their properties are similar to type III gold alloys
- Copper containing Ag-Pd alloys contains Ag, 60%, Pd, 25%, and Cu, 15%. The properties of the alloys resemble type IV gold alloys

- These alloys have greater potential for tarnish and corrosion
- These alloys are *not* used for metal ceramic restorations but to fabricate all metal restorations.

## Discoloration of Porcelain by Silver

Porcelain with greater sodium content is said to exhibit a more intense discoloration because of rapid silver diffusion in sodium containing glass. This process is called as *greening*. Although discoloration can be green, yellow-green, yellow-orange and brown in color. The intensity of discoloration is more at the cervical area as in this region localization of silver concentration is high because of surface diffusion from the marginal metal **(Fig. 23.11)**. In some porcelain, the discoloration effect is highly minimized because of conversion of silver oxide to silver ions by porcelain with higher affinity for oxygen.

> **CLINICAL SIGNIFICANCE**
>
> A ceramic conditioner can be used to reduce the discoloration by providing barrier between the alloy and porcelain.

## Alloys for Ultralow Fusing Porcelain

High gold alloys are used as alloys for ultralow fusing porcelains as the sintering temperature of these porcelains is below 850°C.

# BASE METAL ALLOYS

## Introduction

Base metal casting alloys were introduced in early 1970s because of the rapid fluctuating prices of gold and other noble metals. Due to this popularity of base metals alloys for use in cast metal and metal-ceramic restorations increased manifold. Most of the base metal alloys are based on nickel and chromium. Other base metal alloys are cobalt-chromium and iron-based alloys.

## Classification of Base Metal Alloys

According to O' Brien, based on their use, they are classified as follows (**Flowchart 23.1**):
- *Removable partial denture (Fig. 23.12):*
  - Cobalt-chromium
  - Cobalt-chromium-nickel
  - Nickel-chromium
  - Titanium.
- *Fixed partial dentures:*
  - Nickel chromium—either with beryllium or without beryllium
  - Cobalt-chromium
  - Titanium.
- *Surgical implants:*
  - Cobalt-chromium-molybdenum
  - Nickel-chromium-cobalt.

### Composition of Nickel Chromium Alloys for Crowns and Metal Ceramic Prosthesis

- Ni, 61–81% by wt.
- Cr, 11–27%
- Mo, 2–4%
- Al, 2.5–4%
- Fe, 0.1–0.4%
- Be, 0.5–1.5%
- Cu, 0.13–1.5%
- Mn, 0.14–3%
- Si, 0.2–1.1%.

### Composition of Cobalt Chromium Alloys

- Co, 53–67%
- Cr, 25–32%
- Mo, 2–6%.

## Base Metal Alloys used for Metal-ceramic Restorations

Chromium containing alloys are commonly used as substructures for metal-ceramic prosthesis. Commonly used alloys are:
- Nickel-chromium alloys—with or without beryllium
- Cobalt-chromium alloys.

### Nickel-Chromium Alloys

- Most commonly used alloy for metal-ceramic restorations (**Fig. 23.13**).

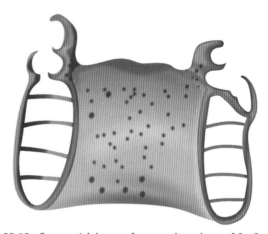

**Fig. 23.12:** Cast partial denture framework made up of Co-Cr alloy.

**Flowchart 23.1:** Flowchart explaining classification of base metal alloys.

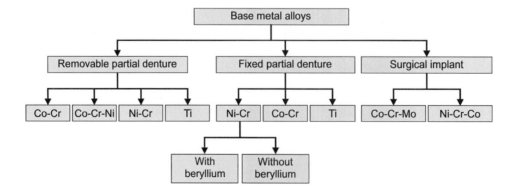

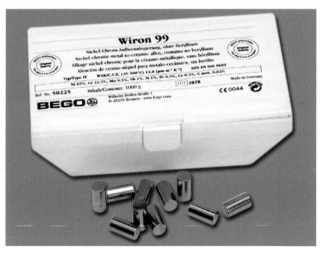

**Fig. 23.13:** Nickel-chromium alloy pellets used for metal-ceramic restorations.

- *Composition:*
  - Ni, 62.8% and Cr, 11–22%
  - Small amounts of Mo, Al, Mg, Si, Co, Ga, Fe, and Zr
  - Be, 0.5–2% may or may not be present.
- These alloys can be easily etched electrochemically. The etched surface forms larger surface area for bonding with resin cements **(Fig. 23.14)**
- Molybdenum reduces the thermal expansion coefficient.
- Aluminum increases strength and hardness
- Beryllium enhances castability by reducing melting temperature of the alloy and acts as grain refiner.

### Cobalt-Chromium Alloys

Cobalt-chromium alloy contains 53–65% cobalt, 27–32% chromium, 2–6% molybdenum and minor amounts of tungsten, iron, copper, silicon, tin, manganese and ruthenium.

### Properties

Physical and mechanical properties of base metal alloys have been given in **Table 23.8**.

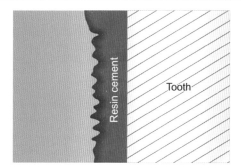

**Fig. 23.14:** Alloy surface can be etched electrochemically to create large surface area for resin cement.

- Nickel-chromium alloys have *highest elastic modulus* among all dental alloys (207 GPa). These alloys are twice as stiff as the gold alloys. This allows the cross-sectional thickness of the restoration to be thin and provides more space for porcelain veneer without compromising on the strength
- They have *meting range* between 1,232°C and 1,454°C.
- These alloys can be *polished* to high luster. They are white in color
- They are lighter as compared to gold alloys with *densities* slightly greater than 8 g/cm$^3$
- They have *high hardness and tensile strength* which allow casting of alloy in thin sections. Also, it helps in fabrication of long span FPDs
- The percent elongation of alloys containing chromium is 2–3%
- The metal-ceramic bond of base metal alloy is having comparable strength as that of noble metal alloys. They have adequate oxide layer which is necessary for proper porcelain bonding
- *Coefficient of thermal expansion* of Ni-Cr alloy is similar to the porcelain which helps in preventing cracking during sintering
- Nickel-chromium-beryllium alloys provide better bonding to porcelain than nickel chromium alloys
- *Beryllium* aids in increasing fluidity, controls surface oxidation, improves casting performance and results

| Base metal alloy | Tensile strength (MPa) | Yield strength (MPa) | Modulus of elasticity (GPa) | Elongation (%) | Density (g/cm³) |
|---|---|---|---|---|---|
| Nickel-chromium alloy | | | | | |
| Ni-Cr-Be | 778–1355 | 325–838 | 165–210 | 3–23.9 | 7.9 |
| Ni-Cr | 539–919 | 180–858 | 141–248 | 32.6 | 7.9–8.7 |
| Cobalt-chromium | | | | | |
| Co-Cr-Mo | 655–889 | 390–644 | 155–240 | 1.5–10 | 8.5 |
| Co-Cr-Ni | 685 | 470 | 198 | 8 | 7.5–8.5 |
| Co-Ni-Cr-Mo | 795–1,007 | 240–655 | 232 | 50–70 | 9.2 |

**Table 23.8:** Physical and mechanical properties of base metal alloys.

in more reliable and better porcelain-metal bond. It increases castability by lowering the melting range of the alloy and acts as grain refiner

- Bonding of porcelain to metal in non-beryllium containing alloys is inhibited by the thick oxides that deposits on the underlying cast framework
- Nickel chromium alloys have *high sag resistance* which is superior to all noble metal alloys
- They form *corrosion resistant layer* of chromium oxide on the surface
- These alloys have higher *casting shrinkage* than gold alloys. To compensate for this greater mold expansion is needed
- It has *low cost* as compared to noble and high noble alloys
- *Biocompatibility* of nickel containing alloys is controversial. Some studies have reported high incidence of allergic reactions in some patients
- High incidence of respiratory cancer is prevalent in people exposed to occupation exposure to nickel
- Beryllium is found to be mutagen and in different forms found to carcinogenic.

## Surface Preparation of Casting for Better Bonding

- Surface preparation of substrate casting is critical. The porcelain bearing surface of the casting is ground and finished using ceramic-bonded aluminum oxide stones
- After finishing the framework is sand blasted with fine grit aluminum oxide **(Fig. 23.15)**.

## *Advantages*

- Has high strength, stiffness and hardness
- Forms highly corrosion resistance layer

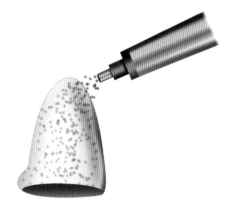

**Fig. 23.15:** Metal coping is sandblasted with fine grit aluminum oxide.

- Has high sag resistance
- Relatively inexpensive.

## *Disadvantages*

- Technique sensitive
- High hardness makes occlusal adjustment difficult and time consuming
- High hardness and strength requires high speed laboratory equipment and special abrasive disks and stones for grinding and finishing.

## Base Metal Alloys for Removable Partial Dentures

Base metal alloys containing substantial amount of chromium are used for construction of removable partial denture frameworks, metal denture bases and periodontal splints.

## *Cobalt-Chromium*

- Most commonly used alloy for constructing removable partial denture frameworks
- Haynes patented the cobalt chromium alloy in 1907
- First used in dentistry in 1929 and marketed as Vitallium (Co-Cr-Mo)
- *Venable* and *Stuck* in mid-1930s found that Vitallium had superior resistance to bodily fluids and had no effect on the surrounding hard or soft tissues. *Dr Strock* in 1939, first placed the Venable screws made of Co-Cr-Mo alloy in the human bone. These were the first implant which showed some evidence of bond growth. Though these "implants" soon failed.
  - *Composition:*
    - Co—60%, and Cr, 25–30%
    - Small amounts of Mo, Mg, Al, W, Fe, Ga, Si, C, and Pt
- Small quantity of manganese and silicon increases the flow of molten metal
- Mo, tungsten and carbon improves hardening and strength of the alloy
- Chromium content should not be more than 30% because this makes the alloy difficult to cast and increases brittleness of the alloy
- Cobalt increases the elastic modulus and strength
- Molybdenum is added to lower the coefficient of thermal expansion and increases corrosion resistance
- Tungsten improves corrosion resistance and decreases Cr-depleted intermetallic areas
- Nickel improves ductility but reduces the hardness of the alloy.

- Co-Cr alloy exhibit nonhomogenous microstructure which is similar to Ni-Cr base metal alloys
- Heat treatment of Co-Cr alloys reduces yield strength and ductility of the alloys
- O'Connor et al. in 1996 found that castability of Co-Cr alloy was in the range of Ni-Cr alloy without Be. But coefficient of thermal expansion of Co-Cr alloy is not that compatible as the Ni-Cr alloy.

### Nickel-Chromium Alloys

- *Composition*:
  - Ni, 70%, Cr, 16% and Al, 2%
  - Be, 0.5%—lowers melting range, improves flow and grain structure.
  - Small amounts of Mo, tungsten, Mg, Co, Si, and C
- Aluminum and nickel form an intermetallic compound that increases the hardness and strength of the alloy.

### Properties

- *Melting range:* Melting range of these alloys is between 1,399°C and 1,454°C
- *Polishability:* These alloys can be polished to high luster and is silvery white in color
- *Density:* Chromium containing alloys are lighter than the gold alloys. Density varies between 8 g/cm³ and 9 g/cm³. Lightweight materials are useful in fabricating large and bulky removable partial dentures
- *Casting shrinkage:* Linear casting shrinkage is high between 2.05% and 2.33%
- *Hardness:* Cobalt-chromium alloys are about 10 times harder than the type IV gold alloys. VHN is 370
- *Tensile strength:* The ultimate tensile strength ranges between 621 MPa and 828 MPa
- *Modulus of elasticity:* Stiffness of cast base metal alloys is almost twice that of cast gold alloys. The modulus of elasticity is almost 207 GPa
- *Elongation:* These alloys are brittle in nature and exhibit elongation of 1–2%
- *Corrosion resistance:* Surface of the alloys is made passive by spontaneous development of thin, transparent layer of chromium oxide. All chromium containing alloys are attacked by chlorine.

### Drawbacks

- Clasps made of cast metal have tendency to break after short duration of use due to fatigue
- If the cast metal framework requires minor adjustment, it becomes difficult to trim because of its high hardness, strength and low elongation

- High hardness of the alloys can cause abrasion of the opposing natural tooth or restorations.

## TITANIUM AND ITS ALLOYS

Commercially pure (CP) titanium and its alloys are used as an alternative to chromium containing alloys because of its excellent biocompatibility, low cost, low density, high corrosion resistance and favorable mechanical properties. It is not classified as noble or precious or base metal alloys because of its excellent biocompatibility. Titanium was synthetically extracted using *Kroll process* in 1936.

### Applications (Fig. 23.16)

- Used for cast metal prosthesis
- As metal ceramic prosthesis
- Dental implants
- Removable partial denture frameworks
- Bar superstructures
- Orthodontic wires.

### Composition

Commercially pure titanium is composed of:

- Titanium: 99.9%
- Oxygen: 0.18–0.40%
- Iron: 0.2–0.5%
- Nitrogen: 0.03–0.05%
- Carbon: 0.1%
- Hydrogen: 0.015%.

| Classification of Titanium Alloys |
|---|
| Commercially pure titanium comes in four grades according to American Society for Testing and Materials (ASTM). It is based on different allowable oxygen and iron content. <br> • *Grade I:* It is purest and softest form. Its tensile strength is 240 MPa. Composed of Ti. 99%; N, 0.03%; C, 0.08%; H, 0.015%; Fe, 0.20; and O, 0.18 <br> • *Grade II:* Composed of Ti, 99; N, 0.03; C, 0.08; H, 0.015; Fe, 0.30; and O, 0.25 <br> • *Grade III:* Composed of Ti, 99, N, 0.05; C, 0.08; H, 0.015; Fe, 0.03; and O, 0.35 <br> • *Grade IV:* Composed of Ti, 99; N, 0.05; N, 0.08; C, 0.015; Fe, 0.50; and O, 0.40. |

### Properties

- *Melting point:* Titanium has melting point of 1,668°C. It has highest melting temperature of all the alloys used for melting ceramic restorations and it possesses high sag resistance

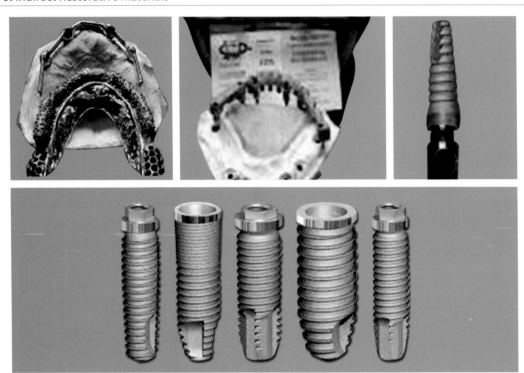

**Fig. 23.16:** Uses of titanium and its alloys.

- *Casting:* It is difficult to cast titanium and its alloys because of high casting temperature which is about 2,000°C, rapid oxidation and reaction with investment during casting
- Titanium is melted in special casting machines with argon atmosphere with compatible casting investment. Recently, CAD/CAM (computer aided design/computer aided milling) technology is used to fabricate titanium crowns and copings. This method completely eliminates the problems of castings **(Fig. 23.17)**
- Titanium reacts with investment and forms very hard α *case* which is 150 μ thick on the surface of casting. The surface treatment of casting is done using caustic NaOH-based solutions or silicon nitride coatings to increase the bond between it and porcelain. Low expansion dental porcelains are used for bonding to titanium
- *Structure:* Commercially pure titanium has *hexagonal closed packed* lattice structure. This lattice configuration is called as α *(alpha) phase*. This phase persists till the temperature of 885°C. At his temperature lattice configuration changes to *body centered cubic* structure and it is called as β *(beta) phase*. This structure transformation gives four different phase combinations of titanium alloys which are α, near α, α-β, and β phase **(Fig. 23.18)**.
- Aluminum, carbon, nitrogen, oxygen, gallium and tin are commonly added α *phase stabilizers to* α-β

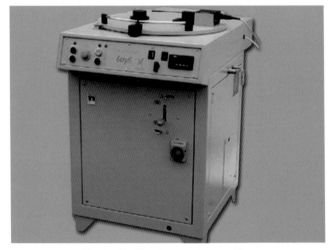

**Fig. 23.17:** Titanium casting machine.

*phase.* Molybdenum, cobalt, nickel, niobium, copper, palladium, tantalum and vanadium are common β *phase stabilizers for* α-β *and* β *phases.* The most common alloys used are CP titanium, Ti 6, Al-4V and Ti-Mo orthodontic wires
- Titanium frameworks are mainly β phase and are stronger but they are less ductile than the dominant α phase

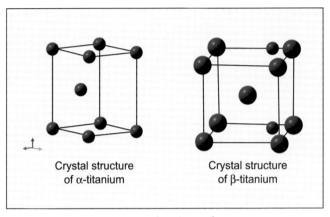

Crystal structure of α-titanium        Crystal structure of β-titanium

**Fig. 23.18:** Crystal structure of titanium.

- *Strength:* Tensile strength of pure titanium is 250 MPa. Addition of oxygen or iron increases the strength and reduces the ductility
- *Hardness:* Vickers hardness of cast CP titanium is 210.

- *Elastic modulus:* Of CP titanium is 117 GPa. It is comparable to tooth enamel and gold alloys
- *Density:* It is light weight metal as compared to base metal alloys. Its density is 4.1 g/cm$^3$
- *Biocompatibility:* It has excellent biocompatibility with both soft and hard tissues
- *Coefficient of thermal expansion:* It has low coefficient of thermal expansion of $9.4 \times 10^{-6}/°C$
- *Corrosion resistance:* It is highly resistant to tarnish and corrosion. Thin passivating layer of 10 μm thick is formed spontaneously to provide corrosion resistance. If this film is abraded or scratched, repassivation occurs almost instantaneously. As oxidation of titanium increases above 900°C, ultralow fusing porcelains are recommended
- *Metal ceramic restorations:* Porcelain fusion temperature should be controlled to below 800°C to prevent phase transition from α to β phase. Special low expansion porcelain should be used and sintering should take place in argon atmosphere for better metal ceramic bond. Titanium and alloys are recommended for nickel sensitive patients.

## TEST YOURSELF

### Essay Questions

1. Classify dental casting alloys. Describe the precious metal alloys in detail.
2. Classify casting alloys used for metal-ceramic restorations. Discuss base metal alloys used for casting metal-ceramic restorations.
3. What are noble metal alloys? Discuss in detail palladium silver alloys.

### Short Notes

1. Ideal requirements of casting alloys.
2. High noble alloys.
3. Noble alloys.
4. Co-Cr alloys.
5. Ni-Cr alloys.
6. Titanium alloys.
7. Bonding of porcelain to metal.
8. Greening effect.

### Multiple Choice Questions

1. High noble metal alloys should contain minimum how much of gold?
   A. 40%
   B. 60%
   C. 75%
   D. 90%
2. Noble metal elements include all of the following, *except*:
   A. Platinum
   B. Palladium
   C. Gold
   D. Silver
3. Which of the following metals should be added to casting alloy to promote oxide formation for chemical bonding of porcelain to metal structure at high temperature?
   A. Lead or beryllium
   B. Indium or tin
   C. Silver or copper
   D. Cobalt or chromium
4. Which type of metal is formed by casting into an ingot or bar and can be changed in different form?
   A. Transformed metal
   B. Stainless steel
   C. Wrought metal
   D. Milled metal
5. Which metal can be added in high noble alloys to increase strength?
   A. Cobalt or chromium
   B. Nickel or beryllium

C. Silver or copper

D. Iron or aluminum

6. Fusion temperature of dental gold casting alloy can be reduced by adding:
   A. Copper
   B. Silver
   C. Platinum
   D. Zinc.

7. Co-Cr alloys as compared to gold alloys have:
   A. Same yield strength, higher elastic modulus and hardness
   B. High yield strength, low modulus of elasticity and hardness
   C. Low yield strength, high modulus of elasticity and hardness
   D. Low yield strength, low modulus of elasticity and hardness

8. Small increase in one of the following constituent can produce drastic change in physical properties of the base metal alloys:
   A. Carbon
   B. Cobalt
   C. Nickel
   D. Molybdenum

9. Cast gold alloy in comparison to base metal alloy have higher value in which of the following property:
   A. Specific gravity
   B. Modulus of elasticity
   C. Hardness
   D. Strength

10. The property which allows gold alloys to be burnished is:
    A. Resilience
    B. Percent elongation
    C. Rigidity
    D. Surface hardness

11. Softening heat treatment of gold alloys is also called as:
    A. Solution hardening
    B. Age hardening
    C. Work hardening
    D. All of the above

12. If in gold alloys content of gold is increased then:
    A. Percent elongation increases
    B. Hardness increases
    C. Corrosion resistance reduces
    D. None of the above

13. Gold alloys with high percent elongation is best used for:
    A. Single crown
    B. Fixed partial dentures
    C. Inlays
    D. Cast framework

14. Passivating layer on Co-Cr alloy is:
    A. Chromium carbide
    B. Ferric oxide
    C. Cobalt oxide
    D. Chromium oxide

## ANSWERS

| | | | |
|---|---|---|---|
| 1. A | 2. D | 3. B | 4. C |
| 5. C | 6. B | 7. A | 8. A |
| 9. A | 10. B | 11. A | 12. A |
| 13. C | 14. D | | |

## BIBLIOGRAPHY

1. Ansavice KJ. Phillip's Science of Dental Materials. 11th edition. St. Louis: WB Saunders; 2003.
2. Anusavice KJ. Noble metal alloys for metal-ceramic restoration. Dent Clin North Am. 1985;29:789-803.
3. Asgar K, Allan FC. Microstructure and physical properties of alloys for partial denture castings. J Dent Res. 1968;47:189-97.
4. Baran GR. Selection criteria for base metal alloys for use with porcelain. Dent Clin North Am. 1985;29:779-87.
5. Baran GR. The metallurgy of Ni-Cr alloys for fixed prosthodontics. J Prosthet Dent. 1983;50:639-50.
6. Brantley WA, Cai Z, Papazoglou E, et al. X-ray diffraction studies of oxidized high-palladium alloys. Dent Mater. 1996;12:333-41.
7. Brantley WA, Laub LW. Metal selection. In: Rosensteil SF, Land MF, Fujimoto J (Eds). Contemporoary Fixed Prosthodontics, 4th edition. St. Louis: Elsevier; 2006. pp. 599-609.
8. Bridgeport DA, Brantley WA, Herman PF. Cobalt-chromium and nickel-chromium alloys for removable prosthodontics, Part I: Mechanical properties. J Prosthodont. 1993;2:144-50.
9. Cai Z, Bunce N, Nunn ME, et al. Porcelain adherence to dental cast CP titanium: effects of surface modifications. Biomaterials. 2001;22:979-86.
10. Civjan S, Hugel EF, Marsden JE. Characteristics of two gold alloys used in fabrication of porcelain-fused-to-metal restorations. J Am Dent Assoc. 1972;85:1309-15.
11. Craig RG, Powers JM. Restorative Dental Materials, 11th edition. St. Louis: Mosby; 2002.
12. Fairhurst CW, Anusavice KJ, Hashinger DT, et al. SW. Thermal expansion of dental alloys and porcelains. J Biomed Mat Res. 1980;14:435-46.
13. Givan DA. Precious metals in dentistry. Dent Clin North Am. 2007;51:591-601.
14. Herö H, Syverud M, Gjönnes J, et al. Ductility and structure of some cobalt-base dental casting alloys. Biomaterials. 1984;5:201-8.
15. Leinfelder KF, O'Brien WJ, Taylor DF. Hardening of dental gold alloys. J Dent Res. 1972;51:900-10.
16. Leinfelder KF. An evaluation of casting alloys used for restorative procedures. J Am Dent Assoc. 1997;128:37-45.
17. Mackert JR, Ringle RD, Fairhurst CW. High temperature behavior of a Pd-Ag alloy for porcelain. J Dent Res. 1983;52:1229-35.

18. McCracken M. Dental implant materials: commercially pure titanium and titanium alloys. J Prosthodont. 1999;8:40-3.

19. McLean JW, Hughes TH. The reinforcement of dental porcelain with ceramic oxides. Br Dent J. 1965;119:251-67.

20. Moffa JP. Biocompatibility of nickel based dental alloys. CDAJ. 1984;12:45-51.

21. Morris HF, Asgar K. Physical properties and microstructure of four new commercial partial denture alloys. J Prosthet Dent. 1975;33:36-46.

22. Morris HF. Properties of cobalt-chromium metal ceramic alloys after heat treatment. J Prosthet Dent. 1990;63:426-33.

23. O'Brien WJ. Dental Materials and their Selection, 3rd edition. Chicago: Qunitessence Publishing Co. Inc.; 2002.

24. O'Connor RP, Mackert JR Jr, Myers ML, et al. Castability, opaque masking, and porcelain bonding of 17 porcelain-fused-to-metal alloys. J Prosthet Dent. 1996;75:367-74.

25. Ohkubo C, Hanatani S, Hasoi T. Present status of titanium removable dentures—a review of the literature. J Oral Rehabil. 2008;35:706-14.

26. Papazoglou E, Brantley WA, Carr AB, et al. Porcelain adherence to high-palladium alloys. J Prosthet Dent. 1993;70:386-94.

27. Papazoglou E, Brantley WA, Johnston WM. Evaluation of high-temperature distortion of high-palladium metal-ceramic crowns. J Prosthet Dent. 2001;85:133-40.

28. Roach M. Base metal alloys used for dental restorations and implants. Dent Clin North Am. 2007;51:603-27.

29. Setcos JC, Babaei-Mahani A, Silvio LD, et al. The safety of nickel containing dental alloys. Dent Mater. 2006;22:1163-8.

30. Shillenburg HT, Hobo S, Fisher DW. Preparation, design and margin distortion in porcelain fused to metal restorations. J Prosthet Dent. 1973;29:276-84.

31. Tai Y, DeLong R, Goodkind RJ, et al. Leaching of nickel, chromium, and beryllium ions from base metal alloy in an artificial oral environment. J Prosthet Dent. 1992;68:692-7.

32. Togaya T, Suzuki M, Tsutsumi S, et al. An application of pure titanium to the metal porcelain system. Dent Mater J. 1983;2:210-9.

33. Venable CS, Struck WG. Electrolysis controlling factor in the use of metals in treating fractures. J Am Med Assoc. 1938;111:1349-52.

34. Watanabe I, Kiyosue S, Ohkubo C, et al. Machinability of cast commercial titanium alloys. J Biomed Mater Res. 2002;63:760-4.

35. Wataha JC, Hanks CT. Biological effects of palladium and risk of using palladium in dental casting alloys. J Oral Rehabil. 1996;23:309-20.

36. Wataha JC, Messer RL. Casting alloys. Dent Clin North Am. 2004;48:499-512.

37. Wataha JC. Alloys for prosthodontic restorations. J Prosthet Dent. 2002;87:351-63.

38. Winkler S, Morris HF, Monteiro JM. Changes in mechanical properties and microstructure following heat treatment of nickel-chromium base alloy. J Prosthet Dent. 1984;52:821-7.

39. Wu Q, Brantley WA, Mitchell JC, Vermilyea SG, Xiao J, Guo W. Heat-treatment behavior of high-palladium dental alloys. Cells Mater. 1997;7:161-74.

# Casting Procedures and Casting Defects

*'Without your involvement you can't succeed. With your involvement you can't fail.'*
*—APJ Abdul Kalam*

## INTRODUCTION

Casting is a procedure to convert a wax pattern of the restorations to replicate into a metallic replica. This process is widely used in dentistry to fabricate various fixed restorations. Most of the dental castings are done using the Lost wax technique. Although this technique was used for centuries but it was known to the world when WH Taggart introduced this technique using a casting machine in 1907. This procedure is favored widely as it is convenient and inexpensive to fabricate fairly accurate dimensionally stable casting.

Lost wax casting procedure is briefly described as follows **(Fig. 24.1)**. The success of the procedure depends on how each step is accomplished.

- Tooth is prepared in the mouth to receive cast restoration
- Final impression is made of the prepared tooth using appropriate impression material. Usually for cast restoration elastomeric impression materials are preferred
- Most commonly gypsum (die stone) is poured into the impression to form a master cast, which is exact replica of the dental arch
- Prepared die is sectioned
- Wax pattern is fabricated using inlay wax on the die to simulate the lost tooth structure

- Sprue is attached to the wax pattern
- Wax pattern along with the sprue is removed from the die and is attached to the sprue former in the casting ring
- Casting ring is lined with a casting liner
- Casting ring with the pattern is poured with investment material
- Investment material is allowed to set
- Wax is eliminated by process of burnout in a furnace forming an empty mold
- Casting is done in a casting machine using an appropriate metal alloy by forcing the molten metal into the empty mold
- Casting is allowed to cool and then is divested
- Casting is cleaned
- Sprue is removed and the casting is finished and polished
- The finished cast restoration is then cemented on the prepared tooth.

## FABRICATION OF WAX PATTERN

Wax pattern fabrication is convenient as it is inexpensive, quick, reversible and customized. It can be made by two methods—indirect and direct methods.

## Direct Method

The wax pattern is directly prepared on the tooth in the mouth. Wax used for this purpose should be sufficiently heated to have adequate flow and plasticity so that it can reproduce the details of the cavity or prepared tooth. Wax pattern made by this method is prone to undesirable and unavoidable induced stresses **(Fig. 24.2)**.

## Indirect Method

In this method, the wax pattern is formed over the die prepared after pouring the impression. This method is used for all types of restorations. The wax pattern fabrication by this method is much more convenient and easy to manipulate. Inorder to prevent sticking of the wax to the die, lubricant is used. Some technicians recommend the use of spacer on the stone die to allow space for the cement in the final restoration. The thickness of spacer varies between 10 and 30 μm. Inlay pattern wax is melted over alcohol flame and is added over the die in small increments. After addition of each increment cooling is allowed to reduce distortion because of shrinkage. The wax is used to produce the anatomy of the tooth and pattern appears to simulate the natural tooth. The wax pattern is inspected for accurate fit with tight junctions at the margins **(Fig. 24.3)**.

**CLINICAL SIGNIFICANCE**

Pattern should not be cooled or heated too rapidly as it has greater tendency to distort. However, even after taking all precautions, still wax patterns may show relaxation of internal stress. Therefore, it is recommended that wax patterns should be invested as soon as possible. Storage of wax patterns for long should be avoided.

## REMOVAL OF WAX PATTERN

Wax pattern fabricated on the master die is removed in line with the path of withdrawal from the die. The wax pattern should not be forced out or removed in any other path. Unnecessary force may break or distort the pattern. Master die should be lubricated before wax pattern fabrication to facilitate its removal.

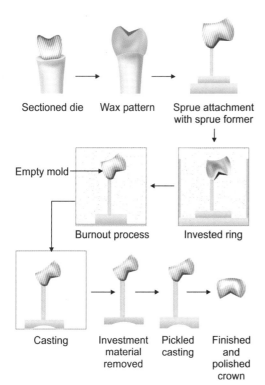

**Fig. 24.1:** Lost wax technique.

Sectioned die → Wax pattern → Sprue attachment with sprue former

Empty mold → Burnout process ← Invested ring

Casting → Investment material removed → Pickled casting → Finished and polished crown

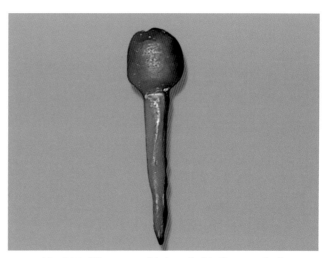

**Fig. 24.2:** Wax pattern fabricated with direct method.

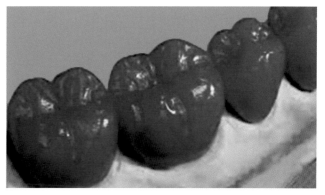

**Fig. 24.3:** Wax pattern made with indirect method.

# SPRUING THE WAX PATTERN

Proper sprue design and technique of spruing is critical for the success of cast restoration. Design of the sprue varies depending on the type of alloy used, type of restoration being casted and the type of casting machine (**Fig. 24.4**).

## Rationale

- To provide channel for elimination of wax during burnout
- To fix pattern in the space such that mold can be formed
- To provide channel for ingress of molten metal to reach the empty mold
- To compensate for alloy shrinkage during solidification.

## Requirements of a Sprue

- Should allow molten wax to escape from the mold
- Should allow molten metal to flow smoothly
- Should allow metal to be molten state until it fills the mold completely
- Should provide reservoir of molten metal which compensates for alloy shrinkage during solidification.

## Types of Sprues

- *Based on the type of material:*
  - *Hollow metal sprue:* Often hollow to increase contact surface area and to strengthen the attachment between the sprue and pattern.
  - *Round wax sprue:* Most preferred for casting as they melt at the same rate as the pattern and allows easy escape of the molten wax.
  - *Plastic sprue:* Soften at higher temperature than wax temperature and may result in roughened casting.
- *Based on the design:*
  - Prefabricated sprue
  - Custom-made sprue
- *Based on type of spruing (**Fig. 24.5**):*
  - *Direct spruing:* It provides direct connection between the wax pattern and the sprue base
  - *Indirect spruing:* In this reservoir or connector, bar is placed between the pattern and the sprue base.

## Sprue Diameter

Diameter of the sprue is selected as the same size as the thickest area of the wax pattern. For a small pattern, small diameter sprue is used whereas for large pattern, larger sprue is required. If the sprue is too thin as compared to the pattern, the area will solidify before the casting itself and result in localized shrinkage porosity. A 2.5 mm diameter sprue is recommended for molar and metal ceramic patterns. A 2.0 mm diameter sprue is recommended for premolars and partial veneer restorations.

## Sprue Position

Spure should be ideally attached to the point of greatest bulk of the pattern which is away from margins and the occlusal contacts (**Fig. 24.6**). Usually, largest noncentric cusp is used to reduce subsequent grinding of the occlusal anatomy and contact areas. The point of attachment should be smooth to minimize turbulence and should allow molten metal to be directed to all parts of the mold. Apart from the occlusal surface, some clinician prefer to attach the sprue at the proximal wall or just below the non-functional cusp.

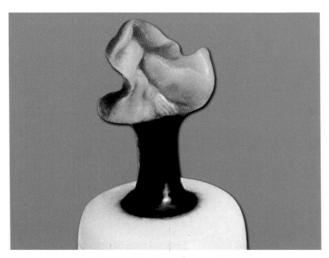

**Fig. 24.4:** Spruing of wax pattern.

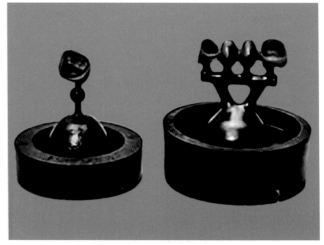

**Fig. 24.5:** Types of spruing.

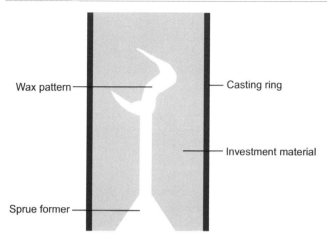

**Fig. 24.6:** Sprue should be attached to the greatest bulk of the wax pattern.

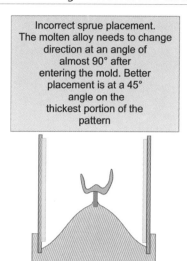

**Fig. 24.7:** Incorrect placement of sprue leads to casting failure.

## Sprue Attachment

Point of attachment of the sprue to the wax pattern should be flared for high density gold alloys and should be restricted for low density alloys. Sprue should be attached to the wax pattern at the largest cross-sectional area. The molten alloy should be allowed to flow from thick section to the surrounding thin areas rather than the reverse **(Fig. 24.7)**. This sequence reduces the risk of turbulence of the molten alloy. The sprue should be long enough to position the wax pattern in the casting ring properly. The wax pattern should be positioned within 6 mm of the trailing end of the casting ring.

### CLINICAL SIGNIFICANCE

Wax sprues are preferred over the plastic sprues. If plastic sprues are used then two stage burn-out process is recommended because plastic spures soften at temperature above the melting range of inlay pattern wax.

Sprues can be attached either directly or indirectly. In direct wax spruing, sprue provides direct channel between the wax pattern and the crucible former whereas in Indirect spruing a reservoir or connector bar is positioned between the pattern and the crucible former. Indirect spruing is usually used for fixed partial dentures and multiple single units and direct spruing is preferred for single wax patterns.

A reservoir is attached to the sprue to prevent localized shrinkage porosity. When the molten metal alloy fills the empty mold, then the pattern area of the mold should solidify first and the reservoir area should solidify last. The reservoir helps in furnishing molten alloy into the mold since it solidifies in the end.

## Sprue Length

The length of the sprue should be long enough to position the pattern in the casting ring within 6 mm of trailing end and yet should be short enough so that molten alloy does not solidifies before it fills the mold. In cases of phosphate-bonded investment, it is possible to position the wax pattern within 3–4 mm of the top of the investment. For gypsum bonded investment, the wax pattern should be within 6 mm from the open end of casting ring **(Fig. 24.8)**. If sprue is short, the wax pattern is too far to permit the gases to escape adequately and to allow the molten metal alloy to flow into the mold completely **(Fig. 24.9)**. If these gases are not allowed to escape then it can result in porosity in the casting. For accuracy in casting the wax pattern should, be positioned as close to the center of the ring as possible.

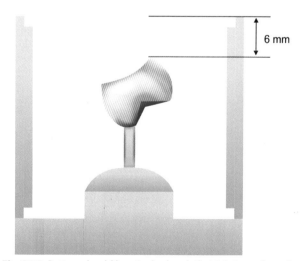

**Fig. 24.8:** Pattern should be attached such that it is 6 mm from the end of the casting.

### Sprue Direction

Sprue should not be attached at right angle to the broad flat surface of the pattern to avoid turbulence and porosity. The sprues should be attached at an angle of 45° angle to the proximal area for satisfactory casting **(Fig. 24.10)**. The sprue should be attached away from delicate part of the wax pattern because the molten alloy tends to abrade or fracture the investment in this portion and will result in casting failure.

## CRUCIBLE FORMER OR SPRUE FORMER

Sprue is attached to the sprue former or crucible former which is usually made of rubber. This forms the base of the casting during investment. The casting ring and the sprue former provides a seal so that investment material does not flow out. It helps in confining the investment material within

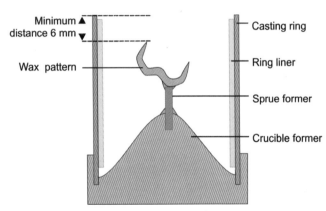

**Fig. 24.9:** Correct length of the sprue.

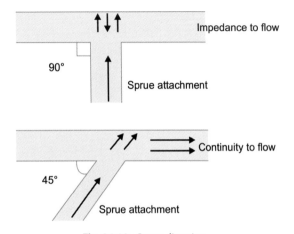

**Fig. 24.10:** Sprue direction.

the casting ring. The shape of the sprue former depends on the type of casting machine used. Mostly the sprue former is high enough to allow the use of short sprue and to allow the pattern to be positioned near the end of the casting ring **(Fig. 24.11)**.

## CASTING RING LINER

Casting ring helps in confining the investment in place during setting and restricts the expansion of the mold. Casting ring is lined by a ring liner to allow greater expansion. In the past, *asbestos ring liner* was material of choice but its use is discouraged because of its carcinogenic potential. Currently, two *nonasbestos ring liners* are used which are *aluminosilicate ceramic liner* and the *cellulose (paper) liner*. The rationale behind using casting ring liner is to allow the hardening investment material to expand during setting.

### CLINICAL SIGNIFICANCE

If casting liner was not used, the investment material would not expand outwards as it is completely constrained by metal ring. This would push the investment backwards into the wax pattern resulting in cavity (mold) of the same size or smaller as the wax pattern. During casting because of casting shrinkage, it will result in undersized casting. Therefore, moist soft ring liner is used with the hardening investment to result in a cavity (mold) which is larger than the wax pattern when the investment material is completely set.

The casting liner of appropriate size is cut so that it fits the inside of the casting ring without overlapping **(Fig. 24.12)**. The liner can be wet or left dry for use. Dry casting liner is avoided as it will absorb water from the investment material and will reduce setting expansion. In the wet technique, the casting ring with liner is immersed in water and excess water is shaken off. Liner should not be squeezed as this will lead to removal of variable amount of water

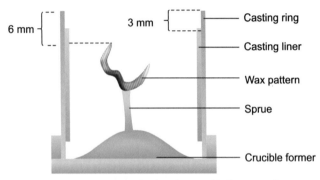

**Fig. 24.11:** Wax pattern attached to the crucible former with sprue is ready for investing.

resulting in non-uniform expansion. Ceramic liner unlike cellulose liner have network of fibers to retain water on the surface. The thickness of liner should not be less than 1 mm for adequate expansion. Casting ring liner aids in providing greater normal setting expansion and semi-hygroscopic expansion. The ring liner should be placed short of the ends of the ring in order to produce uniform expansion.

### CLINICAL SIGNIFICANCE

If the casting ring liner is flushed with ends of the ring then the longitudinal and hygroscopic setting expansion is not restricted. There is greater expansion in unrestricted longitudinal direction than in the radial direction, i.e towards the center of the ring. Therefore, it is desirable to restrict longitudinal expansion by placing the ring liner short of the ends of the ring.

Since the casting ring liners are products made of paper, they are completely burned out during the burnout process. Thicker casting liner or using two layers of casting liners provides greater semi-hygroscopic and normal setting expansion than single liner.

### Ringless Casting Technique

This technique is used with high strength, phosphate bonded investment material. In ringless casting, paper or a plastic casting ring is used to permit unrestricted setting expansion **(Fig. 24.13)**.

## INVESTING PROCEDURE

The wax pattern is cleaned of oil, debris or grease. Wax pattern cleaner or diluted synthetic detergent (surfactant) is used to reduce surface tension of wax (hydrophobic) and allows better wetting of the investment material (hydrophilic) to the pattern. Appropriate amount of liquid and investment powder are mixed in prescribed ratio until all the powder is wet. Then mechanical mixing under vacuum is done to remove air bubbles created during mixing. The mixed material is quickly painted using a thin brush in and around the wax pattern. Then the remaining investment is vibrated slowly into the casting ring. For vacuum investing, same instruments used for mixing are also used for investing.

With vacuum investing, the texture of the cast surface is smoother producing accurate details and has better tensile strength. It also, produces highly reduced surface imperfections. For vacuum mixing special equipment consisting of plastic bowl and metallic mixing blades are used. The casting ring with the sprue former and wax pattern is connected to the top part of the vacuum mixer. Such arrangement is made so that the investment material flows directly into the open end of the casting ring whereas the entire assembly remains under vacuum **(Fig. 24.14)**.

### CLINICAL SIGNIFICANCE

During investment procedure excessive vibration should be avoided because it can dislodge small wax patterns from the sprue former resulting in miscast or it can cause the solid to settle at the bottom and the watery investment to come up and can surround the pattern resulting in surface roughness of the casting.

For hygroscopic expansion, the casting ring is immediately placed in water bath at 37°C with the crucible former facing downwards. The hygroscopic expansion produces the total setting expansion of 1.5% which is more than twice that achieved by normal setting. Likewise to achieve thermal expansion the invested casting ring

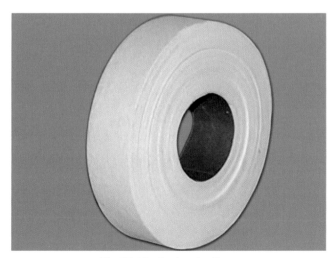

**Fig. 24.12:** Casting ring liner.

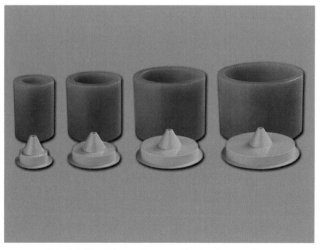

**Fig. 24.13:** Silicone ring used for ringless casting.

is allowed to bench set undisturbed for the time period recommended by the manufacturer.

*Carbon containing* investments are used for gold alloys and metal ceramic alloys. A *noncarbon investment* is used for carbon sensitive alloys like silver palladium, nickel chromium or cobalt chromium alloys.

## Wax Elimination or Burnout Procedure

Once the investment material is completely set, it should be transferred to the burnout furnace. Before that the crucible former and any metallic sprue former is removed without damaging the mold. The mold is checked carefully for any debris which is removed with a brush. After removal of the rubber spure former, the ring consists of attached wax pattern with a sprue which is completely surrounded by investment material. The invested ring is then placed into a burnout furnace at 500°C for Gypsum-bonded investment in hygroscopic technique and 700°C in thermal expansion technique. For the phosphate, bonded investment-the temperature varies between 700°C and 1030°C, depending on the type of alloy used. The temperature setting is more critical in gypsum bonded as they have tendency of investment decomposition. Burnout process should begin when the investment material is still wet because water trapped in the investment pores reduces the absorption of gases. Heating should be gradual to allow steam to escape without cracking of the mold. The ring should always be placed downward in the ceramic tray so that easy escape of molten gases such as carbon monoxide is allowed. The gases also escape through various pores in the invested mold **(Fig. 24.15)**. Burnout temperature and time recommended for various investment material is summarized in **Table 24.1**.

## Precautions During Wax Burn-Out Process

- The casting ring should be kept in the burnout furnace at the room temperature and then the temperature is gradually increased to the maximum. The casting ring should not be heated rapidly because this causes flaking of the mold walls. Placing the ring suddenly at high temperature causes temperature difference between the outer and the inner layer of the investment resulting in cracking. Investment containing cristobalite which has high thermal expansion and low inversion temperature are highly prone for cracking.
- Usually the casting ring is left in the burnout furnace for 45–90 minutes depending on the type of investment, type of expansion and the type of alloy used.
- The burnout temperature should be maintained for extended period of time to compensate for the drop in temperature when the casting ring is removed from the furnace just before casting.

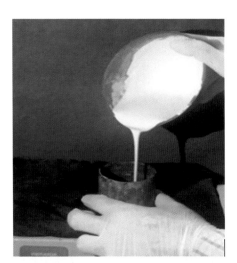

**Fig. 24.14:** Pouring of investment material.

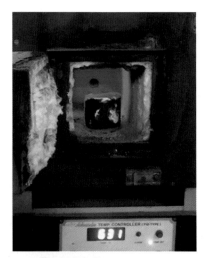

**Fig. 24.15:** Burnout process.

**Table 24.1:** Burnout temperatures, time and type of expansion of various casting investment materials.

| Type of investment | Time | Maximum temperature | Type of expansion |
| --- | --- | --- | --- |
| Gypsum bonded | 1 hour | 500°C/ 900°F | Hygroscopic |
| Gypsum bonded | 1 hour | 700°C/1200°F | Thermal |
| Phosphate bonded | 45 minutes | 700°C–1030°C | Thermal |
| Ethyl silicate bonded | | 1090–1180°C | Thermal |

## Time Between Burnout Process and Casting

The investment contracts as it cools. In normal conditions about 1 minute time is allowed between removal of the casting ring from the burnout furnace and casting. This short duration does not cause contraction of the mold when the casting ring is removed from the burnout furnace and taken for casting. However, in cases of high heat technique slight time lapse is critical. Therefore to prevent heat loss during transfer the casting ring is maintained at the maximum temperature in the burnout furnace. This is called as 'Heat soaking.'

Even in low heat technique, it is advisable to cast as soon as the casting ring is removed from the burnout furnace to minimize any contraction in the mold. Metal tongs are used to transfer the casting ring from the burnout furnace to the casting machine

## LOW HEAT TECHNIQUE

Alloys with high gold content (Noble metal alloys) uses the low heat hygroscopic technique. In this technique compensatory expansion is achieved by—(i). Placing the casting ring in water bath at 37°C, (ii). The warm water enters the investment mold from top and increases hygroscopic expansion, and (iii) Thermal expansion is achieved at 500°C. This technique has following advantages:
- As the temperature is less there is less degradation of investment material.
- Cooler surfaces gives smoother casting
- The mold can be directly placed in the furnace at 500°C.
The invested mold are placed in burnout furnace for 60–90 minutes. Additional time may be required to eliminate residual fine carbon. If this is not eliminated it may result in back-pressure porosity. Newer Noble metal alloys may require slightly greater amount of expansion. This increased expansion can be achieved by:
- Increasing the water bath temperature to 40°C
- Using double layers of casting ring liners
- Increasing the burnout temperature in the range of 600–650°C.

## HIGH HEAT TECHNIQUE

This technique is employed in casting metal alloys (base metal alloys or those used for metal ceramic prosthesis) in Gypsum-bonded and Phosphate-bonded investment materials. High heat technique requires greater expansion than the high noble or noble metal alloys. The total expansion obtained from this technique includes setting expansion (0.7%) and thermal expansion (1.25%) which is about 2 % or more. As alloys used for metal ceramic prosthesis have higher melting and solidification temperature, greater expansion is required for casting. The normal burnout temperature for phosphate-bonded investment varies between 750°C to 1030°C. The temperature is slowly increased to 315°C and thereafter, it is rapidly increased to maximum. The holding time for maximum temperature is 30 minutes.

## Casting Crucibles

The casting metal alloys are placed and melted in a crucible before the process of casting **(Fig. 24.16)**. The casting crucible should fulfill the following requirements:
- Should not contaminate the alloy by reacting with it
- Should be able to withstand high casting temperature and molten metal
Various kinds of crucibles used for different types of alloys are depicted in **Table 24.2.**

### Types of Casting Crucibles

- *Clay crucible:* Used for high noble and noble alloys
- *Carbon crucible:* Used for high noble alloys and high fusing, gold based metal ceramic alloys
- Silica or *Quartz crucible:* Used for high fusing alloys of any type. Any alloy with high melting temperature which is sensitive to carbon contamination. Also useful for alloys with high palladium content such as palladium silver alloys for metal ceramic copings. Carbon crucibles should not be used for silver palladium, nickel-chromium, cobalt chromium alloys.
- *Zirconia-alumina crucible:* Used for any type of high fusing alloys **(Fig. 24.17)**.

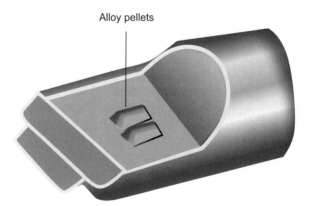

Alloy pellets

**Fig. 24.16:** Alloy pellets are placed in casting crucible.

**Table 24. 2:** Types of crucibles used for different types of alloys.

| Type of crucibles | Type of alloy |
| --- | --- |
| Clay | High noble and noble alloys |
| Carbon | High noble, high fusing gold-based alloys |
| Silica or quartz | High fusing alloys |
| Zirconia-Alumina | High fusing alloys |

## CASTING

### Definition

*Casting is process in which an object is formed by the solidification of a fluid that has been poured or injected into the mold.* **-GPT 8th Edition**

### Casting Machines

- *Torch melting/centrifugal casting machine:* Alloy melted by flame torch and casting is done using centrifugal force.
- *Electrical resistance:* Alloy is melted by electrical resistance and is cast into the mold centrifugally by motor or spring action.
- *Induction melting machine:* Alloy is melted by induction machine and is cast into the mold centrifugally by motor or spring action.
- *Vacuum-or pressure-assisted casting machine:* Alloy is vacuum arc melted and casting is done by pressure in an argon atmosphere.

### Torch Melting/Centrifugal Casting Machine

In this casting machine, a torch flame is used to melt the alloy in a glazed ceramic crucible. The torch flame is generated from a mixture of propane and air, natural gas and air, acetylene and air or acetylene and oxygen. The spring in the casting machine is wound for 2–5 turns depending on the particular machine and the desired speed of the casting rotation. The casting ring is ensured in proper position. Once the heated alloy reaches the casting temperature, the lever is released and the spring triggers rotary motion to complete the casting. Hydrostatic pressure develops along the casting as the mold is filled by the molten alloy. Pressure gradient from the tip of the casting to the bottom is sharp and parabolic in form. This machine is used for casting gold alloys **(Fig. 24.18)**.

### Electrical Resistance-heated Casting Machine

In this type of casting machine, the electric current is passed through resistance heating conductor to melt the metal alloy. The alloy is placed in a graphite or

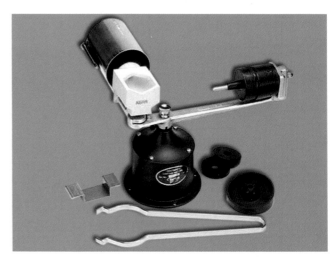

**Fig. 24.18:** Centrifugal casting machine.

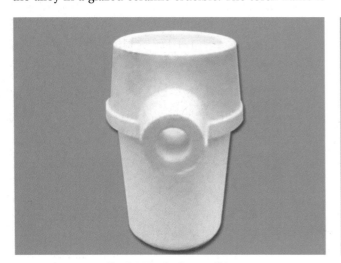

**Fig. 24.17:** Casting crucible.

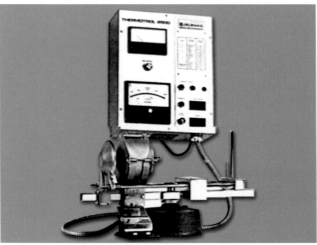

**Fig. 24.19:** Electrical resistance—heat-casting machine.

ceramic crucible and is contacting the casting ring. This arrangement is advantageous for alloys melted for metal ceramic restorations because the alloy button remains molten for longer period of time and solidification occurs gradually till the completion of casting. This ensures lesser chances of casting failure. Carbon crucible should be avoided for melting high palladium alloys, palladium silver alloy and base metal alloys because of contamination problem **(Fig. 24.19)**.

## Induction Melting Machine

Induction-casting machine is the most commonly used casting machine to melt high fusing alloys such as metal ceramic alloys or base metal alloys. In this type of casting machine, the metal alloy is melted in the crucible by producing magnetic field. The crucible is surrounded by water cooled metal tubing inorder to reduce excess heat buildup. Alternating current (AC) flows through the primary winding coil to generate variable magnetic field in the area of the alloy. The alloy is melted till it reaches the casting temperature. This molten alloy is forced into the empty mold using a centrifugal force by air pressure or vacuum to complete the casting **(Figs. 24.20 A and B)**. This machine is commonly used to cast base metal alloys but not used for noble metal alloys.

## Direct Current Arc Melting Machine

This method of melting is usually employed to melt industrial-grade alloys such as steel. Arc melting is accomplished by passing a direct current between two electrodes namely, the alloy metal and the tungsten. This method is used to produce high temperature and is used to melt high fusing metals or alloys such as titanium. Caution should be taken as in this method, there is very high risk of overheating of the alloys and damage may occur after few seconds of prolonged heating **(Fig. 24.21)**. Tungsten electrode is water cooled inorder to reduce temperature build-up.

## Vacuum or Pressure-assisted Casting Machine

In this machine, the alloy is melted to the casting temperature and is drawn into the evacuated mold by gravity or vacuum. The molten alloy is forced into the empty mold using additional pressure. When *titanium and titanium alloys* are casted, vacuum arc heated argon pressure-casting machine is required **(Fig. 24.22)**.

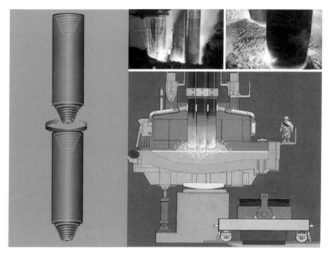

**Fig. 24.21:** Direct current arc-melting machine.

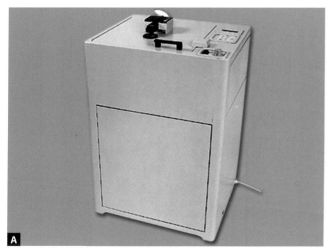

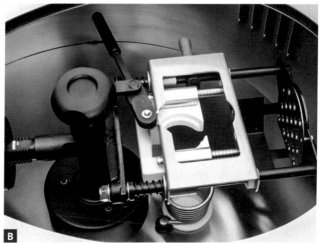

**Figs. 24.20 A and B:** Induction-casting machine.

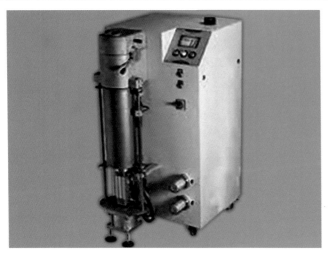

**Fig. 24.22:** Vacuum- or pressure-assisted casting machine.

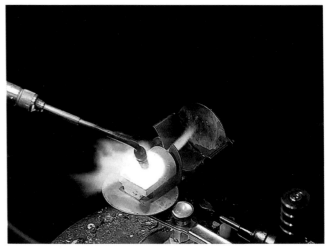

**Fig. 24.23:** Torch melting of high noble alloys.

## Casting Procedure for Noble Metal Alloys

As soon as the invested ring is removed from the burnout furnace, the molten alloy should be centrifuged into the mold within 30 seconds. Clean crucible is placed in its bracket on the arm of the casting machine. Crucible used for base metal alloys cannot be used for noble alloys. Casting alloy pellets are placed in the inner sidewall of the crucible which should be sufficient to fill the mold, sprue and the crucible former to ensure sharp and complete detail of the casting. The fuel commonly used for the torch melting is mixture of natural gas or artificial gas and air, although oxygen air and acetylene can also be used. Care should be taken to obtain a nonluminous brush flame. The gas air blow pipe is adjusted to produce a conical flame **(Fig. 24.23)**.

## Zones of Conical Flame **(Fig. 24.24)**

*Mixing zone:* It is a cool and colorless cone which directly emanates from the nozzle. Here zone and gas are mixed before combustion. No heat is present in this zone.

*Combustion zone:* It is a greenish blue zone in which partial combustion takes place. It is an oxidizing zone which should be kept away from the molten alloy during fusion.

*Reducing zone:* It is the dim blue zone which is the hottest area in the flame. This zone is the **only zone** used for heating

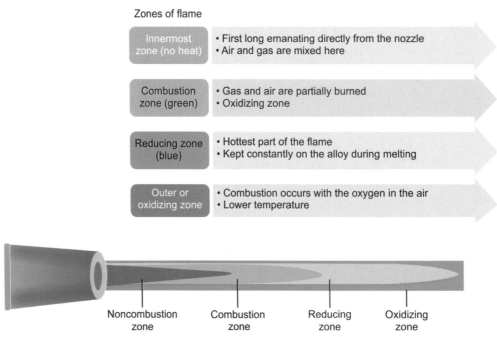

**Fig. 24.24:** Zones of flame.

the casting alloys. The zone should be constantly kept over the alloy to be melted. When this zone is in contact with the gold alloy, the surface appears bright and mirror like.

*Oxidizing zone:* It is the outermost zone in which combustion occurs with the oxygen in the air. This zone should never be used to melt the alloy as it has lower temperature than the reducing zone and also it oxidizes the alloy. If this zone contacts the metal, the surface appears dull.

A small amount of flux can be added to the warmed metal to increase the fluidity of the alloy and prevents oxidation. Borax can be used as a flux which help in preventing oxidation and dissolve any oxides that are formed. The alloy when heated first appears spongy and then small globules are formed. Later the molten alloy becomes spheroidal shaped. As soon as the proper temperature is achieved the casting procedure should be carried out immediately. The blowpipe is kept on the alloy and the counterweight is applied with the other hand until the pin drops. This allows the machine to spin, thus forcing the molten alloy into the mold with centrifugal force.

## Melting of Base Metal Alloys

Base metal alloys, titanium and titanium alloys are melted in special induction melting machines, vacuum melting or arc melting units. Care is taken to minimize the risk of oxidation and interaction of the investment with the molten alloys.

## Cleaning the Casting

Once the casting of noble metal alloys is solidified, the ring is removed and quenched in water immediately as the button appears dull red. This leaves the cast metal in an annealed state (softened) which allows easy removal from the investment. The advantages of the annealed state is easy finishing, polishing and burnishing of the casting.

### *Rationale Behind Quenching*

- The heated investment when comes in contact with water undergoes violent reaction causing granular investment to crumble with ease.
- Once the noble metal alloy is annealed it can be easily finished, polished or burnished.

However, base metal alloy or metal ceramic alloys should not be quenched but allowed to cool. In such castings since phosphate bonded investment material is used cleaning and recovery of casting is difficult. Investment from the base metal and metal ceramic casting is removed by sandblasting with fine alumina particles **(Fig. 24.25)**. Acid should never be used to clean base metal alloys.

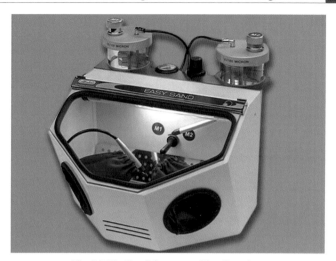

**Fig. 24.25:** Sandblaster used for divesting.

Once the casting is completely divested, the sprues are removed from the casting using abrasive disks mounted in a handpiece and the casting is cleaned or pickled. The cleaned casting is finished and polished using different types of abrasives.

## Pickling

After the investment material is removed, the casting appears dark because of oxides and tarnish. The surface film so formed is removed by pickling process.

*Pickling is defined as 'a solution or bath for preserving or cleaning.'*

*—GPT 8th Edition*

In this process, the discolored casting is heated in an acid **(Fig. 24.26)**. For gypsum-bonded investment casting, the best Pickling agent is 50% hydrochloric acid solution. Hydrochloric acid helps in removing the oxide coating and aids in removal of any residual investment material.

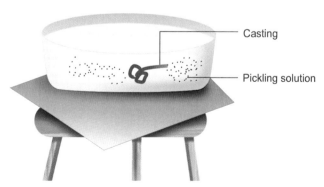

**Fig. 24.26:** Pickling of the casting.

But fumes of hydrochloric acids are health hazard and should be vented through a fume hood. As an alternative, sulfuric acid can be used more appropriately. For pickling, casting should be placed in a test tube or dish and acid should be poured over it. The pickling solution should be heated but not boiled and should be changed frequently.

> **CLINICAL SIGNIFICANCE**
> Pickling is not recommended for gold based, palladium-based metal ceramic alloys and base metal alloys.

Abrasive-blasting devices are more preferred for cleaning the surface of the casting because of health and environmental hazards associated with pickling solutions.

## LAWS OF CASTINGS

The entire process of investing and casting is complex involving multiple steps. Any deviation from the basic principles will lead to defect in the casting. There are certain fundamental principles in casting which should be strictly followed. The laws of casting are given below:

1. **Law 1—Spruing**—Sprue should be attached to the thickest part of the wax pattern (**Figs. 24.27 and 25.28**). The heated molten alloy should flow from the reservoir, i.e area of greater volume to area of lesser volume.
   Defect—can cause incomplete casting, short-rounded margins.
2. **Law 2—Orientation**—Single or multiple wax patterns should be oriented in the ring such that all the restoration margins should face the trailing edge of the ring when it is placed in the casting machine. To identify such an orientation, a drop of wax is added on the crucible former and the patterns are fixed towards this side.
   Defects—short margins and incomplete casting.

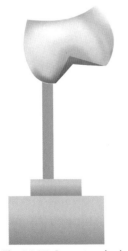 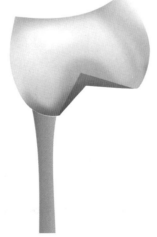

**Fig. 24.27:** Sprue attached to largest non-centric cusp.    **Fig. 24.28:** Point of attachment should be flared for high density alloy.

3. **Law 3—Pattern position**—place the wax pattern in the 'cold zone' of the investment mold and the reservoir is place in the 'heat center' of the casting ring. Heat center is towards the center of the ring and the cold zone is the area along the periphery of the casting ring.
   Defect—shrinkage porosity
4. **Law 4—Shrinkage**—A reservoir should have sufficient molten alloy to accommodate the shrinkage that occurs within the restoration. As the molten alloy solidifies, it shrinks and creates a vacuum. This vacuum (void) should be able to extract additional metal from the adjacent source which is the reservoir.
   Defect—suck back porosity
5. **Law 5—Button**—Button obtained after casting shows whether there was a proper casting of the wax pattern. Button should not be re-casted if a runner bar or internal reservoir was used. This can be counterproductive as it can draw the heated alloy away from the bar and shift the heat center which will reduce the amount of metal to the restoration.
   Defect—porosity in restoration, suck back porosity, potential distortion during porcelain firing.
6. **Law 6—Turbulence**—Pathway of the flow of molten metal alloy should be smooth, gradual and without impediments. Turbulence can be minimized if not totally eliminated by avoiding sharp turns or acute angles during sprue attachments. Turbulence can occlude air in the casting.
   Defect—voids in casting, surface pitting.
7. **Law 7—Length of casting ring**—the length and diameter of the casting ring should be selected such that it is adequate to accommodate the patterns to be invested. There should be a gap of ¼ inch between two patterns and ¼ inch from the trail end of the ring. There should be a gap of 3/8 inch between the ring liner and the wax pattern. If there is too little investment especially towards the top of the ring, there are chances that the molten alloy can break through the mold. Again if too much of investment is there, then the pattern will be closer to the heat center and there will not be impairment to escape of gases.
   Defect—mold fracture, casting fins, shrinkage porosity.
8. **Law 8—Surface tension**—wax pattern wettability to the investment material should increase by reducing the surface tension. Debubblizer is sprayed to reduce the surface tension. Use of too much debubblizer can result in formation of surface film that can dilute or weaken the investment.
   Defect—fins on the casting.
9. **Law 9—Investment**—Investment materials should be mixed in proper water powder ratio. Two factors should be considered—(i). Concentration of the special liquid,

(ii) Total volume of the liquid. If the mix is too thick it will result in too much expansion and if it is too thin it will lead to less expansion.

Defect—ill fitting casting.

10. **Law 10—Air entrapment**—The investment material should be mixed using a vacuum mixer. This removes air and gaseous byproducts which gets entrapped during hand manipulation. Vacuum mixed investment allows more uniform expansion.

　　Defect—distortion of casting, small nodules on the casting.

11. **Law 11—Setting time**—Before the burnout process, the casting investment should be allowed to completely set. If the investment material is not completely set, it can result in weak mold which will be unable to withstand pressure and expansion produced by the formation of steam in early stages of heating. Most of the investments require 1 hour for complete setting.

　　Defect—cracking of mold, fins on casting.

12. **Law 12—Wax elimination**—Correct wax elimination method should be selected for particular type of alloy used. Plastic sprues should undergo two stage wax elimination procedure. Heat soaking is recommended to ensure all plastic patterns are melted out.

　　Defect—short margins, cracked fins, cracks in molds.

13. **Law 13—Heat source**—The selected heat source should be capable of melting the alloy to sufficient fluidity. Inaccurate placement of heat source can prevent the molten alloy to completely fill the mold **(Fig. 24.29)**. Too much heating can burn off minor alloying elements. Most of the base metals do not pool together but heating high noble and noble alloys can result in pooling and forming one molten mass.

　　Defect—rough casting, investment breakdown, short margins.

14. **Law 14—Reducing zone of flame**—Use the reducing zone of the flame when melting the alloy **(Fig. 24.30)**. An improperly adjusted flame can add carbon or oxygen to the alloy during melting.

　　Defect—gas inclusion porosity, alteration in properties of the molten alloy

15. **Law 15—Force**—Adequate force should be applied to force the molten alloy into the heated mold. Low density alloys require greater force than the higher density alloys **(Fig. 24.31)**.

　　Defect—short margins, incomplete casting, mold fracture, fins on casting

16. **Law 16—Margins**—casting should be done towards the margins of the wax patterns. The heated casting ring should be placed in the crucible using the orientation dot as the guide such that the patterns face the trail edge.

　　Defect – short margins, incomplete castings.

17. **Law 17—Quenching**—do not quench the casting ring immediately after casting. Always allow the investment and the casted alloy to cool to room temperature. Uneven cooling and shrinkage between the alloy and investment can apply tensile forces on the casting.

　　Defect—hot tears in the restoration.

## CASTING DEFECTS

Casting of metal alloys is a complex procedure which involves multiple steps. Any shortcoming in one of the step can lead to failure in the casting. Defects in casting can occur if there is any discrepancy in any of the steps starting from impression making to the final process of casting.

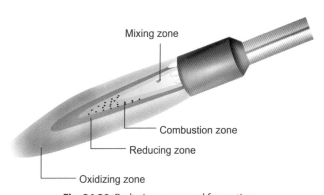

**Fig. 24.30:** Reducing zone used for casting.

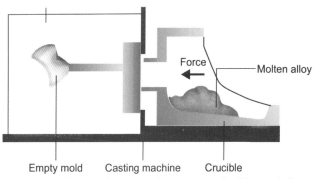

**Fig. 24.31:** Schematic diagram to show casting of noble metal alloys.

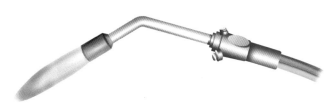

**Fig. 24.29:** Heat source used for casting.

## Classification of Casting Defects

- Distortion
- Surface roughness and irregularities
- Porosity
- Incomplete casting.

### Distortion

The distortion of casting is related to distortion of the wax pattern. This can occur during the direct technique when the wax pattern is removed from the oral cavity. Distortion can occur due to thermal changes, relaxation of internal stresses, improper handling at the time of removal of pattern or during storage.

#### Causes

- Improper manipulation of wax
- Delayed investing of pattern
- Heating of pattern during spruing results in distortion
- If casting is overheated during soldering process, it results in warping or melting of the margins.

#### Remedy

- Pattern should be invested as soon as possible to reduced warpage.
- Proper manipulation of wax. Wax should be added in small increments to minimize incorporation of residual stress.
- Proper handling of wax pattern during removal. Wax pattern should be removed along the path of insertion without damaging the margins. For this separating media is applied on the surface of die to ensure complete separation of the wax pattern.
- If storage of pattern is necessary then it should be stored in refrigerator but not more than 30 minutes.
  - Use of hard wax rather than soft wax for pattern fabrication as soft wax is more susceptible to temperature change.

### Surface Roughness, Irregularities and Discoloration

Surface roughness is defined as relatively finely spaced surface imperfections whose height, width and direction establish the predominant surface pattern.

Surface irregularities are isolated imperfections such as nodules and scratches which are not characteristics of the entire surface area.

Surface discoloration is due to breakdown products such as sulfur compounds which contaminates the casting. Also, any discrepancy in temperature or heating time can result in incomplete reaction which can lead to formation of carbon residue contaminating the alloy.

Surface roughness usually occurs because of breakdown of the investment at excessive burnout temperature or due to excessive heating of the casting alloy.

#### Causes

*Air bubbles:* Air bubbles attached to the surface of the wax pattern during investing forms small nodules on the casting **(Fig. 24.32)**.

#### Remedy

These air bubbles can best be avoided by using vacuum investing technique. Wetting agent can aid in preventing collection of air bubbles on the surface of the pattern. But it is not a certain remedy.

#### Water Films

If the wax pattern slightly moves or is vibrated after investing, it may result in formation of water film irregularly over the surface of pattern and investment material. This can result in surface irregularities on the surface. Too high L/P ratio can also cause surface irregularities.

*Remedy:*
- Proper use of wetting agent can prevent such irregularities.
- Use of proper L/P ratio.

#### Rapid Heating Rates

Rapid heating of the investment leads to flaking resulting in fins in the casting **(Fig. 24.33)**.

*Remedy:*
Mold should be heated gradually. Greater the bulk of the investment, more slowly, it should be heated.

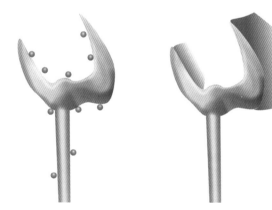

**Fig. 24.32:** Small nodules on casting.    **Fig. 24.33:** Fins on the casting.

## Underheating

If the mold is underheated, there are chances of incomplete elimination of the wax **(Fig. 24.34)**.

*Remedy:* Proper heating of the mold is recommended.

## W/P Ratio

Greater the W/P ratio, rougher the casting. If the ratio is small, the investment is too thick to be applied to the pattern.

*Remedy:* Water and powder should be mixed accurately and should be vacuum invested.

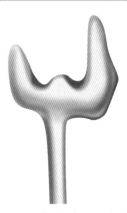
**Fig. 24.34:** Incomplete wax elimination results in rounded casting.

## Prolonged Heating

Prolonged heating of the casting leads to disintegration of gypsum-bonded investment and the walls of the investment are roughened. Sulfur compounds released from the investment can contaminate the casting **(Fig. 24.35)**.

*Remedy:* Mold should be heated to the accurate casting temperature and casting should be done immediately.

## Temperature of the Alloy

If the alloy is heated to very high temperature before casting, it will result in surface roughness of the casting.

*Remedy:* Temperature should be accurately controlled.

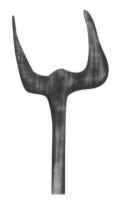
**Fig. 24.35:** Black roughened casting due to prolonged heating.

## Casting Pressure

If the casting pressure is too high, then it will result in rough casting

*Remedy:* In air pressure-casting machine, the gauge pressure should be 0.10–0.14 MPa for smaller casting.

## Position of Pattern

If several patterns are invested in the same ring, they should not be close to each other and should not be in the same plane.

*Remedy:* Spacing between the patterns should not be less than 3 mm.

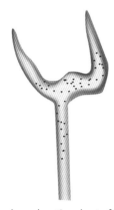
**Fig. 24.36:** Roughened casting due to foreign particles.

## Foreign Particles

If foreign particles enter the mold, it causes surface roughness and can also create surface voids. They form sharp well-defined deficiencies. If flux enters the mold with the metal, it shows bright appearing concavities **(Fig. 24.36)**.

*Remedy:* Crucible former should be clean before investing.

## Porosity

Porosities can be of two types—(1) internal and (2) external. Internal porosity weakens the casting and external porosity can lead to discoloration and can even cause secondary caries or periodontal disease.

**Classification of Porosity**

*Classification of porosities of noble metal casting alloys:*
- Based on solidification shrinkage
  - Localized shrinkage porosity
  - Microporosity
    - Suck back porosity
- Based on trapped gases
  - Pinhole porosity
  - Gas inclusions
  - Subsurface porosity
    - Back pressure porosity
- Based on residual air trapped in the mold.

### Shrinkage Spot or Localized Shrinkage Porosity

This type of porosity occurs because of improper flow of molten metal and its premature solidification. Molten Noble metal alloy as it starts to solidify it starts shrinking linearly at the rate of 1.25%. Because of this shrinkage more molten metal should be fed to the empty space to compensate this shrinkage. This excess molten metal is provided through the reservoir. If the sprue diameter is small or there is inadequate reservoir, the sprue will solidify first leaving behind the porosity created through shrinkage. This localized shrinkage porosity usually occurs at sprue – casting junction **(Fig. 24.37)**.

*Causes*
- Sprue diameter is too small or narrow
- Mold temperature is too low.

*Remedy*
- Sprue should be used of correct thickness

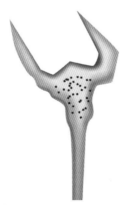

**Fig. 24.37:** Localized shrinkage porosity occurs at sprue casting junction.

- Sprue should be attached to the thickest portion of the wax pattern
- Sprue should be flared at the point of attachment or reservoir should be placed close to the pattern
- Temperature of the mold should not be too high or low.

### Suck Back Porosity

This type porosity is a variation of localized shrinkage porosity. This porosity occurs as an external void on the internal surface of crown opposite to the attachment of the sprue. A hot spot is formed by molten metal impinging on the mold wall near the sprue when the sprue is attached at right angle to the wax pattern. This Hot spot area has higher localized mold temperature and retains heat for longer duration then rest of the mold. This causes the local area to freeze at the end and results in suck back porosity. It frequently occurs at the sharp occlusoaxial or incisoaxial line angle which is not well rounded **(Fig. 24.38)**.

*Remedy:*
- This porosity can be eliminated by flaring the point of sprue attachment
- *By reducing the temperature difference between the mold and the molten alloy:* By attaching the sprue at proper angulation.

### Microporosity

It occurs when there is rapid solidification, if the mold or casting temperature is too low. Because of this there is formation of small, irregular microvoids called as microporosities. It is particularly evident in fine grain alloy castings.

*Remedy:* Casting temperature should be properly controlled.

### Pinhole Porosity

In molten state many metal alloys dissolve or occlude gases. Metals such as copper, gold and silver dissolve oxygen

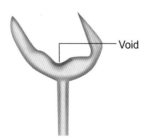

**Fig. 24.38:** Suck back porosity.

whereas molten palladium and platinum has high affinity for hydrogen gas and oxygen. These gases on solidification are expelled causing tiny voids called pinhole porosity **(Fig. 24.39)**.

### Gas Inclusion Porosities

These are also spherical voids which are much larger than the pinhole porosity. These are also due to dissolved gases in the molten metal. All castings are likely to have certain amount of porosities, but they should be kept to minimum as they can adversely affect the physical properties of the casting. These gas inclusions can also be caused by poorly adjusted torch flame, i.e. use of mixing or oxidizing flame rather than the reducing flame. Castings contaminated by gases are black in color and are difficult to clean.

*Remedy:*
- These porosities can be minimized by pre-melting the gold alloy in a graphite crucible or a graphite block.
- By proper adjustment of the torch flame and using the reducing zone of the flame for melting.

### Subsurface Porosity

The exact cause of this type of porosity is not clear. This type of porosity may be due to gas bubbles incorporated at the mold wall as the molten alloy first freezes. If the temperature of the mold or the alloy is too high, it will cause the first portion of the alloy which contacts the mold to solidify first and form a thin layer. The alloy which flows behind this layer shrinks on solidification and pulls away creating a subsurface porosity. This porosity can also occur, if short thick sprue is used.

*Remedy*
- By controlling the rate at which the molten metal enters the mold.
- By using longer sprue.

- By controlling the alloy or mold temperature.

### Back Pressure Porosity

This type of porosity is produced in the dental castings due to inability of the gases in the mold to escape during the casting procedure. The entrapment of air in the mold creates increased pressure in the mold and prevents the molten alloy to completely fill the mold resulting in porous casting with rounded incomplete margins. To minimize this, the wax pattern should not be placed more than 6–8 mm away from the end of the casting ring **(Fig. 24.40)**.

*Remedy:*
- Use of proper burnout temperature
- Adequate casting pressure
- Proper L/P ratio
- Using investment with adequate pores
- Pattern should not be more than 6 mm away from the end of the casting ring
- Proper spure diameter, length, direction and flaring is necessary.

### Incomplete Casting

Partial or no casting occurs most commonly due to inability of the molten alloy to fill the mold because of inadequate venting of the investment and too high viscosity of the molten metal. If there is insufficient casting pressure, then air cannot be vented quickly and the molten alloy does not fill the mold before it solidifies.

Another common cause of incomplete casting is incomplete elimination of wax residues from the mold. The pores in the investment are blocked because of this and therefore air cannot be vented out completely. This will result in shiny rounded margins which are due to the reducing atmosphere formed by carbon monoxide left by the residual wax **(Fig. 24.41)**.

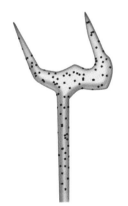

**Fig. 24.39:** Pin hole porosity.

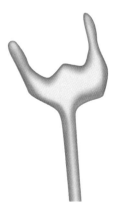

**Fig. 24.40 :** Rounded incomplete margins due to back pressure porosity.

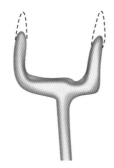

**Fig. 24.41:** Incomplete casting.

*Possible Reasons for Incomplete Castings*

- Inadequate casting pressure
- Too low casting or mold temperature
- Too viscous molten alloy
- Incomplete wax elimination
- Lower L/P ratio
- Back pressure due to incomplete air venting
- Premature solidification of the alloy
- Improper positioning of the sprues.

## TEST YOURSELF

### Essay Questions

1. Discuss in detail the casting procedure starting from the investment stage to the removal of casting.
2. Classify casting defects. Describe each of them with causes and methods to prevent them.
3. Discuss various Laws of casting.
4. Describe in detail porosities in casting.
5. Describe various zones used for melting the metal alloy.
6. Define casting. Write briefly about various casting machines used for dental casting.

### Short Notes

1. Localized shrinkage porosity.
2. Pin hole porosity.
3. Suck back porosity.
4. Sprue.
5. Casting ring liner.
6. Pickling.
7. Reservoir.
8. Casting crucible.

### Multiple Choice Questions

1. Suck back porosity in the casting can be eliminated by
   A. Increasing the mold–metal temperature differential
   B. Increasing the flow of molten metal
   C. Flaring the point of the sprue attachment
   D. None of the above
2. Back pressure porosity can be rectified by:
   A. Vacuum investing the wax pattern
   B. Reducing the mold and casting temperature
   C. Using proper technique of the burnout temperature of the casting pressure
   D. All of the above
3. Main function of asbestos in casting ring is:
   A. Absorb moisture from investment
   B. Aid in expansion of investment
   C. To prevent fracture of investment
   D. Allow escape of trapped air
4. Ceramic liner should have thickness of:
   A. 0.6 mm
   B. 0.8 mm
   C. 1 mm
   D. 2 mm
5. The zone of oxy-acetylene flame used for melting the alloy is:
   A. Combustion zone
   B. Oxidizing zone
   C. Reducing zone
   D. All of the above
6. High heat technique utilizes temperature for thermal expansion at:
   A. 900°F
   B. 1200°F
   C. 1500°F
   D. 1800°F
7. Simultaneous nucleation of solid grains and bubbles results in:
   A. Subsurface porosity
   B. Back pressure porosity
   C. Suck back porosity
   D. Pin hole porosity.
8. In contrast to low heat investments, high heat investments:
   A. Cannot be heated beyond 750°C
   B. Are used for PFM alloys
   C. Undergo greater expansion
   D. Are made with gypsum
9. The amount of bubbles in an investment can be reduced by:
   A. Reducing water powder ratio
   B. Mixing investment under vacuum
   C. Increasing water powder ratio
   D. Investing under water

10. The rationale of burnout process does not include:
    A. Increase the density of investment material
    B. Expand the investment material
    C. Vaporize the wax pattern from the mold
    D. Increase the temperature of the investment

## ANSWERS

| | | | | | | | |
|---|---|---|---|---|---|---|---|
| 1. C | | 2. D | | 3. B | | 4. C | |
| 5. C | | 6. B | | 7. A | | 8. B and C | |
| 9. B | | 10. A | | | | | |

## BIBLIOGRAPHY

1. Ansavice KJ. Phillips's Science of Dental Materials. 11th edition. St. Louis, Saunders, 2003.
2. Asgar K, Arfaei AH. Castability of crown and bridge alloys. J Prosthet Dent. 1985;54:60.
3. Craig RG, Powers JM. Restorative Dental Materials. 11th edn. St Louis, Mosby Inc., 2002.
4. Davis DR, Nguyen JH, Grey BL. Ring volume/ring liner ratio and effective setting expansion. Int J Prosthodont. 1992;5:403-8.
5. Davis DR. Potential health hazard of ceramic ring lining material. J Prosthet Dent. 1987;57:362-9.
6. Donovan TE, White LE. Evaluation of an improved centrifugal casting machine. J Prosthet Dent. 1985; 53:609.
7. Dootz ER, Asgar K. Solidification patterns of single crowns and three unit bridge castings. Quint Dent Technol. 1986;10:299-305.
8. Eames WB, MacNamara JF. Evaluation of casting machines for ability to cast sharp margins. Oper Dent. 1978;3:137.
9. Earnshaw R, Morey EF. The fit of gold alloy full crown castings made with ceramic casting ring liners. J Dent Res. 1992;71:1865-70.
10. Earnshaw R. The effect of casting ring liners on the potential expansion of a gypsum bonded investment. J Dent Res. 1988;67:1366-70.
11. Johnson A. The effect of five investing techniques on air bubble entrapment and casting nodules. Int J Prosthodont. 1992;5:424-33.
12. Mackert JR. An expert system for analysis of casting failures. Int J Prosthodont. 1988;1:268.
13. Naylor WP, Moore BK, Phillips RW. A topographical assessment of casting ring liners using scanning electron microscopy (SEM). Quint Dent Technol. 1987;11:413.
14. Nielson JP, Ollerman R. Suck-back porosity. Quint Dent Technol. 1976;1:61-5.
15. Nielson JP. Pressure distribution in centrifugal dental casting. J Dent Res. 1978;57:261-9.
16. O'Brien WJ, Nielson JP. Decomposition of gypsum investments in the presence of carbon. J Dent Res. 1959;38:541-7.
17. Phillips RW. Relative merits of vacuum investing of small castings as compared to conventional methods. J Dent Res. 1947;26:343-52.
18. Shillingburg HT, Hobo S, Whitsett LD et al. Fundamentals of Fixed Prosthodontics, 3rd edn. Carol Stream, IL, Qunitessence Publishing Co. Inc, 1997.
19. Tuccillo JJ, Nielson JP. Sprue design for cast gold alloys. Dent Lab Rev. 1964;39:14.
20. Vaidyanathan TK, Schulman A, Nielson JP, et al. Correlation between macroscopic porosity location and liquid metal pressure in centrifugal casting technique. J Dent Res. 1981;60:59-66.
21. Verret RG, Duke ES. The effect of sprue attachment design on the castability and porosity. J Prosthet Dent. 1989;61:418-24.
22. Wagner AW. Causes and cures for porosities in dental casting. Qunit Dent Technol. 1979;3:57.
23. Eames WB, O'Neil SJ, Monteiro J, et al. Techniques to improve the seating of the castings. J Am Dent Assoc. 1978;96:432-7.
24. Ito M, Kuroiwa A, Nagasawa S, et al. Effect of wax melting range and investment liquid concentration on the accuracy of a three-quarter crown casting. J Prosthet Dent. 2002;87:56-7.
25. Ito M, Yamagishi T, Oshida Y, et al. Effect of selected physical properties of waxes on investments and casting shrinkage. J Prosthet Dent. 1996;75:211-6.
26. Stevens L. The effect of early heating on the expansion of phsopahte bonded investment. Aust Dent J. 1983;28:366-9.
27. Zeltser C, Lewinstein I, Grajower R. Fit of crown wax patterns after removal from the die. J Proshet Dent. 1985;53:344-6.

*'You are designed for accomplishment, engineered for success and endowed with the seeds of greatness.'*
—*Zig Zagler*

## INTRODUCTION

During the 20th century efforts were made to search for alternative alloy to the gold alloys because of the increased cost of gold. Many modern alloy systems do not include precious metals and are referred to as base metal alloys. Wrought metal alloys are cold worked cast metal alloys that can be plastically deformed to alter shape of the structure.

## DEFINITION

*Wrought metal is defined as cold worked metal that has been plastically deformed to alter the shape of the structure and certain mechanical properties (strength, hardness and ductility).*

Wrought alloys are formed when a cast metal alloy or pure metal is permanently deformed due to any reason. Deformation of these alloys results in alteration in its microstructure having properties which are different from the cast metal alloy or pure metal. These alloys show significant differences in their hardness, proportional limit and ductility.

## USES

- Orthodontic wires and appliances
- Clasps for removable partial dentures
- Endodontic files and reamers
- Crowns used in pedodontics
- Surgical instruments.

Common wrought alloys used in dentistry are stainless steel, cobalt-chromium-nickel alloys, nickel-titanium and β-titanium. Some wrought alloys having limited application in dentistry are wrought noble metal alloys, wrought commercially pure titanium in dental implants. Wrought alloys exhibit properties and microstructure which are not associated with the same alloy when casted. Wrought alloys are commonly used for manufacturing orthodontic wires.

## DEFORMATION OF THE METAL ALLOY

Plastic deformation of the metal alloy occurs when the stress induced by the applied force extends beyond the proportional limit. Even after removal of force the metal alloy does not regain its original shape. During deformation of metal alloy number of changes occur at the atomic level.

## IMPERFECTIONS IN CRYSTAL STRUCTURE

During crystallization of the molten metal or alloy into the solid state, crystals grow randomly by atomic diffusion. This

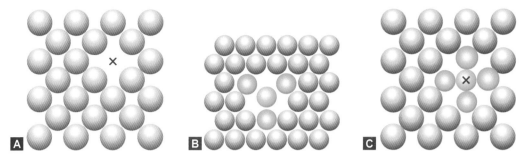

**Figs 25.1A to C:** Diagram showing point defect: (A) Vacancy; (B) Trivacancy; and (C) Interstitial atom.

leads to formation of structural imperfections throughout the crystal structure. The crystal imperfection is due to change in lattice positions of the atoms. Displaced, missing or extra atoms can lead to formation of "point defects". Likewise if the change occurs in plane of atoms in the crystal then it is called as "line defect". Crystal imperfection can also be due to change in the boundaries between the crystals.

## Point Defects

If in a crystal lattice one atom is missing in the structural arrangement then it is called as "vacancy" or "vacant" atom. If two or three such atoms are missing then it is referred to as divacancy or trivacancy respectively. These point defects occur at a given temperature when the crystal structure is in the equilibrium state. Vacancy is primary point defect which allows atomic diffusion to take place during crystallization **(Figs 25.1A to C)**.

## Line Defects (Dislocations)

As mentioned above if the change in crystal structure occurs along the edge or plane of the atoms then it is called as "line defect" or "dislocation". Simplest type of line defect is called as Edge dislocation which is located at the edge of the half plane and is symbolized as ($\perp$) **(Fig. 25.2)**.

When sufficiently large shear stress is applied between the upper and lower faces of the crystal structure of a metal. The interatomic bonds near the edge dislocation easily break and newer bonds are formed with the next row allowing the dislocation to move one interatomic distance forward. The plane along which the edge dislocation moves is called as "slip plane" **(Fig. 25.3)**. Continuous application of shear stress will move the dislocation forward until it reaches the boundary of the crystal structure. At the boundary it can be observed that atomic planes on one side of the slip plane are displaced one interatomic spacing as compared to the other side of the slip plane. The direction in which the slip planes have been displaced is called as "slip direction". The combination of both the slip plane and slip direction is called as "slip system".

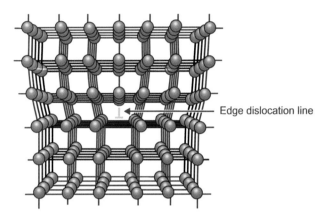

**Fig. 25.2:** Edge dislocation in cubic crystal.

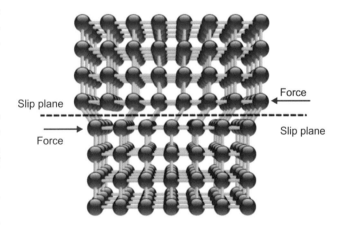

**Fig. 25.3:** Diagram showing slip plane.

### CLINICAL SIGNIFICANCE

Number of slip systems in a metal or alloy signifies the inherent ability of the metal to plastically deform. Metal or alloy with face centered cubic (FCC) structure has largest number of slip systems. Metals having FCC structure such as gold, silver, copper, palladium, platinum and nickel are highly ductile.

Metals having body centered cubic (BCC) structure have comparatively less slip systems than the FCC. These metals show lesser ductility. Likewise if the metals such as zinc which have hexagonal close packed (HCP) structure then they have very few slip systems in comparison to FCC and BCC structure. These metals show very low ductility in comparison to the above mentioned crystal structure.

Shear stress required to cause permanent deformation in a metal crystal structure having edge dislocations is much less than that required by crystal structure of the polycrystalline metal. In metal containing edge dislocation one row of atomic bonds in one plane needs to be broken at a time whereas in polycrystalline metal crystal structure, all rows of atomic bonds in two planes need to be broken with greater force. In the present discussion, proportional limit in a stress-strain plot will indicate the onset of significant movement of dislocations. When stress exceeds the proportional limit there is permanent deformation which occurs in the metal crystal because of dislocation movement and slip between the atomic planes.

## DISLOCATION MOVEMENT IN POLYCRYSTALLINE ALLOYS

In a pure metal crystal movement of the dislocation along its slip plane is relatively smoother with less interference as compared to movement of dislocations in a polycrystalline metal alloy structure. This is because metal alloys have multiple phases such as solid solutions and precipitates in addition to dislocations found in pure metal crystal structure. Therefore, to allow dislocation movement in a polycrystalline alloy, increased stress is required.

In a solid solution alloy there is local distortion around the solute atoms in the lattice structure. Due to this there will be hindrance in the movement of the dislocation along the slip planes. Apart from this there are precipitates which can be coherent or incoherent depending on the continuity of the atomic bonds with the solution matrix **(Fig. 25.4)**.

In coherent precipitate the atomic bonds are continuous with the interface of solution matrix whereas in incoherent precipitates the atomic bonds are not continuous with the interface of surface matrix. Greater stress is required for movement of dislocation through the coherent and incoherent precipitates. Although dislocations around the incoherent precipitates loop around these particles.

Ductile metals can permanently deform under mechanical stress at temperature below their recrystallization temperature (cold working). It can create large number of point defects and dislocations which can interact with each other inhibiting their movements. In these metals after cold working greater amount of stress will be required to allow movement of dislocations. Cold working also shows alteration of shape of the grains. Dislocation movement is difficult if it has to move from one grain to another grain especially when it is misaligned (Fig. 25.5).

Grain boundary represents the end of the slip planes where dislocations does not move further and starts to accumulate there. As the size of the grain becomes smaller, boundary area due to accumulation will increase further impeding the movement of dislocations. Grain size can be controlled by adding a grain refiner or by rapidly cooling or quenching. For movement of the dislocations along the slip planes greater amount of stress is needed. Since proportional limit of such alloys is increased, the above mentioned methods are also mechanism of increasing strength of the alloy. These mechanisms are strain hardening, grain refinement strengthening and solid solution strengthening.

### CLINICAL SIGNIFICANCE

In wrought alloys (cold worked) the hardness, proportional limit and yield strength increases whereas the modulus of elasticity of the alloy remains the same and the ductility decreases.

If the cold working process is continued, eventually the wrought alloy will fracture. This is due to development

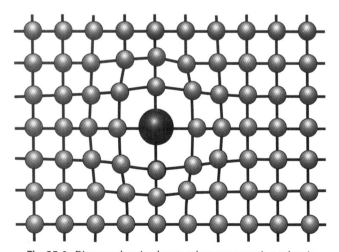

**Fig. 25.4:** Diagram showing larger sphere representing solute in solid solution alloy.

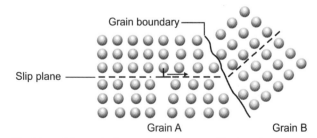

**Fig. 25.5:** Schematic diagram to show spatial lattice of two grains adjacent to each other.

of microcracks formation at the site of fracture initiation. Microcracks can result from accumulation of dislocations at the grain boundaries between two microstructural phases. Alloys may also undergo brittle or ductile fracture because of variations in factors such as composition, microstructure, temperature and strain rate. For example, rotary endodontic file made of carbon steel can show brittle fracture because of torsional loading due to coalescence of microvoids.

## TWINNING

Twinning is the alternate method of permanent deformation in metals where dislocation movement is not involved. It occurs when two separate crystals share some of the same crystal lattice points in a symmetrical manner. This results in an intergrowth of these crystals in different configurations. Twin boundary separates both these crystals and this boundary is called as "twinning plane" **(Fig. 25.6)**. A portion of the crystal which has lattice orientation which is different than the original orientation is called as "twin". On X-ray crystallography both these crystals look identical on the either side of the boundary. The stress required to twin a crystal is greater than that required for slip system.

Slip system is considered to be normal deformation mechanism whereas twinning is preferred mechanism at high strain rate and low temperature. Plastic deformation in twinning occurs by just reorientation of the lattice structure, i.e. only atoms in the lattice move but their relative position to each other remains the same. Whereas in slip system, deformation occurs when position of the atoms relative to each other has changed **(Fig. 25.7)**.

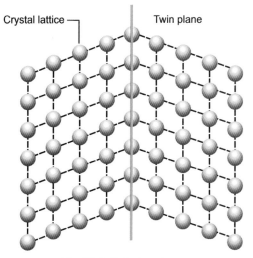

**Fig. 25.6:** Twinning plane.

**CLINICAL SIGNIFICANCE**

In dentistry, twinning is observed in alpha titanium alloys which are used in manufacture of dental implants. It is also the mechanism of reversible transformation between the austenitic and martensitic structure in nickel-titanium orthodontic wires.

## EFFECTS OF ANNEALING ON COLD WORKED METAL

The properties of cold worked metal such as strain hardening, reduced ductility, increased dislocation density and distorted grains can be reversed by annealing process. Greater and more severe the degree of cold working, faster the effects of annealing is reversed.

*Annealing can be defined* as "controlled heating and cooling process designed to produce desired properties of the metal". This process is done to soften metals so as to increase their plastic deformation potential, to stabilize shape and to increase machinability. Annealing is process in which higher temperature will be required if the melting point of the metal is high.

The process of annealing takes place in three stages namely, recovery, recrystallization and grain growth **(Fig. 25.8)**.

## RECOVERY

- In this stage when the metal is heated it initiates atomic diffusion and the properties of the cold worked metal tend to disappear before any significant change is observed.

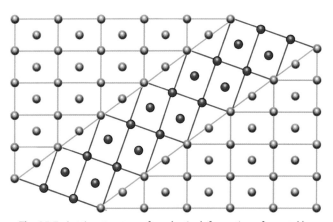

**Fig. 25.7:** Lattice structure after plastic deformation of a metal by twinning under tension.

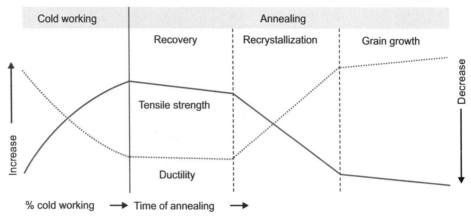

**Fig. 25.8:** Effect of annealing on cold worked metal.

- There is very slight decrease in tensile strength but the ductility of the alloy remains the same.
- Cold worked metal possess residual stresses which tends to relax during machining of the metal resulting in warping. This tendency of warping can be eliminated by subjecting the cold worked metal to the heat treatment in which recovery occurs.

**CLINICAL SIGNIFICANCE**

Orthodontic appliances fabricated by bending wires are subjected to annealing process to relieve stress. The heat treatment during this process helps in stabilizing the configuration of the appliance and permits exact determination of force that an appliance will be able to deliver in the mouth.

- The heat treatment should be given in the recovery temperature stage and not at higher temperature
- This heat treatment aids in eliminating the residual stresses in the appliance and makes it more resistant to fracture.

## RECRYSTALLIZATION

- The next stage in annealing process after recovery is recrystallization
- In this stage severely cold worked metal is subjected to heat treatment beyond the recovery stage. There is rapid change at the microstructural level where atoms are rearranged in lower energy configuration
- The old deformed grains disappear completely and are replaced by new strain free grains
- These new grains are gathered in the most severely cold worked region of the metal. After the completion of recrystallization, the metal becomes soft and ductile. It resembles the same structure as it was before cold working
- If the orthodontic appliance needs to be heat treated for stress relief, recrystallization stage should be

avoided as the alloy becomes soft and has reduced resilience
- Cold working of the metal is necessary for recrystallization stage of annealing to occur.

**Classification of Orthodontic Wires**

Based on the type of material used:

*Orthodontic wires:*
- Stainless steel
- Cobalt-chromium-nickel.

*Titanium alloys:*
- Nickel-titanium
- Beta-titanium.

## GRAIN GROWTH

- If the cold working is more severe greater numbers of nuclei are formed during recrystallization stage. The grain size of the recrystallized metal varies between fine and fairly coarse grain
- If the recrystallized metal is annealed further then grain growth stage of annealing occurs as larger grains starts consuming the smaller ones to limit the grain boundary area
- Grain growth ceases to occur once coarse grains are formed
- Grain size of the cast alloy is unaffected by the prolonged annealing near the solidus temperature as impurity atoms or secondary phases which are formed at the grain boundary immobilizes it and prevents their migration during annealing
- Formation of larger grain size is disadvantageous as it has low proportional limit and substantial local permanent deformation. This weakness can result in fracture of alloy which is used in thin diameter.

## IDEAL REQUIREMENTS FOR ORTHODONTIC WIRES

- Should have *low stiffness* to give better control during movement of teeth and to produce lighter forces
- Should be *highly formidable*, i.e. it should be easily shaped, bent and altered into complex configuration without fracturing
- Should have *large springback action*, i.e. the wire can be deflected over longer distance without getting permanently deformed
- Should be *tough* to withstand the functional forces without distorting or fracturing
- Should have *low coefficient of friction*
- Should be *biocompatible*
- Should be highly corrosion resistant.

## FACTORS CONSIDERED DURING SELECTION OF WIRES

- Force delivery characteristics—depends on composition and structure of the wires, wire segment geometry
- Elastic working range
- Corrosion resistance
- Biocompatibility
- Cost
- Ease of joining the parts to fabricate complex appliances.

## MANUFACTURING OF ORTHODONTIC WIRES

1. *Melting and casting*: The raw metal ore is melted using an electric furnace for several hours to form ingots. These ingots are then shaped so that wires or sheet can be extracted from them.
2. *Drawing*: The metal ingot is drawn into the desired shape by placing in a die and applying pull or push force.
3. *Annealing*: During the drawing the metal is cold worked and therefore, it is subjected to annealing process, i.e. it is heated and cooled under controlled condition. This helps in removing stress from metal by recrystallization

means. The process aids in improving strength and flexibility of the wire.
4. *Finishing*: The annealed wires are then subjected to finishing process by using various abrasives.

## CARBON STEEL

- This type of steel has limited use in dentistry
- It is iron-carbon binary alloy which contain less than 2.1% carbon **(Fig. 25.9)**
- Based on three possible crystal structures, carbon steel are of three types: (1) ferrite, (2) austenite and (3) martensite
- *Ferrite* is a BCC structure which is stabilized at temperatures below 912°C. It contains carbon atoms in interstitial sites between the iron atoms. The solubility in this structure is very less and it can be maximum of 0.02% at 723°C
- *Austenite* is a FCC structure which is stabilized between 912°C and 1394°C. In this phase also carbon atoms are interstitially located between the iron atoms. When plain carbon steel which contains 0.8% carbon are cooled slowly in this phase it undergoes solid state eutectoid transformation at 723°C resulting in microstructural constituent called as *pearlite*. It contains alternate fine scale lamellae of ferrite and iron carbide ($Fe_3C$) called as *cementite* or *carbide*. Iron carbide has an orthorhombic crystal structure and has greater hardness and rigidity than austenite or ferrite
- *Martensite*: This is formed when austenitic structure is rapidly cooled (quenched) it undergoes spontaneous transformation to a body-centered tetragonal (BCT) structure. The sequence of iron atoms are highly distorted by the carbon atoms resulting in very hard, strong and brittle alloys. Cutting edge of the carbon steel instruments is made of martensitic structure as it provides high hardness and permits grinding of the sharp edge. Martensite is a metastable phase and it decomposes to form ferrite and carbide when heated to higher temperature. The hardness of carbon steel can be reduced by *tempering process* but it is balanced by increase in toughness **(Fig. 25.10)**.

---

### Classification of Wrought Alloys

- Wrought noble metal alloys
- Wrought base metal alloys
  - Carbon steel
  - Stainless steel
  - Cobalt-chromium-nickel alloys
  - Nickel-titanium
  - Beta-titanium alloys.

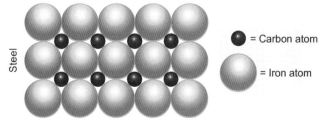

Steel

= Carbon atom

= Iron atom

**Fig. 25.9:** Carbon steel.

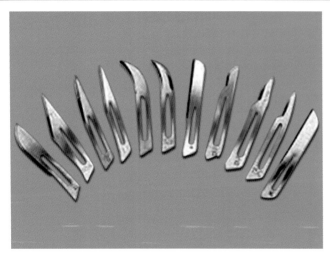

**Fig. 25.10:** Cutting blades made of martensite carbon steel.

## STAINLESS STEEL

Stainless steel is formed by adding 12–30% chromium to carbon steel. It is highly resistant to tarnish and corrosion because of the formation of passivating layer of chromium oxide. If this layer is disrupted in mechanical or chemical means it is formed again in an oxidizing environment.

### Historical Background

*1912: Sherman* introduced vanadium surgical steel which had elasticity and ductility. However, vanadium steel possessed poor biocompatibility.

*1912: Harry Brearley* of UK accidentally discovered steel while searching corrosion resistant alloy for gun barrels.

*1919:* Steel first introduced to dentistry by *E Hauptmeyer* of Germany. He named it "Wipla" meaning platinum.

*1924:* 18–8 stainless steel invented by *WH Hatfield.*

*1926:* 18–8 austenitic stainless steel was introduced which was much stronger and had greater corrosion resistance. *Strauss* in 1926, added 2–4% molybdenum to 18–8 steel and it had even greater resistance to acidic and chloride environment. Later, carbon content in this alloy was lowered to 0.08% and was called 316 stainless steel.

*1929:* Stainless steel used to manufacture orthodontic wires.

*1930: E Angle* used stainless steel as ligature wire.

*1937:* Study showed stainless steel wire is an efficient and effective material for orthodontic treatment.

### Manufacturing of Stainless Steel

Several ores of iron such as hematite, limonite and siderite are converted to iron using blast furnace. Iron is either collected at the bottom in the solid state as pig iron or is transferred in the molten state to manufacture steel.

**Commonly used methods for manufacturing steels are:**
- Bessemer process
- Open-hearth process
- Heroult electric arc furnace.

### Uses **(Fig. 25.11)**

- Commonly used as orthodontic wires and appliances
- Stainless steel crowns used in pediatric dentistry
- Magnetic connectors and clips
- Dental implants
- Surgical instruments.

### Classification of Stainless Steel

Based on the type of crystal structure formed by iron atoms, stainless steel is of three types **(Table 25.1):**
1. Ferritic stainless steel
2. Martensitic stainless steel
3. Austenitic stainless steel.

### Ferritic Stainless Steel

- Composed of Cr: 11.5–27%, Ni: 0, C: 0.20 maximum and Fe: balance. Si, P, S, Mn, tantalum and niobium are present in small amounts
- It has BCC crystal structure which is stable up to 912°C They have good corrosion resistance but are low in strength
- Low strength is because they cannot be heat hardened or work hardened as temperature change induces no phase change in the solid state
- Has low cost and has number of industrial uses but have limited use in dentistry.

**Table 25.1:** Composition of three different types of stainless steel.

| Type of space lattice | Chromium% | Nickel% | Carbon% |
|---|---|---|---|
| Ferritic (BCC) | 11.5–27 | 0 | 0.2 max |
| Austenitic (FCC) | 16–26 | 7–22 | 0.25 max |
| Martensitic (BCT) | 11.5–17 | 0–25 | 0.15–1.2 |

*Abbreviations:* BCC: base-centered cubic; FCC: face centered cubic; BCT: body-centered tetragonal.

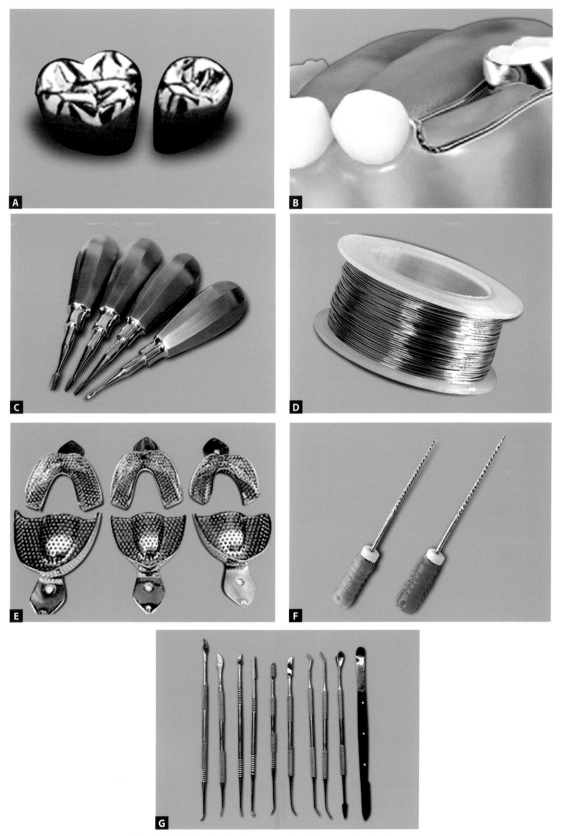

**Figs. 25.11A to G:** Various uses of stainless steel in dentistry.

## Martensitic Stainless Steel

- *Composition*, Cr: 11.5–17%, Ni: 0–2.5%, C: 0.15–1.20 and Fe: balance. Si, P, S, Mn, tantalum and niobium are present in small amounts.

  It is formed when austenite steel is transformed into the martensite steel. The transformation occurs when a heated austenite steel is subjected to rapid cooling (quenching). This rapid cooling traps carbon atoms within the crystal structure forming a BCT structure
- They have BCT crystal structure
- They can be heat hardened as the plain carbon steel
- They are popularly used for surgical and cutting instruments because of higher strength and hardness
- Yield strength of this type of steel varies between 500–1900 MPa
- Hardness varies between 230 BHN and 600 BHN (Brinell hardness number)
- Corrosion resistance of martensitic steel is least among the types of stainless steel
- Corrosion resistance and ductility which is only 2% is further reduced by hardening heat treatment.

## Austenitic Stainless Steel

- *Composition*, Cr: 16–26%, Ni: 7–22%, C: 0.25 maximum, and Fe: balance. Si, P, S, Mn, tantalum and niobium are present in small amounts
- They are the most corrosion resistant stainless steel and have FCC structure. It is stable at temperature between 912°C and 1394°C
- They are commonly used as orthodontic wires, endodontic instruments, crowns in pedodontics, magnetic connectors and clips and dental implants
- Type 302 and type 304 of the AISI series is most commonly used and are referred to as 18–8 stainless steel. This type is commonly used in orthodontic stainless steel wires and bands
- Composition of type 302 steel is Cr: 17–19%, Ni: 8–10%, C: 0.15 % maximum, Mn: 2%
- Composition of type 304 steel is Cr: 18–20%, Ni: 8–12%, C: 0.08% maximum, Mn: 2%
- Another type 316 L (low carbon) is commonly used to fabricate dental implants and is composed of Cr: 16–18% , Ni: 10–14%, Mo: 2–3%, C: 0.03% maximum and Mn: 2%
- 18–8 stainless steel is extensively used in dentistry. Hand drawn arch wires used in orthodontics were introduced in 1929
- Currently austenitic steel are used for orthodontic wires and appliances because of lower cost, good mechanical properties and adequate corrosion resistance **(Fig. 25.12)**

- Austenite phase in orthodontic wires is metastable and the cold working creates BCC martensitic structures. The BCC structure in ferrite and martensitic are ferromagnetic at room temperature and austenitic structure is nonmagnetic **(Fig. 25.13)**
- This type of steel is preferred over ferritic stainless steel in dental use because of following reasons:
  - Possess greater ductility and can be cold—worked without fracturing
  - Can attain substantial strength during cold working
  - Can be easily welded
  - Can overcome sensitization process
  - Are easy to shape and form.

## Function of Each Constituent of Alloy

- Nickel helps in stabilizing the homogenous mass at low temperature
- Chromium forms the passivating layer of chromium oxide. This layer protects steel from tarnish and corrosion
- Carbon imparts strength and hardness. The total carbon content should not be more than 0.2% as greater content

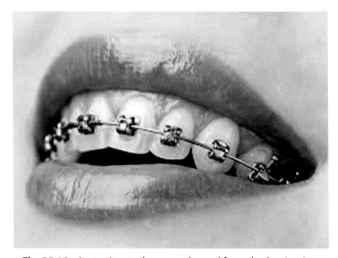

**Fig. 25.12:** Austenite steel commonly used for orthodontic wires.

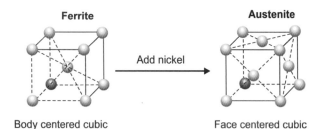

**Fig. 25.13:** Body-centered cubic (BCC) structure of ferrite changes to face centered cubic (FCC) structure of austenite steel by adding nickel.

will lead to formation of carbon carbide which will be susceptible to corrosion
- Silicon provides resistance to corrosion
- Phosphorous reduces the sintering temperature.

## Properties of Austenitic Steel

### Sensitization

Austenitic stainless steel may lose its corrosion resistance if it is heated between 400°C and 900°C. The exact temperature depends on the amount of carbon content. The reduction in corrosion resistance is due to the precipitation of chromium-iron carbide at the grain boundaries at high temperatures. The carbon atoms rapidly diffuses at the grain boundary to combine with chromium and iron atoms to form $(CrFe)_4C$ and thus loses corrosion resistance. Formation of a $(CrFe)_4C$ is most rapid at 650°C. Areas which are near the grain boundary have reduced corrosion resistance because chromium is more depleted in these areas. Stainless steel is susceptible to intragranular corrosion **(Fig. 25.14)**.

*Methods to minimize sensitization:*
- To reduce carbon content—so that carbide precipitation does not occur. But this method is not economically feasible
- Heat treatment—if the stainless steel is severely cold worked and then heat treated within the sensitization temperature range, $(CrFe)_4C$ forms at the dislocations which are located in the slip planes within the bulk grains. With this carbides are more uniformly distributed rather than concentrating at grain boundary.

### Stabilization

This is a method of preventing sensitization by introducing one or more elements in austenitic steel which form carbide precipitates preferring over chromium. Such elements are niobium or titanium with tantalum. This method of reducing sensitization is called as stabilization. This method

is not used for orthodontic stainless steel wires as this will add to the cost.

*Advantages:*
- Can withstand functional forces due to high stiffness
- It is highly ductile and malleable and can be easily drawn into wires or beaten to sheets
- Can be cold worked without the risk of fracture which increases the strength of the metal
- It has good formability and due to this reason number of steel wires can be twisted or braided together to form multistranded arch wires. Twisted or braided wires can produce large elastic deflection with low force.
- Good corrosion resistance
- Have adequate strength to resist distortion
- Are biocompatible
- Are economical and easily available
- As they have smooth surface the stainless steel brackets produce less friction than nonmetal brackets.

*Disadvantages:*
- Have lower springback action than Ni-Ti wires
- Require frequent activations as they have high stiffness
- Difficult to solder because if temperature is raised above 500°C, its corrosion resistance is compromised
- As it deliver greater force than arch wires made of other alloys, it causes greater discomfort.

## Mechanical Properties of Orthodontic Wires

- *Elastic modulus* of stainless steel orthodontic wires is 180 GPa. It is twice that of gold but is lower than the Co-Cr-Ni wires
- *Yield strength* is 1600 MPa and the ultimate tensile strength is 2100 MPa. Strength and hardness of stainless steel increases if the cross-section of the wire is decreased as greater cold working will be required to form a smaller wire
- 18–8 stainless steel orthodontic wires are stronger than Cobalt-chromium-nickel wires, titanium-molybdenum (Ti-Mo), and nickel-titanium (Ni-Ti) wires
- *Formability* is defined as the ability to bend the wire into the configuration desired by the clinician. 18–8 stainless steel wires have excellent formability. Numbers of 90° cold bends without fracture are five for 18–8 stainless steel. It indicates the comparative formability of the orthodontic wires
- *Resiliency* refers to the workability of the wire acting as a spring. Stainless steel have favorable resiliency as compared to gold wires
- *Flexibility or springback* is defined as the materials maximum elastic deflection and is the ratio of the yield strength over the modulus of elasticity. The springback of stainless steel wires is slightly more than that of the gold wires but is lesser than the Ti-Mo and Ni-Ti wires

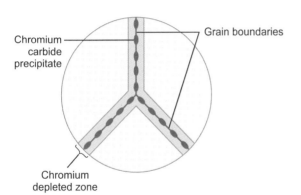

**Fig. 25.14:** Sensitization in austenitic stainless steel.

- *Joinability* is the ability of the wire to be joined, i.e. weld or solder to attachments. Soldering of stainless steel wires is possible but at times can be difficult. This difficulty can be reduced by using low fusing solders and by reducing the time of soldering or welding to the minimum.

### Recovery Heat Treatment

- During manufacturing process of the stainless steel wires, the material is cold worked which reduces its ductility
- A recovery heat treatment is recommended to increase the elastic properties by heating the material between 400°C and 500°C to relieve the residual stresses
- This heat treatment promotes the recovery annealing stage, which eliminates the residual stresses produced during manufacturing process
- With this heat treatment, elastic modulus is increased by 10% and springback improves from 0.0060–0.0094% to 0.0065–0.0099%.

### Braided and Twisted Wires (Figs. 25.15A and B)

- Very small diameter stainless steel wires are braided or twisted together by manufacturers to form round or rectangular cross-section wires of 0.4–0.6 mm
- The bending mechanics for multistranded orthodontic wires is much complex. These wires are able to sustain large elastic deflections in bending and such wires apply much lower forces for a given deflection.

### Soldering and Welding of Stainless Steel Wires

- Low fusing solder is recommended for soldering stainless steel wire so as to minimize carbide precipitation and substantial softening of the wire

- Silver solder are used instead of gold solder
- Soldering of orthodontic wires occurs between 620°C and 665°C
- Fluorides are used as soldering flux to dissolve the passivating surface film of chromium oxide
- Orthodontic bands and brackets are joined by welding process. Flat surface of bands and brackets are usually joined by spot welding. A large electric current is passed through the electrode to flow through the overlapped band material at a spot which require welding. There is production of intense localized heating resulting in fusion of the overlapped metal. The joint area which is welded is susceptible to corrosion because of the loss of the passivating layer caused due to sensitization.

### *Advantages of Stainless Steel Wires*

- Lowest cost of wire alloys
- Highly biocompatible
- Excellent formability for fabrication into orthodontic appliances
- Can be soldered and welded.

### *Disadvantages of Stainless Steel Wires*

- Have high force delivery
- Have relatively low springback in bending compared to β-titanium and nickel-titanium alloys
- Can be susceptible to intergranular corrosion after heating to required temperature for soldering.

## COBALT-CHROMIUM-NICKEL ALLOYS

Orthodontic wires and appliances made of Co-Cr-Ni alloys were first marketed in 1950s. These alloys were originally developed as watch springs and was called as *Elgiloy*. Later

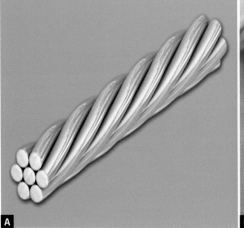
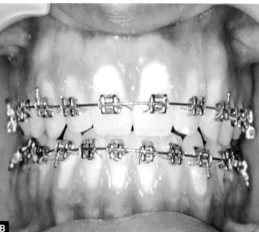

**Figs. 25.15A and B:** Braided and twisted orthodontic wires.

on these alloys were used in dental use. They have superior fatigue resistance and longer resilience as compared to stainless steel wires. This alloy can be cold worked, solution hardened as well as precipitation hardened. One manufacturer markets Elgiloy wires into four different tempers—(1) soft, (2) ductile, (3) semiresilient and (4) resilient. But the most commonly and widely used Elgiloy is the soft temper (Elgiloy blue) which is easily manipulated and heat treated to achieve increased resilience **(Fig. 25.16)**. Study by Ingram and colleagues (1986) showed that Co-Cr-Ni wires showed less ductility before heat treatment as compared to after heat treatment. The alloy showed increased ductility and mechanical properties which were comparable to stainless steel after heat treatment.

## Composition

Co: 40%, Cr: 20%, Ni: 15%, Fe: 15.8%, Mo: 7%, Mn: 2%, C: 0.16% and Be: 0.04%. Composition of Elgiloy is similar to that of the Co-Cr-Ni casting alloy.

## Properties of Elgiloy

- Has excellent tarnish and corrosion resistance
- Can be subjected to soldering and welding similar to the stainless steel wires
- Can be cold worked, solution hardened and precipitation hardened
- As with stainless steel wires heat treatment between 900°C and 1200°C has increased its ductility
- Heat treated Co-Cr-Ni wires have similar mechanical and springback properties as the stainless steel wires
- Have superior fatigue resistance and resilience as compared to stainless steel
- The modulus of elasticity is 184 GPa.

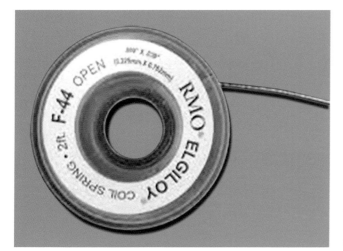

**Fig. 25.16:** Elgiloy wire.

- The yield strength of the alloy is 1400 MPa and the ultimate tensile strength is 1700 MPa
- Springback for Elgiloy blue wire is 0.0045–0.0065 and is increased to 0.0054–0.0074 after heat treatment
- Formability of Elgiloy blue wire is 8, i.e. eight number of 90° cold bends can be given without fracture.

## Uses

- Orthodontic wires and appliances
- Blade and subperiosteal implants made with Co-Cr-Ni-Mo wrought forgings
- Bone plates and screws made with Co-Cr-Ni-Mo wrought forgings
- Quad helix appliances.

## Advantages

- Relatively lower cost than nitinol and β-titanium wires
- Excellent biocompatibility
- Outstanding formability
- Can be soldered and welded
- Excellent corrosion resistance.

## Disadvantages

- Has high elastic force delivery
- Lower springback than stainless steel.

## NICKEL-TITANIUM ALLOYS

Nickel-titanium alloy was first developed by *Buehler* at *Naval Ordnance Laboratory* in 1962 and called it *nitinol*. This alloy was first used in dentistry by *Andreason* in 1970 as orthodontic wire. The term *nitinol* is derived from nickel (Ni), titanium (Ti) and Naval Ordnance Laboratory (NOL) where it was first developed. Nitinol currently represents family of alloys with minor variations in the percentage of nickel and titanium of bulk compositions.

## Uses

- Orthodontic wires
- Crowns and fixed partial dentures
- Endodontic instruments
- Blade implants
- Bone plates.

## Properties

- Ni-Ti wires have modulus of elasticity as 40 GPa. Very low elastic modulus results in very low orthodontic forces
- Springback for Ni-Ti wires is much greater as compared to stainless steel and Elgiloy. This high springback value

permits the wire to use low forces to perform large deflections

- It has yield strength of 430 MPa and ultimate tensile strength as 1500 MPa
- Formability of Ni-Ti wires is 2, i.e. two number of 90° cold bends can be given without fracture. It shows low formability as compared to stainless steel and Elgiloy wires. It readily fractures if bend sharply
- It possesses highest resilience as compared to stainless steel and Elgiloy wires, i.e. it can apply greater moving force for tooth alignment
- It possesses high ductility and is capable of undergoing substantial work hardening
- It shows shape memory and superelasticity of the material
- Soldering and welding of these wire is not possible because of temperature induced microstructural changes
- They have relatively rough surfaces which can result in high value archwire-bracket friction prolonging the treatment time
- Mixed corrosion has been found in nitinol wires when exposed to 1% saline solution. Selective leaching of Ni ions has also been reported in some studies. This can result in inflammatory tissue response in hypersensitive patients.

### Orthodontic Wire Alloys: Superelasticity and Shape Memory

- *Composition,* Ni: 55%, Ti: 45% and small amounts of Co, Cu and Cr
- It is an equiatomic intermetallic compound
- The Ni-Ti intermetallic compound exists in different crystal structures. The *austenitic Ni-Ti phase* has complex ordered BCC structure and *martensitic Ni-Ti* phase have distorted, monoclinic, triclinic or hexagonal structure
- Between the transformation of martensitic Ni-Ti and austenitic phase, an intermediate phase is formed called as the *R phase*. This phase has rhombohedral crystal structure
- Originally nitinol wire was made of predominantly heavily work hardened martensitic alloy and had Vickers hardness of 430 VHN
- Orthodontic wires having *superelasticity* were introduced in mid-1980s. These wires consist of substantial amount of austenitic Ni-Ti structures at room temperature. The superelasticity phenomenon occurs when stress is applied to the austenitic Ni-Ti phase to the point of plastic deformation in order to convert it into martensitic Ni-Ti structures. During this phase transformation the stress does not increase with the increased strain up to 8% and is called as superelasticity

- Orthodontic nitinol wires also possess the *shape memory effect*. The shape of the wire is originally established when the wire is heated at temperature near 480°C. If this wire (arch wire) is manipulated by the clinician and placed into the brackets which are bonded onto the malpositioned teeth, then exposure of this wire to lower transformation temperature cause this wire to return to its original shape, thereby promoting tooth movement. Shape memory effect occurs when the stable BCC austenitic structure transforms into twinned martensitic hexagonal structure
- Orthodontic wires with shape memory effect have superior springback with superelastic and nonsuperelastic wires **(Fig. 25.17)**.

### *Advantages*

- Force delivery is lowest in comparison to other orthodontic wires
- Excellent springback
- Superelastic and shape memory effect
- Superelastic alloys can be heat treated by clinician to vary force delivery characteristics.

### *Disadvantages*

- Costly
- Has rough surface
- Cannot make sharp bends. Difficult to make permanent bends
- Lowest in vitro corrosion resistance
- Concerns about Ni ion release.
- When exposed to saline shows less corrosion resistance than 18-8 stainless steel.

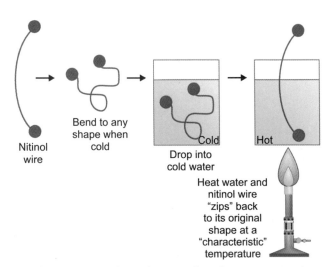

**Fig. 25.17:** Nitinol wires have excellent shape memory and superelasticity.

## Nickel-Titanium Endodontic Instruments

Nickel-titanium endodontic instrument consists of Ni: 56% and Ti: 44%. The superelastic property is most desirable for endodontic instrument. These alloys can change their structure from austenitic (base centered cubic) to martensitic (close packed hexagonal) as function of stress during root canal preparation. The superelastic property of Ni-Ti wire permits deformation of 8% strain in endodontic instruments with complete recovery whereas recovery in stainless steel instrument is less than 1%.

Ni-Ti endodontic instruments have higher strength and lower modulus of elasticity which is beneficial in preparing curved root canals **(Figs. 25.18A and B)**. These files have also been used to make rotary endodontic files. These files are manufactured by machining rather than by twisting tapered wire blanks. The edges of the cutting flutes on some nickel-titanium instruments are characterized by substantial permanent deformation referred to as *rollover*.

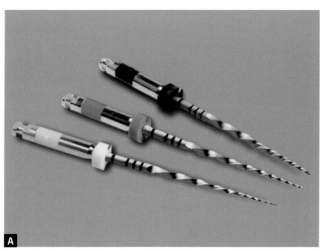

**A**

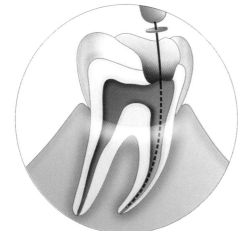

**B**

**Figs. 25.18A and B:** Ni-Ti wires used for endodontic instrumentation.

Due to cyclic fatigue Ni-Ti instruments have tendency to fracture.

## BETA-TITANIUM ALLOYS

Pure titanium has different crystallographic forms at different temperatures. Stable form below 885°C is α-titanium which is an HCP structure whereas at higher temperature stable form is β-titanium which is a BCC structure. Elements like aluminum, carbon, oxygen and nitrogen aids in stabilizing α-titanium structure and certain elements such as vanadium, molybdenum and tantalum stabilizes the β-titanium structure.

### CLINICAL SIGNIFICANCE

The α-titanium structure is not used as orthodontic wires because of difficulties in fabrication and lower formability than β-titanium structures.

### Beta-Titanium Orthodontic Wires

*Burstone* and *Goldberg* introduced the β-titanium Ti-Mo wires in 1980.

### Composition

Ti: 79%, Mo: 11%, Zr: 6% and Sn: 4%.
Molybdenum is added to stabilize the BCC β-titanium structure to room temperature, increasing its formability. These alloy referred to as titanium-molybdenum alloy (TMA).

### Properties

- Elastic modulus of β-titanium wires is 70 GPa. They have relatively low stiffness but are now available in higher range of stiffness values.
- Yield strength varies between 860 and 1200 MPa.
- *Springback* of β-titanium is much greater than the stainless steel and Elgiloy wires and similar to the nitinol wires.
- Beta-titanium wires can be highly cold worked and they have *high formability*. They can be readily bent into different orthodontic configurations. They have highest formability of any orthodontic wires **(Fig. 25.19)**.
- These are the only orthodontic wires which can be *welded*. The wires can be readily joined by electrical resistance welding units. Adequate heat is necessary to show minimum distortion of the original cold worked microstructure. Insufficient or overheating will lead to failure of the joint.
- These alloys have *excellent corrosion resistance* and environment stability. This is due to the formation of

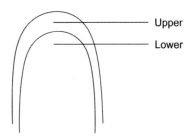

**Fig. 25.19:** Beta-titanium used as archwire material in orthodontics.

passive $TiO_2$ film. This alloy is free of Ni and can be used in Ni-sensitive patients

- Surface roughness of these wires is much greater than the stainless steel and the Elgiloy wires. This roughness can cause increased sliding friction with the metal bracket. To reduce this bracket friction *nitrogen ion implantation* technique is employed. Although recent study claims that there was no significant difference in the rate of space closure on using ion-implanted TMA, conventional TMA (non-ion implanted) and stainless steel wires
- They can be highly cold worked and are only wires which are Ni-free alternative among orthodontic wires
- They do not show signs of pitting corrosion.

*Advantages*

- Intermediate force delivery between stainless steel, Elgiloy and nitinol
- Excellent formability
- Excellent springback characteristics
- Excellent biocompatibility.

*Disadvantages*

- Costly

- High archwire-bracket friction with original TMA (reduced for nitrogen ion implanted TMA).

## WROUGHT NOBLE METAL ALLOYS

Wrought noble metal alloys currently have very limited use in dentistry. However, in the past they have been used to fabricate the removable partial denture clasps, orthodontic appliances, retention pins for restorations and endodontic posts.

Wrought wire clasps for removable partial dentures are joined by means of soldering. These clasps have greater flexibility and strength as compared to cast clasps of similar composition.

Types of noble alloy wires:

- *Type I*: Consists of at least 75% of gold, platinum and palladium.
- *Type II*: Consists of at least 65% gold, platinum and palladium.

### Properties

- Elastic modulus of these wires is about 100–120 GPa. It increases by 5% following hardening heat treatment
- Heat treatments to strengthen or soften the wrought alloys are similar to gold casting alloys
- *Platinum-gold-palladium (P-G-P)* wires are used for endodontic posts and for clasps to which removable partial denture framework can be casted. It consists of Au: 25–30, Pt: 40–50, Pd: 25–30 and Cu: 16–17%. The fusion temperature of these wires is increased for these wires
- *Palladium-silver-copper (P-S-C)* wires are also used for dental applications. The fusion temperature for these wires is higher than those for the gold alloy wires but lower than the PGP wires.

## TEST YOURSELF

### Essay Questions

1. What are wrought alloys? Classify and write in detail about nitinol wires.
2. Classify stainless steel wires. Describe each type in detail.

### Short Notes

1. Superelasticity.
2. Springback action.
3. Austenite steel.
4. Slip system.
5. Twinning.

6. Beta-titanium wires.
7. Cobalt-chromium-nickel wires.
8. Sensitization and stabilization.
9. Dislocations.
10. Effects of annealing of cold worked metal.

### Multiple Choice Questions

1. Wrought alloys are:
   A. Heat treated
   B. Heat softened
   C. Cold worked during fabrication
   D. With fine grain structures

2. The process by which fibrous wrought gold alloy structure is gradually lost and results in crystalline structure is called as:
   A. Recrystallization
   B. Work hardening
   C. Heat treatment
   D. Solid solution transformation
3. Cold working or work hardening results in all of the following *except*:
   A. Increase in hardness
   B. Increase in yield strength
   C. Increase in ductility
   D. Increase in ultimate tensile strength
4. Elevation of temperature above crystallization temperature results in.
   A. Decrease in grain size
   B. Grain growth
   C. Increased strength
   D. Increased proportional limit
5. Recrystallization of metal is affected by:
   A. Time and temperature
   B. Initial grain size of the alloy
   C. Composition of the alloy
   D. All of the above
6. Softening heat treatment is also called as:
   A. Annealing
   B. Work hardening
   C. Age hardening
   D. All of the above
7. A gold alloy when given heat softened treatment results in the formation of:
   A. Intermetallic compound
   B. Eutectic mixture
   C. Peritectic mixture
   D. Solid solution
8. Tempering of metal
   A. Increases hardness and toughness
   B. Increases hardness but reduces toughness
   C. Decreases hardness but increases toughness
   D. Decreases both hardness and toughness
9. Stainless steel with least corrosive resistance:
   A. Ferritic
   B. Austenitic
   C. Martensitic
   D. Cementitic
10. Passivation of chrome cobalt nickel alloy is due to the formation of:
    A. Chromium oxide
    B. Cobalt oxide
    C. Chromium carbide
    D. Iron oxide
11. Stainless steel with least strength is:
    A. Ferritic
    B. Austenitic
    C. Martensitic
    D. Cementitic
12. Titanium alloys for implants has following composition:
    A. Titanium, aluminum and vanadium
    B. Titanium, chromium and cobalt
    C. Nickel, titanium and chromium
    D. Nickel, titanium and cobalt
13. Maximum number of bends can be given in the following:
    A. Stainless steel
    B. Cr-Co-Ni
    C. Ni-Ti
    D. Beta titanium
14. Shape memory of nitinol wire is due to:
    A. Change from austenitic to martensitic
    B. Change from martensitic to austenitic
    C. Change from ferritic to austenitic
    D. Change from martensitic to ferritic
15. Alloy with highest elastic activation range is:
    A. Beta titanium
    B. Nitinol
    C. Stainless steel
    D. Cr-Co-Ni
16. Modulus of elasticity is highest for which of the following:
    A. Beta titanium
    B. Nitinol
    C. Stainless steel
    D. Cr-Co-Ni

## ANSWERS

| | | | |
|---|---|---|---|
| 1. C | 2. A | 3. C | 4. B |
| 5. D | 6. A | 7. D | 8. C |
| 9. C | 10. A | 11. A | 12. A |
| 13. B | 14. A | 15. A | 16. D |

## BIBLIOGRAPHY

1. Andreasen GF, Morrow RE. Laboratory and clinical analyses of nitinol wire. Am J Orthod. 1978;73:142-51.
2. Angolkar PV, Kapila S, Duncanson MG Jr, Nanda RS. Evaluation of friction between ceramic brackets and orthodontic wires of four alloys. Am J Orthod Dentofacial Orthop. 1990;98:499-506.
3. Anusavice KJ. Phillips' Science of Dental Materials, 11th edition. St. Louis: Saunders, 2003.
4. Asgharnia MK, Brantley WA. Comparison of bending and tension tests for orthodontic wires. Am J Orthod. 1986;89:228-36.
5. Bass JK, Fine H, Cisneros GJ. Nickel hypersensitivity in the orthodontic patient. Am J Orthod Dentofacial Orthop. 1993;103:280-5.

6. Brantley WA. Comments on stiffness measurements for orthodontic wires. J Dent Res. 1976;55:705.

7. Brantley WA. Orthodontic wires. In: Brantley WA, Eliades T, (Eds). Orthodontic Wires: Scientific and Clinical Aspects. Stuttgart, Germany: Thieme; 2001.

8. Brantley WA, Augat WS, Myers CL, Winders RV. Bending deformation studies of orthodontic wires. J Dent Res. 1978;57:609-15.

9. Brantley WA, Luebke FL, Mitchell JC. Performance of engine-driven rotary endodontic instruments with a superimposed bending deflection: V. Gates Glidden and Peeso drills. J Endod. 1994;20:241-5.

10. Bryant ST, Thompson SA, al-Omari MA, Dummer PM. Shaping ability of Profile rotary nickel-titanium instrument with ISO sized tips in simulated root canals: Part 1. Int Endod J. 1998;31:275-81.

11. Burstone CJ, Goldberg AJ. Beta titanium: a new orthodontic alloy. Am J Orthod. 1980;77:121-32.

12. Burstone CJ, Goldberg AJ. Maximum forces and deflections from orthodontic appliances. Am J Orthod. 1983;84:95-103.

13. Craig RG, Powers JM. Restorative dental materials, 11th edition. St. Louis (MO): Mosby: 2002.

14. Drake SR, Wayne DM, Powers JM, Asgar K. Mechanical properties of orthodontic wires in tension, bending and torsion. Am J Orthod. 1982;82:206-10.

15. Fillmore GM, Tomlinson JL. Heat treatment of cobalt chromium alloys of various tempers. Angle Orhtod. 1979;49:126-30.

16. Goldberg J, Burstone CJ. An evaluation of beta titanium alloys for use in orthodontic appliances. J Dent Res. 1979;58:593-9.

17. Harris EF, Newman SM, Nicholson JA. Nitinol arch wire in a simulated oral environment: changes in mechanical properties. Am J Orthod Dentofacial Orthop. 1988;93:508-13.

18. Hildebrand HF, Veron C, Martin P. Nickel, chromium, cobalt dental alloys and allergic reactions: an overview. Biomaterials. 1989;10:545-8.

19. Iijima M, Brantley WA, Yuasa T, Kawashima I, Mizoguchi I. Joining characteristics of beta-titanium wires with electrical resistance welding. J Biomed Mater Res B Appl Biomater. 2008;85:378-84.

20. Ingram SB Jr, Gipe DP, Smith RJ. Comparative range of orthodontic wires. Am J Orthod Dentofacial Orthop. 1986;90:296-307.

21. Johnson E. Relative stiffness of beta titanium archwires. Angle Orthod. 2003;73:259-69.

22. Kapila S, Angolkar PV, Duncanson MG Jr, Nanda RS. Evaluation of friction between edgewise stainless steel brackets and orthodontic wires of four alloys. Am J Orthod Dentofacial Orthop. 1990;98:117-26.

23. Kapila S, Sachdeva R. Mechanical properties and clinical applications of orthodontic wires. Am J Orhod Dentofacial Orthop. 1989;69:183-94.

24. Kim H, Johnson JW. Corrosion of stainless steel, nickel-titanium coated nickel-titanium and titanium orthodontic wires. Angle Orthod. 1999;69:39-44.

25. Kula K, Phillips C, Gibilaro A, Proffit WR. Effect of ion implantation of TMA archwires on the rate of orthodontic sliding space closure. Am J Orthod Dentofacial Orthop. 1998;114:577-80.

26. Kusy RP, Greenberg AR. Effects of composition and cross section on the elastic properties of orthodontic wires. Angle Orthod. 1981;51:325-41.

27. Kusy RP. A review of contemporary archwires: their properties and characteristics. Angle Orthod. 1997;67:197-207.

28. Kusy RP. Orthodontic biomaterials: from the past to the present. Angle Orthod. 2002;71:501-12.

29. Kusy RP. The future of orthodontic materials: the long-term view. Am J Orthod Dentofacial Orthop. 1998;113:91-5.

30. Lin MC, Lin SC, Lee TH, Huang HH. Surface analysis and corrosion resistance of different stainless steel orthodontic brackets in artificial saliva. Angle Orthod. 2006;76:322-9.

31. Lopez I, Goldberg J, Burstone CJ. Bending characteristics of nitinol wire. Am J Orthod. 1979; 75: 569-75.

32. Marinello CP, Luthy H, Scharer P. Influence of heat treatment on the surface texture of an etched cast nickel-chromium base alloy: an evaluation by profilometric records. J Prosthet Dent. 1986;56:431-5.

33. Miura R, Mogi M, Ohura Y, Hamanaka H. The super-elastic property of the Japanese NiTi alloy wire for the use in orthodontics. Am J Orthod Dentofacial Orhtop. 1986;90:1-10.

34. Oh KT, Kim YS, Park YS, D, Kim KN. Properties of super stainless steels for orthodontic applications. J Biomed Mater Res B Appl Biomater. 2004; 69:183-94.

35. Roach MD, Wolan JT, Parsell DE, Bumgardner JD. Use of X-ray photoelectron spectroscopy and cyclic polarization to evaluate the corrosion behavior of six nickel-chromium alloys before and after porcelain-fused-to-metal firing. J Prosthet Dent. 2000;84:623-34.

36. Sarkar NK, Redmond W, Schwaninger B, Goldberg AJ. The chloride corrosion behavior of four orthodontic wires. J Oral Rehabil. 1983;10:121-8.

37. Staffolani N, Damiani F, Lilli C, Guerra M, Staffolani NJ, Belcastro S, et al. Ion release from orthodontic appliances. J Dent. 1999;27:449-54.

38. Takahashi J, Okazaki M, Kimura H, Furuta Y. Casting properties of NI-Ti shape memory alloy. J Biomed Mater Res. 1984;18:427-34.

39. Thompson SA. An overview of nickel-titanium alloys used in dentistry. Int Endod J. 2000;33:297-310.

40. Tschernitschek H, Borchers L, Geurtsen W. Nonalloyed titanium as a bioinert metal—a review. Quintessence Int. 2005;36:523-30.

41. Walia H, Brantley WA, Gerstein H. An initial investigation of the bending and torsional properties of nitinol root canal files. J Endod. 1988;14:346-51.

42. Wataha JC, Messer RL. Casting alloys. Dent Clin North Am. 2004;48:499-512.

43. Watanabe I, Kiyosue S, Ohkubo C, Aoki T, Okabe T. Machinability of cast commercial titanium alloys. J Biomed Mater Res. 2002;63:760-4.

44. Wilson DF, Goldberg AJ. Alternative beta-titanium alloys for orthodontic wires. Dent Mater. 1987;3:337-41.

45. Winkler S, Morris HF, Monteiro JM. Changes in mechanical properties and microstructure following heat treatment of nickel-chromium base alloy. J Prosthet Dent. 1984;52:821-7.

# Soldering and Welding

*'Action makes more fortune than caution.'*

—*Marquis de Vauvernargues*

## INTRODUCTION

Metal joining procedures are often used in fabrication of the dental appliances. These metal joining procedures can be soldering, brazing and welding. Soldering and brazing are similar terms, both require a filler metal which joins the two substrate metals. The main difference between soldering and brazing is that in brazing the filler metal has melting temperature above 450° C whereas in soldering the melting temperature is below 450° C. However, welding is the process of joining the metal surfaces locally by fusing usually without requiring a filler metal.

## DEFINITIONS

*Soldering: Process of joining two or more metal components by melting a filler material between them at a temperature below their solidus temperature and filling the gap between them using a molten metal with a temperature below 450° C.*

*Brazing: "Process of joining two or more metal components by melting a filler material between them at a temperature below their solidus temperature and filling the gap between them using a molten metal with a temperature above 450° C."*
— *GPT 8th Ednition*

The term "solder" is derived from latin word "solidare" meaning "to make solid". Soldering process requires a filler metal to join or "make solid".

## HISTORICAL BACKGROUND

- *Evidence of soldering dates back some 5000 years back*: Early Mesopotamian civilization
- *4000 years ago*: Tin was discovered which was used for soldering
- *3000 years ago*: Swords used by Sumerians were soldered (joined)
- *2000 years ago*: Romans used lead and tin to join water pipes
- *Medieval age*: Alcohol flame was used to soften metals
- *1921*: First electric and mass producing soldering iron was introduced
- *1971*: Blow pipes were invented to aid in soldering.

## TYPES OF SOLDERING

The process of soldering can be of three types:
1. Soft soldering
2. Hard soldering
3. Brazing.

### Soft Soldering

This process involves joining of two metals with a filler metal having a very low melting temperature which is usually less than 350° C. Since heat generated is low it is commonly used in electronic industry because excessive heat will damage the electronic parts. To produce heat for melting the filler metal small electric gun or iron is sufficient. This type of soldering is not used in dentistry because the strength of the joint is less which is not suitable to be used in load bearing areas. Also, the joint lacks corrosion resistance. Most commonly used filler metal used is made of lead-tin alloy.

### Hard Soldering

The melting point of filler metal used is less than 450° C. This type of soldering is commonly used in dentistry as it produces the solder joint which has adequate strength. The heat source required to generate heat to melt the alloy is provided by gas torch. Apart from dentistry, hard soldering can also be used in jewelry and refrigeration industry.

### Brazing

In this process two metal substrates are joined by a filler metal having melting temperature of more than 450° C. As the melting temperature is high it required special equipment such as carbon arc torch to melt the alloy. Special eye wear is indicated when using this technique for metal joining. High melting alloys can be joined using this technique.

## COMPONENTS OF DENTAL SOLDERING (FIG. 26.1)

The process of soldering has followings components:
- Substrate metal
- Filler metal/solder
- Flux
- Antiflux
- Heat source.

### Substrate Metal

- Substrate metal also called as basis metal
- It is the pure metal or alloy which is prepared to be joined by another substrate metal or alloy
- For the process of soldering the surface of the substrate metal should be thoroughly cleaned to allow intimate contact with the molten filler metal

- The composition of the substrate metal determines the type of oxide produced during heating and the type of flux to be used to reduce the oxide formation
- Critical factors which determine the wettability of the substrate with the molten solder alloy are the composition and the cleanliness of the substrate metal.

### Soldering Filler Metal

- Soldering filler metal should be compatible with the substrate metal but the composition need not be the same. The filler metal bonds with the substrate metals by capillary action. It flows into the surface of the substrate metal and binds with a mechanical joint
- Flow temperature of the filler metal should be at least 55.6°C lower than the solidus temperature of the substrate metal. (Solidus temperature is that temperature at which the alloy begins to melt, whereas liquidus temperature is that temperature above which the alloy is completely molten and free flowing)
- Flow temperature refers to the temperature at which the filler metal flows and wet the substrate metal creating a bond. It can vary depending on the type of substrate metal, flux and the ambient atmosphere
- For pre-soldering, high melting range solder is used to prevent sag deformation of the partial denture and remelting of the solder when porcelain is fired
- Time and temperature are two critical parameters in soldering process. If flow temperature of the filler metal is not too high, still soldering can occur if the temperature is kept constant for sufficient time. The metal joining occurs due to diffusion
- For adequate joint strength the filler metal should sufficiently wet the surface of the substrate metal
- Substrate metals with oxides have poor wetting characteristics and the molten filler metal will not adequately spread on the oxide layer of the substrate metals. Therefore to have good wettability the oxide layer from the substrate metals should be removed
- Another important property of filler metal to produce good metal bond is its fluidity.

### CLINICAL SIGNIFICANCE
The molten filler metal should flow freely in the gap between the substrate metals. Any hindrance to this flow will compromise in the soldered joint.

## IDEAL REQUIREMENTS OF A DENTAL SOLDER

- Should melt at lower temperature than that of the substrate metal
- Should be as strong as the substrate metal

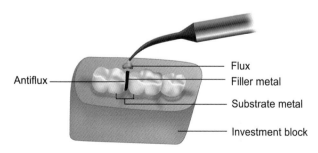

**Fig. 26.1:** Components of soldering.

- When melted, it should be wet and flow freely over the parent metal. High fusing solder have low surface tension and flow easily through narrow gaps as compared to low fusing solder which flow poorly through narrow gap
- Color should match that of metal being joined
- It should be resistant to tarnish and corrosion
- Should resist pitting during heating and application.

## Classification of Solder

- Based on the melting range of alloy
  - Soft solders
  - Hard solders
  - Very hard/brazing solders
- Based on the type of metal
  - Precious metal solders
  - Nonprecious metal solders.

## Soft Solders

- These are called soft solders because they have a low melting range of about 260° C and primarily consist of soft lead
- They are made of lead-tin eutectic alloy which are in ratio of 40:60
- These solders do not require specialized equipment to melt. A small electric gun is sufficient to melt the solder
- The joint is weak and lack corrosion resistance
- This type of solder is commonly used for plumbing work and sometimes also referred to as "plumbers solder"
- Other soft solders are tin-silver, zinc-tin, cadmium-silver.

## Hard Solders

- Hard solders have melting range less than 450° C. They possess higher strength and hardness

- A gas torch is usually adequate to melt the alloy
- Two commonly used hard solders are:
  1. Gold solders
  2. Silver solders.

*Gold solder (Fig. 26.2):* Composition of both gold and silver solders is described in **Table 26.1.**
- *Gold:* Proportions of gold is determined by its fineness. Makes the alloy highly corrosion resistant
- *Silver:* Improves wetting of gold solder. It also whitens the alloy
- *Copper:* It improves strength of solder, lowers the fusion temperature and makes it amenable to age hardening
- *Tin and zinc:* Lowers the fusion temperature of the solder
- *Nickel:* Added instead of copper in order to whiten the alloy.

*Silver solder (Fig. 26.3):* Less commonly used in dentistry. They are used when a low fusing solder is required for soldering operations on stainless steel or other base metal alloys. The formation of silver-copper eutectic is responsible for the low melting range of this type of solder. The corrosion resistance is inferior to that of gold solders. Although they have strength which is comparable to the gold solders.

**Table 26.1**  Composition of both gold and silver solder.

| Gold solder | Silver solder |
| --- | --- |
| Gold: 65–81% | Silver: 10–80% |
| Silver: 8–16% | Copper: 15–50% |
| Copper: 7–16% | Zinc: 4–35% |
| Tin: 2–4% | Cadmium—traces |
| Zinc: 2–3% | Tin and phosphorous—traces |

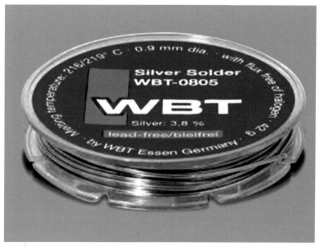

**Fig. 26.2:** Gold solder.                    **Fig. 26.3:** Silver solder.

*Brazing solders:* These solders require very high temperature to melt which is higher than 450°C. The soldered joint have good strength and the joint is usually as strong as the substrate metal. These solders require specialized equipment to generate heat to melt the solder metal.

## Soldering Flux

- The term flux means "flow"
- Flux is used to eliminate any oxide coating on the surface metal surface when the filler metal is molten and is ready to flow into place
- Most of the currently available fluxes incorporate two or more types in their composition
- Fluxes usually have temperature ranges for optimum performance. Thus, flux made for presoldering alloys will not be suitable for postsoldering alloys and vice versa.

### Classification of Flux

*Based on their purpose of use:*
- *Type I (surface protection):* This type of flux covers the surface of the metal and does not allow the formation of oxides by preventing access to oxygen
- *Type II (reducing agent):* This type reduces any oxides which are formed and expose the clean surface of metal
- *Type III (solvent):* It helps in dissolving any oxides which are present.

*Based on their pH:*
- Acidic fluxes
- Basic fluxes
- Neutral fluxes.

*Based on their source:*
- *Organic (e.g. rosin fluxes):* Used in soft soldering procedures which require low temperature
- *Inorganic:* Can be halogenides or acid-based fluxes.

*Commonly used dental fluxes are:*
- *Boric and borate compounds:* Used with noble metal alloys. They behave as protective fluxes by forming low temperature glass. They also act as reducing fluxes for low stability oxides such as copper oxide. Borax flux is manufactured from dehydrated borax, silica and boric acid
- *Fluoride fluxes:* Used with base metal alloys and are usually combined with borates. They help to dissolve the more stable chromium, nickel and cobalt oxides. Fluoride dissolves any oxide which comes in contact by acting as solvent. Fluoride flux consists of potassium fluoride, boric acid, borax glass and sodium carbonate.

Sometimes combination of fluxes can be used depending on the requirement.

### Function of Each Ingredient of Flux

- *Potassium fluoride:* It aids in dissolving the passivating surface film formed by chromium which prevents the solder from wetting the metal
- *Boric acid:* It helps in lowering the fusion temperature of the solder
- *Borax glass:* It helps in forming a protective layer on the surface of the metal
- *Silica:* It keeps the molten flux on the surface
- *Charcoal:* It acts as reducing agent.

### Manipulation

- Fluxes are usually painted on the surface of the substrate metal or are fused on the surface of the filler metal (**Fig. 26.4**)
- Flow of excess flux should be avoided as this will lead to formation of weakened joint
- At the same time if too little flux is used it will burnout and will be ineffective
- Also, if residual flux is covered with porcelain, it will lead to its discoloration or air bubble entrapment
- Flux forms glass during the soldering process by combining with the metal oxides. This glass is removed by sandblasting with alumina abrasive particles followed by boiling in water for 5 minutes
- It is important to remove excess flux entrapped in the filler metal as it can lead to formation of weakened joint
- After soldering process, the investment material is divested and the joint area is sandblasted using alumina particles. Thereafter, the joint is kept in boiling water for 5 minutes.

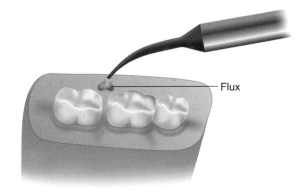

**Fig. 26.4:** Flux part is applied to the solder joint.

## Antiflux

- It is a substance such as graphite which prevents flow of molten solder on areas coated by the substance and helps in confining solder to the work area
- It is applied on the surface before flux or the solder is applied
- *Graphite* is removed at high temperature
- Therefore, at high temperature suspension of *rouge or calcium carbonate* in alcohol is used.

## Heat Sources

It is the important part of soldering process. Heat sources are usually of following types: (i) flame soldering, (ii) oven soldering, (iii) infrared soldering, and (iv) laser welding.

### Flame Soldering

- Commonly heat is applied through gas—air or gas-oxygen torch **(Fig. 26.5)**
- Type of torch is selected on the basis of type of fuel used
- The flame should generate sufficient temperature to raise the temperature of the substrate metal and filler metal to the soldering temperature
- Lower the heat content of the fuel, more fuel is burned for longer period of time to generate the required total heat
- Some of the commonly used fuel used to melt dental casting alloys along with its heat content (Table 26.2).

### Hydrogen
- Heat content of hydrogen gas is the least and thus heating would be slow

- There is considerable loss of heat to air, soldering investment and other parts of casting
- Hydrogen gas is not suitable to join substrate metal for pre-soldering.

### Natural Gas
- Heat content of natural gas is four times that of hydrogen gas
- Available natural gas is nonuniform in composition and usually has water vapor in it
- Water vapor cools the flame and uses some of the heat content.

### Acetylene
- It has the highest flame temperature and its heat content is higher than the hydrogen or natural gas
- The temperature can vary from one part of the flame to another is by 100° C
- Because of this variation, the positioning of the torch is critical to ensure proper zone of the flame
- Also, it is a very unstable gas which readily decomposes to carbon and hydrogen
- Carbon release can incorporate into nickel and palladium-based alloys leading to inferior mechanical properties of the alloys
- Hydrogen is absorbed by palladium-based alloys and can lead to increase casting porosity.

**CLINICAL SIGNIFICANCE**

If the flame is not adjusted properly, it may extinguish the torch with the associated release of carbon from the tip of the torch **(Fig. 26.6).**

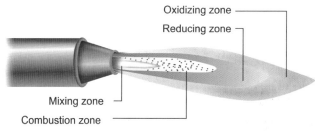

**Fig. 26.5:** Gas air torch commonly used for soldering.

| Table 26.2: Commonly used fuel gases. | | |
|---|---|---|
| *Type of fuel* | *Flame temperature (°C)* | *Heat content (BTU/ft³)* |
| Hydrogen | 2,660 | 275 |
| Natural gas | 2,680 | 1,000 |
| Propane | 2,850 | 2,385 |
| Acetylene | 3,140 | 1,448 |

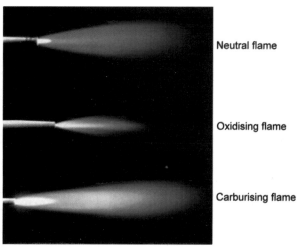

**Fig. 26.6:** Oxyacetylene flame.

*Propane*
- It is considered best fuel gas because it has highest heat content and has good flame temperature
- Butane which has similar properties can also be used in place of propane
- Both these gases have uniform quality of gas which is water free.

## Oven Soldering

- The surfaces of the metal substrate is first coated with flux and then the filler metal is introduced between the substrate metal
- The entire assembly is placed in the furnace which provides high heat to melt the filler metal
- Here, less heat is lost to the environment and other parts of the casting as the assembly is enclosed in the furnace **(Fig. 26.7)**.

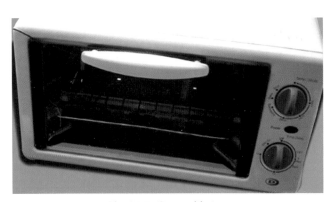

**Fig. 26.7:** Oven soldering.

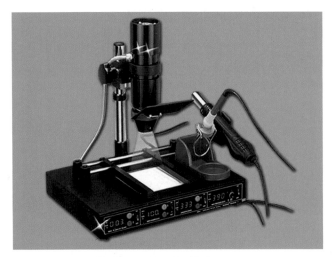

**Fig. 26.8:** Infrared soldering unit.

## Infrared Soldering

- Can be used for low ceramic connectors as well as preceramic solder joint
- Here infrared light is used as the heat source
- Solder assembly should be placed accurately in relation to the focal point of the reflector which concentrates heat
- Joints have similar strength as the conventional soldering **(Fig. 26.8)**.

## Soldering Investment

- The investment used for soldering should not expand as much as that used for casting because soldering process is done at a lower temperature than casting
- Gypsum-bonded investment containing quartz is used to solder gold alloys whereas phosphate-bonded investments are used for high fusing solder **(Fig. 26.9)**.

## PROPERTIES OF DENTAL SOLDERS

- *Fusion temperature*: Melting range of gold solders vary between 545–870° C and silver solder melt in the range of 600–700° C. The fusion temperature of the solder should be at least 50° C less than the parent metal
- *Mechanical properties*: Gold solders have sufficient strength and hardness and is comparable to cast gold alloys. The tensile strength of gold solder varies between 250–630 MPa. Silver solders have comparable mechanical properties as the gold solder
- *Corrosion resistance*: Gold solder have better corrosion and tarnish resistance as compared to silver solder. Tarnish and corrosion resistance increases with the gold content in the solder. However, as there is difference

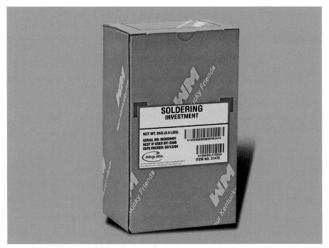

**Fig. 26.9:** Soldering investment.

between the composition of solder and its parts, the joint area is prone to galvanic corrosion

- *Wetting properties*: A solder should have good flow in order to adequately wet the patent metal for better joining. Gold flow of filler metal is dependent on the interfacial energies between the parent metal, solder and the flux.

## TECHNIQUE OF SOLDERING

- *Free hand soldering*: The parts are assembled and held in contact manually while the heat and solder are applied. For example, soldering of orthodontic appliances. Orthodontics use needle thin flame torches to heat the joint area and the soldering is done without using an investment
- *Investment soldering*: The parts to be joined are positioned in the soldering type of investment. The hardened investment holds it in position while the heat and solder are applied. This type of soldering is recommended to solder parts for fixed partial dentures or joining clasp of cast partial dentures.

### Steps in Soldering Procedure

- Selection of solder
- Cleaning and preparing surface of the parts to be joined
- Assembly of the parts to be joined in soldering investment
- Application of flux
- Preheating the parts
- Placement of solder

- Heating the solder by controlling proper temperature and time
- Cooling of assembly followed by quenching in water.

## SOLDERING PROCEDURE (FIG. 26.10)

- *Cleanliness*: Substrate metal parts which are to be joined are cleaned. Cleaning is a prime requisite for soldering because it aids in proper wetting of the surface to achieve bonding
- *Occlusal indexing:* It is important to accurately maintain the relationship of the parts to be joined until the prosthesis is embedded in the soldering investment. Materials which give highly accurate indexing are autopolymerizing acrylic resin (Duralay), stone, sticky wax, 4 META adhesive resin and zinc oxide eugenol. Excess bulk of the resin index should be avoided as it will reduce accuracy because of additional polymerization shrinkage **(Fig. 26.11)**
- *Gap between parts*: Gap width of 0.012 inch is recommended for strength. If the gap is too wide, the

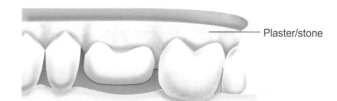

Plaster/stone

**Fig. 26.11:** Occlusal index used to maintain relationships of the parts.

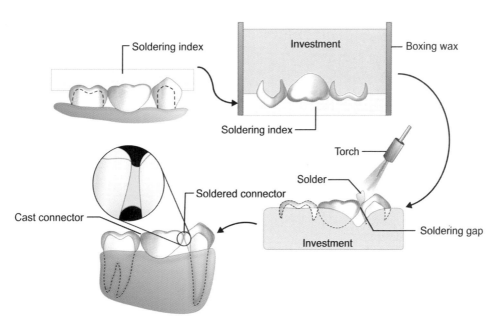

**Fig. 26.10:** Schematic diagram to explain soldering procedure.

joint strength will be influenced by the strength of the filler metal. If the gap is too small, strength will be influenced by flux inclusions, porosity due to incomplete flow of filler metal or both. Gap width of 0.008 inch is considered as optimum as is determined by inserting a business card between the parts **(Fig. 26.12)**

- *Soldering investment*: Casting to be soldered is boxed using boxing wax, and soldering investment is mixed and vibrated into the boxed area. Before pouring the investment material the gap is covered by triangular-shaped utility wax. Investment is allowed to set for one hour and then boxing wax is removed. The indexed wax is softened and then removed using heavy laboratory knife **(Fig. 26.13)**
- *Application of flux*: Flux paste is applied when the casting is still warm. The paste will melt and will be drawn over the entire solder joint by capillary action
- *Preheating of the parts*: It is done in order to ensure even heating. Preheating of casting is done for 10–15 minutes
- *Selection of solder proper color, fusion temperature and flow*
- *Flame-reducing or neutral*: Portion of the flame used to heat the soldering assembly is at the tip of the reducing zone as it produces the most efficient burning process and the maximum heat.

**CLINICAL SIGNIFICANCE**

Blowpipe is obliquely aimed as it results in more even heating and minimum distortion.

- On heating, solder will flow through the joint and flame should not be removed until the soldering process is completed. This helps in providing protection from oxidation at the soldering temperature **(Fig. 26.14)**
- *Temperature*: Lowest temperature which is sufficient to produce sound solder joint should be used. The heat provided to the substrate metal should be sufficient to reach the flow temperature of the filler metal
- *Time*: Flame should be maintained in position long enough until filler metal has flowed completely into the concentration. Longer time increases the possibility of diffusion between the substrate metal and the filler metal whereas shorter time leads to incomplete filling of the joint area.

# WELDING

*It is the process to unite or fuse two pieces by hammering, compression or by rendering soft by heat with the addition of a fusible material.*

*—GPT 8th Edition*

## Indications

- Used to joint flat structures like orthodontic bands and brackets
- Used to weld pediatric band and appliances
- Used to joint wrought clasp and repair broken metal partial dentures.

## Types

- Spot welding
- Laser welding

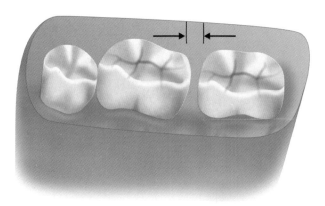

**Fig. 26.12:** Gap width of 0.012 inch is recommended for strength.

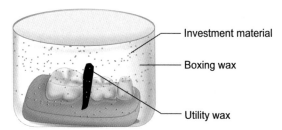

**Fig. 26.13:** Soldering investment is mixed and vibrated into the boxed area.

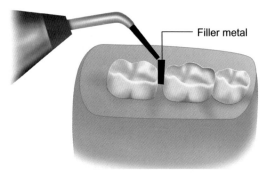

**Fig. 26.14:** Filler metal melted with gas oxygen torch.

- Plasma arc welding
- Tungsten inert gas welding.

## Spot Welding

Welding is done by passing an electric current through the pieces to be joined. The wire or band which is to be welded is held together between the copper electrodes. These pieces are also simultaneously pressed together. The resistance of the metal to flow of current causes intense localized heating and fusion of the metal. The combined heat and pressure fuses the metals into a single piece. For proper welding, sufficient voltage and duration is applied by using copper electrodes. Spot welding is commonly used in orthodontics to weld bands and wire (**Figs. 26.15 and 26.16**).

## Laser Welding

- Laser welding introduced to dentistry in 1970s
- A laser generates a coherent, high intensity pulse of light which is focused
- Types of dental lasers available are—Dentaurum Dental laser DL 2002, Haas Laser LKS and the Heraeus Haas Laser 44 P
- It is helpful in joining cast titanium components
- Individual titanium parts are precisely aligned in a laser welding unit
- Laser welding and plasma welding is performed in an argon gas atmosphere
- The laser unit consists of a box containing laser tips, argon gas source and a stereomicroscope with lens for precise alignment of the laser beam with the titanium components
- To ensure metal is melted in a small area, the time duration and intensity of the pulse should be controlled.

- One of the benefits of laser welding is that the joint will be composed of same pure titanium as the substrate components. Thus, having excellent biocompatibility and avoiding the chances of galvanic corrosion effects in the prosthesis
- Maximum penetration depth of the laser welding unit is 2.5 mm
- As small amount of heat is generated, the substrate metal parts can be hand held during the welding process
- The welding procedure is monitored by high magnification video (**Fig. 26.17**).

*Advantages:*
- Lower heat generation
- No oxide formation because of the inert argon atmosphere.

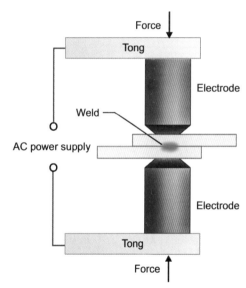

**Fig. 26.16:** Spot welding.

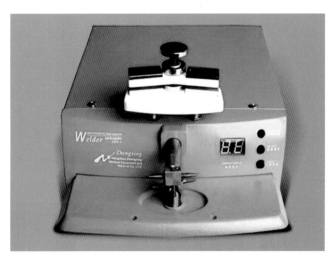

**Fig. 26.15:** Dental spot welder.

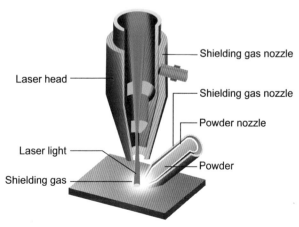

**Fig. 26.17:** Laser welding.

- Joint made of the same pure titanium as the components, thus reducing the risk of galvanic corrosion.

## Pressure Arc Welding

- *Pressure arc welding* and *Tungsten inert gas welding* follow similar technique **(Figs. 26.18 and 26.19)**
- In both techniques, the heating materials are joined by an arc established between the non-consumable tungsten electrode and the part to be welded
- The electrode and the area to be welded are protected by using an inert gas which may be argon or helium
- The primary difference between both these techniques is that in pressure arc welding the constrictor torch is used to concentrate the electric arc.

*Advantages:*
- Welding of superior quality and excellent finish
- Welding can be done in any position because thickness can be controlled
- Excellent control of weld area
- Less time consuming.

*Disadvantages:*
- Large heat is produced which can cause microstructural transformation
- Difficulty to weld butt type joint
- Chances of porosity due to argon gas.

## Pressure Welding

- Pressure welding is useful in welding thin gold foils together by applying pressure by hand
- As pure gold is highly malleable, pressure welding by hand is possible

- Pure gold does not have surface oxides but have adsorbed gases on the surface
- Absorbed gases are removed by degassing procedure and the exposed surfaces are compressed together before surface gases are adsorbed
- Gold foils can also be pressure welded by using gold foil condensers to form gold restorations **(Fig. 26.20)**.

## Cast Joining Technique

- Alternate method of joining cast components of fixed partial denture
- This technique was first proposed by *Weiss* and *Munyon* (1980)
- Cast components are held together by mechanical retention
- Joint area is ground to make space of at least 1 mm
- Mechanical undercuts are prepared at the interphase **(Fig. 26.21)**.

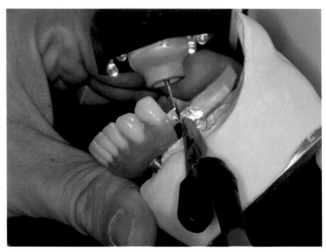

**Fig. 26.19:** Tungsten inert gas welding.

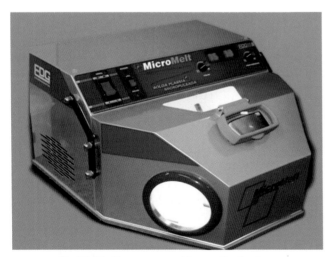

**Fig. 26.18:** Pressure arc welder used in dentistry.

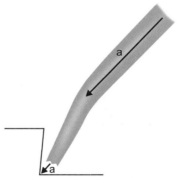

**Fig. 26.20:** Gold foils can be pressure welded with foil condensers (a= line of force remains parallel with the shaft or handle of condenser).

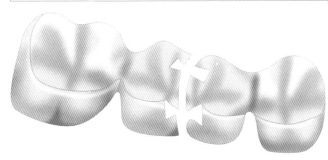

**Fig. 26.21:** Cast components held by mechanical retention.

## Technique of Welding

Welding process requires the following steps:
- Clean the surface of the substrate metal to be welded
- Appropriate electrode is selected for welding of substrate metal. A broad electrode is selected for thin metal surface and a narrow electrode is selected for thick surface of metal. The surfaces of the electrodes should be clean, smooth, and perpendicular to the long axis
- Welding machine is adjusted following the manufacturer's instructions.

- The substrate metal surface is inserted between the electrodes. The electric current is passed through the parts. Heat and pressure generated helps in joining the substrate metal parts together. This process is called as "spot welding".

### Advantages

- Easy to manipulate
- Solder or flux is not required
- Flat surfaces are easily joined
- Less chances of failure at the joint
- Joint is strong
- Heat generation is very less and therefore can be done with hand.

### Failure in Welding

- If the surfaces to be welded are not clean
- If proper electrodes are not selected for given metal
- If electrode ends do not contact the evenly with the surfaces to be joined.

---

# TEST YOURSELF

## Essay Questions

1. Define soldering and brazing. Describe each components of soldering.
2. Define welding. Describe different types of welding used in dentistry.
3. Describe various heat sources used for melting metal alloys for soldering process.

## Short Notes

1. Spot welding.
2. Laser welding.
3. Plasma welding.
4. Brazing.
5. Investment soldering.
6. Solder.
7. Flux.
8. Filler metal.
9. Gold solder.

## Multiple Choice Questions

1. Width of gap between substrate metal units is:
   A. 0.1 inch
   B. 0.01 inch
   C. 0.001 inch
   D. 0.24 inch
2. The solder used for soldering two metal alloy parts should have:
   A. Fusion temperature below the fusion temperature of both the alloys
   B. Fusion temperature above the fusion temperature of both the alloys
   C. Fusion temperature equal to the either of the alloys
   D. None of the above
3. Gap between substrate metal units in soldering is because of:
   A. To increase strength of the solder and the solder parts
   B. Allow flow of the solder and allow expansion of the soldered parts
   C. To increase the esthetics and to achieve better contact
   D. All of the above
4. The reason for failure of the abutment retainers to seat after soldering is related to:
   A. Lack of parallelism between the abutments
   B. Dimensional changes in the metal during soldering
   C. Failure to correctly position the retainers during soldering
   D. Failure of the temporary restoration to maintain proper tooth position

5. To be biologically and functionally acceptable, the soldering joint between the pontics and the connector in a fixed partial denture should be:
   A. Longer cervico-occlusally as well as wider buccolingually
   B. Longer cervico-occlusally but narrower buccolingually
   C. Short cervico-occlusally and narrower buccolingually
   D. Shorter cervico-gingivally but wider buccolingually

6. The primary purpose of flux is:
   A. To prevent oxidation of the metal during melting
   B. To increase the melting point of the flux
   C. To prevent contamination of the metal and the liner
   D. All of the above

7. Which of the following is not used as flux material
   A. Borax
   B. Boric acid
   C. Potassium fluoride
   D. Magnesium carbonate

8. Brazing is another term for:
   A. Soldering
   B. Welding
   C. Soldering and welding
   D. None of the above

9. The purpose of flux used in soldering is:
   A. Lower the melting point of the solder
   B. Make the solder harden quickly
   C. Prevent the solder from flowing to areas where the solder is not needed
   D. Remove oxides from the surfaces of the metal units to be soldered so that the solder can flow and wet the surfaces better

10. Solder can be used in all of the following, *except*:
    A. Joining a wire loop to a band to make a space retainer
    B. Joining pontic to the retainer
    C. Adding contact to the crown
    D. Repairing the hole in the occlusal surface of a crown discovered at the time of oral examination.

## ANSWERS

| | | | |
|---|---|---|---|
| 1. C | 2. A | 3. B | 4. C |
| 5. B | 6. A | 7. D | 8. A |
| 9. D | 10. D | | |

## BIBLIOGRAPHY

1. Anusavice KJ. Phillips' Science of Dental Materials, 11th edition. St. Louis: Saunders, Elsevier, 2003.
2. Craig RG, Powers JM. Restorative Dental Materials, 11th edition. St. Louis: Mosby Inc., 2002.
3. Kaylakie WG, Brukl CE. Comparative tensile strengths of non-noble dental alloy solders. J Prosthet Dent. 1985;53:455-62.
4. Monday JL, Asgar K. Tensile strength comparison of presoldered and postsoldered joints. J Prosthet Dent. 1986;55:23-7.
5. Rasmussen EJ, Goodkind RJ, Gerberich WW. An investigation of tensile strength of dental solder joints. J Prosthet Dent. 1979;41:418-23.

# Section 7

# Endodontic and Preventive Materials

# Endodontic Materials

*'The secret of success is constancy of purpose.'*

*—Benjamin Disraeli*

## INTRODUCTION

Endodontics is that branch of dentistry which deals with the morphology, physiology and pathology of dental pulp and the periradicular tissues. Success of endodontic treatment requires the usage of large number of endodontic materials which are well tested through scientific investigation, clinical trials and time. Some of the commonly used and recent endodontic materials are discussed in this section.

## IRRIGATING MATERIALS

Irrigation of the root canal during instrumentation is essential part of endodontic treatment. This process ensures the canal is free of tissues, bacterial and bacterial products and dentinal debris. They also serve as lubricants for metallic instrumentation used in the canal. Thoroughly irrigated canal provides a favorable environment for successful obturation and ultimate clinical success.

### Rationale

The primary function of irrigation of root canal is:
- To flush out organic debris and tissue fragments from the root canal
- To dissolve the organic tissues especially from lateral and accessory canals
- To provide antibacterial action and be effective against the bacteria lodged deep within the canal
- To provide lubrication during root canal instrumentation.

### Factors Affecting the Efficacy of the Irrigating Materials

- *Type of pulpal tissue*: The pulp tissue to be removed can be necrotic, vital or chemically fixed. It is easier to remove necrotic pulp as compared to the vital pulp tissues
- *Diameter and curvature of the root canal*: In larger diameter and straighter canals, irrigants can better penetrate to the maximum depth of the root canal as compared to the curved canal
- *Volume of the irrigant*: Greater the volume of the irrigant greater will be the cleaning of the canals
- *Temperature of the irrigant*: Warmer irrigant increases the efficacy of the irrigant. Tissue dissolving efficacy of 0.5% sodium hypochlorite at 45°C is same as that of the 5.25% hypochlorite at 20°C
- *Technique and extent of canal instrumentation*: Cleaning and shaping of the root canal is done together. Proper shaping will allow better cleaning of the canal

- *Concentration of the irrigant*: Sodium hypochlorite when used at higher concentration has better efficacy then when used at concentration of 0.5%
- *Length and time of contact*: The irrigant should be left in the root canal for adequate time period to show maximum efficacy
- *Depth of the irrigating needle*: Needle of the irrigating solution should go as apical in the canal as possible for maximum efficacy. The needle should be inserted at least 1.5 mm short of the working length to achieve better debridement
- *Surface tension of the irrigant*: Greater the surface tension of the irrigant, greater will be wettability of the canal
- *Type and gauge of the needle*: Larger diameter needle will deliver greater amount of irrigant as compared to narrower diameter needle.

### Classification of Irrigating Materials

Irrigation materials can be classified on the basis of their action as:
1. *Flushing action*: Normal saline, distilled water and anesthetic solutions
2. *Antibacterial*: Sodium hypochlorite, chlorhexidine, mixture of tetracycline, acid and detergent (MTAD), electrochemically activated water
3. *Chelating*: Ethylenediaminetetraacetic acid (EDTA)
4. *Tissue dissolving*: Sodium hypochlorite
5. *Bubbling*: Hydrogen peroxide and sodium hypochlorite.

### Sterile Solution

- Sterile saline when used as irrigant relies totally on the physical flushing action of irrigation to remove debris
- It is highly biocompatible as compared to other irrigants
- It does not possess the antibacterial effect or tissue dissolving ability
- Its use has reduced completely over period of time.

### Sodium Hypochlorite Solution *(Fig. 27.1)*

- It is the most commonly used endodontic irrigant
- *Dakin* in 1915 first recommended it to be used for debridement of infected wound
- It is used in the concentration of 1–5.25% for effective antimicrobial properties
- It has broad spectrum antimicrobial effect and is effective against bacteria, fungi, spores and viruses
- It is important to replenish sodium hypochlorite frequently as its antimicrobial property depends on availability of free chlorine from dissolution of hypochlorite

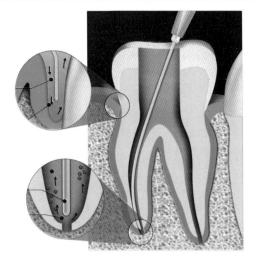

**Fig. 27.1:** Sodium hypochlorite used as root canal irrigant.

- The success of sodium hypochlorite as endodontic irrigant depends on preparation of the canal to remove gross debris and enlargement of the canal so that the solution can penetrate the apical portion
- It is usually supplied as 5.25% concentration.

### CLINICAL SIGNIFICANCE

During irrigation, the solution should not penetrate past the apical foramen into the periradicular tissues as it can result in severe pain, periapical bleeding and swelling.

- Irrigation should be done slowly with light pressure using nonbinding needle **(Fig. 27.2)**
- Its ability to dissolve tissue and its antimicrobial effect is enhanced at elevated temperatures.

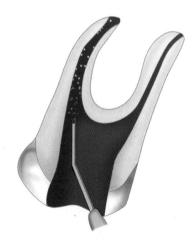

**Fig. 27.2:** Irrigation should be done slowly to remove gross-debris using light pressure.

- Gutta-percha points can be sterilized by soaking in sodium hypochlorite solution for 1 minute at 1% concentration and for 5 minutes at 0.5% concentration.

## Mechanism of Action

Sodium hypochlorite shows antibacterial and tissue dissolving property. Its action can be observed as following types:

- *Saponification reaction*: It dissolved organic tissues and fat solvent. It degrades the fatty acids into salts (soap) and glycerol (alcohol) thereby reducing the surface tension of the remaining solution
- *Neutralizing action*: It neutralizes amino acids forming salt and water
- *Chloramination reaction*: Hypochlorous acid and hypochlorite ions are responsible for amino acid degradation and hydrolysis. When this acid contacts the organic tissues it releases chlorine which has strong antimicrobial action.

### Chlorhexidine Gluconate

- It is biguanide which is an antibacterial material that can be used as endodontic irrigant
- It is commonly used as plaque controlling agent in the concentration of 0.2%
- For its use as endodontic irrigant, it should be used in the concentration of 2%
- Although it has antibacterial quality but it does not have ability to dissolve tissue remnants as hypochlorite solution neither it can remove the smear layer
- It can be used as an adjunct to sodium hypochlorite solution as effectiveness of chlorhexidine as sole irrigant is not suitable.

### Hydrogen Peroxide

It can also be used as endodontic irrigant, but it is less effective than sodium hypochlorite solution because of its ability to dissolve necrotic tissues. It is used in the concentration of 3% and it acts by bubbling out the debris. It mildly disinfects the canal.

**CLINICAL SIGNIFICANCE**

However, it should never be used as the last irrigant because of its ability to combine with the pulp debris and blood to form gas. This gas when released causes continuous pain and swelling. It is therefore not used nowadays because of the above mentioned disadvantages.

## CHELATING AGENTS

Chelating agents are used to remove the smear layer which is formed along the canal wall during instrumentation. Smear layer is 1–2 μm thick layer which is composed of organic and inorganic components formed from cutting and scrapping action of the endodontic files. Removal of the smear layer permits better adaptation of the sealer to the canal wall and this aid in improving adhesion and sealing of the canal. Bacteria may also be part of smear layer.

### Ethylenediaminetetraacetic Acid

- It is a chelating material which has ability of removing smear layer when used along with the sodium hypochlorite solution
- Apart from removal of smear layer it facilitates loosening of calcific obstruction in the root canal **(Fig. 27.3)**
- Sodium hypochlorite is required to dissolve the organic portion of the smear layer and then irrigation with EDTA removes the inorganic portion of the smear layer
- On removal of smear layer, there is increase in the diameter of the dentinal tubules
- About 17% of EDTA is used as effective chelating agent in endodontics
- These products improves instrumentation with rotary Ni-Ti files or conventional files by lubrication
- Root canal irrigation with 17% EDTA for 1 minute followed by final rinse with sodium hypochlorite is the most commonly used method to remove the smear layer
- It has no antibacterial effect.

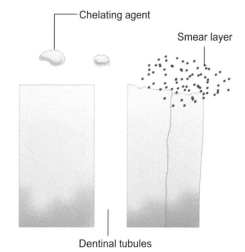

**Fig. 27.3:** Chelating agent is used to remove smear layer and open dentinal tubules.

- It removes smear layer and softens dentin. The extent of demineralization depends on the exposure time
- The optimal working time of EDTA is 15 minutes after which no more chelating action takes place due to buffering action of the dentin
- For example, RC-Prep (Premier), Glyde (Dentsply) **(Fig. 27.4)**.

## MIXTURE OF TETRACYCLINE, ACID AND DETERGENT (FIG. 27.5)

- Mixture of tetracycline, acid and detergent is a chelating agent which is used as an alternative to EDTA for removing the smear layer. It disinfects the root canal and removes the smear layer. It is a mixture of tetracycline isomer, an acid (citric acid) and a detergent
- Mineral trioxide aggregate dentin (MTAD)(Biopure, Dentsply, Oklahoma) are shown to be less cytotoxic than eugenol, 3% $H_2O_2$, Ca (OH)$_2$ paste and 5.25% sodium hypochlorite solution

- M Torabinejad first formulated MTAD. It is composed of 3% doxycycline, 4.25% citric acid and 0.5% Tween 80, a polysorbate 80 detergent. Doxycycline has antibacterial action. It chelates with dentin to provide sustained release which is more lethal for Gram-positive bacteria. It acts by inhibiting protein synthesis of bacteria by reversibly binding with 30S ribosomal subunits. Citric acid and detergent are used to remove the smear layer whereas the detergent acts as a lubricant
- It is used as a final rinsing solution after the use of sodium hypochlorite. After its use sealer is applied and obturation is done. For final irrigation, 1 mL of MTAD is recommended to be placed for 5 minutes and thereafter rinsing with 4 mL of MTAD as final rinse
- It results in complete removal of the smear layer without significantly changing the dentinal tubules
- MTAD is contraindicated in pregnant patient, lactating mothers and in children below 8 years
- On comparing with EDTA, it is found to result in cleaner dentinal tubules in the apical portion and showed lesser erosion of the tubules **(Table 27.1)**.

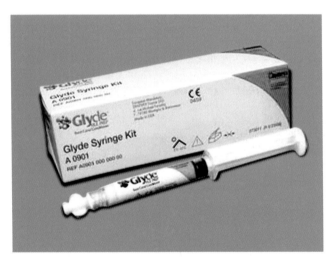

**Fig. 27.4:** Glyde—root canal conditioning agent.

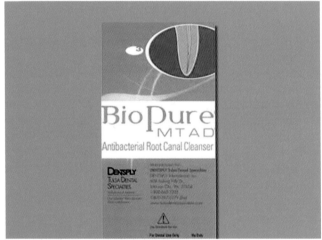

**Fig. 27.5:** MTAD—antibacterial root canal cleanser.

**Table 27.1:** Comparison of intracanal irrigants.

| Properties | MTAD | EDTA | Sodium hypochlorite |
|---|---|---|---|
| Antimicrobial activity | Present | Absent | Present |
| Smear layer removal | Present | Present | Absent |
| Dentin conditioning | Present | Present | Absent |
| Positive effect on sealing of root canal | Present | Present/absent | Absent |
| Time for application | 5 minutes | 1 minute | 40 minutes |
| Biocompatibility | Present | Present | Absent |
| Pulp dissolving capacity | Present | Present/absent | Present |

Abbreviations: MTAD, mineral trioxide aggregate dentin; EDTA, ethylenediaminetetraacetic acid.

# INTRACANAL MEDICAMENTS

Biomechanical shaping and cleaning of the root canal is accepted principle of endodontic treatment. This procedure involves the use of antimicrobial irrigant to remove microorganisms from the canal. But in cases of nonvital pulp, certain viable bacteria are retained. To eliminate or reduce the bacterial count in such canals, intracanal medicaments are used **(Figs. 27.6A to C)**.

## Ideal Requirements for Intracanal Medicaments

- Should eliminate any remaining bacteria after root canal instrumentation
- Should neutralize tissue debris and make canal inert.
- Should act as barrier against leakage from temporary filling material
- Should dry persistently wet canal
- Should reduce inflammation of the periapical tissues.

### Classification of Intracanal Medicaments

1. Phenolic agents
2. *Halogens*:
   - Iodine compounds
   - Iodine potassium iodide
   - Sodium hypochlorite.
3. *Nonphenolic biocides*:
   - Alcohols (e.g. ethanol)
   - Aldehydes (e.g. formaldehydes and glutaraldehydes)
   - Biguanides (e.g. chlorhexidine)
   - Quaternary ammonium compounds.
4. Calcium hydroxide
5. Corticosteroids
6. Antibiotics.

## Volatile Medicaments

Medicaments such as *metacresylacetate, camphorated monochlorophenol* (CMCP) and *formocresol* were used as intracanal medicaments. These materials showed strong antibacterial qualities. The duration of action of such medicaments was for short period of time. Toxic effects of these materials to the vital tissue and potential distribution of these materials to the body have been well-documented.

# CAMPHORATED MONOCHLOROPHENOL

This type of intracanal medicament was first developed by Walkhoff in 1891. It is composed of two parts of parachlorophenol and three parts of gum camphor. It has wide antibacterial spectrum and is effective against fungi. Parachlorophenol is antibacterial agent whereas camphor acts as a vehicle which reduces the irritating effect of parachlorophenol. It is placed with the help of cotton pellet which is squeezed dried **(Fig. 27.7)**.

### CLINICAL SIGNIFICANCE

Care should be taken that this material does not pass beyond the periapical tissues as it can cause pain and flare up.

## Iodine Potassium Iodide

It is a type of disinfectant which acts as an oxidizing agent by reacting with free sulfhydryl groups of bacterial enzymes, cleaving disulfide bonds. It has high antibacterial activity and has low toxicity. It is formed by mixing 4 g of potassium iodide with 2 g of iodine in 94 cc of distilled water.

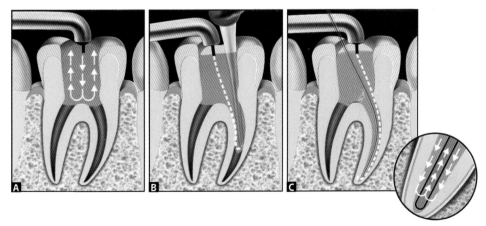

**Figs. 27.6A to C:** Intracanal medicaments are used to remove microorganisms from the canal.

## Formaldehyde (**Fig. 27.8**)

Formaldehyde in the form of "formocresol" is extensively used in endodontic treatment. Despite to be known to have high toxicity, mutagenicity and has carcinogenic potential, it is still used because it is a nonspecific bacterial medicament which is effective against both the anaerobic and aerobic microorganisms (bactericidal) present in the root canal. Formocresol was developed by Buckley in 1906. It is composed of formaldehyde 19%, cresol 35%, water 46% and glycerin. It shows both protein coagulating effect of phenolic compounds and alkylating effect of formaldehyde. It is used in pulpotomy to fix the retained pulp tissues. A damp cotton pellet of formocresol when placed in contact with the pulp tissue in the pulp chamber leads to persistent inflammatory reaction (**Fig. 27.9**).

## Calcium Hydroxide

- This material has been successfully used in dentistry for past 90 years in procedures such as pulp capping, apexification, etc.
- Hermann first introduced calcium hydroxide to endodontics in 1930s
- It is the most common, scientific and popular intracanal medicament (**Fig. 27.10**)
- When used as intracanal medicament, calcium hydroxide powder is mixed with sterile water, saline or anesthetic
- Commercial preparations of calcium hydroxide are also available.

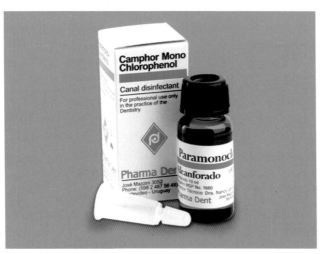

**Fig. 27.7:** Camphorated monochlorophenol (CMCP).

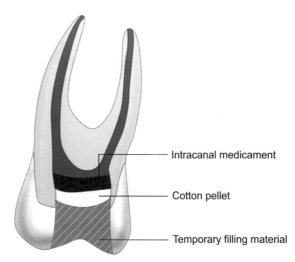

**Fig. 27.9:** Use of intracanal medicament.

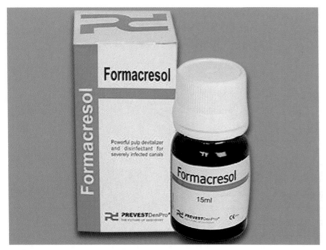

**Fig. 27.8:** Formocresol.

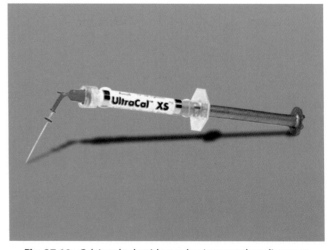

**Fig. 27.10:** Calcium hydroxide used as intracanal medicament.

## Classification of Calcium Hydroxide

- *According to the setting time calcium hydroxide is classified as*:
  - *Fast setting (chemical cure)*: It is used as sub-base or cavity liner. Its setting reaction is accelerated in presence of water
  - *Controlled setting (light cure)*: Indicated in cases of direct or indirect pulp capping
  - *Slow setting*: Used as temporary sealing material
  - *Nonsetting*: Used as intracanal medicament.
- *According to the type of availability*:
  - Powder is mixed with different vehicles
  - As single paste system
  - As two paste system.

*Properties*

- pH of calcium hydroxide is 12.5 which contributes to its antibacterial and biologic properties. High pH aids in destruction of the bacterial cell membranes and protein structures
- Antibacterial property of calcium hydroxide is due to the release of hydroxyl ions which results in highly alkaline environment. Rate of diffusion of hydroxyl ions is slow in the root canal because of its buffering capacity with the dentin. Release of hydroxyl ions also depends on the vehicle which carries calcium hydroxide. Various vehicles used are water, glycerin, polyethylene glycol or propylene glycol. Water-based vehicles show greater degree of solubility and require multiple dressings as compared to other vehicles. Other medicaments such CMCP and 0.12% chlorhexidine can be combined to produce synergistic results
- It has shown to dissolve the necrotic pulp tissues
- It is highly biocompatible as it has been successfully used for pulp capping and apexification for years.

### CLINICAL SIGNIFICANCE

In cases of accidentally exposing pulp during cavity preparation, calcium hydroxide is directly applied as bandage over the bleeding tissue to promote dentin bridge formation in order to preserve the vitality of the pulp.

- It is difficult to completely remove calcium hydroxide from the root canal even after copious irrigation
- Has strength
- Has high solubility.

## CORTICOSTEROIDS

Corticosteroids have been applied topically and has been used as anti-inflammatory agent in the root canal. Corticosteroids are not used alone but as mixture with the antibiotics in the paste from. Apart from anti-inflammatory effect they are found to inhibit root resorption.

## ANTIBIOTICS

This material has been successfully used in dentistry for past 60 years in procedures such as pulp capping, apexification, etc.

Antibiotics use in endodontic treatment was reported by Grossman in 1951. He used an antibiotic paste called as PBSC (penicillin, bacitracin, streptomycin and caprylate sodium). This mixture of antibiotics targeted specific microorganisms such as penicillin was used to target Gram-positive bacterias, streptomycin targeted Gram-negative bacterias, bacitracin targeted penicillin-resistant strains and caprylate sodium targeted yeast. Later caprylate sodium was replaced by nystatin which is widely used as antifungal agent.

Two commonly used antibiotic pastes used as intracanal medicament in endodontic treatment are:
1. Ledermix paste
2. Septomixine forte paste.

*Ledermix paste* composed of demeclocycline HCl (3.2% concentration) and triamcinolone acetonide (corticosteroid in the concentration of 1%). Later it was replaced by broad spectrum antibiotics which is tetracycline. The drawback of using this paste was that if it was left in the pulp chamber it has tendency to stain the tooth to brownish color due to presence of tetracycline.

*Septomixine forte paste* composed of neomycin, polymyxin B sulfate and dexamethasone 0.05% (corticosteroid). Both the antibiotics used in this paste were found to be ineffective to the flora which is commonly seen in the root canal.

Other antibiotics used are clindamycin which was found to be effective against microorganism found in the root canal.

*Triple antibiotic paste* consisting of metronidazole, ciprofloxacin and minocycline have been found to be highly effective against multiple microorganisms present in the root canal. However, minocycline was found to cause staining in the tooth.

## PLACEMENT OF INTRACANAL MEDICAMENT

Intracanal medicaments have been applied in very small quantity using cotton pellet. Minimal quantity ensures easy removal of the medicament. Medicaments such as calcium hydroxide are applied by means of syringe. The advantage of using the syringe is that desired quantity of intracanal medicament reaches close to the apex of the root canal.

At the time of obturation of the root canal, the intracanal medicament should be removed completely. Copious irrigation of the canal helps in removal of the intracanal medicaments.

## ROOT CANAL SEALER

Root canal sealers (ADA specification no. 57, ISO specification no. 6876:2001) are used to cement the gutta-percha or core material to provide a fluid-tight seal or hermetic seal of the canal space. It is used to lubricate the cones during lateral compaction and to fill voids and intricate ramifications of the canal system.

### Ideal Requirement of a Root Canal Sealer (Grossman, 1988)

- It should be tacky when mixed and should adhere to the core material (usually gutta-percha) and the canal wall.
- Should provide a hermetic seal, i.e. should maintain a fluid-tight seal of the canal **(Fig. 27.11)**
- Should be radiopaque to aid in visualization and evaluation of obturation of the lateral canals and apical ramifications
- It should not shrink on setting because any shrinkage will create gaps at the dentin interface or within the core materials thus breaking the seal
- It should not stain the tooth structure because any leaching of the components of the sealer will discolor the crown
- Should be bacteriostatic.

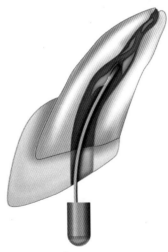

**Fig. 27.11:** Root canal sealer is applied to lubricate gutta-percha cones and provide fluid-tight seal.

- Reduced setting time in order to provide sufficient working time to allow placement of the obturation material into the canal
- It should be insoluble in oral fluids as dissolution will compromise the hermetic seal
- It should be tissue tolerant as biocompatibility of the sealer will promote periradicular repair
- Should be soluble in solvent if required to remove the filling.

### Classification of Root Canal Sealer

Based on the type of the material used root canal sealers can be classified as the following:
- Zinc-oxide eugenol-based
- Calcium hydroxide-based
- Glass ionomer-based
- Resin-based
- Silicone-based
- Mineral trioxide aggregate (MTA)-based.

#### Zinc-oxide Eugenol-based

- This type is the most commonly used and oldest root canal sealer
- They are gold standard by which other sealers are compared
- Components of powder are mixed with eugenol to form sealer
- For example, pulp canal sealer (SybronEndo), Intrafil (SS White), Endofil (Dentsply).

*Composition*
- *Rickert's formula (1931):* Also called as Kerr's sealer was first developed by Dixon and Rickert in 1931.
    - *Powder:*
        - Zinc-oxide: 41.2%
        - Precipitated silver: 30%
        - White resin: 16%
        - Thymol iodide: 12.8%
    - *Liquid:*
        - Clove oil: 78%
        - Canada balsam: 22%
- *Grossman's formula (1958):*
    - *Powder:*
        - Zinc-oxide: 42%
        - Staybelite resin: 27%
        - Bismuth subcarbonate: 15%
        - Barium sulfate: 15% increases radiopacity
        - Sodium borate: 1%
    - *Liquid:* Eugenol.

This formula is considered standard by which other root canal sealers are compared. Resin is added to improve the adhesive quality of the sealer. It can also react with zinc to produce matrix-stabilized zinc-resinate that aids in reducing the solubility of the sealer **(Fig. 27.12)**.

The ratio of bismuth subcarbonate and sodium borate controls the working and setting times of the sealer.

### Setting Reaction

When powder is mixed with eugenol it forms zinc eugenolate crystals embedded with zinc-oxide. Free eugenol is present as the material sets and reduces as the setting process continues. These sealers have adequate working time and sets faster in presence of humidity and mouth temperature. Smaller particle size increases the setting time whereas vigorous and longer spatulation reduces the setting time.

### Calcium Hydroxide-based Sealers

These sealers were developed to take advantage of biocompatibility and possible bioactivity of calcium hydroxide when placed in contact with the vital pulp or apexification. But for this bioactivity, the calcium hydroxide should dissociate into calcium and hydroxyl ions. This will lead to compromised sealing ability of the sealer. It has proved to provide short-term sealing ability but long-term sealing ability remains questionable **(Fig. 27.13)**.

*Sealapex composition:*
- *Base:*
  - Zinc oxide
  - Calcium hydroxide
  - Butyl benzene
  - Sulfonamide
  - Zinc stearate

- *Catalyst:*
  - Barium sulfate
  - Titanium dioxide
  - Isobutyl salicylate.

### Polymer-based Sealers

Polymers used as endodontic sealers are epoxy resins and polyketone compound **(Fig. 27.14)**. Epoxy resin material shows good handling characteristics and adhesion to dentin but has significant toxicity in the unset form. But after 24 hours, epoxy resin sealers show the least toxicity of endodontic sealers.

Polyketone sealers are resin reinforced chelate which is formed between zinc-oxide and diketone. This material has tacky consistency and so the handling of this material

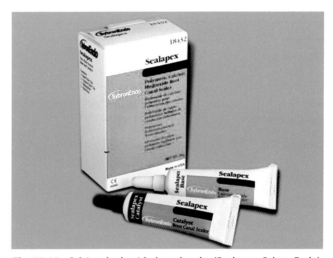

**Fig. 27.13:** Calcium hydroxide-based sealer (Sealapex–SybronEndo).

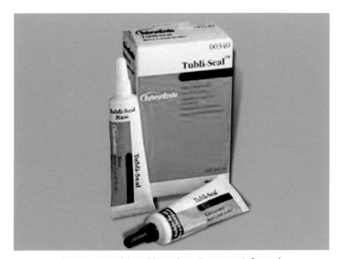

**Fig. 27.12:** Tubliseal based on Grossman's formula.

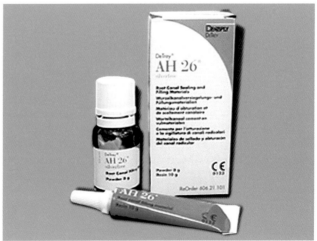

**Fig. 27.14:** Polymer-based sealers.

is difficult. Though, they show good adhesion to dentin and have low solubility. They have been reported to show elevated level of cellular toxicity.

### AH 26 Composition

First developed by Schroeder in 1957
- *Powder*:
  - Bismuth oxide
  - Hexamethylenetetramine
  - Silver powder
  - Titanium oxide
- *Liquid*: Bisphenol diglycidyl ether.

### Glass Ionomer Sealers

One of the major advantages of glass ionomer sealer is its chemical bonding with the dentin. They improve the seal and aids in strengthening the root against fracture. Canals obturated with gutta-percha using glass ionomer sealer have shown greater resistance to fracture than other sealers.

These sealers have excellent biocompatibility, but they are more viscous and have shorter working time. Retreatment is difficult because of its hardness and relative insolubility.

*Ketac Endo:* This glass ionomer-based sealer was first developed by Ray and Seltzer in 1991.
- *Powder*:
  - Calcium aluminum lanthanum fluorosilicate glass
  - Calcium volframate
  - Silicic acid
  - Pigments.
- *Liquid*:
  - Polyethylene polycarbonic acid
  - Copolymer of tartaric acid
  - Water.

## SILICONE-BASED SEALERS

### Lee Endofill

It is injectable silicone-based root canal sealer. It can be used along with the obturating material like gutta-percha or can be used alone as a sealant. Once cured it becomes pink rubbery solid resembling gutta-percha. It is easy to remove in cases of retreatment. Its primary drawback is that it shrinks on setting.

### Composition

- *Base*:
  - Hydroxyl terminated dimethyl polysiloxane
  - Undecylenic acid
  - Benzyl alcohol
  - Hydrophobic amorphous silica bismuth subnitrate
- *Catalyst*:
  - Tetraethyl orthosilicate
  - Polydimethylsiloxane.

## OBTURATING MATERIALS

Successful endodontic treatment comprises of proper cleaning, shaping and three dimensional obturation of the root canal. The materials which are used to fill the root canal three-dimensionally are called as obturating materials (ADA specification no. 78, ISO specification no. 6877: 2006).

### Ideal Requirement

- Should be able to seal the root canal three dimensionally
- Should provide hermetic seal when used with sealer, which should be impervious to moisture
- Should be easy to manipulate
- Should be easy to remove in case of retreatment
- Should be nonirritating, non-carcinogenic and non-mutagenic
- Should be radiopaque
- Should be biocompatible
- Should be easily sterilizable
- Should be dimensionally stable
- Should be bacteriostatic
- Should not stain the tooth or leach in the canal.

### Classification of Obturating Materials

Based on the type of material used for obturation:
1. *Metals*:
   - Silver points
   - Stainless steel files
   - Titanium wires.
2. *Plastics*:
   - Gutta-percha
   - Resilon.
3. *Pastes*:
   - Mineral trioxide aggregate
   - Zinc oxide eugenol
   - Calcium hydroxide paste
   - Iodoform paste
   - Chloropercha
   - Eucapercha
   - $N_2$
   - Biocalex.

### Silver Cones

Silver cones were first used by *Jasper* in 1941 as obturating material in root canal treatment. The uses of silver cones were common during 1940–1960 due to its bactericidal property. This material is no more used now because of its disadvantages such as lack of adequate seal, poor retrievability, improper debridement and poor corrosion resistance.

## Advantages

- Can be used in narrow and curved canal
- Has bactericidal property
- Has greater rigidity than gutta-percha points.

## Disadvantages

- Retrievability is very difficult in cases of retreatment
- Poor corrosion resistance
- Chances of poor lateral seal
- Postpreparation is difficult.

## GUTTA-PERCHA

It is one of the oldest dental materials which is currently used as root canal filling material. It is produced from the juices of trees of the sapodilla family in Malaysia, Indonesia and Brazil. This material is an isomer of natural rubber called trans-polyisoprene. They are harder, less elastic and have greater brittleness than natural rubber. They usually occur in two forms, i.e. (1) alpha phase and the (2) beta phase. Alpha phase is a naturally occurring form of gutta-percha and if this is heated to 65°C, it melts to form amorphous form. This amorphous material is cooled rapidly to recrystallizes forming the beta phase. This phase (beta) is commonly used in endodontics.

### Historical Development

- *1656 AD*: *John Tradescant* referred to gutta-percha as "mazer wood" which is a pliable material that was warmed in water and molded in different shapes
- *1842*: *William Montgomerie*, a medical officer in Indian service, introduced gutta-percha into practical use in the West. He was the first to appreciate the potential of this material in medicine
- *1843*: *Jose D'Almeida* of Singapore presented gutta-percha to the Royal Asiatic Society of England
- *1847*: *Asa Hill* first used gutta-percha in dentistry by mixing with carbonate of lime and quartz and calling it as "Hills Stopping"
- *1848*: Gutta-percha first used as insulating material for underground telegraph lines
- *1850s*: Gutta-percha used for number of items such as threads, surgical instrument, carpets or golf balls
- *1867*: *GA Bowman* reported to use of gutta-percha as root canal filling material

- *1887*: *SS White* Company started manufacturing of gutta-percha points
- *1914*: Callahan used rosins to soften and dissolute gutta-percha during obturation
- *1942*: *CW Bunn* reported the existence of crystalline form of gutta-percha in two phases–(1) alpha phase and (2) beta phase. Beta phase of gutta-percha is commonly used as obturating material in endodontics
- *1958*: *Ingle* and *Levine* advocated standardization of endodontic instruments
- *1959*: *Ingle* and *Levine* introduced standardized gutta-percha cones for obturation of root canal

### Classification of Gutta-Percha

1. *Based on types of phases*:
   - Alpha
   - Beta
   - Gamma
2. *Based on the sizes*:
   - Standardized gutta-percha
   - Nonstandardized gutta-percha
3. *Based on degree of taper*: 0.02, 0.04 and 0.06
4. *Based on the method of use*:
   - Thermoplasticized gutta-percha
   - Chemically softened gutta-percha
   - Cold gutta-percha
5. *Based on the type of calibration*:
   - Calibrated gutta-percha
   - Noncalibrated gutta-percha
6. *Based on incorporation of medicament*:
   - Medicated gutta-percha
   - Nonmedicated gutta-percha.

### Composition

It consists of 25% of organic component (gutta-percha, waxes and resins) and 75% of inorganic component (zinc-oxide and metal sulfates).

- *Gutta-percha*: 19–22%—acts as matrix
- *Zinc-oxide*: 59–75%—filler.

In small amounts:

- *Metal sulfates*: 1–18%—gives radiopacity
- *Waxes*: 1–4%—provides plasticity
- Resins
- Coloring agents
- Antioxidants.

### Supplied As

- Gutta-percha cones or pellets of various dimensions which are sterilized by irradiation by the manufacturer. They can be available in both standardized and nonstandardized sizes (**Fig. 27.15**)

- The nonstandardized forms can be of three types—(1) medium, (2) medium-fine, or (3) fine-fine.
- Thermoplasticized gutta-percha available as:
  - Solid core system
  - Injectable system.
  For example, Obtura III **(Fig. 27.16)**, Calamus, Ultrafil 3D
- Gutta-percha can also be medicated with iodoform, chlorhexidine, calcium hydroxide or tetracycline.

## Uses

- As obturating material **(Fig. 27.17)**
- For tracing a sinus tract
- For thermal pulp testing
- As temporary stopping in inlay cavity.

*Use of gutta-percha in obturation of root canals:*
- Gutta-percha alone cannot be used as to provide hermetic seal to a root canal as it does not have any adhesive quality
- It requires sealer to provide a seal of the canal-gutta-percha interface **(Fig. 27.18)**
- It is applied to the root canal with some condensation pressure
- Lateral condensation force is applied with the help of spreaders or vertical condensation force is applied with the help of plugger
- Pluggers are long, slightly tapered, metallic instruments with flattened or blunt tips which are designed to compact gutta-percha and sealer vertically
- Both these methods are used to provide better adaptation of the gutta-percha into the root canals.

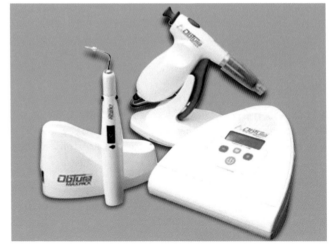

**Fig. 27.16:** Obtura III system.

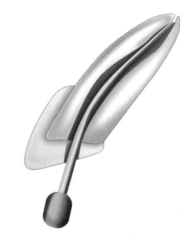

**Fig. 27.17:** Gutta-percha points used for obturation of root canal.

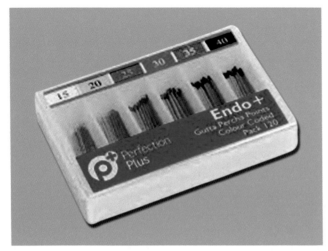

**Fig. 27.15:** Gutta-percha cones supplied in various sizes.

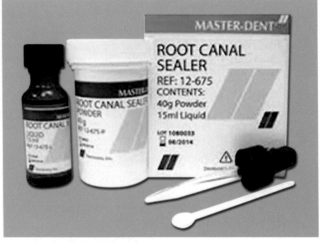

**Fig. 27.18:** Root canal sealer.

## Storage

Prolonged storage of gutta-percha makes them brittle especially when exposed to raised temperature, air and direct light. This is because of the conversion of cones from beta phase to naturally occurring alpha phase due to oxidation of the cones. Refrigeration is advised if stored for long duration. Long-term stored cones can be rejuvenated by immersing in hot water at 55°C for approximately 1–2 seconds and then immediately placed in cold water. This process converts the cones to usable beta phase.

### Disinfection of Gutta-percha Cones

The gutta-percha cones are disinfected by immersing in 5.25% sodium hypochlorite solution for 1 minute. Just before using them for obturation they are immersed in 60% ethyl alcohol to remove the crystallized sodium hypochlorite.

## Removal of Gutta-percha

Gutta-percha is usually removed during retreatment or postspace preparation. This is accomplished using rotary Ni-Ti files, using solvents such as chloroform or using heated instrument. Other solvents used are xylene, halothane, orange wood oil and rectified turpentine oil.

*Advantages:*
- Are inert and biocompatible
- Are thermoplastic and when heated can take any shape
- Can be easily removed
- Can be disinfected.

*Disadvantages:*
- Thermoplastic or chemically softened gutta-percha shrinks and can lead to microleakage

- Lack adhesiveness
- Lacks rigidity.

## RESILON

- This is recently introduced thermoplastic synthetic polymer which is based on principle of chemical bonding of the root canal filling material to the canal wall **(Fig. 27.19)**
- This polymer is based on polymers of polyester containing bioactive glass and radiopaque fillers
- It shows great potential for improving both the apical and the coronal seal of the canal.

### Composition

- *Filler 70%*: Calcium hydroxide, barium sulfate, barium glass and silica
- *Sealant*: Epiphany root canal sealant which is a dual cure dentin resin composite sealer.

### Supplied As

Master cones and accessory cones similar to gutta-percha points **(Fig. 27.20)**. They are also available as pellets which are used in backfilling with thermoplastic techniques.

### Procedure

- The root canal surface is etched and primed to achieve chemical bond as in other dentin bonding agents
- The dentin surface is rinsed with 17% EDTA to remove the smear layer
- Surface is dried but not desiccated and epiphany primer is applied. This primer is self-etching
- Then root canal sealer is applied in the canal.

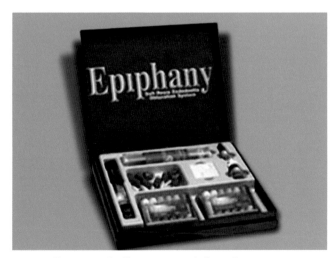

**Fig. 27.19:** Resilon—root canal obturating system.

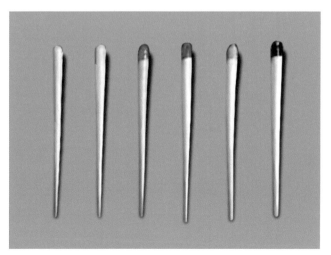

**Fig. 27.20:** Color-coded Resilon points.

- Resilon core is then filled into the canal. Resilon-Epiphany system forms Monoblock
- After root canal is obturated, it is light cured for 40 seconds. The coronal 2 mm of the canal is cured with this and the remaining canal is self-cured in 15–30 minutes
- If the root canal filling needs to be removed, it can be easily softened and dissolved by chloroform.

## RETROGRADE FILLING MATERIAL

- The rationale behind retrograde filling is to hermetically seal the canal such that bacteria or their toxins do not percolate from root canal space into the periradicular tissues
- It is done when surgical root canal therapy is done
- This type of procedure is indicated when nonsurgical method fails or cannot be performed. In this method, the root apex of the tooth is resected and a retrograde filling is done **(Fig. 27.21)**
- Commonly used retrograde filling materials include—amalgam, MTA and reinforced zinc-oxide eugenol.

### Amalgam

- Traditionally, this was one of the most commonly used retrograde filling materials
- It provided acceptable apical seal and functioned well in the periapical environment
- But effects of mercury in periapical tissues, leakage of amalgam retrofils and concern of corrosion products lead to the search of alternative retrograde filling material.

### Reinforced Zinc-oxide Eugenol

- Reinforced zinc-oxide eugenol materials such as IRM and Super EBA are used.

- It has adequate strength and showed higher success rate than amalgam
- Biocompatibility of freshly set material is questionable because of the presence of eugenol
- Although studies have suggested acceptable long-term biocompatibility for both these materials.

### Mineral Trioxide Aggregate (**Fig. 27.22**)

- Mineral trioxide aggregate is popularly used as retrograde filling material
- This material was developed in 1995 at Loma Linda University by Dr Torabinejad and Dr Dean White
- It has composition similar to Portland cement. This material initially was gray in color later in the year 2002 white MTA (Pro Root) was developed.

#### Composition

- *Powder*: Contains 75% of Portland cement
    - Tricalcium silicate: 45–75%
    - Dicalcium silicate: 7–32%
    - Tricalcium aluminate: 0–13%
    - Bismuth or tantalum oxide: 20–35%
    - Calcium sulfate dihydrate: 2–10%
    - Tetracalcium aluminoferrite: 0–18%.
- *Liquid*: Viscous aqueous solution of water soluble polymer.

#### Setting Reaction

When MTA powder is mixed with sterile water in the ratio of 3:1 (powder:liquid). It behaves as hydraulic cement which when mixed with water gradually or instantly sets in air or water. The set material contains hydrated compound which increases in strength with time. Initial setting occurs in 3–4 hours and with time further maturation occurs. The set

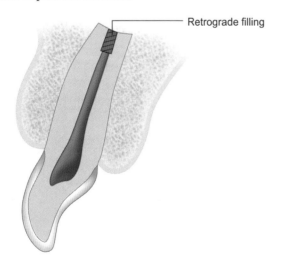

**Fig. 27.21:** Retrograde filling done after resecting the apical root portion.

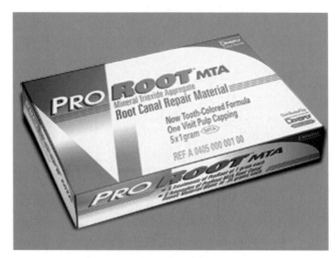

**Fig. 27.22:** Mineral trioxide aggregate.

cement contains interlocking cubic and needle-like crystals which forms the basic framework. The spaces between the cubic crystals are filled by needle-like crystals.

### Properties

- It sets in the presence of moisture and hardening time of 2 hours 45 minutes to 4 hours
- It is a biocompatible material with excellent sealing ability and dentinogenic activity
- Mineral trioxide aggregate showed significantly less leakage than amalgam, Super EBA (modified ZnOE cement) or IBM (intermediate restorative material). Studies have also shown less marginal gap and better adaptation in the root end than the amalgam, Super EBA and IRM
- Compressive strength after 2 hours is 40 MPa and increases up to 68 MPa after 21 days
- Setting expansion is less than 0.1%
- During setting MTA slightly expands resulting in better adaptation to the cavity walls showing better sealing properties
- Antibacterial and antifungal properties. MTA forms calcium hydroxide which has high alkaline pH and has good antibacterial properties
- Biocompatible as it nonmutagenic or carcinogenic
- It does not react with any other restorative material
- It is capable of producing cementum by activating cementoblasts
- It has ability to induce formation of dentin bridges as calcium hydroxide paste
- Mineral trioxide aggregate should be stored in dry place and should be tightly closed after use
- It can also be used to repair perforations, as direct pulp capping agent, to layer pulp stumps for apexogenesis and to close open apices in apexification.

### Indications

- Apexification
- Root canal filling
- Perforation repair
- Internal bleaching
- Pulpotomy, pulp capping agent
- Resorption repair.

### Advantages

- Provides good biologic seal
- Induces osteogenesis—high pH induces hard tissue formation
- Superior sealing ability to most of the available retrograde materials

- Cementoinductive and cementoconductive properties
- Hydrophilic—requires moisture to set
- Radiopacity
- Compressive strength increases as it matures. Its strength is 40 MPa at 24 hours and 67.3 MPa after 21 days
- Good adaptation of MTA to the tooth margins because of setting expansion.

### Disadvantages

- Initially difficult to manipulate when soft
- Has long setting time
- Can lead to discoloration due to the presence of manganese and iron
- Cost is high
- Difficult to remove after the material completely sets
- No known solvent material.

## CALCIUM ENRICHED MIXTURE

Calcium enriched mixture (CEM) is water based cement which primarily consists of calcium oxide introduced in 2006. CEM cement releases both calcium and phosphorous ions resulting in the formation of hydroxyapatite on the surface. It shows antibacterial properties similar to calcium hydroxide and greater than MTA. Its sealing ability is comparable to MTA. It induces hard tissue formation over the resected root end. Moreover, it is economical and it exhibit surface properties similar to the surrounding dentin.

## DIAKET

Diaket is a polyvinyl resin—reinforced chelate which is formed between zinc oxide and diketone. It is used as root canal sealer and retrograde filling material. When this material is mixed in ratio of two to three parts of powder to one part of liquid it produces firm consistency mixture having adequate working time (4 minutes 30 seconds). It is radiopaque and has sealing ability is greater than amalgam, glass ionomer, EBA cement and intermediate restorative material.

## POLYMETHYLMETHACRYLATE BONE CEMENT

Recently introduced material which shows promise to be used as retrograde filling material. PMMA bone cement is supplied in the form of powder and liquid. It shows excellent interlocking between the soft and the hard tissues of the bone. However, its drawbacks are that methyl methacrylate (MMA) monomer may show toxicity and the heat released during polymerization may harm the adjacent tissues.

# TEST YOURSELF

## Essay Questions

1. Classify root canal irrigants. Write in detail about sodium hypochlorite.
2. Enumerate various intracanal medicaments. Write briefly about each.
3. Discuss the importance of using calcium hydroxide in endodontic treatment.
4. Classify various root canal sealer. Write briefly about any two of them.
5. Classify various obturating materials. Discuss in detail use of gutta-percha as ideal obturating material.
6. Describe the use of mineral trioxide aggregate (MTA) as retrograde filling material.

## Short Notes

1. Grossmann sealer.
2. EDTA.
3. MTAD.
4. Resilon.
5. Chlorhexidine.

## Multiple Choice Questions

1. Gutta-percha is sterilized by:
   A. Glass bead sterilizer
   B. Sodium hypochlorite solution 55%
   C. Moist heat
   D. Dry heat.
2. Most commonly used solution for root canal irrigant is:
   A. EDTA
   B. Sodium hypochlorite
   C. Hydrogen peroxide
   D. Saline solution
3. Sodium hypochlorite acts:
   A. As lubricant during instrumentation
   B. By dissolving organic pulp remnants
   C. As bleaching and antiseptic agent
   D. All of the above
4. Gutta-percha can be softened by:
   A. Alcohol and chloroform
   B. Xylene and chloroform
   C. Eugenol and chloroform
   D. Ethyl chloride and eugenol
5. Formocresol produces tissue fixation and:
   A. Coagulative necrosis
   B. Liquefaction necrosis
   C. Caseous necrosis
   D. Does not produce necrosis

6. Concentration of EDTA utilized during biomechanical preparation is:
   A. 20% at pH 7.4
   B. 15% at pH 5
   C. 15% at pH 7.3
   D. 25% at pH 7.4
7. Gutta-percha cones should not be used for root canal filling of:
   A. Primary teeth
   B. Permanent last molars
   C. Teeth with wide root canals
   D. Teeth with curved roots
8. Gutta-percha when used as a root canal filler as:
   A. Seals dentinal tubules
   B. Prevents staining of the tooth
   C. Is inert and only serves to fill the space left vacant by the pulp
   D. It interacts with periapical tissues and assists in healing
9. Effective action of irrigating solution depends on:
   A. Chelating action
   B. Volume of the solution
   C. Aspiration of the solution
   D. Antimicrobial action
10. Filling of choice for primary root canals:
    A. ZOE
    B. Calcium hydroxide
    C. Gutta-percha
    D. Chlorpercha
11. Discoloration of endodontically treated tooth results from:
    A. Improper debridement
    B. Sealer cement left in pulp chamber
    C. Obturating material
    D. All of the above

---

## ANSWERS

| 1. B | 2. B | 3. D | 4. B |
|------|------|------|------|
| 5. A | 6. C | 7. A | 8. C |
| 9. B | 10. A | 11. D | |

---

## BIBLIOGRAPHY

1. Cleggs MS, Vertucci FJ, Walker C, et al. The effect of exposure to irrigant solutions on apical dentin biofilms in vitro. J Endod. 2006;32:434-7.
2. Dorn SO, Gartner AH. Retrograde filling materials: a retrospective success-failure study of amalgam, EBA, and IRM. J Endod. 1990;16:391-3.

3. Friedman CE, Sandrik JL, Heuer MA, et al. Composition and physical properties of gutta-percha endodontic filling materials. J Endod. 1977;3:304-8.

4. Gatewood RS. Endodontic materials. Dent Clin N Am. 2007;51:695-712.

5. Goodman A, Schilder H, Aldrich W. The thermomechanical properties of gutta-percha II. The history and chemistry of gutta-percha. Oral Surg Oral Med Oral Pathol. 1974;37:954-61.

6. Grossman L. Endodontic practice, 11th edition. Philadelphia: Lea and Feebiger; 1988. pp. 255.

7. Gutman JL, Milas VB. History. In: Cohen S, Burns RC (Eds). Pathways of the Pulp, 3rd edition. St. Louis (MO): The CV Mosby Company; 1984. pp. 823-42.

8. Gutmann JL, Witherspoon DE. Obturation of the cleaned and shaped root canal system. In: Cohen S, Burns RC (Eds). Pathways of the Pulp, 8th edition. St. Louis: Mosby; 2002.

9. Spangberg I. Instruments, materials and devices. In: Cohen S, Burns RC (Eds). Pathways of Pulp, 8th edition. St. Louis: Mosby; 2002. pp.545-6.

10. Torabinejad M, Chivian N. Clinical applications of mineral trioxide aggregate. J Endod. 1999;25:197-205.

11. Torabinejad M, Cho Y, Khademi AA, et al. S. The effect of various concentrations of sodium hypochlorite on the ability of MTAD to remove the smear layer. J Endod. 2003;29:233-9.

12. Torabinejad M, Falah RA, Kettering JD, et al. Bacterial leakage of mineral trioxide aggregate as a root-end filling material. J Endod. 1995;21:109-12.

13. Torabinejad M, Khademi AA, Babagoli J, Cho Y, Johnson WB, Bozhilov K, et al. A new solution for removal of the smear layer. J Endod. 2003;29:170-5.

14. Torabinejad M, Watson TF, Pitt Ford TR. Sealing ability of a mineral trioxide aggregate when used as a root end filling material. J Endod. 1993;19:591-5.

15. Tronstad L, Barnett F, Flax M. Solubility and biocompatibility of calcium hydroxide containing root canal sealers. Endod Dent Traumatol. 1988;4:155.

16. Wadachi R, Araki K, Suda H. Effect of calcium hydroxide on the dissolution of soft tissue on the root canal wall. J Endod. 1998;24:326-30.

17. Zmener O, Dominquez FV. Tissue response to a glass ionomer used as an endodontic cement. Oral Surg Oral Med Oral Pathol. 1983;56:198-205.

# Preventive and Bleaching Materials

*'No steam or gas drives anything until it is confined. No Niagara is ever turned into light and power until it is tunneled. No life ever grows until it is focussed, dedicated and disciplined.'*

—*Harry Emerson Fosdick*

## INTRODUCTION

The concept of prevention has changed since the time of GV Black's principle—"extension for prevention". The current concept is based on complete elimination of both primary and secondary caries as well as reducing minimum tooth structure for a given restoration. It is well documented that fluoridation helps in prevention of dental caries by demineralization of tooth enamel. This chapter will focus on various preventive dental materials which includes fluoride containing resins, fluoride-releasing resins, pit and fissure sealants, glass ionomers, other fluoridated agents and mouth guards. It also includes various tooth bleaching materials commonly used in dentistry.

## DENTAL PLAQUE

*Dental plaque is defined as the soft deposits that form the biofilms adhering to the tooth surface or other hard surfaces in the oral cavity, including removable and fixed restorations.*

Dental plaque is primarily composed of microorganisms. It is observed that more than 325 different species microorganism are found in plaque. Prevention of dental plaque is one of the most important needs to control oral disease in general population.

Measures for plaque control are using antiplaque agents which are in form of mechanical aids and chemical form.

## ANTIPLAQUE AGENTS

ADA specification No. 68.

### Classification of Dental Plaque Control Aids

**Mechanical Plaque Control Aids**
- *Toothbrushes*:
  - Manual toothbrush
  - Electric/powered toothbrush.
- Tooth paste
- *Interdental cleaning aids*:
  - Dental floss
  - Wooden tips
  - Interdental brushes—proxabrush, unitufted brush and miniature bottle brush.
- *Oral irrigation devices*: Waterpik.

**Chemical Plaque Control Agents**
- *Agents directed toward supragingival plaque control*:
  - Enzymes
  - *Antiseptics*:
    - Bisbiguanide antiseptics
    - Quaternary ammonium compound
    - Phenolic compounds
    - Other antiseptics
    - Metal ions
    - Oxygenating solutions
    - Fluorides.

- *Agents used for subgingival plaque control:*
  - Keyes technique
  - Antiseptics
- Plaque disclosing agents.

# BISBIGUANIDE ANTISEPTICS

## Chlorhexidine

Chlorhexidine (CHX) is an effective antimicrobial agent which was first developed by Imperial Chemical Industries in UK in 1940s. It was only in 1954 that it was marketed as an antiseptic to be used for skin wounds. Initially, it was used in dentistry for presurgical disinfection of the mouth and later it was used as antiplaque agent **(Fig. 28.1)**.

### Uses

- As adjunct to oral hygiene maintenance
- During professional prophylaxis
- In patients with jaw fixation
- In physically and mentally handicapped patients.

### Mechanism of Action

Chlorhexidine binds to the oral mucosa through the mucinous layer coating on it and is retained in the oral cavity for hours. It adsorbs to the carboxyl group of the mucosal surface and it gradually displaces calcium from the sulfate group of the plaque thereby disrupting its structure.

### Properties

- *High substantivity*: Ability of the substance to be retained and bind to the soft and hard tissues
- Potent antibacterial agent
- Antiplaque agent.

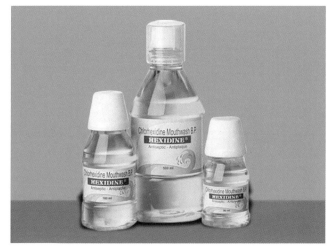

**Fig. 28.1:** Chlorhexidine mouthwash.

### Supplied As

- *Mouth rinse*: Used in concentration of 0.2–0.12%. Studies reveal when mouth rinse with concentration of 0.2% and 0.12% are used in equal doses there is no significant difference in their efficacy
- *Gels*: 0.1% CHX gels
- Sprays: Available in 0.1% and 0.2%.

### Side Effects

- Brown staining of teeth with long-term use
- Bitter taste
- Burning sensation of the mucosa
- Discoloration of teeth, tongue and restoration
- Dry mouth
- Epithelial desquamation.

# DEMINERALIZATION AND REMINERALIZATION CYCLE (FIG. 28.2)

Tooth enamel is a unique mineralized substance, which continuously undergoes demineralization and remineralization. It is the equilibrium between the two processes which keep the teeth strong and healthy. Demineralization occurs when the pH of the saliva drops below 5.5 (critical pH) and the mineral ions (calcium and phosphate ions) are released from the tooth enamel into the plaque and saliva. The tooth enamel containing apatite crystals is dissolved by organic acids (lactic and acetic) which is produced by the cellular action of the plaque bacteria on the dietary carbohydrates.

Remineralization occurs when the pH of the saliva increases resulting in deposition of calcium, phosphate and fluoride ions from the saliva and the plaque. It forms more acid resistant fluorapatite crystals. These crystals are larger in size and provides more favorable surface to volume ratio. Thus these larger apatite crystals are more resistant to enamel breakdown by the acid attack.

## Types of Remineralization Agents

- Traditional agents, e.g. fluorides
- Contemporary agents, e.g. casein phosphopeptide-amorphous calcium phosphate (CPP-ACP) complex.

## Ideal Requirements for Remineralization Agents

- Should be capable of diffusing into the subsurface layer of enamel
- Should increase remineralization potential of saliva
- Should resists calculus formation
- Should be capable of use in acidic environment'
- Should not deliver excess calcium to the tooth surface.

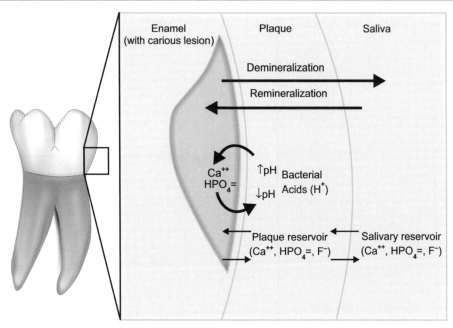

**Fig. 28.2:** Demineralization and remineralization cycle.

## FLUORIDE

Fluoride is a naturally occurring mineral which can be found in well water, food which has absorbed fluoride, in various dental products, etc. The accepted optimal level of fluoride in drinking water ranges between 0.7 and 1 parts per million (ppm). Excessive consumption of fluoride can lead to *fluorosis*. The severity of fluorosis can vary from small white spots or bands to mottled enamel with severe pitting **(Fig. 28.3)**.

Recent studies have shown that topical application of fluoride provide greatest anticariogenic benefits. Through this application fluoride present in the saliva surrounding the tooth structure is incorporated into the surface of enamel crystals during remineralization to form *fluorapatite*. This makes the tooth more resistant to acids produced by cariogenic bacteria. Fluoride has been shown to interfere with the essential enzyme activity of the bacteria and cause their death **(Fig. 28.4)**.

All fluoride products should be used as directed and should be kept away from small children for safety purposes. If a child consumes excessive fluoride than prescribed, then vomiting should be induced and milk containing magnesia should be given in order to tie-up fluoride. Cow's milk can also be given to slow the absorption of fluoride in the stomach.

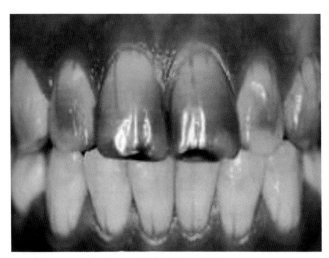

**Fig. 28.3:** Fluorosis.

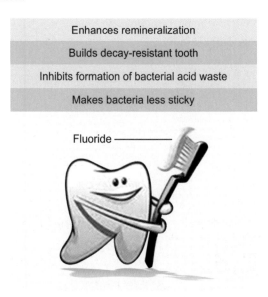

**Fig. 28.4:** Functions of fluoride.

**Table 28.1:** Comparison of various modes of delivery of fluorides.

| Modes of delivery | Fluoride product | Fluoride content (ppm) | Frequency of use | Precautions | Common brands |
|---|---|---|---|---|---|
| In-office treatment | 1.23% APF gel | 12,300 | Every 6 months | GIT upset, vomiting if swallowed, may etch esthetic restorations, not used in children below 3 years | Nupro APF gel (Dentsply), Minute gel (Oral B), Fluoridex foam (discuss dental) |
| | 2% NaF | 9,000 | Every 6 months | GIT upset, vomiting on swallowing, not used for children below 3 years | Neutra-foam (Oral B), NuproNeutral (Dentsply), Denticare Topical Foam (Medicom) |
| Home use | 1.1% NaF gel or toothpaste | 5000 | Daily | Not used for children below 6 years | Prevident (Colgate), NeutraCare (Oral B) |
| | 0.4% SnF2 gel | 900 | Daily | Not used for children below 6 years, may cause tooth staining | Gel-Kam (Colgate), Stop (Oral B), Perio Plus (Discus dental), Denticare gel (Medicom) |
| | 0.2% NaF rinse | 900 | Weekly | Not used for children below 6 years | Fluorinse (Oral B), Prevident Dental rinse (Colgate) |
| Over the counter home use | 0.05% NaF rinse | 250 | Daily | Not used for children below 6 years | Fluorigard (Colgate), ACT (Johnson and Johnson) |
| | 0.24% NaF toothpaste | 1,100 | Daily | Not used for children below 6 years | Various brands |
| | 0.8% MFP toothpaste | 1,100 | Daily | Use pea sized amount for children below 6 years | Various brands |

*Abbreviation*: GIT, gastrointestinal tract

## Modes of Delivery (**Table 28.1**)

*Systemic route (ingested fluoride)*: Fluoride can be ingested through drinking water where fluoride may be present naturally or supplied. A part of systemically ingested fluoride is available in the oral cavity in form of saliva (**Fig. 28.5**).

*Topical route (in-office fluoride application):* Patients with high caries index or children with newly erupted permanent teeth are indicated for professional application of fluorides. Topical fluorides gels or foam are applied by means of disposable trays for a period of 1–4 minutes. Caries reduction of 20–26% is seen in patients when topical fluorides are applied for one to two times per year. Acidulated phosphate fluoride (APF) is often used for children as it contains 12,300 ppm fluoride and has good enamel uptake. Topical fluoride commonly recommended for adults is 2% neutral sodium fluoride which contains 9,000 ppm of fluoride. Unlike APF gels it does not etch porcelain or composite restorations.

**CLINICAL SIGNIFICANCE**

Fluoride varnishes in form of 5% sodium fluoride are directly applied to the surface of the teeth. These varnishes are useful for treatment of early dental caries (**Fig. 28.6**).

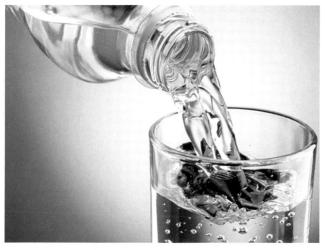

**Fig. 28.5:** Water fluoridation.

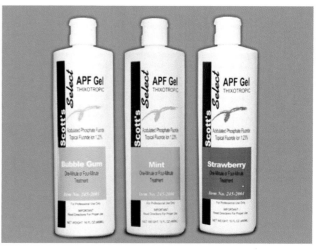

**Fig. 28.6:** APF gels used for in-office fluoride applications.

*Self-applied topical gels:* Such application is recommended for patients who are at moderately to high risk of dental caries. Orthodontic patients or xerostomic patients are indicated for self-applied fluoride gels. These gels are available as 1.1% neutral sodium fluoride and 0.4% stannous fluoride. Although stannous fluoride causes staining of the surface of teeth and delivers less fluoride to the teeth. Mode of delivery of self-applied gels are either through brushing or by using custom tray.

### CLINICAL SIGNIFICANCE

The application through custom tray is more effective than brushing as saliva dilutes the gel on application **(Fig. 28.7)**.

*Over-the-counter fluoride rinses:* Daily fluoride rinses have shown to reduce caries incidence by 28%. Fluoride rinses are available as 0.05% of sodium fluoride. The patient is instructed to rinse for 20–30 seconds, thereafter spit the excess and not eat or drink for at least 30 minutes. Fluoride rinses are recommended just before the bedtime as residual fluoride can remain in saliva during sleep.

*Fluoride containing toothpaste:* Toothpastes containing sodium monofluorophosphate (MFP) and sodium fluoride are shown to be more effective and stable chemically than stannous fluoride. The fluoride content of most toothpastes are 1,000 ppm.

### CLINICAL SIGNIFICANCE

*Fluoride containing prophylaxis paste:* Fluoride is added to the prophylaxis paste in order to compensate for the lost fluoride during polishing. Since these pastes contain pumice as the abrasive agent, some amount of fluoride is removed during stain removal.

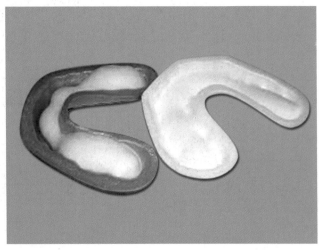

**Fig. 28.7:** Fluoride foams are applied using custom trays.

## Casein Phosphopeptide-Amorphous Calcium Phosphate

Casein phosphopeptide-amorphous calcium phosphate is a milk protein which aids in remineralization of the teeth and helps in prevention of caries. This complex protein was first developed by E Reynolds and coworkers at the University of Melbourne. A specific phosphoprotein is derived from bovine milk and is combined with the nanoparticles of amorphous calcium phosphate. The availability of calcium and phosphate bound by casein phosphopeptide (CPP) increases when the pH reduces (acidic).

### Mechanism of Action

Casein phosphopeptide forms nanoclusters with amorphous calcium phosphate producing a pool of calcium and phosphate ions which maintain super saturation of these ions in saliva. By buffering action the levels of calcium and phosphate ions in the plaque is increased thereby reducing the process of demineralization and increasing remineralization.

### Indications

- Used to remineralize early carious lesions
- Used to counteract the action of acids in cases of erosion
- Used to reduce dentin hypersensitivity as it has ability to block dentinal tubules
- Used alone or combination with fluoride can be used as prophylactic agent before bonding orthodontic brackets.

### CLINICAL SIGNIFICANCE

When used with glass ionomer cement (GIC), it increases the microtensile bond strength by the incorporation of CPP-ACP nanoparticles in the cross-linked matrix (*Mazzaoui* et al. 2003).

### Supplied As

- Tooth cream (GC Tooth Mousse™)
- Chewing Gum (Recaldent Gum, Trident White) **(Fig. 28.8)**
- Mouth rinses
- Tooth pastes
- Lozenges
- Energy drinks
- Sprays.

## Evidence of Preventive Role of CPP-ACP in Dental Caries

*Christos and George 2007* found in the in vitro study on human teeth that CPP-ACP agent when present reduces demineralization and increases remineralization. They used

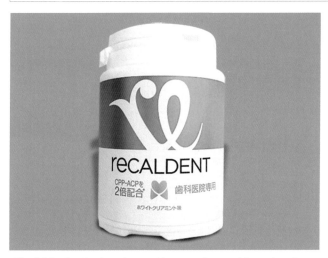

**Fig. 28.8:** Casein phosphopeptide-amorphous calcium phosphate (CPP-ACP) chewing gum.

multiple internal reflection—Fourier transform infrared spectroscopy for their analysis.

### CPP-ACFP (GC Tooth Mousse Plus)

Casein phosphopeptide has the ability to bind with fluoride apart from calcium phosphate. There is a synergistic effect when CPP-ACP complex binds with fluoride. CPP-ACFP (fluoride containing) has higher remineralization effect than CPP-ACP used alone.

CPP-ACFP is formed by adding 900 ppm of 0.2% sodium fluoride. On remineralization, the majority of mineral formed is fluorapatite which is highly acid resistant to acid attack as compared to hydroxyapatite. CPP has ability to adhere to 25 calcium ions, 15 phosphate ions and 5 fluoride ions per molecule. In this way, CPP can act as an efficient delivery system for fluoride. Studies show that CPP-ACFP provided better remineralization than CPP-ACP used alone. **(Fig. 28.9).**

## BETA TRICALCIUM PHOSPHATE

Tricalcium phosphate exists in two forms—(1) alpha and (2) beta. The beta form of tricalcium phosphate is more stable and less soluble than the alpha form. It is capable of providing increased availability of calcium ions. At the time of manufacturing process a protective barrier is formed around the calcium ions to allow it to coexist with fluoride ions. When the toothpaste comes in contact with the saliva on brushing, this barrier breaks releasing calcium, phosphate and fluoride ions. The tooth absorbs these ions and increases the remineralization process. However, the effect of remineralization cannot be compared to CPP-ACP or fluoride as the level of evidence is still in preliminary stage **(Fig. 28.10)**.

## PIT AND FISSURE SEALANTS

*Pits and fissures* (ADA specification no. 39, ISO specification no. 6874:2005) are usually deep, narrow channels in the enamel surface that can extend close to the dentinoenamel junction. They have tendency of collecting food debris and bacteria and have high susceptibility to dental caries. Pit and fissure sealants provide a conservative method of protecting pits and fissures by preventing bacteria and food debris from entering them.

*Pit and fissure sealants* are unfilled or lightly filled resins which are used to seal the noncarious pits and fissures of deciduous and permanent teeth.

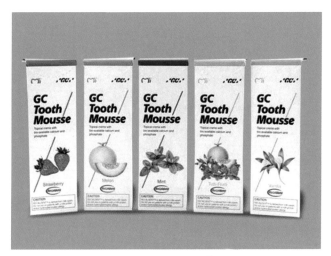

**Fig. 28.9:** CPP-ACFP (GC Tooth Mousse).

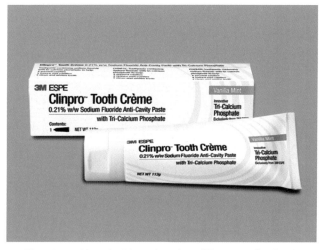

**Fig. 28.10:** Beta-tricalcium phosphate (Clinpro tooth crème).

## Rationale

It is used to prevent dental caries in pits and fissures which are susceptible for carious lesions more often in deciduous and young permanent teeth **(Fig. 28.11)**.

## Indications

- Deep pits and fissures in deciduous molars and permanent molars and premolars
- Deep pits in maxillary central and lateral incisors.

## Composition

Pit and fissure sealants are similar to composite resins chemically. They are resin which is usually composed of either bisphenol A-glycidyl methacrylate (bis-GMA) or urethane dimethacrylate (UDMA).

Polymerization can occur by chemical reaction (chemical/self-cure) or by light activation (light cure). Currently most of the available pit and fissure sealants are light cure. Some of the filler particles used in sealants are radiopaque which allow them to be seen in radiographs. Polymerization results in formation of highly cross-linked polymer networks.

Glass ionomer restorative material containing fluorides have also been used as pit and fissure sealants. Their major drawback was faster wearing and chipping with time. However, in order to achieve optimum retention and fluoride release, filled resin sealants containing fluorides are developed. In these sealants, fluoride is released at very fast rate in the first week after placement and thereafter it becomes constant.

## Supplied As

Light cure materials are supplied as single paste system whereas self-cure are supplied as two paste system (initiator and accelerator) **(Fig. 28.12)**.

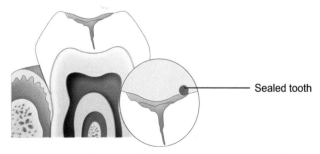

**Fig. 28.11:** Pit and fissure sealants used to seal deep pits and fissures.

## Working Time and Setting Time

- For self-cure sealants—setting time is 2 minutes from start of mixing of both the pastes. Working time is 90 seconds
- For light cure sealants—40 seconds of light curing is needed on each tooth to polymerize. The light tip should be placed as close to the resin as possible to maximize light intensity.

## Manipulation (Figs 28.13A to F)

- Tooth surface is cleaned with pumice to remove any surface debris. Wash and dry
- Isolate the tooth (e.g. cotton rolls and rubber dam)
- The cleaned surface is microscopically roughened by acid etching technique (37% phosphoric acid) for 30–60 seconds
- After etching, the surface is rinsed and air dried
- The tooth is thoroughly isolated
- Dispense sealant in a tray. In case of self-cure mix for 15–20 seconds
- Sealant is applied to the etched surface
- In case of light cure sealant, cure for 40 seconds with the light source
- Sealant is inspected for complete coverage
- Occlusion is checked and excessive sealant is removed
- The restoration is finally finished and polished.

## *Wear Resistance*

Pit and fissure sealants have a tendency to wear against opposing occlusion. The sealants containing no organic filler particles will wear faster than those containing filler particles.

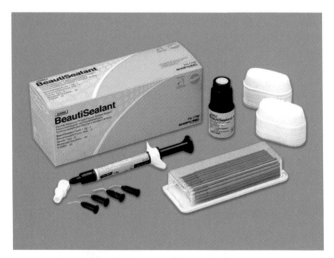

**Fig. 28.12:** Pit and fissure sealant.

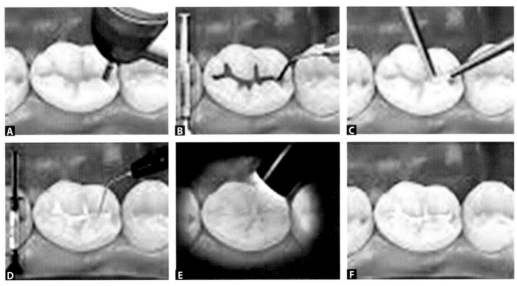

**Figs. 28.13A to F:** Steps in application of pit and fissure sealants.

## PREVENTIVE RESIN RESTORATIONS

The preventive resin restorations (PRR) are composite resins which are placed after minimal excavation where there is incipient lesion in the pits or fissures of the tooth. The deep pit or fissure is first filled with glass ionomer and then the occlusal surface is filled with the sealant. These restorations are commonly done in premolars and molars. PRR are found to be much more conservative than amalgam restorations where pits and fissures are prepared and included in the cavity design **(Fig. 28.14)**.

## DESENSITIZING AGENTS

Dental sensitivity to hot, cold or sweet food is one of the most common complain given by the patient visiting a dentist. The materials which are professionally applied or available over-the-counter (OTC) are used to reduce or eliminate sensitivity are called as *desensitizing agents*.

### Causes of Sensitivity

According to the hydrodynamic theory of dentin sensitivity, the tooth is said to be sensitive when dentinal tubules are exposed to the oral cavity. When stimulus such as cold or hot food causes the dentinal fluid to move, it deforms the sensitive nerve endings located at the junction of pulp and dentin causing acute, sharp pain **(Fig. 28.15)**.

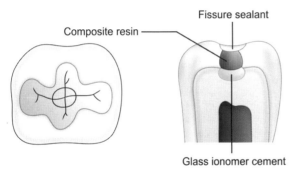

**Fig. 28.14:** Preventive resin restoration.

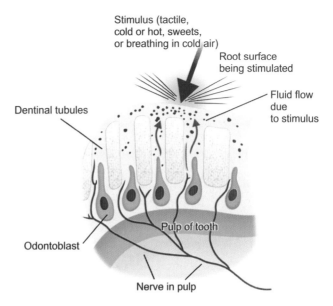

**Fig. 28.15:** Hydrodynamic theory to explain teeth sensitivity.

*The common causes of tooth sensitivity are as:*
- Root caries
- Cervical abrasion due to faulty brushing
- Erosion by acids
- Abfraction associated with bruxism
- Scaling and root planning
- Leakage of restoration on the root
- Cracked tooth.

### Mechanism of Action

Most of the desensitizing agents act by blocking or plugging the open dentinal tubules to reduce sensitivity. The tubules can be blocked chemically or mechanically depending on the type of agents used. Some agents such as potassium nitrate are used in toothpastes and act by passing through the dentinal tubules to the pulp and soothing the pulp. Some agents are used at the time of placement of restoration or after scaling and root planning. It is seen after bleaching procedure the teeth become sensitive. Some manufacturers have added chemicals such as potassium nitrate or fluoride to reduce sensitivity during bleaching **(Fig. 28.16)**.

### Types of Desensitizing Agents

On the basis of uses, the desensitizing agents can be classified as **(Table 28.2)**:
- Fluoride varnishes and gels

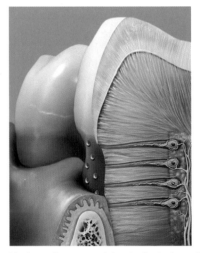

**Fig. 28.16:** Blocking the exposed dentinal tubules reduces tooth sensitivity.

- Toothpastes
- Inorganic salt solutions
- Resin primers and bonding agents.

## MOUTH GUARDS AND SPLINTS

*Mouth guards or mouth protectors* (ADA specification no. 99) are routinely used to protect the dentition from direct or indirect trauma. The Center for Disease Control and

| **Table 28.2:** Various desensitizing agents. | | | |
|---|---|---|---|
| Types of desensitizing agent **(Figs. 28.17A to D)** | Common brand | Active ingredient | Duration of effectiveness |
| Toothpastes | • Sensodyne (Block Drug)<br>• Sensodyne F (Block Drug)<br>• Colgate Sensitive (Colgate)<br>• Thermoseal (ICPA) | • Strontium chloride<br>• Potassium nitrate<br>• Potassium nitrate<br>• Potassium nitrate and sodium monofluorophosphate | Several days/ weeks |
| Fluoride gel/varnish | • Gel-Kam (Colgate)<br>• Prevident (Colgate)<br>• Duraphat (Colgate)<br>• Fluor Protector (Vivadent) | • 0.4% stannous fluoride<br>• 1.1% sodium fluoride<br>• Sodium, stannous and strontium fluoride<br>• Fluoride varnish compound | Several days/week |
| Inorganic salts | • Sensodyne Sealant (Block Drug)<br>• Protect (Butler)<br>• Ultra EZ (Ultradent)<br>• Desensitize (DenMat)<br>• Relief (Discus Dental) | • Ferric oxalate<br>• Potassium oxalate<br>• 3% potassium nitrate and 0.11% sodium fluoride<br>• 5% potassium nitrate<br>• Potassium nitrate | Immediate/ repeated applications |
| Resin agents | • Gluma desensitizer (Kulzer)<br>• Gluma comfort bond and desensitizer (Kulzer)<br>• Seal and Protect (Caulk/Dentsply)<br>• All-Bond DS (BISCO)<br>• Clearfil SE bond (J Morita)<br>• Hurriseal (Beutlich)<br>• Microprime (Danville materials) | • 5% Glutaraldehyde, 35% HEMA<br>• GLUMA 4 Meta-resin<br>• Prime and bond NT with 7% filler<br>• NTG-GMA and BPDM primers<br>• Phosphate monomers (self-etching)<br>• HEMA, 0.5% sodium fluoride, benzalkonium chloride<br>• HEMA, 0.5% sodium fluoride, benzalkonium chloride | Immediate effect |

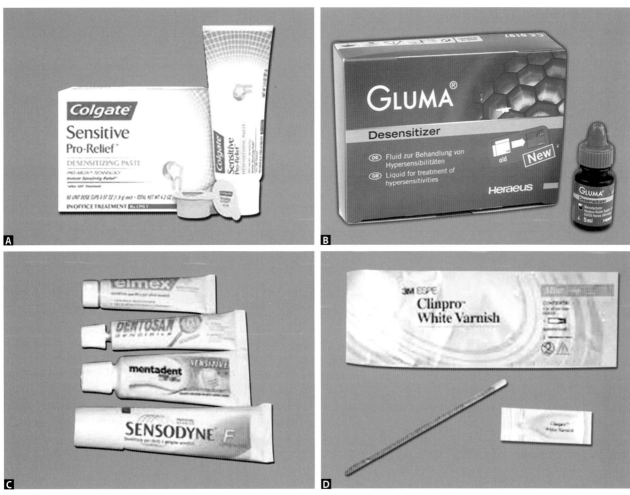

**Figs. 28.17A to D:** Commonly used desensitizing agents.

Prevention mandates the participants to wear mouth guards in all contact or semicontact sports. Most sportsperson wear mouth guards for safety of their dentition from trauma.

Apart from sports dentist recommend mouth guards in patient with parafunctional habits such as bruxism. These mouth guards are referred to as *night guards*.

### Sports Mouth Guards

Sports mouth guards can be custom made in laboratory or can be purchased OTC (Over-the-counter). The OTC mouth guards are of two types: (i) stock type (ii) hand adapted soft material.

The stock type is available in different sizes and is uncomfortable to wear as they do not fit accurately. The hand made one are made of flexible thermoplastic material which are softened in hot water and then hand adapted in the mouth. The excess material is cut with sharp scissors. These mouth guards are again very difficult to adapt and use **(Fig. 28.18)**.

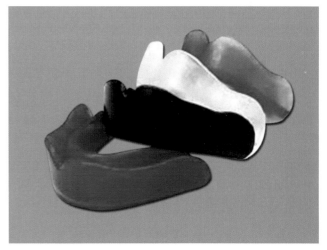

**Fig. 28.18:** Stock type mouth guard.

Custom made mouth guards are the most accurately fitting and well tolerated by the patient. Primary cast is made after pouring impression of the mouth. The casts

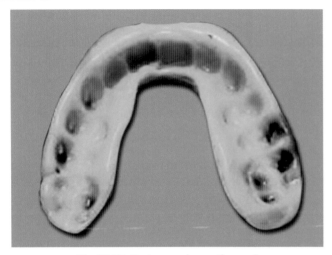

**Fig. 28.19:** Custom made mouth guard.

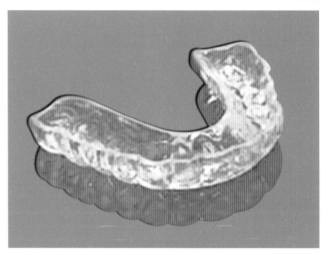

**Fig. 28.20:** Custom made night guard.

are trimmed horseshoe shaped. A thermoplastic material is heated and vacuum adapted to the cast. After adaption the vinyl material is allowed to cool. The excess material is trimmed with heavy duty scissors. The advantages with this type of mouth guard are excellent fit and more comfort of use to the patient **(Fig. 28.19)**.

### Night Guards

Night guards are recommended for Bruxism patients, i.e. who grind their teeth during sleep in the night. This guard helps in preventing wear of teeth. They protect the incisal and occlusal surfaces from wearing or chipping or fracturing of the cusp. There are two types of materials which are used to fabricate night guards: (1) hard acrylics (methyl methacrylate resin and monomer), (2) thermoplastic sheets of polyvinyl or polyethylene material **(Fig. 28.20)**.

## BLEACHING MATERIALS

Tooth bleaching (ADA specification no. 136) is a procedure of whitening the teeth by removing intrinsic or extrinsic stains. It can be done as an *in-office* procedure or as home bleach procedure.

### Composition

The main ingredients of the bleaching agents are:
- Hydrogen peroxide in varying concentrations
- Carbamide peroxide
- Urea peroxide
- Nonhydrogen peroxide system containing sodium chloride, oxygen and natrium fluoride.
- Potassium nitrate or fluoride to reduce sensitivity.

### Mechanism of Action

The bleaching agents occur when hydrogen peroxide or nonperoxide bleaching material penetrates the enamel to the dentin and oxidizes the pigments in the dentin resulting in the lighter shades. The process can be accelerated by applying low intensity heat or high intensity light such as conventional curing light, laser beam or high intensity plasma arc light.

### Types of Stain

Stains on the tooth surface can be of two types: (1) Extrinsic stains (2) Intrinsic stains.
1. *Extrinsic stains:* Discoloration on the surface of the tooth. It can be removed by ultrasonic scaling and polishing.
2. *Intrinsic stains:* Stains incorporated inside the tooth structure. It cannot be removed by conventional ultrasonic scaling. It may require bleaching process to remove such stains.

### Causes of Staining

- *Extrinsic stains:*
  - *Poor oral hygiene:* Yellow, brown, green or black stains
  - *Tobacco products:* Yellow brown, black stains
  - Tea, coffee, foods: Brown to black stains
- *Intrinsic stains:* Drugs induced during tooth development
  - Tetracycline stains: Brown, gray, black bands
  - Fluoride stains: White bands, brown spots or bands.

*Drug induced after tooth development: Minocycline:* Brown, gray stains.

*Conditions during tooth formation:*
- *Blood disorder (purpura):* Red, brown and purple
- *Trauma:* Blue, black and brown.

*Pulpal changes:*
- *Obliteration of root canal:* Yellow
- Pulpal necrosis with hemorrhage
- Pulpal necrosis without hemorrhage.

*Causes in nonvital teeth:*
- *Trauma during pulp extirpation:* Gray and black
- *Tissue remnants in pulp chamber:* Brown, gray and black
- *Restorative dental materials:* Brown, gray and black
- *Endodontic materials:* Gray and black.

*Combination of intrinsic and extrinsic stains:*
- *Aging:* Yellow stains
- *Fluorosis:* White, brown stains.

## Classification of Bleaching

- *In-office bleaching:*
  - Bleaching of vital teeth
  - Bleaching of nonvital teeth.
- Home bleaching.

### In-office Bleaching *(Fig. 28.21)*

*Bleaching of vital teeth*: Various bleaching agents are used in varying concentration to bleach vital teeth in the clinic. Commonly used bleaching agents are 35% hydrogen peroxide and 35% carbamide peroxide. Use of 35% carbamide peroxide is more effective and controllable than the liquid hydrogen peroxide. Recently, *power bleach technique* is introduced. The advantages of this technique are that bleaching can be done is single appointment and is less dependent on patient compliance. In this technique; light cure unit, plasma arc light or lasers are used to bleach in 45 minutes to 1 hour. To protect the gingiva, petrolatum jelly or light cured material is applied. Currently bleaching gels or mixed paste has color indicators which show completion of the oxygenating cycle. Application of gels can be repeated till desired results are achieved.

*Procedure*
- Teeth are cleaned with pumice paste
- Preoperative photograph is taken. Starting shade of the teeth is recorded
- Gel or jelly is applied over the gingiva and interdental papilla for protection following the manufacturer's instructions
- Rubber dam is placed to isolate the teeth
- Bleaching gel is applied to the tooth surface. Light or heat is applied according to the manufacturer's instructions
- After completion the gel is rinsed off and wiped with gauze piece
- Shade is checked and if desired result not achieved the procedure should be repeated.

*Bleaching of nonvital teeth:* In a nonvital tooth, the necrotic breakdown products or hemoglobin of the blood in the pulp can escape into the surrounding dentinal tubules causing tooth discoloration. The restoration over the endodontic access cavity is removed. The tooth is isolated with rubber dam to protect the gingiva or oral soft tissues from damage. A seal is established at the base of the endodontic access preparation to prevent the bleaching solution to leak into the periodontal ligament. This can cause external resorption of the tooth. A 30% hydrogen peroxide solution is placed in the pulp chamber with saturated cotton pellet. Heat is applied over the pellet to activate the peroxide. Another technique is called the *walking bleach* in which the bleaching gel [mixture of sodium perborate monohydrate and Superoxol (30% hydrogen peroxide)] is sealed into the pulp chamber with temporary restoration. Patient is recalled after 2–5 days, once the bleaching paste is oxidized and bleaches the tooth. The bleaching solution is removed from the chamber and is replaced with composite or amalgam restoration.

### Home Bleaching or Night Guard Bleaching **(Fig. 28.22)**

Home bleaching is an effective and cost-effective method of bleaching of the teeth. Bleaching agent commonly used as home bleach is 10–16% carbamide peroxide with neutral pH in the form of viscous gel. The bleaching gel is placed in custom made thin plastic tray which may or may

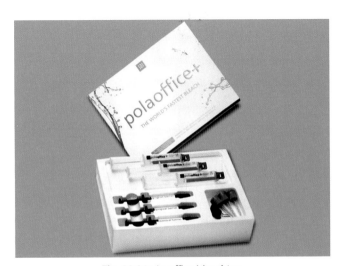

**Fig. 28.21:** In-office bleaching.

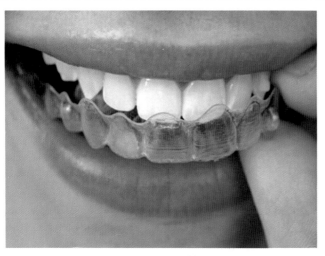

**Fig. 28.22:** Night guard bleaching.

not have reservoirs to hold the bleaching gel. Duration of use can vary from few hours to maximum overnight wearing depending on the patient needs. The home bleach procedure is usually recommended for 2 weeks but may be prolonged in cases with tetracycline stains. It may be not possible to remove all the tetracycline stains with these bleaching agents. Home bleaching is as effective as the in-office bleaching.

### Drawbacks of Bleaching

- Tooth sensitivity—can be reduced by decreasing duration of bleaching
- Irritation of gingiva, soft tissues—can be reduced by protecting the gums or soft tissues with jelly before applying bleaching gels.

## TEST YOURSELF

### Essay Questions

1. Classify various sources of fluoride. Discuss in detail systemic fluorides.
2. Describe various fluoride application procedures.
3. Classify various mechanical and chemical aids in plaque control. Write in detail about chlorhexidine.
4. Classify pit and fissure sealants. Write about light cure resin sealants.

### Short Notes

1. Preventive resin restorations.
2. Sodium fluoride.
3. Home bleaching.
4. Vital bleaching.
5. Methods of remineralization.
6. CPP-ACP complex.
7. APF gels.
8. Desensitizing agents.

### Multiple Choice Questions

1. High level of fluoride in found naturally in:
   A. Tea
   B. Coffee
   C. Raw seafood
   D. Beans
2. The main purpose of mouth guard is:
   A. To use as bleaching tray
   B. To protect the teeth and supporting structures during contact sports
   C. To use as tray for fluoride application
   D. To keep teeth in alignment after orthodontic retainers
3. Custom made mouth guards and splints are made of:
   A. Composite resin
   B. Tray acrylic
   C. Thermoplastic sheet of resilient plastic or hard processed acrylic resin
   D. Plastic material softened by boiling
4. Bleaching of teeth:
   A. Removes only extrinsic stains only
   B. Make teeth soft
   C. Can cause sensitivity of teeth
   D. Removes only intrinsic stains only
5. Primary purpose of most desensitizing agent is:
   A. To plug the openings of the exposed dentinal tubules
   B. To occlude the opening in the tooth enamel
   C. When added in toothpaste reduces burning sensation to gingiva
   D. Applied before prophylaxis
6. Bleaching acts:
   A. By removing surface stains
   B. By penetrating both enamel and dentin and by oxidizing the stains
   C. By forming a white coating on the tooth surface
   D. By sealing surface porosities on the tooth
7. Pit and fissure sealant is:
   A. Indicated for all permanent molars
   B. Unfilled or lightly filled resins
   C. Used for protecting from smooth surface caries
   D. Permanent and do not require replacement

8. Preventive resin restoration is:
   A. Indicated for an incipient lesion
   B. Extensive caries on molars
   C. Deep groove in caries free molar tooth
   D. Recurrent decay around an existing amalgam

## ANSWERS

| 1. A | 2. B | 3. C | 4. C |
|------|------|------|------|
| 5. A | 6. B | 7. B | 8. A |

## BIBLIOGRAPHY

1. Baum L, Phillips RW, Lund MR. Prevention of dental disease. Textbook of Operative Dentistry, 3rd edition. Philadelphia: WB Saunders; 1995.
2. Bird D, Robinson D. Preventive, restorative and cosmetic dentistry. Torres and Ehrlich Modern Dental Assisting, 6th edition. Philadelphia: WB Saunders; 1999.
3. Ferracane JL. Materials in Dentistry—Principles and Applications, 2nd edition. Philadelphia: Lippincott Williams and Wilkins; 2001.
4. Gladwin MA, Bagby MD. Tooth bleaching: oral appliances. In: Clinical Aspects of Dental Materials. Philadelphia: Lippincott Williams and Wilkins; 2000.
5. Gupta R, Prakash V. CPP-ACP complex as a new adjunctive agent for remineralization: a review. Oral Health Prev Dent. 2011;9:151-65.
6. Hatrick CD, Eakle WS, Bird WF. Dental materials—Clinical Application for Dental Assistants and Dental Hygienists, 1st edition. Philadelphia: WB Saunders; 2003.
7. Haywood VB. Current status and recommendation for dentist-prescribed, at home tooth whitening. Contemp Esthet Rest Pract. 1999;3:2-9.
8. Kugel G. Effective tooth bleaching in 5 days: using a combined in-office and at-home bleaching system. Compend Contin Educ Dent. 1997;18:378-83.
9. Leinfelder KF. Ask the expert. Anything new in pit and fissure sealants? J Am Dent Assoc. 1999;130:533-4.
10. Mandel JD. Chemotherapeutic agents for controlling plaque and gingivitis. J Clin Periodontol. 1988;15:488-98.
11. Reynold E, Cai F, Cochrane NJ, Shen P, Walker GD, Morgan MV, et al. Fluoride and casein phosphopeptide-amorphous calcium phosphate. J Dent Res. 2008;87:344-8.
12. Reynold EC. Remineralization of enamel subsurface lesions by casein phosphopeptide-stabilized calcium phosphate solutions. J Dent Res. 1997;76:1587-95.
13. Reynold EC. The prevention of subsurface demineralization of bovine enamel and change in plaque composition by casein in an intra-oral model. J Dent Res. 1987;66:1120-7.
14. Reynolds EC. Anticariogenic complexes of amorphous calcium phosphate stabilized by casein phosphopeptides: a review. Spec Care Dentist. 1998;18:8-16.
15. Ripa LW, Wolff MS. Preventive resin restorations: indications, technique, and success. Quintessence Int. 1992;5:302-15.
16. Simonsen RJ. Retention and effectiveness of dental sealant after 15 years. J Am Dent Assoc. 1991;122:34-42.
17. Ten Case JM, Featherstone JDB. Mechanistic aspects of the interactions between fluoride and dental enamel. Crit Rev Oral Biol Med. 1991;2:283-96.

# Section 8

## Recent Trends in Dental Materials

# Dental Implant Materials

ADA Specification No. 40

*'Innovation distinguishes between a leader and a follower.'*

*—Steve Jobs*

## INTRODUCTION

Throughout history human beings have attempted replacement of teeth with artificial substitute. In the past, extracted teeth, wood, ivory, dry bone, gold, gold wires and other materials have been used as replacement. Biocompatibility was one of the major issues for failure of the treatment. Over past four or five decades, implants made of titanium and its alloys have gained wide popularity and acceptability as they have shown highly predictable results. The high rate of success and clinical longevity of dental implants have allowed larger number of patient the benefits of fixed restorations. Dental implant treatment has become highly attractive treatment option because of its predictability, relative simplicity and minimal invasiveness. Multiple investigations have revealed more than 90% success rate of implants both in maxilla and mandible. It is important to have basic knowledge of implant materials and their applications as implant treatment is one of the most sought after treatment option for treating edentulous and partially edentulous patients.

## HISTORICAL CONSIDERATIONS

- *936–1013 AD*: *Albucasis de Condue* used ox bone to replace missing teeth
- *1800*: *Pierre Fauchard* and *John Hunter* advocated tooth transplantations

- *1809*: *Maggiolo* fixed gold roots to pivot teeth by using springs
- *1887*: Harris-shaped platinum post-coated with lead like tooth root and implanted into the socket
- *1895*: *Bonwell* used gold or iridium tubes implanted into bone to restore a single tooth or to support complete denture prosthesis
- *1898*: *Payne* implanted silver capsule as foundation to received porcelain crown which was cemented later
- *1905*: *Scholl* developed porcelain corrugated root implant
- *1913*: *Greenfield* advocated the use of hollow basket implant made from meshwork of 24-gauge iridium-platinum wires soldered with 24 karat gold
- *1937*: *Venable, AE Strock* and *Beach* analyzed the effects of metals on bone. They advocated the use of inert, biocompatible metal called as "Vitallium"
- *1940*: *Dahl* first developed the subperiosteal implants
- *1947*: *Formiggini* developed single helix wire spiral implant made from tantalum or stainless steel
- *1948*: *Goldberg* and *Gershkoff* devised the first viable subperiosteal implant
- *1952*: *Branemark* developed threaded implant design made of pure titanium. He extensively studied the physiological, mechanical, biological and functional aspect
- *1963*: *Linkow* designed and developed the hollow basket implants with vents and screw heads

- *1965*: *Branemark* first placed dental implant in human bone
- *1977*: *Branemark* coined the term osseointegration.

## DEFINITION

*Dental* implant is defined as *a prosthetic device made of alloplastic materials implanted into the oral tissues beneath the mucosal and/or periosteal layer, and on/or within the bone to provide retention and support for a fixed or removable dental prosthesis.*

## CLASSIFICATION OF DENTAL IMPLANTS

### Based on the Type of Material Used

#### Metals and Alloys

- Stainless steel
- Cobalt-chromium-molybdenum based
- Titanium and its alloys
- Surface-coated titanium
- Other metals and alloys.

#### Ceramics

- Tricalcium phosphate
- Hydroxyapatite
- Aluminum oxide
- Calcium aluminates.

#### Polymers and Composite

- Polymethyl methacrylate
- Polytetrafluoroethylene
- Polyethylene
- Silicone rubber
- Polysulfone.

#### Carbons

- Polycrystalline glassy carbon (vitreous)
- Carbon silicon.

### Based on the Design of Implants

#### Subperiosteal Implants

This type of device first developed by Dahl (1940) and then modified by Berman (1951). It is a framework which derives its support by resting over the bony ridge without penetrating it. It is used for restoration of partially and completely edentulous jaws where there is insufficient bone support for endosseous implant placement. This type of design is obsolete and is very rarely used **(Fig. 29.1)**.

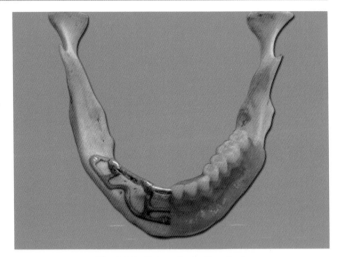

**Fig. 29.1:** Subperiosteal implant.

*Disadvantages*
- Retrievability of implant is difficult
- Excessive bone loss
- Rejection of implant is high
- Limited success rate.

#### Transosteal Implants

Also called as *Staple bone implant, transmandibular implant (TMI) and mandibular staple implants.* As the name suggests these implants penetrate both the superior and inferior cortical plates covering the entire thickness of the mandible. Transosteal implants were first developed in Germany in 1920s, popularized by Small (1968). *Bosker* in 1982 developed the TMI which were made of gold alloys **(Fig. 29.2)**.

#### Endosteal Implants

They are the most commonly used implants for restoring partially and completely edentulous jaws. These implants are most successful and frequently used because of high

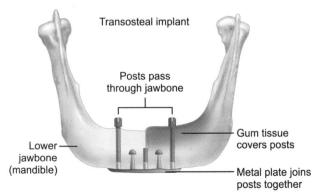

**Fig. 29.2:** Transosteal implant.

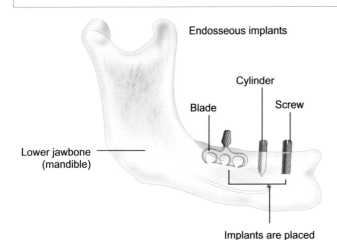

**Fig. 29.3:** Endosteal implants.

success rate. Endosseous implants only transect one cortical plate. These implants lie within the bone. They are of three types—(1) root form implants, (2) plate form implants and ramus frame type implants **(Fig. 29.3)**.

Blade implants were placed after cutting a groove into the bony ridge. These implants usually have holes in them so that bone could grow through it and hold the implant for extra stability. Such implants were not used for single tooth replacement because of its large size.

---

**CLINICAL SIGNIFICANCE**

Root form implants are most successful and effective implants as they are surrounded by bone. After placement, the implants are allowed to heal so that new bone forms and implants are osseointegrated.

---

### Epithelial Implants

It is the type of implant which is placed in the oral mucosa. In this type, oral mucosa is used as the attachment site for the metal inserts.

### Based on their Reaction to Bone

#### Bioactive

Ability of the implant to simulate bone formation, through ion exchange with host tissues they form chemical bonds between the host tissues and bioactive material, e.g. hydroxyapatite and tricalcium phosphate.

#### Bioinert

These materials do not bond directly to the bone but are mechanically held in contact to the bone. Bone grows and fills in through this particular material and holds them in position, e.g. zirconium oxide and aluminum oxide.

### Based on the Mechanism of Attachment

- *Osseointegration*: It is the process in which living bony tissue is integrated with an implant material without any intervening fibrous connective tissues **(Fig. 29.4)**.
- *Fibrointegration*: In this implant attachment was through the low differentiated fibrous tissues. This process is also called as *pseudo-periodontium* **(Fig. 29.5)**.

### Based on the Surface Treatments

- Hydroxyapatite coated
- Plasma sprayed
- Blasted or etched with other biomaterials
- Electropolished
- Machined.

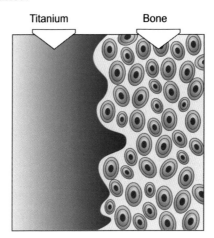

**Fig. 29.4:** Osseointegration.

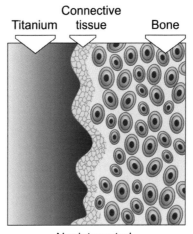

**Fig. 29.5:** Fibrointegration.

## Based on the Macroscopic Design

- Hollow design
- Cylindrical or conical design
- Threaded design.

# INDICATIONS AND CONTRAINDICATIONS

## Indications

- Patient unable to wear removable partial or complete dentures
- Free end distal extension without any posterior abutment
- Number and location of the natural abutment is unfavorable
- To avoid preparation of sound or minimally restored teeth to receive fixed partial denture in single edentulous space
- Presence of adequate bone height, width, length, contour and density.

## Contraindications

### Absolute Contraindications

- Acute and terminal illness
- Pregnancy
- Uncontrolled metabolic disorders
- Bone and soft tissue infection.

### Relative Contraindications

- Patient on radiotherapy
- Uncontrolled diabetic
- Parafunctional habits
- HIV
- Bisphosphonate usage either orally or intravenous
- Patient with unrealistic expectation
- Poor patient motivation and oral hygiene
- Inadequately trained clinician
- Poor patient compliance.

## Advantages

- Aids in preserving bone
- Enhances masticatory efficiency
- Helps in maintaining proper vertical dimension
- Immune to dental caries
- High level of predictability
- Improves esthetics and phonetics
- Increases retention and stability of the prosthetic restoration.

## Disadvantages

- Initial treatment cost is high
- Patient to undergo a surgical procedure
- Procedure depends on availability of bone and clinicians skills.
- Limited scope in placement in medically compromised patient.

## Uses

- Dental implants are used to replace missing tooth or teeth by anchoring prosthesis to the jawbone
- Can be used to anchor extraoral prosthesis.

# CONCEPT OF OSSEOINTEGRATION

*PI Branemark* coined the term "osseointegration" in 1977. According to him, osseointegration can be defined as the direct structural and functional connection between organized, living bone and the surface of a load bearing implant without intervening soft tissue between the implant and the bone.

*Definition: Osseointegration is defined as the apparent direct attachment or connection of osseous tissue to an inert, alloplastic material without intervening connective tissues.*

*Rationale:* To achieve direct contact between the bone and the implant without any fibrous tissues between the two interfaces.

## Mechanism of Attachment

- During placement of the implant there should be good contact between the bone and the implant surface to ensure good primary stability
- Blood clot forms at the osteotomy site, which is replaced by bone over a period of time
- Initial clot formation is followed by proliferation and differentiation of numerous phagocytes and undifferentiated mesenchymal cells from adjacent periosteum
- Initial bone trauma leads to resorption of the bone which will decrease the primary stability which was initially achieved
- This necrotic bone is replaced by initial woven bone formation
- Quality of bone and its volume that contacts the implant determines its initial stability. This stability should be maintained for the bone to form over a period of time
- After the critical period of 2 weeks, the bone formation takes place and the level of bone contact and implant stability is enhanced

- Depending on the initial stability and the quality of bone, single stage or two stage surgery is done
- In single stage implant procedure, the primary stability is good and the implants can be loaded immediately whereas in the two stage procedure implants are submerged till it attains adequate stability. After 3–4 months, the implants are uncovered and then loaded
- Greater osseointegration is observed in cortical bone with good blood supply than in the cancellous bone
- The degree of osseointegration increases with time and function
- Greater forces applied to the implant may lead to apical movement of the bone margins resulting in some loss of osseointegration.

*Factors influencing osseointegration are:*

- *Biocompatibility and implant design*: Commercially pure titanium (cp Ti) implants are the most commonly used material to establish osseointegration. The implant design influences greatly the initial stability and its function. The design parameters are:
  - *Implant length*: Commonly used implant lengths are between 8 mm and 15 mm which correspond closely to the natural root length
  - *Implant diameter*: For adequate implant strength at least 3.25 mm diameter implants are used. Most commonly used diameter is 4 mm. Implant diameter rather length influences the amount of force distributed to the surrounding bone
  - *Implant shape*: Implant shapes such as hollow cylinders, hollow screws, solid cylinders or solid screws influence the amount of osseointegration and this provides initial stability. Alteration in the size or pitch of the threads can influence the initial stability of implants
  - *Surface characteristics*: Degree of roughness influences the osseointegration. Surface treatment like grit blasting, etching, plasma sprayed or hydroxyapatite coating improves osseointegration by increasing the bone to implant contact.
- *Bone factors*: Quality and quantity of bone greatly influences the stability of implant during placement. Well-formed cortical and dense trabecular bone with good blood supply is most desirable for implant placement. Quality of bone is influenced by factors such as infection, smoking or irradiation which reduces blood supply to the bone
- *Loading factors*: Sufficient time for healing should be given to the implant before loading. Ideally 6 months for maxilla and 4 months for mandible is recommended
- *Prosthetic considerations*: Properly planned occlusal loading will help in increased bone to implant contact

and long-term osseointegration. The functional loading conditions depend on the following:

- *Type of occlusal factors*: Shallow cuspal inclines and reduced loading during lateral excursion results in lesser load transfer to the surrounding bone
- *Type of prosthetic reconstruction*: It may vary from a single tooth replacement to full arch reconstruction or implant supported overdentures
- *Number, location and design of implants*: The greater number of implants will distribute the functional forces over the larger surface area, thereby reducing the amount of load per area
- Similarly, location and design of implants influences osseointegration of dental implants
- *Patient habits*: Any parafunctional habits will drastically influence the prognosis of the treatment
- *Design and properties of implant connectors*: Rigid connectors which are having passive fit help in distributing load between the multiple implants and also provide good splinting.

## Surface Treatment of Implants

As mentioned earlier surface characteristics of implants is critical for osseointegration. There are various methods of surface treatment of implants.

Methods of surface treatments:

- *Ablative procedures*: It involves the removal of material from the surface of a material through:
  - Acid etching
  - Grit blasting
  - Anodizing
  - Sandblasted and acid-etched (SLA) surface.
- *Additive procedure*: It involves creating a layer by addition of material through:
  - Plasma spray
  - Porous sintering
  - Sputter deposition
  - Electrophoretic deposition
  - Biomimetic precipitation
  - Soluble gel coating.

### Acid Etching

The surface of implant is pitted by means of acid etching process. Strong acids, such as hydrochloric acid (HCl), nitric acid (HNO$_3$) and sulfuric acid (H$_2$SO$_4$) are used for this purpose. The roughness achieved by acid etching depends on the type of acid, immersion time of implant, bulk, and surface topography. Minimum roughness achieved from this process is in the range of 0.3–1 μm (Sa value). *The Sa value refers to the mean height of peaks and pits on the surface.* Roughness on the surface of implant by acid etching is believed to improve osseointegration.

**CLINICAL SIGNIFICANCE**

Etched surface increases the surface area which aids in improving the mechanical interlocking of bone with implant.

### Grit Blasting

This process is done by blasting the surface of implants with small particles of aluminum trioxide and titanium dioxide. As grit blast hits the surface of implants, it forms craters which cause roughness.

**CLINICAL SIGNIFICANCE**

The roughened implant surface promotes adhesion, proliferation and differentiation of osteoblasts, and therefore increases osseointegration. The Sa value is in the range of 0.5–2.0 μm.

### Anodization

Anodization of titanium implant surface results in partial crystalline and phosphate enriched microstructural topography. The roughness achieved helps in improving bone growth due to mechanical interlocking thereby increasing osseointegration. This method shows greater bone implant contact ratio and higher overall clinical success rate.

### Sandblasted and Acid-etched Surfaces

Currently available dental implants are both SLA to increase the surface roughness. SLA surface shows increased hydrophilicity of the implant surface because of minimal carbon contamination. SLA active implants show greater healing, increased osseointegration and stability.

### Plasma Spraying

Hydroxyapatite crystals are most commonly used material to plasma spray the implant surface to increase the bioactivity of the implants. Through this method calcium phosphate layer is deposited on the surface of the implant. Thickness of the coating is in the range of 100–300 μm. There is about six times increase in the surface area using this method. The average roughness is in the range of 5 ± 1 μm. Hydroxyapatite coated surface shows greater bone implant surface contact. However, there is possibility of microbial infection, thickness of coating is nonuniform and the long-term adhesion of the hydroxyapatite coating is questionable.

### Porous Sintering

It is the method of incorporating porosity on the surface of implant by sintering metal powder. The porous layer on the surface aids in increased retention due to improved ingrowth of bone into these porous layer. Currently, greater roughness is sought by laser sintering method which helps in improving long-term performance.

### Sputter Deposition

It is one of the methods of depositing bioceramic thin films of calcium phosphate on the implant surface. It helps in improving adhesion of the substrate and bioceramic material. This method is time consuming.

### Biomimetic Precipitation

The implant surface is biomimetically precipitated with calcium phosphate to promote early bone growth on the porous surface. Through this technique thick layer of hydroxyapatite coating is formed which is 20–25 μm thick.

**CLINICAL SIGNIFICANCE**

Coatings of these materials greatly improves osseo-integration and have higher torque value for removal compared to uncoated titanium implants.

## HEALING PROCESS IN IMPLANTS

The healing process around the dental implant is similar to the process that occurs for primary bone. The healing process in implants occurs in three phases namely:
1. Osteophyllic phase
2. Osteoconductive phase
3. Osteoadaptive phase.

### Osteophyllic Phase

- After osteotomy procedure when the rough surface implant is placed, blood is present between the surface and bone which subsequently forms a clot
- At this time only small portion of implant is in contact with bone and the rest of the surface is exposed to extracellular fluid and cells
- During the initial implant-bone interaction, cytokines are released which increases collagen synthesis and regulate bone metabolism
- While inflammatory phase is active, there is vascular ingrowth from the surrounding vital bone starting from the third day
- Vascular network matures in the first 3 weeks after implant placement.

- There is cellular differentiation, proliferation and activation which occurs during this phase
- Ossification occurs from the first week itself when the osteoblasts cells migrate from the endosteal surface of the trabecular bone and inner surface of buccal and lingual cortical bone
- This phase lasts for 1 month.

### Osteoconductive Phase

- During this phase as the osteoblasts spreads along the metal surface to deposit the osteoid
- Initially, immature connective tissue matrix in the form of thin woven bone is laid down which is called the *footplate*
- Fibrocartilaginous callus matures into the bone callus similar to the endochondral ossification of bone
- This phase occurs for the next 3 months
- After 4 months of implant placement, maximum surface area of implant is covered by bone
- At the end of this phase, a steady state is reached and there is no more formation of bone.

### Osteoadaptive Phase

- This final phase occurs after 4 months of implant placement
- In this phase, remodeling of bone occurs even after the implants are exposed and loaded
- After loading, the bone surrounding the implant thickens in response to the load transmitted to the implant
- Reorganization of the vascular pattern is observed during this phase
- About 4–8 months of healing period is recommended for adequate osseointegration depending on the quality of the bone.

## COMPONENTS OF DENTAL IMPLANTS (FIGS. 29.6 AND 29.7)

Parts of all the implant systems are usually similar.

*Implant body or fixture:* It is a component that actually engages the bone. Usually, the fixture is made of titanium or alloys. They can be having different implant surface such as threaded, perforated, nonthreaded, plasma sprayed or coated. Plasma sprayed or coated implants are used to increase attachment of bone.

*Cover screw:* It is a screw that is placed in the implant during healing.

*Healing cap or gingival former:* It is a dome-shaped screw which is placed after the stage II surgery. It projects from the soft tissues into the oral cavity. They help in enhancing soft tissue esthetics by developing papilla and marginal gingiva.

*Transmucosal abutment:* It provides a connection between the implant fixture and the prosthesis that will be fabricated. It can be straight or angled and it eventually supports the prosthesis directly. Abutment can engage either an internal or external hexagon on the fixture that serves as the antirotational device.

### Classification of Abutments

- *Based on angulation*:
  - Straight
  - Angled abutment.
- *Based on the type of material used*:
  - Titanium
  - Zirconia
  - Gold alloy.
- *Based on the fabrication process*:
  - Custom made
  - Prefabricated: (a) Hollow abutments and (b) solid abutment
  - Computer-aided design/computer-aided manufacturing (CAD/CAM) based.

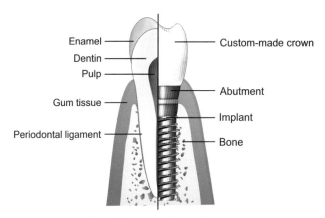

**Fig. 29.6:** Parts of dental implant.

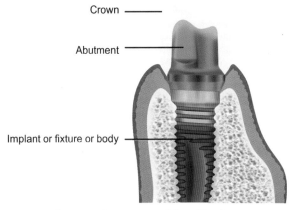

**Fig. 29.7:** Components of dental implants.

## Implant Abutment Connection

*Prosthesis:* It is attached to the abutment with the help of screw, cement or precision attachment.

*Impression post:* It is any device which is used to register the portion of dental implant or dental implant abutment relative to the adjacent oral structures. These impression post are then connected with the laboratory analog and the impression is poured with gypsum.

*Laboratory analog:* This component is machined to exactly simulate the implant. It is screwed into the impression post after it is removed from the mouth and placed back in the impression before pouring into the stone cast.

*Waxing sleeve:* It can be a plastic pattern or metal component which is casted to eventually become part of the prosthesis.

## SUCCESS CRITERIA OF IMPLANTS

The minimum success criteria proposed by Albrektsson et al. (1986) are:
- Implant should be immobile when tested clinically
- No peri-implant radiolucency on radiographic evaluation
- Radiographic vertical bone loss around implant after 1 year in function should not be less than 0.2 mm per annum
- Success rate after 5 years of service should be at least 85% and after 10 years, it should be 80%.

   Success of implant is characterized by absence of signs and symptoms such as pain, paresthesia, infections, neuropathies or violation of the inferior dental canal.

## IMPLANT MATERIALS

### Stainless Steel

- Used in the form of surgical austenitic steel with 18% chromium, 8% nickel and 0.05% iron-carbon
- Chromium imparts corrosion resistance and nickel helps in stabilizing the austenitic structure
- Alloy mostly used in wrought and heat treated from which has high strength
- They were used to fabricate ramus blade, ramus frame, stabilizer pins and some mucosal inserts
- Currently not used because of nickel sensitivity and its susceptibility to crevice and pitting corrosion.

### Advantages

- Has high strength and ductility and thus is resistant to brittle fracture
- Easily available
- Low cost and ease of fabrication.

### Disadvantages

- Allergic potential of nickel
- Susceptibility to pitting and crevice corrosion.

### Cobalt-chromium-molybdenum Alloy

- Used in as cast or cast and annealed condition
- Used in fabrication of custom made implant designs such as subperiosteal frames
- Composed of cobalt 63%, chromium 30% and molybdenum 5% and small amounts of carbon, manganese and nickel
- Cobalt provides continuous phase for basic properties
- Chromium provides corrosion resistance by formation of passivating layer (chromium oxide)
- Molybdenum provides strength and stabilizes the structure
- Carbon acts as hardener
- Ductility of the alloy can be improved by reducing the carbon content
- *Vitallium* was introduced by *Venable* in 1930s but was found to produce chronic inflammation with fibrous encapsulation resulting in the mobility of the implants
- *Ticonium* is an alloy made of Ni, Cr, Mo and Be alloy which was also used as dental implant material but had reduced biocompatibility.

### Advantages

- Good strength and high modulus of elasticity
- Low cost
- High corrosion resistance
- Low ductility.

### Disadvantages

- Ductility is least and therefore bending should be avoided
- Technique sensitive during fabrication
- Critical to use all the elements in proper concentration.

### Titanium and Alloys

- Titanium and titanium alloys are the most commonly used material used for dental implant fabrication owing to its high strength, high corrosion resistance, low specific gravity and high heat resistance. Its high strength is because of closely packed hexagonal crystal lattice structure. Its high corrosion resistance is because of formation of stable, passive oxide layer **(Fig. 29.8)**
- Commercially pure titanium consists of 99% titanium and 0.5% oxygen and minor amounts of impurities such

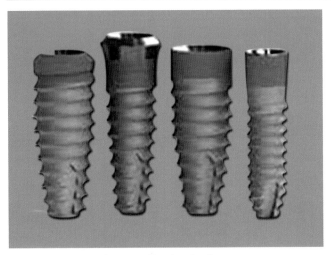

**Fig. 29.8:** Titanium implants.

as nitrogen, hydrogen and carbon. It is a highly reactive material which oxidizes (passivates) on contact with air or normal tissue fluids to form a passivating layer of titanium oxide. Since the passivating layer minimizes biocorrosion, this property is desirable for implant devices. With the formation of titanium oxide, titanium or its alloy is highly corrosion resistant. The titanium oxide layer nevertheless releases titanium ions slowly when it comes in contact with electrolyte such as blood or saliva.

---

**CLINICAL IMPORTANCE**

When a cut surface of titanium is exposed to atmosphere, a passivating layer of thickness 10 Å forms on the surface within millisecond.

---

- Any abrasion or scratch on the surface during placement of implant *repassivates in vivo* through surface controlled oxidation kinetics. The passivating property of titanium and its alloy is further enhanced by treating it with nitric acid to form a thick and durable layer on the surface
- Density of titanium is 4.5 g/cm³ and is therefore 40% lighter than steel
- Modulus of elasticity (97 GN/m²) is one-half that of steel but is 5–10 times more than that of compact bone
- It has a high strength to weight ratio.

*Titanium Alloys*

- Most common alloy of titanium used in implant dentistry is titanium-aluminum-vanadium (Ti-6Al-4V) alloy
- This alloy contains 90% titanium, 6% aluminum and 4% vanadium by weight

- The mechanical properties of the titanium alloy are better than the cp Ti
- Titanium alloy has 60% greater strength than pure titanium and it more costly
- Both cp Ti and titanium alloys have *excellent corrosion resistance*
- The passivating layer of titanium oxide has a *high dielectric property* which is responsible to make the surface of the implant more reactive to the biomolecules through the increased electrostatic forces. It therefore, helps in osseointegration
- Titanium-based materials have high fatigue strength (500–700 MPa).

**Other Metals and Alloys**

- Early implants were made of metal such as tantalum, platinum, gold, palladium and its alloys
- Recently tungsten, hafnium and zirconium have been used
- Gold, platinum and palladium have low strength
- Gold and platinum are costly and have limited use in dental implants.

**Vitreous Carbon Implant**

- Carbon and carbon compounds were first used in dental implantology in 1960s
- Vitreous carbon is highly biocompatible and is inert in nature
- Composed of carbon body with an internal 316 L stainless steel post
- Modulus of elasticity of carbon is comparable with the bone and dentin
- Carbon is brittle in nature and does not possess sufficient strength to tolerate physiologic loads within the oral environment. It has relatively low compressive strength
- Due to loading, microcracks become evident on the body of implant and this creates internal pathways for biological fluids on the stainless steel post
- This leads to corrosion of the implant body resulting in the inflammation of the surrounding tissues
- Inflammation results in severe bone loss leading to ultimate failure of the implant.

**Carbon Silicon Compounds**

- Carbon compounds are chemically inert and lack ductility (brittle). They are susceptible to mechanical fracture on rapid high magnitude mechanical loading
- They are good conductors of heat and electricity
- Ceramic and carbon compounds are used as coatings on metallic and ceramic materials

- Carbon silicon compounds have silicon rich layer along the surface region
- This material should be handled with extreme care as carbon surface are easily susceptible to contamination during manipulation and placement
- For good bone adaptation, the surface should be extremely clean.

### Polymers and Composites

- Synthetic polymers are commonly used in implant dentistry because of its favorable mechanical properties
- Some of the polymeric biomaterials are polytetrafluoroethylene, polyethylene terephthalate, polyethyl methacrylate
- They have low rigidity and reduced strength but have higher elongation to fracture and therefore used in areas of bony defects
- They are helpful in transfer of forces to soft and hard tissues
- These materials cannot be autoclaved or dry heat sterilized. Mostly they are sterilized by gamma irradiation
- These materials should be soaked in sterile water or saline as they have electrostatic surface charge which is capable of attracting dust particles
- Since, they have relatively low mechanical strength they have limited application in tooth root replacement systems
- They are used as components in dental implants. For example, IMZ implants has intramobile element made of polyoxymethylene which acts as internal shock absorber **(Fig. 29.9)**.

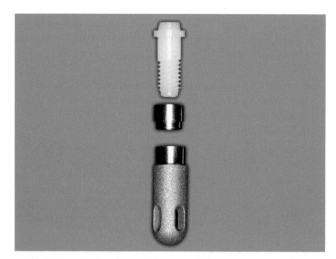

**Fig. 29.9:** IMZ implants with intramobile component made of polyoxymethylene.

## BONE AUGMENTATION MATERIALS

Replacement of bone is a complex phenomenon and sometimes can be quiet challenging. Mature compact bone is composed of 30% organic matrix and 70% calcium salts. 90% of the organic matrix is composed of collagen fibers and rest forms ground substance which is composed of chondroitin sulfate and hyaluronic acid.

## MECHANISM OF BONE AUGMENTATION

There are primarily three mechanisms by which bone regeneration occurs when bone graft material is used:
1. Osteogenesis
2. Osteoinduction
3. Osteoconduction

### Osteogenesis

*It is defined as development of bone, formation of bone.*

*—GPT, 8th Edition.*

- This process involves formation and development of bone with the help of viable cells in the graft material.
- Osteogenic cells help in formation of bone in the soft tissues and initiates active bone growth in bony areas **(Fig. 29.10)**.
- For example, autogenous graft.

### Osteoinduction

*It is defined as the capability of chemicals, procedures, etc. to induce bone formation through the differentiation and recruitment of osteoblasts.*

*—GPT, 8th Edition*

- This process involves in stimulating osteogenesis by inducing osteoblasts from the surrounding tissues to

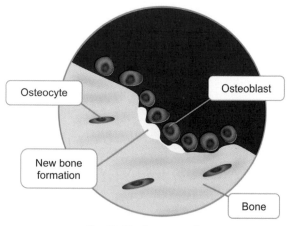

**Fig. 29.10:** Osteogenesis.

form bone by providing a biologic stimulus such as proteins or growth factors
- It aids in formation of bone even in those sites where usually bone is not present.

## Osteoconduction

- This process involves in providing scaffold or physical matrix for growth of new bone
- These graft materials themselves do not produce bone, but they aid in providing matrix for new bone formation
- They require existing bone or differentiated mesenchymal cells for formation of bone
- For example, alloplast materials.

*Ideal requirement of bone graft materials:*

- It should be biocompatible
- It should be easy to fabricate
- It should be shaped intraoperatively
- It should be inexpensive
- It should be osteoinductive, osteoconductive
- It should be sterilized
- It should possess marginal integrity over longer duration.

### Classification of Bone Augmentation Materials

On the basis of the type of materials used.
- Bone grafts
- Bone graft substitutes (with or without biological constituents).

#### Bone Grafts

- Autogenous graft
- Allografts
- Xenografts.

#### Bone Graft Substitutes

- *Ceramics*:
  - Calcium phosphates
  - Bioactive glasses and glass ceramics
  - Calcium sulfates
  - Calcium aluminates.
- *Polymers*:
  - Polymethyl methacrylate
  - Lactic/glycolic acid.
- *Natural materials*:
  - Collagen
  - Demineralized bone matrix
  - Bone morphogenic proteins.

## BONE GRAFTS

Bone grafts are used to augment bone in the areas which are deficient of bone. These grafts can be of the following types:
- Autogenous graft
- Allograft
- Alloplasts, xenograft.

### Autogenous Bone Graft

- It is also called as *autografts*
- These bone graft materials are transferred from one site to another site within the same individual
- They are considered *gold standard* by which all other graft material is compared as they possess all the desirable properties
- Because of *absence of antigenicity* they have excellent biocompatibility
- They can be cortical or cancellous or combination of both
- *Cancellous grafts* revascularize faster because of their spongy nature as compared to the cortical graft. Revascularization starts from 5th day onward.

**CLINICAL SIGNIFICANCE**

This type of graft is weak initially but thereafter continues to regain strength.

- In *cortical grafts* considerable resorption occurs because of the osteoclastic activity before osteoblastic bone formation

**CLINICAL SIGNIFICANCE**

Cortical grafts are stronger initially but weaken over a period of time, thereafter regaining its strength.

- Grafted autogenous bone heals into growing bone by all three mechanisms of bone formation
- Autogenous grafts can be harvested from both *intraoral site* and *extraoral sites* depending on the requirements
- For smaller defects intraoral sites are preferred. Common intraoral sites are chin, retromolar area, ramus of the mandible, third molar area
- Common extraoral site is iliac crest, and rib crest
- Bone harvesting is done using trephine burs or surgical bone traps
- Graft when placed into the defect should be stable and closely adapted
- Graft stability is enhanced by using a membrane, e.g. GBR (guided bone regeneration).

### Limitations

- Need for second operative site
- Difficulty in obtaining adequate amount of graft material
- Morbidity associated with the graft material.

## Allograft

- Also called as *allogenic, homologous* or *homografts* (**Figs 29.11A and B**)
- Graft material obtained from *another individual* of the *same* species
- This type of graft material closely matches the recipient in architecture and constituting elements
- Graft material is harvested from cadavers and is processed and sterilized
- They are available in different shapes such as particulate, thin cortical plates, sheets or large blocks of bone
- The mechanism of bone regeneration is primarily osteoconduction
- This type of bone acts as scaffold for bone regeneration and is resorbable
- Allografts are available as demineralized freeze-dried bone allografts (DFDBAs), mineralized freeze dried bone allograft (FDBA).

### Limitations

- Problem of antigenicity
- Potential for transmission of diseases.

## Xenografts

- Also called as *heterografts* or *xenogeneic* grafts
- These graft materials are derived from *different species*
- Usually they are bovine in origin
- Bovine bone mineral grafts can be used for onlay grafting procedures
- They can be used along with barrier membranes in augmenting infrabony pockets.

- It can be used in rebuilding atrophic alveolar ridges when supported with titanium meshes
- Successful use in sinus elevation procedure has been well documented
- Bio-Oss is bovine bone in which the organic component is completely removed to form a mineralized bone architecture.

### Limitations

- These are nonimmunogenic
- Chances of trans-species infection.

## BONE GRAFT SUBSTITUTES

These are alloplastic material. These are synthetically derived materials which are inert with very limited or negligible osteoinductive activity (**Figs. 29.12A to E**).

- These materials can be resorbable or nonresorbable
- They are supplied as various pore sizes or particle sizes
- They can be combined with bioactive proteins to provide osteoinduction
- For example, hydroxyapatite, coral and algae derived hydroxyapatite, calcium phosphates, calcium sulfate, collagen and polymers.

*Benefits of alloplasts:*
- Absence of antigenicity
- Potential for disease transmission is negligible
- Abundant supply.

## Ceramics

The most commonly used bioactive materials in implant dentistry are ceramic-based materials.

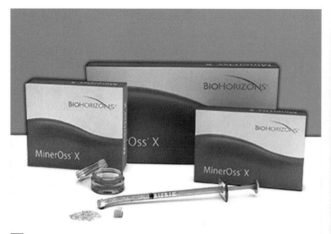

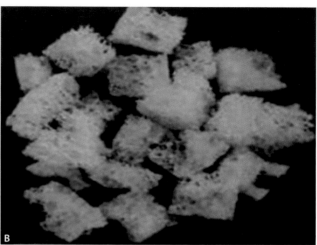

**Figs. 29.11A and B:** Allograft materials.

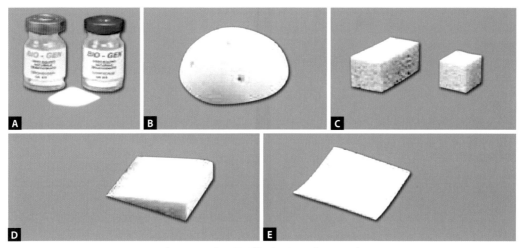

**Figs. 29.12A to E:** Alloplastic graft materials.

## Classification of Ceramics as Bone Graft Substitutes

Ceramic materials can be divided into two types:
1. *Bioactive ceramics,* e.g. hydroxyapatite, bioglass, beta tricalcium phosphate, etc.—these materials exhibit chemical contact with the host bone.
2. *Bioinert ceramics,* e.g. aluminum oxide, titanium oxide, etc.—these materials do not bond directly to the bone but are mechanically held in contact with the host bone.

### General Properties

- The ceramic biomaterials are osteoconductive materials where new bone formation occurs along their surfaces
- They are alloplastic graft materials
- These materials are used in augmentation of the resorbed ridges and reconstruction of the osseous defects
- They provide a scaffold or matrix to enhance new bone formation. These materials themselves are not capable of forming new bone
- They have excellent biocompatibility
- They exhibit good compressive strength and poor tensile strength similar to the property of the bone
- On account of poor tensile strength their use is limited to low stress bearing regions
- They are available in different shapes, sizes and textures and the particles can be amorphous or crystalline
- *Aluminum oxides* are considered as *gold standard* for ceramic implants due to its inertness and no evidence of ion release. *Zirconia* has also shown high inertness but possess less wettability than aluminum oxide. These ceramic implant materials are *not bioactive* as they do not promote bone formation. They have high strength, stiffness and hardness. Most commonly used as subperiosteal or transosteal implants.

### Hydroxyapatite

- *Calcium phosphates* are most commonly and successfully used as bone augmenting and grafting material
- Commonly used calcium phosphates are *hydroxyapatite and tricalcium phosphates.* These materials are *bioactive* as they aid in formation of new bone and promotes bond between the implant and the bone
- Hydroxyapatite is mineral which is primarily inorganic having composition similar to bone and teeth **(Fig. 29.13)**:
    - Chemical formula is $Ca_{10}(PO_4)_6(OH)_2$
    - Bovine derived hydroxyapatites are highly biocompatible and readily bonds with adjacent hard and soft tissues
    - Its mechanism of bone regeneration is osteoconduction. They are bioactive and biodegradable ceramics
    - Its physical and chemical properties determine the clinical application and the rate of resorption.

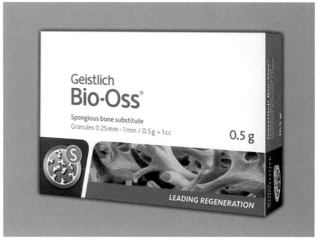

**Fig. 29.13:** Hydroxyapatite crystals.

- As compared to smaller particles, large particles resorps slowly and are present for longer duration at the augmentation site
- Similarly, an amorphous graft resorbs faster as compared to the crystalline grafts
- Limitation of porous ceramics is that their strength decreases as the porosity of the graft increases
- Hydroxyapatite crystals are used for augmenting alveolar ridges and for filling osseous defects
- Solid dense bone particles possess high compressive strength but are brittle and are therefore used in low stress bearing areas.

## Bio-Oss

- It is bovine derived inorganic bone matrix material. Bovine bone is chemically treated to remove its organic component **(Fig. 29.14)**
- Mechanism of bone regeneration is osteoconduction. It undergoes physiologic remodeling to get incorporated in the surrounding bone.

### CLINICAL SIGNIFICANCE

For smaller defects, it can be used alone. It is commonly used in treating periodontal defects, in dehiscence and fenestrations around the implant and in small sinus osteotomies.

For treating large defects, it is combined with autogenous bone for successful augmentation. It is commonly used in sinus lift procedures.

- Pepgen-15 (P15) is a synthetic peptide which mimics the cell binding capacity of type I collagen. Studies show the materials coated with P-15 shows enhanced bone formation in shorter period of time as compared to inorganic bovine bone and DFDBA material.

## Bioglass

- They comprise of calcium and phosphate salts (CaO and $P_2O_5$) similar to that found in bone and teeth and have sodium salts with silicon ($Na_2O$ and $SiO_2$) which aids in mineralization of the bone **(Fig. 29.15)**
- These are bioactive ceramics as they stimulate formation of new bone
- The bioactivity level of bioglass is high; therefore the process of osteogenesis starts soon after implantation
- Mechanism of bone regeneration is osteoinductive. They are brittle in nature and are used in low stress bearing areas
- They are primarily used for ridge augmentation or bony defects
- Their interfacial bond strength with metal and other ceramic substrates are weak and are subjected to dissolution
- However, they have unique property to bond both with the bone and the soft connective tissues
- PerioGlas is a synthetic particulate form of BioGlass that is used to treat the infrabony defects.

## Tricalcium Phosphates

- It is similar to hydroxyapatite **(Fig. 29.16)**
- Mechanism of bone regeneration is osteoconductive and provides a scaffold that is needed for deposition of new bone
- They can be combined with osteogenic or osteoinductive material to improve handling characteristics of graft during placement
- They have been shown to have no adverse effect on cell morphology, viability and cell count
- For example, Cerasorb is a beta-tricalcium phosphate material.

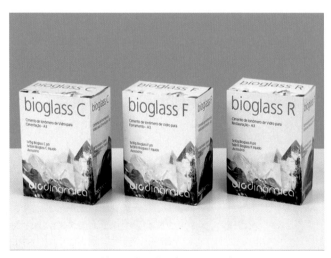

**Fig. 29.14:** Bio-Oss graft material.    **Fig. 29.15:** Bioglass material.

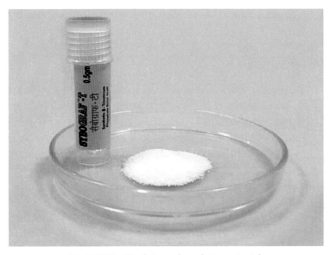

**Fig. 29.16:** Tricalcium phosphate material.

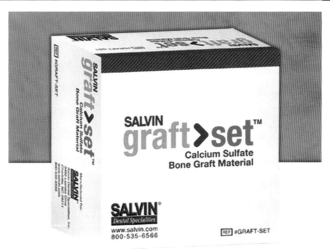

**Fig. 29.17:** Calcium sulfate bone graft material.

## Calcium Sulfate

- Commonly used along with DFDBA for bone regeneration **(Fig. 29.17)**
- When medical grade calcium sulfate is mixed with DFDBA using a diluent it forms a moldable plaster which can be molded in desired shape in presence of blood
- They are used immediately after implant placement around the implants
- As they are adhesive in nature, sutures are not required. It dissolves in approximately 30 days without causing any inflammatory reaction.

### Advantages of Bioactive Materials

- Are highly biocompatible
- Composition similar to bone
- Capable of bonding to both the hard and soft tissues
- Minimal thermal and electrical conductivity
- Possess similar modulus of elasticity as the bone
- Has similar color to the bone.

### Disadvantages of Bioactive Materials

- Has low tensile strength and shear strength and use limited to low stress bearing areas
- Has relatively low attachment strength
- Solubilities are variable depending on the product and its clinical application.

## BIOCOMPATIBILITY OF DENTAL IMPLANTS

- Biocompatibility of synthetic substances which are used for replacement or augmentation of biological tissues has always been a critical issue

- The critical aspect of biocompatibility is dependent on intrinsic nature of material and its surface properties
- According to ADA provision for accepting dental implant materials are—adequate strength, ease of fabrication and sterilization without degrading of material, biocompatible, free from defects and minimum two clinical trials each with minimum 50 human subjects conducted for 3 years
- Metallic implant materials are more susceptible to electrochemical degradation than ceramics
- Implant materials can corrode and wear resulting in formation of submicron sized debris which may elicit local or systemic biologic response. Local accumulation of debris around the implants can result in metallosis or tissue discoloration
- Implant material should not affect the local tissues and organ function
- Principal factor in selection of implant material is its response to bone
- Therefore, success of dental implants is influenced by surface characteristics of implant, site of placement and implant-bone interface.

## BIOMECHANICS IN DENTAL IMPLANTS

Dental implants are subjected to wide range of complex forces in multiple directions. Complete osseointegration of implant ensures transfer of stresses with minimal relative movement between bone and the implant. Stresses generated are greatly influenced by following factors:
- Masticatory factors—frequency of mastication, amount of bite force, mandibular movements
- Type of support to the prosthesis—implant supported, implant—tissue supported or implant tooth supported

- Properties of the materials—ductility, fracture strength, fatigue, modulus of elasticity, etc.

## Biomechanical Considerations

### Implant Design

- Smooth sided, cylindrical implants results in greater shear stress at the bone implant interface. Shear stress can be reduced by coating the surface with hydroxyapatite or plasma spray
- Whereas tapered implants with a taper not more than 30° provides greater component of compressive load at the bone-implant interface and provides ease of surgical placement
- Threaded implants have unique ability to convert the type of load imposed at the bone implant surface by controlling the thread geometry
- Thread geometry parameters which are of importance are—thread depth, pitch and its shape
- Greater the depth of the thread, greater will the functional surface area of the implant. Similarly if the thread pitch is greater, then lesser the number of threads per unit length and thus lesser the functional surface area
- Shape of the thread can be square, V shaped or buttress shaped
- Square threads experiences least amount of shear stress as compared to V-shaped or buttress-shaped threads
- Thread design of implant can influence the bone turnover rate, i.e. the remodeling of bone during occlusal load conditions.

### Length of Implant

- Greater the length of the implant, greater will be the surface area available for function
- Longer implants provide greater stability to lateral loading conditions

- Longer implants are recommended in poor quality bone.

### Diameter of Implant

- Wider diameter implants has greater bone to implant contact with greater surface area. This aids in better stress distribution
- Larger the width of the implant, more closely it is able to match the emergence profile of the natural tooth.

### Number of Implants

- Greater the number of implants, greater will be the distribution of occlusal load and lesser will the stress at the bone implant interface
- More number of implants reduces the cantilever length which reduces the overall stress to the bone.

### Occlusal Loading

- For effective stress distribution, occlusal table should be small and there should be no posterior offset loads. As much as possible forces should be directed along the long axis of the implant bodies
- Bone is ideally suited to bear axially directed compressive force rather than shear or tensile forces. If implant is placed at an angle, there will be greater angled load which will result in greater crestal bone loss
- Premature contact should always be eliminated because it increases the duration and magnitude of occlusal load to the implant body and the surrounding bone
- For a patient with parafunctional habit, occlusal scheme should be selected which will minimize occlusal trauma to the bone
- Occlusal overloading will result in failure of implants because of crestal bone loss, prosthetic failure or peri-implantitis.

---

# TEST YOURSELF

## Essay Questions

1. Classify dental implants. Discuss biocompatibility and biofunctionality of dental implants.
2. Describe various methods of surface treatments of implants.
3. Discuss various ceramic-based materials used in implants.
4. Classify various graft materials. Write in detail autogenous graft materials.
5. Describe the mechanism of bone augmentation.

6. Classify various materials used in implants. Write in detail about titanium and its alloys used in implant.
7. Enumerate parts of implant. Write in detail about abutments.

## Short Notes

1. Osseointegration.
2. Healing in implants.
3. Success criteria of implants.
4. Endosseous implants.
5. Biomechanics of implants.

## Multiple Choice Questions

1. Which of the material is not used as implant material?
   A. Stainless steel
   B. Pure titanium
   C. Nickel-chromium
   D. Cobalt-chromium
2. Which of the following is an acceptable definition of osseointegration?
   A. Bone growth through the hole in the implant by the formation of new bone in intimate contact
   B. Placement of implant directly within a bony structure
   C. Stabilization of an implant by the formation of new bone in intimate contact
   D. Intimate contact between connective tissue and implant resulting in bonding
3. All is true about bioactive implant material, *except*:
   A. Ceramic
   B. Stronger than steel
   C. Chemically bonds to bone
   D. Similar stiffness as bone
4. Hydroxyapatite is coated on the surface of implants to:
   A. To ensure strong union between the implant and the bone
   B. To improve bone growth at the surface of implant
   C. To improve esthetic of metallic implant
   D. To increase biocompatibility of the metal implant
5. The most common metal used in implants is:
   A. Titanium
   B. Stainless steel
   C. Gold
   D. Silver
6. Implants can be used to support which type of prosthesis:
   A. Single crowns
   B. Removable partial dentures
   C. Fixed partial dentures
   D. All of the above
7. Implants are cleaned by:
   A. Carbon steel curettes
   B. Ultrasonic tip
   C. Plastic curettes and scalers
   D. Air polishing system
8. Implant patient should visit dentists for maintenance every:
   A. 3 months
   B. 6 months
   C. 9 months
   D. 12 months

## ANSWERS

| 1. C | 2. C | 3. B | 4. B |
| 5. A | 6. D | 7. C | 8. A |

## BIBLIOGRAPHY

1. Al Ruhaimi KA. Bone graft substitutes: a comparative qualitative histologic review of current osteoconductive grafting materials. Int J Oral Maxillofac Implants. 2001;16:105-14.
2. Al-Sawai AA, Labib H. Success of immediate loading implants compared to conventionally-loaded implants: a literature review. J Investig Clin Dent. 2016;7:217-24.
3. Albrektsson T, Zarb G, Worthington P, Eriksson RA. The long-term efficacy of currently used dental implants: a review and proposed criteria of success. Int J Oral Maxillofac Implants. 1986;1:11-25.
4. Anusavice KJ. Phillips' Science of Dental Materials, 11th edition. St Louis, Missouri: Elsevier Publications; 2004.
5. Baltag I, Watanabe K, Kusakari H, Taguchi N, Miyakawa O, Kobayashi M, et al. Long-term changes of hydroxyapatite coated dental implants. J Biomed Mater Res. 2000;53:76-85.
6. Branemark PI, Zarb GA, Albrektsson T. Tissue integrated Prosthesis: Osseointegration in Clinical Dentistry. Chicago: Quintessence Publishing Co.; 1987.
7. Brunski JB. Biomechanics of oral implants: future research directions. J Dent Educ. 1988;52:755-87.
8. Butz SJ, Huys LW. Long-term success of sinus augmentation using a synthetic alloplast: a 20 patients, 7 years clinical report. Implant Dent. 2005;14:36-42.
9. Ducheyne P. Bioceramics: material characteristics versus in vivo behavior. J Biomed Mater Res App Biomat. 1987;21:219-36.
10. El Ghannam A. Bone reconstruction: from bioceramics to tissue engineering. Expert Rev Med Devices. 2005;2:87-101.
11. Garg AK. Bone biology, harvesting, grafting for dental implants. Rationale and clinical applications. Chicago: Quintessence Publishing Co.; 2004.
12. Grandi T, Garuti G, Guazzi P, et al. Survival and success rates of immediately and early loaded implants: 12-month results from a multicentric randomized clinical study. J Oral Implantol. 2012;38:239-49.
13. Healy KE, Ducheyne P. The mechanisms of passive dissolution of titanium in a model physiological environment. J Biomed Mater Res. 1992;26:319-38.
14. Hoexter DL. Bone regeneration graft materials. J Oral Implantol. 2002;28:290-4.
15. Ichikawa T, Hanawa T, Ukai H, et al. Three-dimensional bone response to commercially pure titanium, hydroxyapatite and calcium-ion-missing titanium in rabbits. Int J Oral Maxillofac Implants. 2000;15:231-8.
16. Jarcho M. Biomaterial aspects of calcium phosphates. Properties and applications. Dent Clin North Am. 1986;30:25-47.
17. Lacefield WR. Materials characteristics for uncoated/ceramic coated implant materials. Adv Dent Res. 1999;13:21-6.
18. Lautenschlager EP, Monaghan P. Titanium and titanium alloys as dental materials. Int Dent J. 1993;43:245-53.
19. Lee JJ, Rouhfar L, Beirne OR. Survival of hydroxyapatite-coated implants: a meta-analytic review. J Oral Maxillofac Surg. 2000;58:1372-9.
20. Lemons J, Natiella J. Biomaterials, biocompatibility, and peri-implant considerations. Dent Clin North Am. 1986;30:3-23.

21. Misch CE, Dietsh F. Bone grafting materials in implant dentistry. Implant Dent. 1993;2:158-67.

22. Precheur HV. Bone graft materials. Dent Clin North Am. 2007;51:729-46.

23. Rangert B, Jemt T, Jörneus L. Forces and moments on Branemark implants. Int J Oral Maxillofac Implants. 1989;4:241-7.

24. Schepers Nej, Ducheyne P, Barbier L, et al. Bioactive glass particles of narrow size range: a new material for the repair of bone defects. Implant Dent. 1993;2:151-6.

25. Skalak R. Biomechanical considerations in osseointegrated prosthesis. J Prosthet Dent. 1983;49:843-9.

26. Smith D. Dental implants: materials and design considerations. Int J Prosthodont. 1993;6:106-17.

27. Sohn BS, Heo SJ, Koak JY, et al. Strain of implants depending on occlusion types in mandibular implant-supported fixed prosthesis. J Adv Prosthodont. 2011;3:1-9.

28. Tagliareni JM, Clarkson E. Basic concepts and techniques of dental implants. Dent Clin North Am. 2015;59:255-64.

29. Thalji G, Bryington M, Kok I, et al. Prosthodontic management of implant therapy. Dent Clin North Am. 2014;58:207-25.

30. Thompson DM, Rohrer MD, Prasad HS. Comparison of bone grafting materials in human extraction sockets: clinical, histologic and histomorphometric evaluations. Implant Dent. 2006;15:89-96.

31. Vult von Steyern P, Kokubo Y, Nilner K. Use of abutment-teeth vs dental implants to support all-ceramic fixed partial dentures: an in-vitro study on fracture strength. Swed Dent. 2005;29:53-60.

32. Zuffetti F, Esposito M, Galli F, et al. A 10-year report from a multicentre randomised controlled trial: Immediate non-occulsal versus early loading of dental implants in partially edentulous patients. Eur J Oral Implantol. 2016;9:219-30.

# Latest Trends in Material Science

*'The real voyage of discovery consists not in seeking new landscapes but in having new eyes.'*

—*Marcel Proust*

## INTRODUCTION

Dental material is an ever-evolving branch of dentistry because of continuous research in this field for a quest to develop an ideal material. Lookout for ideal biomaterial is mainly focused on prevention and treatment of dental caries, periodontal disease and oral cancer. There are number of recent development in dental science which have changed the way dentistry will be practiced in the years to come. It is, therefore, important to have an understanding of the recent trends in material science.

## REQUIREMENTS FOR IDEAL BIOMATERIAL

The focus of ideal biomaterial is to prevent dental caries and periodontal disease. At the same time contribute to rehabilitation of missing, damaged and destroyed hard and soft tissues.

Ideal biomaterial should:

- Be nontoxic, nonirritating to the oral tissues
- Be toxic to microorganism including virus and fungi
- Form excellent seal between the tooth structure and the restorative material
- Be bioactive to simulate in vivo repair or replacement of tissues
- Have similar properties to the tissues to be replaced
- Allow easy manipulation
- Have long clinical success
- Have excellent esthetics.

## SMART MATERIALS

Traditionally materials such as amalgam, composites and cements were designed which did not interact with the oral environment and were passively in contact with the oral structures for years. Change of concept of these "passive" materials with "active materials" started with the realization of the benefit of fluoride releasing materials. Research on these active materials lead to interest in "smart" materials.

*Smart materials are those materials whose properties can be altered in a controlled manner by stimulus such as stress, temperature, moisture, pH, electric or magnetic fields.* Some of "smart materials" available are:

- *Zirconia ceramics*: These ceramic materials transform from a tetragonal to monoclinic crystal form when tensile stress is induced at the crack site resulting in increase in crystal volume and compressive stress which aids in preventing crack propagation
- *Smart composites*: Polymerized with particular wavelength of blue light; another type is composite cement used in orthodontics which change color when polymerized

- *Glass ionomer cement*: This type when desiccated weakens and is easier to remove the orthodontic bands
- *Glass ionomer restoratives*: Increases the release of fluorides when pH in the plaque reduces
- *Nickel-titanium wires*: These are shape memory alloys used in orthodontics
- Glass ionomer cement having thermo-responsive smart behavior—heating or cooling of these materials will result in minimal dimensional change as expected change in dimension will be compensated by the movement of water in or out of the structure
- *Smart sealing materials* help in sealing marginal crevices of the defective restoration with a hydrophilic resin capable of releasing controlled amount of chlorhexidine or other antibacterial agent
- *Smart sealing varnish* helps in controlled release of xylitol or other caries preventive agents
- *Smart anesthesia* will rapidly induce anesthesia when it is applied in the sulcus and an external stimuli can start or stop the anesthetic reaction

## ZIRCONIA IMPLANTS AND ABUTMENTS

The ceramic implant was first placed in US and Germany in 1970s as a joint substitute. Ceramic has been used for manufacturing of dental implants because of its high biocompatibility, inert nature, high strength, low thermal and electrical conductivity and esthetics. Traditionally ceramic materials have limitations because of low ductility and brittleness and their use is confined as calcium phosphate coatings of endosteal and subperiosteal implants and in dental reconstructive surgery.

Recently, yttria stabilized zirconia (Y-TZP) is introduced as endosseous implant material with benefits such as enhanced biocompatibility, increased strength, greater radiopactiy and easier handling at the time of abutment preparation (**Fig. 30.1**). The osseointegration potential of Y-TZP is comparable to that of titanium implants. The zirconia ceramics have better mechanical stability and are well tolerated by bone and soft tissues. Study by Kohal et al. reveals that yttria-partially stabilized zirconia has similar stress distribution as compared to commercially pure Ti implants. Single piece zirconia implants have better clinical acceptability as compared to two piece zirconia implants.

- Zirconia implant abutments are manufactured as replacement to alumina abutments because of enhanced biocompatibility, metal like radiopacity, reduced plaque accumulation and inflammation risk. These abutments are available as either prefabricated or custom made forms. They can be milled in laboratory by CAD-CAM technology. Their primary benefit is esthetics and strength. They are indicated in areas where there is limited gingival tissue height (**Fig. 30.2**).

## LASERS IN DENTISTRY

The term "laser" means "light activation by stimulated emission of radiation".

*Definition: It is a device that transforms light of various frequencies into an intense, small, and nearly nondivergent beam of monochromatic radiation, within the visible range.*
—*GPT 8th Edition*

The use of lasers in dentistry are gaining popularity in the treatment of hard and soft tissues. Some lasers commonly used in dentistry based on their active medium wavelength,

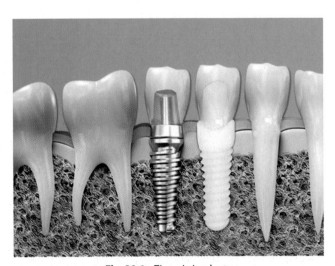

**Fig. 30.1:** Zirconia implants.

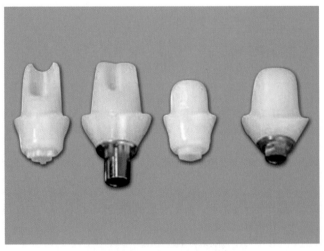

**Fig. 30.2:** Zirconia abutments.

delivery system, emission mode, tissue absorption and clinical applications are argon, diode, neodymium: YAG (neodymium-doped yttrium aluminium garnet), holmium: YAG, $CO_2$ and erbium lasers **(Fig. 30.3)**.

## Historical Development

- *1960*: First laser used
- *1993*: Nd:YAG laser used
- *1993*: Kinetic cavity preparation
- *1994*: $CO_2$ laser and argon lasers introduced
- *1996*: Laser welder
- *1997*: Nd:YAP laser introduced
- *1998*: Er:YAG (erbium-doped yttrium aluminium garnet) laser used.

## Applications of Lasers in Dentistry

### Periodontics

*Nonosseous gingival surgery:*
- Frenectomy
- Gingivectomy

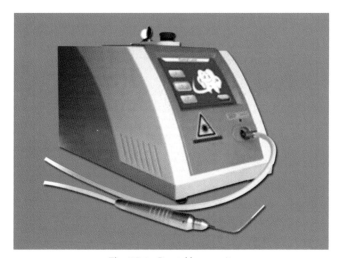

- Free gingival graft procedures
- Gingival depigmentation
- Operculectomy.

*Periodontal regeneration surgery:*
- Osseous recontouring
- Removal of granulomatous tissue
- De-epithelialization.

### Prosthodontics

- Soft tissue or hard tissue removal during crown lengthening procedure **(Figs. 30.4A to C)**
- Creation of site to receive ovate pontic
- Soft tissue contouring during veneer preparation
- Removal of veneers
- Vestibuloplasty
- Management of gingival hyperplasia
- Tuberosity reduction
- Removal of tori
- Soft tissue modifications
- Treatment of epulis fissuratum, denture stomatitis
- Used for welding.

### Implantology

- Second stage surgery
- For treating peri-implantitis cases.

### Oral Surgery

- Biopsy
- Operculectomy
- Apicoectomy
- Treatment of mucositis
- Oral soft tissue pathologies.

### Operative Dentistry and Endodontics

- Caries removal
- Treatment of dental hypersensitivity

**Fig. 30.3:** Dental laser unit.

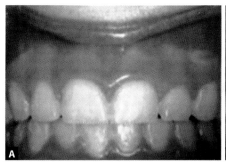
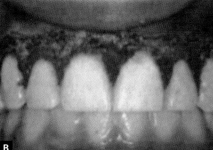
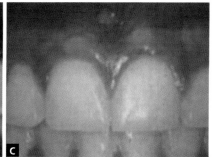

**Figs. 30.4A to C:** Crown lengthening procedure using lasers.

- Cavity preparation
- Teeth bleaching
- Cleaning and shaping of root canal
- Pulp diagnosis through laser Doppler flowmetry
- Endodontic surgery.

### *Advantages of Lasers*

- Provides dry surgical field and increases visibility
- Reduces postoperative swelling, edema and scarring
- Sterilization of the surgical field
- Reduces postoperative pain
- Increased coagulation and reduced mechanical trauma
- Minimizes chances of bacteremia.

### *Disadvantages of Lasers*

- Delayed healing of tissues because of sealing of blood vessels and lymphatics
- Cost of equipment
- Technique sensitive.

## NANOTECHNOLOGY IN DENTISTRY

The word "nano" means 10 to the minus ninth power or one billionth. The concept of nanotechnology was advocated by *Prof Kerie E Drexler*. The word "nano" means "dwarf" in Greek. Nanotechnology is developed at three levels namely, (1) materials, (2) devices and (3) an environment or system. Nanomaterials are the most advanced and developed level.

*Nanodentistry* involves the use of nanomaterial, including tissue engineering and dental nanorobots to maintain comprehensive oral health care.

### CLINICAL SIGNIFICANCE

*Nanorobots* will have potential to induce oral analgesia, desensitize teeth, manipulate teeth to realign and straighten irregular sets of teeth thereby improving longevity of teeth.

There are two approaches in using nanodentistry namely:
1. Bottom-up approach.
2. Top-down approach.

### Bottom-up Approach

#### *Nanoanesthesia*

Administration of local anesthesia is one of the most common procedures in dentistry. Nanoanesthesia is induced by instilling millions of microsized dental robots containing active analgesic component on the oral mucosa. As this anesthesia contacts the tooth surface or mucosal surface, the mobile nanorobots reach the pulp tissue through the dentinal tubules, lamina propria or gingival sulcus. They completely anesthetize the tooth on receiving signals from the clinician. After completion of the procedure the dentist again directs the nanorobots to restore all sensations in the particular tooth by egressing from the tooth via the same pathway as they entered.

### *Dentin Hypersensitivity*

The dentin hypersensitivity is relieved by directing the dental nanorobots to specifically target the exposed dentinal tubules and occlude them.

### *Nanorobotic Dentifrice (Dentifrobots)*

The use of dentifrobots will lead to recognition and destruction of the pathogens that causes tooth caries. They will be delivered by either mouthwash or toothpaste and will inhibit the formation of plaque thereby eliminating halitosis and calculus formation.

### *Tooth Durability*

The tooth durability and its appearance can be improved by replacing the enamel layers with harder materials such as sapphire or diamond. Although these materials improve the properties and esthetics of the tooth but they are brittle and are prone for fracture. They can be made more resistant by incorporating carbon nanotubes.

### *Nanorobots for Orthodontic Treatment*

Commonly called as orthodontic nanorobots which can aid in reducing the time of treatment by rapidly making tooth movement in order to align the teeth **(Fig. 30.5)**.

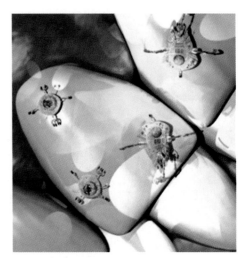

**Fig. 30.5:** Nanorobots in action.

## Decay Resistant Teeth

Nanotechnology can be used to protect any surface or teeth from dental caries. This protection is enabled by polishing teeth with silica which is made from nanoparticles. These materials are about 90,000 times smaller than a grain of sand.

## Top-down Approach

### Nanocomposites

Nanocomposites are nanoparticles which are uniformly present in the resins. These materials have superior mechanical and esthetic properties. As compared to conventional composites they have superior hardness, greater rigidity, greater wear resistance and superior esthetics. Nanocomposites will be restorative material of the future **(Fig. 30.6)**. Currently microhybrid and nanofilled composites have filler particles in the range of 20–600 nm.

### Nanobonds/Nanosolution

These are nanoparticles which are dispersed in the bonding agents uniformly. They have superior bond strength **(Fig. 30.7)**.

### Nanoimpression

These nanoimpression materials are polyvinyl siloxane materials, which are having nanofiller particles. They have superior hydrophilic properties, better flow and greater detail reproduction than the conventional polysiloxane materials **(Fig. 30.8)**.

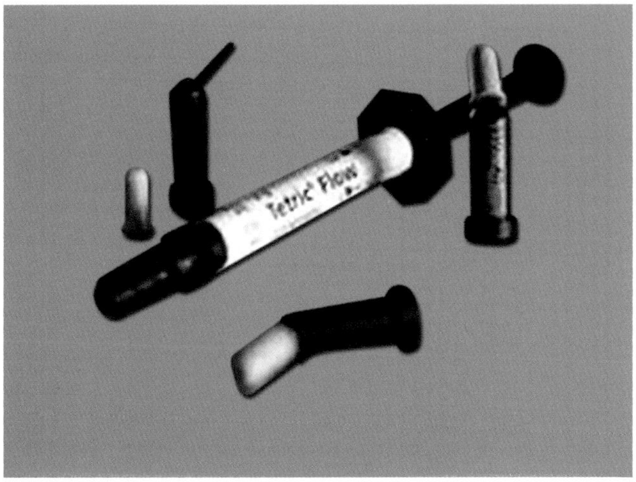

### Nanoneedles

Nanosized suture needles are developed which will aid in surgical procedure for better wound closure.

### Bone Augmentation Materials

Osseous defects can be treated using hydroxyapatite nanoparticles, e.g. Ostim, Vitoss, and NanOss.

### Nanoimplants

Currently endosseous dental implants are introduced whose surface is having nanoscale topography. This surface has capability to alter cellular and tissue response in favor of implant treatment. Presently three nanoscale topography are in use:

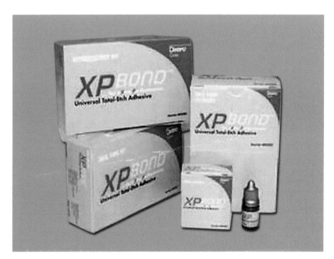

**Fig. 30.7:** Nanosolution used for bonding.

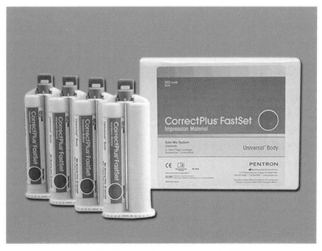

**Fig. 30.8:** Nanoimpression material.

**Fig. 30.6:** Nanocomposites.

1. *Diamond*: It improves hardness, toughness and reduces friction.
2. *Hydroxyapatite*: Increases osteoblast adhesion, proliferation and mineralization.
3. *Graded metalloceramics*: Capable of overcoming adhesion issues.

### Surface Disinfectant

A product developed through nanotechnology called *EcoTrue* is used as surface disinfectant which kills almost 100% HIV viruses and other particles. It is effectively used to sterilize tools and incisions, preventing postoperative infections.

## BIOMIMETIC MATERIALS

Biomimetic refers to the potential ability of the material to mimic nature. It is area of research which deals with study of formation, structure and function of biologically produced substances and materials (e.g. silk and conch shells) and biological mechanisms and processes (such as protein synthesis) for the purpose of synthesizing similar products by artificial mechanisms that mimic natural ones.

*Biomimetic materials:* These are those materials which mimic structures occurring in nature, particularly those that involve self-assembly of components of form, replace, or repair oral tissues (Saunders 2009).

*Natural biomimetic materials* such as alginate (derived from sea weeds) and silk (produced by silkworms) are used as biomaterials.

Collagen is a natural biomimetic material which has triple helix structure and exists in fibril form. It is one of the most commonly found protein materials. It is extensively investigated for its use as biomaterial on account of its cross-linking ability, low antigenicity and high tensile strength. The self-assembling nature of the protein helps in formation of scaffold and assists in guided tissue regeneration. Other proteins such as gelatin is used as a hemostatic agent and fibrinogen is used as tissue sealant.

*Advantages of natural biomimetic material:*
- Do not evoke toxic reactions
- May contain specific protein binding sites and other biochemical signals which help in tissue healing or integration

*Disadvantages of natural biomimetic material:*
- Issue of immunogenicity
- As derived from natural source can be contaminated with microorganisms
- Difficult to sterilize
- Costly.

## SELF-ASSEMBLING MATERIALS

These materials can automatically construct into prespecified biological or non-biological entities. These entities can be derived from polymers, ceramics, metals or composites. Self-assembling occurs in three stages namely, (1) initiation, (2) propagation and (3) termination. Initiation and propagation can be controlled by stimulus such as physical, chemical, mechanical, or biological event or it can be a type of template. Bone graft or soft tissue scaffold materials are type of self-assembling material. The graft materials are in the form of coarse granules which form scaffold and encourage the biological tissues to respond and replace the scaffolding. Materials in future will be having templates of proteins to encourage a particular tissue formation **(Fig. 30.9)**.

## SELF-HEALING MATERIALS

It is also called as self-repairing materials which automatically initiate response to tissue damage or failure. These materials are required to first identify damage and then accordingly repair the damage or failure. All biomaterials have limited life period they undergo degradation gradually through process of corrosion, microleakage, dissolution, erosion or creep. Eventually the material fails and needs replacement. Natural biomaterial such as bone tissues continuously remodels lifelong and is capable of self-healing. On the basis of natural capabilities an epoxy resin with properties similar to resin composite is developed which contains microencapsulated dicyclopentadiene and Grubb's metathesis catalyst. Whenever there is a crack in this epoxy material, microcapsules gets ruptured and release dicyclopentadiene which fills the crack area. It then reacts with Grubb's catalyst to complete its polymerization. Such material has found to be very useful in the process of self-repair and is researched to be used in composite resins as well **(Fig. 30.10)**. Another approach of self-repair is control of cross-linking of polymers by changes in pH.

### CLINICAL SIGNIFICANCE
Self-healing approach in dental biomaterials will be highly useful in increasing clinical durability and improving clinical performance.

## BONE GRAFTING MATERIALS

Bone graft materials are allogenic or xenogenic particles, which act as scaffold for gradual replacement by the patient's bone. Current materials resorb slowly and bone density increases over a period of months before restorative or implant placement can be possible. However for

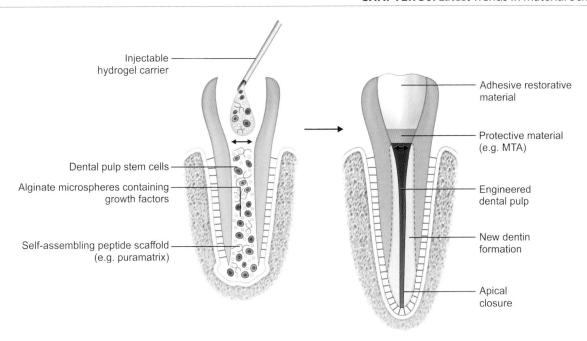

**Fig. 30.9:** Diagram to show use of self-assembling materials to build new tissues.

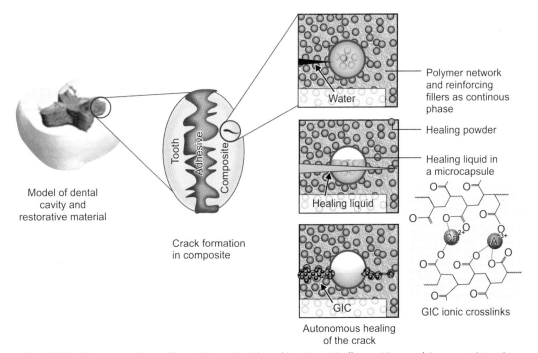

**Fig. 30.10:** Diagram to show self-repairing material used in automatically repairing crack in composite resin.

immediate loading implants faster bone growth simulating materials are needed. PepGen P-15 (Dentsply) is one such material which increases natural bone regeneration in the area of deficient bone. Another material used for sinus augmentation and local alveolar ridge augmentation is

infuse (Medtronic, Minneapolis, MN) which is a collagen sponge with recombinant human bone morphogenetic protein-2.

Bone morphogenetic proteins (BMPs) are growth factors which improve cell interactions and can alter cell behavior.

NovaBone Dental Putty (NovaBone Products, Jacksonville, FL) are used for bone grafting as they provide resorbable scaffold for bone growth.

> **CLINICAL SIGNIFICANCE**
>
> Currently newer formulations of bioactive glasses are developed to initiate osteogenesis and faster bone replacements. These newer graft materials contain more boron and silica than the Bioglass material.

## BIOACTIVE MATERIALS

These materials have the effect on or elicit a response from living tissue, organisms or cell such as inducing the formation of hydroxyapatite. They stimulate reparative dentin formation, are bactericidal and bacteriostatic, help in maintaining pulp vitality, aids in remineralization of adjacent dental tissues, enhance osseointegration on implant surface, improves bond strength and reduce microleakage.

### Uses

- Can act as scaffold and help in regeneration of bone tissues
- Promote tooth remineralization
- Can be used as permanent restorative material
- Helps in occluding dentinal tubules thereby reducing dentinal hypersensitivity
- Can be used as pulp capping agent.

Some of the bioactive materials in use in dentistry are MTA (mineral trioxide aggregate), Acitva Bioactive restorative material, Pulpdent (composite resin which releases greater fluoride than glass ionomers), MTYA1-Ca filler, tetracalcium phosphate, Sol-gel derived bioactive glass (BAG) ceramic containing silver ions, novel endodontic cement (NEC), EndoSequence Root Repair, bioactive $TiO_2$ nanoparticles, etc.

## DETECTION AND TREATMENT OF ORAL CANCER USING NANOTECHNOLOGY

Nanotechnology is used in detection of cancer in early stages which greatly improves the prognosis of the treatment. Nanoparticles which facilitate in the early detection of cancer are nanopores, nanotubes, cantilever and quantum dots **(Fig. 30.11)**.

### Cantilever Array Sensors

As evident the cancer cells produce molecular products, the cantilever sensors are coated with antibodies which

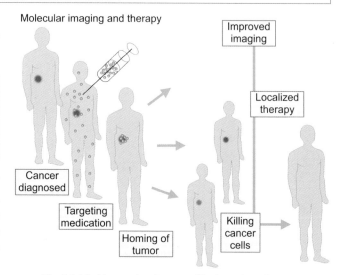

**Fig. 30.11:** Nanotechnology used in detection of cancer.

aids in detecting the presence and concentration of these products.

### Nanopore Devices

These devices aid in detecting error in genetic code which causes cancer.

### Nanotubes

Nanotubes are advanced version of nanopore device which contains carbon rods that are about half the diameter of deoxyribonucleic acid (DNA) molecule. This device not only helps in detecting the altered genetic code but also informs about its precise location. Nanotubes are differentiated from normal cells as they fluoresce under the infrared light whereas the normal cells do not show any reaction. The intensity or wavelength of the emitted Fluorescence light depends on the interaction between the DNA and the DNA disruptor.

### Quantum Dots

Another type of nanoparticles which are used in detection of oral cancer. They consist of tiny crystals which illuminate when stimulated by ultraviolet (UV) light. These particles when injected into the body will drift along until they encounter cancerous lesion. When the cancerous cells come in contact with these dots they will attach to the coating and will glow when stimulated by UV light. The glowing particles enable the clinician to detect cancerous tissues.

### Treatment of Oral Cancer

Nanoparticle dendrimer are used as drug delivery vehicles to target cancer cells. A single unit of dendrimer nanoparticle performs three functions:

1. Detect cancer cell.
2. Kill these cancer cells.
3. Identify cell death.

The nanoparticle dendrimer are basically nanoshells which have a metallic housing and a core made of silica. The amount of heat produced by infrared light to target cancer cells depends on the variable thickness of outer layer. The process of physically selecting the cancer lesions is called as *enhanced permeation retention.*

# TISSUE ENGINEERING

*Tissue engineering is a multidisciplinary approach to replace damaged or lost tissues with new tissues by using biologic materials.*

In the mid-1980s, this concept was first advocated in the United States because there was scarcity of donors for organ transplants. This concept involves placing a biodegradable scaffolds of cells containing growth factors or stem cells into the recipient site to induce growth of new tissues. The growth factors or stem cells helps in regulating the growth of tissues whereas the biodegradable scaffolds provide the necessary microenvironment for their growth.

The rationale behind tissue replacement and reconstruction is to alleviate pain and to restore mechanical stability and function. Currently, the lost tissues are replaced by using autogenous grafts, allografts or alloplasts. But all these materials are having drawbacks and limitations which results in short-term success and may require retreatment. The need is therefore to understand and use tissue engineering for replacing lost tissues in the near future.

## Approaches to Tissue Engineering

There are three major classes which are used in tissue engineering. A common feature in all these approaches are the use of polymeric materials. These are as follows:

1. *Conduction approach*: It uses biomaterials in a passive manner to facilitate growth or regenerative capacity of existing tissues. Polymeric materials used are the barrier membranes. For example, use of barrier membrane in GTR (guided tissue regeneration), Osseointegration of dental implants.
2. *Inductive approach*: This approach involves in activating normal cells next to the defect site by means of specific biological signals to induce growth of new tissues. BMPs or bone morphogenic protein is one such example which is now used widely. BMPs have successfully been used in various clinical trials for regenerating and repairing bone tissues in nonhealing fractures and periodontal diseases. In this approach the polymeric materials used are the BMPs or DNA gene which encodes the protein.

3. *Cell transplantation*: In this approach cells artificially grown in the laboratory are directly transplanted into the recipient site. This approach involves team of specialist including clinician or surgeon, bioengineer and cell biologist.

## Fundamentals of Tissue Engineering

Tissue engineering consists of three basic elements namely, cells, scaffold and biological signaling **(Fig. 30.12)**.

1. *Cells*: Stem cells or morphogens are specialized cells which have capacity of creating differentiated progenies and self-renewal. These cells help in healing and regeneration of tissues.
2. *Scaffolds*: Biodegradable frameworks which provide microenvironment for the cells to proliferate, regenerate and differentiate into new tissues. Depending on the type of tissue to be regenerated the design of scaffold is determined. Some of the materials used for scaffolds are ceramics, natural or synthetic polymers and composites. Research is currently focused on using materials which are biodegradable and bioresorbable. Ideally the scaffold material should resorb after providing a template for tissue regeneration. The rate of biodegradation should be compatible with that of new tissue formation.
3. *Cell signaling*: It is an important element of tissue engineering which governs cell activities and organizes their interactions. These elements should provide a specific biologic signals, which will help the cells to induce growth of new tissues.

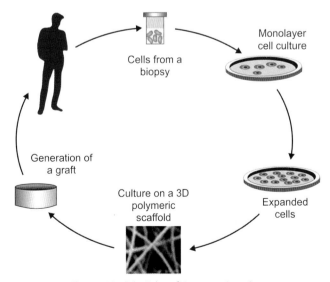

**Fig. 30.12:** Principles of tissue engineering.

## STEM CELLS

These are specialized cells which have unique ability to divide infinitely to produce new cells.

Based on the origin, stem cells are of following types:

*Embryonic stem cells:* Developed from embryos which are fertilized in vitro. These are primitive cells which are grown in the culture medium and not developed from eggs fertilized in the body.

*Embryonic germ cells:* Unlike the embryonic stem cells these cells are collected from the fetus in later stages of its development. The origin of these cells is the gonadal ridge which later on develops into sex organs. These cells have limited capacity to develop into organs as they are in the primitive stage of development.

*Adult stem cells:* These cells develop in the mature organisms are capable of repairing and maintaining the tissues. These cells are routinely used to replace blood and tissues. As they are from the same patient, chances of rejection are very low.

### Dental Stem Cells (Fig. 30.13)

In dentistry, first stem cells were isolated from the pulp tissue of adult third molar and were called as dental pulp stem cells (DPSCs). Although there are various other sites to extract dental stem cells such as dental pulp of deciduous and permanent tooth, apex of developing roots, periodontal ligament and from the dental lamina.

Dental pulp stem cells have shown to differentiate into odontoblasts, adipocytes, chondroblasts, osteoblasts and functionally active neurons. These cells have shown promise in treating various neuronal disorders.

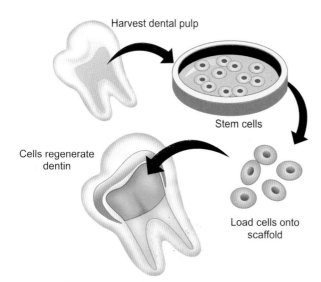

**Fig. 30.13:** Dental stem cells from dental pulp.

Stem cells from human exfoliated deciduous teeth (SHED) over the years have provided an alternative therapy to dental tissue engineering. As compared to other dental stem cells, SHED provides benefits such as:
- Higher proliferative rate
- Retrievability in disposed tissues.

Stem cells banks are available that helps in preserving SHED through cryopreservation. Long-term storage results are still not assessed and require further research.

### Periodontal Ligament Stem Cells

The periodontal ligament is made of specialized cells which are believed to contain progenitor cells which are capable of producing cementoblast like cells, adipocytes and connective tissue rich in collagen fibers.

### Stem Cell Therapies

The technology of bioengineering will be used in future to develop bioengineered filling material which will replace the lost tooth structure due to dental caries. These filling materials will be attached to the existing tooth structure in such a way that it does not directly contact the systemic system of a person thereby minimizing the risk of immune rejection.

### Tooth Regeneration

Tooth regeneration will be ultimate goal in dentistry and may become a reality in the future. It may become a method of replacing missing tooth with cell-based implant rather than the current metallic implants. Biological replacement of tooth will require formation of dental roots, periodontal ligament, pulp tissues and crown portion. This will require interaction of dental epithelial cell and mesenchymal cell progenitor cells as in the natural tooth formation. Still lot of research is required to make total tooth regeneration a reality.

## GREEN DENTISTRY

Green dentistry is an approach which aims at reducing environmental impact of dental practice and which supports and maintains wellness. It helps in protecting the community health and preserving nature. The model of EDA (Eco-Dentistry Association) is adopted on large-scale in the United States of America **(Fig. 30.14)**.

Recommendations from EDA are:
- Reduce waste and pollution
- Save water, energy and money
- Upgrade and use technology like use of digital X-rays, install amalgam separators, install energy efficient

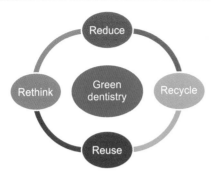

**Fig. 30.14:** Green dentistry.

lamps, use washable coats instead of disposable, use of good evacuation system, etc.

- Support wellness lifestyle
- Focus on four R's—reduce, recycle, reuse and rethink.

## EVIDENCE-BASED DENTISTRY

According to ADA evidence-based dentistry (EBD) is defined as:

*An approach to oral health care that requires the judicious integration of systematic assessments of clinically relevant scientific evidence, relating to the patient's oral and medical condition and history, with the dentist's clinical expertise and the patient's treatment needs and preferences.*

Evidence-based dentistry helps in making decision based on the currently available scientific evidence. It helps in examining and applying the relevant scientific data relating to patient's oral and medical report. It benefits the dentists as they can stay up-to-date with the latest technique and procedures and provide improved treatment to the patient **(Fig. 30.15)**. This concept was first developed by Gordon Guvatt and the Evidence-based Medicine Working Group at McMaster University in Ontario, Canada in 1990s.

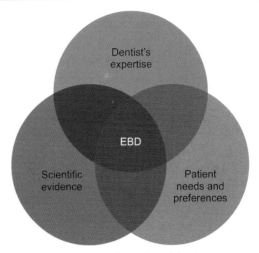

**Fig. 30.15:** Evidence-based dentistry.

Evidence-based dentistry requires the dentists to develop five key skills:

1. Collect information, by putting four part questions to identify the patient problem (P), intervention (I), Comparison (C), and outcomes (O) known as PICO questions.
2. Conduct an efficient computerized search of the literature for the appropriate type and level of evidence.
3. Critically appraise the evidence for validity with an understanding of research methods.
4. Apply the result of the evidence to patient care or practice in consideration for the patient's preferences, values and circumstances.
5. Evaluate the process and your performance through self-evaluation.

Evidence-based dentistry not only helps the dentists but also the patient in obtaining improved care and treatment. In times to come this approach will become necessary to decide the course of treatment in patient care.

## TEST YOURSELF

### Essay Questions

1. Discuss recent trends in dental material science.
2. Describe the role of tissue engineering in dentistry.

### Short Notes

1. Nanotechnology.
2. Smart materials.
3. Self-healing materials.
4. Self-assembling materials.
5. Bone grafting materials.
6. Lasers in dentistry.

7. Green dentistry.
8. Detection of oral cancers using nanotechnology
9. Biomimetic materials.

### Multiple Choice Questions

1. All except one is desirable for ideal biomaterial it should be:
   A. Nontoxic and nonirritating
   B. Nontoxic to microorganisms
   C. Be bioactive to stimulate repair of tissue
   D. Excellent seal between it and the tooth structure

2. Biomimetic materials:
   A. Helps in tissue degeneration
   B. Helps in tissue regeneration
   C. Builds scaffolds
   D. Mimics natural tissues

3. All of the following helps in detection of oral cancer, *except*:
   A. Nanotubes
   B. Quantum dots
   C. Nanopores
   D. Nanoneedles

4. Which are two approaches in nanodentistry:
   A. Bottom-up and top-down
   B. Bottom-down and top-down
   C. Bottom-down and top-up
   D. Bottom-up and top-up

## ANSWERS

| 1. B | 2. B, C and D | 3. D | 4. A |
|------|---------------|------|------|

## BIBLIOGRAPHY

1. Bayne SC. Dental biomaterials: where are we and where are we going? J Dent Educ. 2005;5:15-7.

2. Beuer F, Schweiger J, Edelhof D. Digital dentistry: an overview of recent developments for the CAD/CAM generated restorations. Br Dent J. 2008;204:505-11.

3. Chen FM, Jin Y. Periodontal tissue engineering and regeneration: current approaches and expanding opportunities. Tissue Eng Part B Rev. 2010;16:219-55.

4. Duailibi SE, Duailibi MT, Vacanti JP, Yelick PC. Prospects for tooth regeneration. Periodontol. 2000. 2006;41:177-87.

5. Ferracane JL. Materials in Dentistry: Principles and Applications, 2nd edition. Philadelphia: Lippincott Williams & Wilkins; 2001.

6. Feynman R. There's plenty of room at the bottom. Eng Sci. 1960;23:22-36.

7. Fischer H. Self-repairing material systems—a dream or reality? Nat Sci. 2010;2:873-901.

8. Garcia I, Tabak LA. A view of the future: dentistry and oral health in America. J Am Dent Assoc. 2009;140:44S-48S.

9. Hollister SJ, Murphy WL. Scaffold translation: barriers between concept and clinic. Tissue Eng. 2011;17:459-74.

10. Huang G, Yamaza T, Shea LD, Djouad F, Kuhn NZ, Tuan RS, et al. Stem/progenitor cell-mediated de novo regeneration of dental pulp with newly deposited continuous layer of dentin in an in vivo model. Tissue Eng Part A. 2010;16:605-15.

11. Lemons J, Misch-Dietsh F. Biomaterials for dental implants. In: Misch CE (Ed). Contemporary Implant Dentistry, 3rd edition. St. Louis, Mo, USA: Mosby; 2008. pp.511-42.

12. McCabe JF, Yan Z, Al Naimi OT, Mahmoud G, Rolland SL. Smart materials in dentistry-future prospects. Dent Mater. 2009;28:37-43.

13. Mitra SB, Wu D, Holmes BN. An application of nanotechnology in advanced dental materials. J Am Dent Assoc. 2003;34:1382-90.

14. Mitsiadis TA, Feki A. Papaccio G. Dental pulp stem cells, niches and notch signaling in tooth injury. Adv Dent Res. 2011;23:275.

15. Nakashiawa M, Reddi H. The application of bone morphogenic proteins to dental tissue engineering. Nature Biotech. 2003;21:1025-32.

16. Nammour S. Laser dentistry, current advantages and limits. Photomed Laser Surg. 2012;30:1-4.

17. Ozkurt Z, Kazazoglu E. Clinical success of zirconia in dental applications. J Prosthodont. 2010;19:64-8.

18. Ozkurt Z, Kazazoglu E. Zirconia dental implants: a literature review. J Oral Implantol. 2011;37:367-76.

19. Palmer LC, Newcomb CJ, Kaltz SR, Spoerke ED, Stupp SI. Biomimetic systems for hydroxyapatite mineralization inspired by bone and enamel. Chem Rev. 2008;108:4754-83.

20. Petrovic V, Stefanovic V. Dental tissue—new source for stem cells. Sci World Journal. 2009;9:1167-77.

21. Phillips RW, Keith Moore B. Elements of Dental Materials, 5th edition. Philadelphia:WB Saunders; 1995. pp. 274-8.

22. Rosa V, Della Bonaa A, Cavalcanti BN, Eduardo Nör J. Tissue engineering: from research to dental clinics. Dent Mater. 2012;28:341-8.

23. Sarvanakumar R, Vijaylakshmi R. Nanotechnology in dentistry. Ind J Dent Res. 2006;17:62-5.

24. Slavkin HC, Bartold PM. Challenges and potential in tissue engineering. Periodontol. 2006;41:9-15.

25. Strub JR, Rekow ED, Witkowski S. Computer aided design and fabrication of dental restorations: current systems and future possibilities. J Am Dent Assoc. 2006;137:1289-96.

26. Volponi AA, Pang Y, Sharpe PT. Stem cell biological tooth repair and regeneration. Trends Cell Biol. 2010;20:715-22.

27. Zandparsa R. Dental biomaterials. In: Kutz M (Ed). Biomedical Engineering and Design Handbook, 2nd edition. New York: McGraw-Hill; 2009. pp. 397-420.

28. Zandparsa R. Latest biomaterials and technology in dentistry. Dent Clin North Am. 2014;58:113-34.

# Dental Products Standard Technical Specifications

| ADA No. | Material | Year |
|---|---|---|
| ANSI/ADA Standard No. 1 | Alloy for Dental Amalgam | 2003 (Reaffirmed 2013) |
| ANSI/ADA Standard No. 2 | Dental Gypsum-bonded Casting Investments | 1987 (Reaffirmed 2002) |
| ANSI/ADA Standard No.3 | Dental Impression Compound | 1987 |
| ANSI/ADA Standard No. 4 | Dental Inlay Casting Wax | 1989 (Reaffirmed 2003) |
| ANSI/ADA Standard No. 5 | Dental Casting Gold Alloys | 1988 |
| ANSI/ADA Standard No. 6 | Dental Mercury | 1987 (Reaffirmed 2005) |
| ANSI/ADA Standard No. 7 | Dental Wrought Gold Wire Alloy | 1989 |
| ANSI/ADA Standard No. 8 | Dental Zinc Phosphate Cement | 1987 |
| ANSI/ADA Standard No. 9 | Dental Silicate Cement | 1986 |
| ANSI/ADA Standard No.10 | Denture Rubber (Absolete) | --- |
| ANSI/ADA Standard No. 11 | Agar Impression Materials | 1987 |
| ANSI/ADA Standard No. 12 | Denture Base Polymers | 1987 |
| ANSI/ADA Standard No. 13 | Denture Cold-Curing Repair Resins | 1987 |
| ANSI/ADA Standard No. 14 | Dental Base Metal Casting Alloys | 1989 (Reaffirmed 1998) |
| ANSI/ADA Standard No. 15 | Artificial Teeth for Dental Prostheses | 2008 (Reaffirmed 2013) |
| ANSI/ADA Standard No. 16 | Dental Impression Paste—$ZnO_2$–Eugenol | 1989 (Reaffirmed 1999) |
| ANSI/ADA Standard No. 17 | Denture Base Temporary Relining Resins | 1983 (Reaffirmed 2014) |
| ANSI/ADA Standard No. 18 | Alginate Impression Materials | 1989 |
| ANSI/ADA Standard No. 19 | Dental Elastomeric Impression Materials | 2004 (Reaffirmed 2014) |
| ANSI/ADA Standard No. 20 | Dental Duplicating Material | 1989 (Reaffirmed 1995) |
| ANSI/ADA Standard No. 22 | Intraoral Dental Radiographic Film | 1972 |
| ANSI/ADA Standard No. 23 (with Addendum) | Dental Excavating Burs | 1982 (Reaffirmed 2015) |
| ANSI/ADA Standard No.24 | Dental Base plate Wax | 1991 |
| ANSI/ADA Standard No. 25 | Dental Gypsum Products | 2000 (Reaffirmed 2010) |
| ADA Standard No. 26 | Dental X-ray Equipment | 1991(Reaffirmed 1999) |
| ADA Standard No. 27 | Resin-based Filling Materials | 1993 |
| ANSI/ADA Standard No. 28 | Root Canal Files and Reamers, Type K | 2008 (Reaffirmed 2013) |
| ANSI/ADA Standard No. 30 | Dental Zinc Oxide—Eugenol and Zinc Oxide—Non-Eugenol Cements | 2013 |
| ANSI/ADA Standard No. 31 | Exposure time designation for timers of dental X-ray machines | --- |
| ANSI/ADA Standard No. 32 | Orthodontic Wires | 2006 (Reaffirmed 2010) |
| ANSI/ADA Standard No. 33 | Dental Product Standards Development Vocabulary | 2003 (Reaffirmed 2014) |
| ANSI/ADA Standard No. 34 | Dental Cartridge Syringes | 2013 |

| ADA No. | Material | Year |
|---|---|---|
| ANSI/ADA Standard No. 35 | High Speed Air Driven Hand Pieces | --- |
| ANSI/ADA Standard No. 36 | Diamond Rotary Instruments | --- |
| ANSI/ADA Standard No. 37 | Dental Abrasive Powders | 1986 (Reaffirmed 2015) |
| ANSI/ADA Standard No. 38 | Metal-Ceramic Dental Restorative Systems | 2000 (Reaffirmed 2015) |
| ANSI/ADA Standard No. 39 | Pit and Fissure Sealants | 2006 (Reaffirmed 2011) |
| ANSI/ADA Standard No 40 | Dental Implants | --- |
| ANSI/ADA Standard No. 41 | Recommended Standard Practices for Biological Evaluation of Dental Materials | 2005 |
| ANSI/ADA Standard No. 42 | Dental Phosphate-bonded Casting Investments | 2002 |
| ANSI/ADA Standard No. 43 | Electrically Powered Dental Amalgamators | 1986 (Reaffirmed 2015) |
| ADA Standard No. 44 | Dental Electrosurgical Equipment | 1979 (Reaffirmed 1999) |
| ANSI/ADA Standard No. 46 | Dental Patient Chair | 2004 (Reaffirmed 2014) |
| ANSI/ADA Standard No. 47 | Dental Units | 2006 |
| ANSI/ADA Standard No. 48 | Visible Light Curing Units | 2004 (Reaffirmed 2015) |
| ANSI/ADA Standard No. 48-2 | LED Curing Lights | 2010 (Reaffirmed 2015) |
| ANSI/ADA Standard No. 53 | Polymer-based Crown and Bridge Materials | 2008 (Reaffirmed 2013) |
| ANSI/ADA Standard No. 54 | Double-pointed, Parenteral, Single Use Needles for Dentistry | 1986 (Reaffirmed 2014) |
| ANSI/ADA Standard No. 57 | Endodontic Sealing Material | 2000 (Reaffirmed 2012) |
| ANSI/ADA Standard No. 58 | Root Canal Files, Type H (Hedstrom) | 2010 (Reaffirmed 2015) |
| ANSI/ADA Standard No. 62 | Dental Abrasive Pastes | 2005 (Reaffirmed 2015) |
| ANSI/ADA Standard No. 63 | Root Canal Barbed Broaches and Rasps | 2013 |
| ANSI/ADA Standard No. 69 | Dental Ceramic | 2010 (Reaffirmed 2015) |
| ANSI/ADA Standard No. 70 | Dental X-ray Protective Aprons and Accessory Devices | 1999 (Reaffirmed 2010) |
| ANSI/ADA Standard No. 71 | Root Canal Filling Condensers (Pluggers and Spreaders) | 2008 (Reaffirmed 2013) |
| ANSI/ADA Standard No. 73 | Dental Absorbent Points | 2008 (Reaffirmed 2013) |
| ANSI/ADA Standard No. 74 | Dental Operator's Stool | 2010 (Reaffirmed 2015) |
| ANSI/ADA Standard No. 75 | Resilient Lining Materials for Removable Dentures—Part 1: Short Term Materials | 1997 (Reaffirmed 2014) |
| ANSI/ADA Standard No. 76 | Non-sterile Natural Rubber Latex Gloves for Dentistry | 2005 (Reaffirmed 2015) |
| ANSI/ADA Standard No. 78 | Dental Obturating Cones | 2013 |
| ANSI/ADA Standard No. 80 | Dental Materials—Determination of Color Stability | 2001 (Reaffirmed 2013) |
| ANSI/ADA Standard No. 82 | Dental Reversible/Irreversible Hydrocolloid Impression Material Systems | 1998 (Reaffirmed 2003) |
| ANSI/ADA Standard No. 85 | Part 1—Disposable Prophy Angles | 2004 (Reaffirmed 2009) |
| ANSI/ADA Standard No. 87 | Dental Impression Trays | 1995 (Reaffirmed 2014) |
| ANSI/ADA Standard No. 88 | Dental Brazing Alloys | 2000 (Reaffirmed 2012) |
| ANSI/ADA Standard No. 89 | Dental Operating Lights | 2008 (Reaffirmed 2013) |
| ANSI/ADA Standard No. 91 | Dental Ethyl Silicate-bonded Casting Investment | 1999 |
| ANSI/ADA Standard No. 92 | Dental Phosphate-bonded Refractory Die Materials | 2002 |
| ANSI/ADA Standard No. 93 | Dental Brazing Investments | 2000 |
| ANSI/ADA Standard No. 94 | Dental Compressed Air Quality | 1996 (Reaffirmed 2014) |
| ANSI/ADA Standard No. 95 | Root Canal Enlargers | 2013 |

| ADA No. | Material | Year |
| --- | --- | --- |
| ANSI/ADA Standard No. 96 | Dental Water-based Cements | 2012 |
| ANSI/ADA Standard No. 97 | Corrosion Test Methods | 2002 (Reaffirmed 2013) |
| ANSI/ADA Standard No. 99 | Athletic Mouth Protectors and Materials | 2001 (Reaffirmed 2013) |
| ANSI/ADA Standard No. 100 | Orthodontic Brackets and Tubes | 2012 |
| ANSI/ADA Standard No. 101 | Root Canal Instruments: General Requirements | 2001 (Reaffirmed 2010) |
| ANSI/ADA Standard No. 102 | Non-sterile Nitrile Gloves | 1999 (Reaffirmed 2015) |
| ANSI/ADA Standard No. 103 | Non-sterile Poly Vinyl Chloride Gloves for Dentistry | 2001 (Reaffirmed 2015) |
| ANSI/ADA Standard No. 105 | Orthodontic elastomeric Materials | 2010 (Reaffirmed 2015) |
| ANSI/ADA Standard No. 108 | Amalgam Separators | 2009 |
| ANSI/ADA Standard No. 108:2009 | Addendum | 2011 |
| ANSI/ADA Standard No. 109 | Procedures for Storing Dental Amalgam Waste and Requirements for Amalgam Waste Storage/Shipment Containers | 2006 (Reaffirmed 2012) |
| ANSI/ADA Technical Report No. 110 | Standard Procedures for the Assessment of Laser-induced Effects on Oral Hard and Soft Tissue | 2008 |
| ANSI/ADA Standard No. 113 | Periodontal Curettes, Dental Scalers and Excavators | 2015 |
| ANSI/ADA Standard No. 116 | Oral Rinses | 2010 |
| ANSI/ADA Standard No. 119 | Manual Toothbrushes | 2015 |
| ANSI/ADA Standard No. 120 | Powered Toothbrushes | 2009 (Reaffirmed 2014) |
| ANSI/ADA Standard No. 122 | Dental Casting and Baseplate Waxes | 2007 (Reaffirmed 2013) |
| ANSI/ADA Standard No. 125 | Manual Interdental Brushes | 2012 |
| ANSI/ADA Standard No. 126 | Casting Investments and Refractory Die Materials | 2015 |
| ANSI/ADA Standard No. 127 | Fatigue Testing for Endosseous Dental Implants | 2012 |
| ANSI/ADA Standard No. 128 | Hydrocolloid Impression Materials | 2015 |
| ANSI/ADA Standard No. 130 | Dentifrices-Requirements, Test Methods and Marking | 2013 |
| ANSI/ADA Standard No. 131 | Dental CAD/CAM Machinable Zirconia Blanks | 2015 |
| ANSI/ADA Standard No. 132 | Scanning Accuracy of Dental Chairside and Laboratory CAD/CAM Systems | 2015 |
| ANSI/ADA Standard No. 134 | Metallic Materials for Fixed and Removable Restorations and Appliances | 2013 |
| ANSI/ADA Standard No. 136 | Products for External Tooth Bleaching | 2015 |
| ANSI/ADA Standard No. 137 | Essential Characteristics of Test Methods for the Evaluation of Treatment Methods Intended to Improve or Maintain the Microbiological Quality of Dental Unit Procedural Water | 2014 |
| ANSI/ADA Standard No. 139 | Dental Base Polymers | 2012 |
| ANSI/ADA Standard No. 141 | Dental Duplicating Material | 2013 |
| ANSI/ADA Standard No. 151 | Screening Method for Erosion Potential of Oral Rinses on Dental Hard Tissues | 2015 |
| ANSI/ADA/AAMI Standard ST-40 | Table-Top Dry Heat (Heated Air) Sterilization and Sterility Assurance in Health Care Facilities | 2004 (Reaffirmed 2010) |
| ANSI ADA AAMI Standard ST-55 | Table-top Steam Sterilizers | 2010 |

# Glossary

A

**Abrasive:** A sharp, hard, natural or synthetic substance used for grinding, finishing, or polishing a softer surface.

**Abrasion:** Abnormal wearing of tooth structure through abnormal mechanical process other than mastication.

**Absorption:** The extent to which light is absorbed by the material in an object.

**Accelerator:** A substance that speeds a chemical reaction; also refers to the catalyst in the reaction of impression materials.

**Achromatic:** Entity lacking in hue and saturation, i.e. depicting a series of colors that varies only in lightness or brightness.

**Achromatopsia:** A type of monochromatism in which all colors are perceived as achromatic.

**Acid-base reaction:** Chemical reaction between a compound with replaceable hydrogen ions (acid) and a substance with replaceable hydroxide ions (base) that yields a salt and water; for aqueous cements, the liquid is an acid and the powder is a base.

**Acid-etch technique:** The process of cleaning and roughening a solid surface by exposing it to an acid and thoroughly rinsing the residue to promote micromechanical bonding of an adhesive to the surface.

**Activation:** Process by which sufficient energy is provided to induce an initiator to generate free radicals and cause polymerization to begin.

**Activator:** Source of energy used to activate an initiator and produce free radicals. Three energy sources are currently used to dissociate an initiator into free radicals they are— (I) heat, which supplies thermal energy; (2) an electron donating chemical such as a tertiary amine, which forms a complex and (3) visible light, which supplies energy for photoinitiation in the presence of a photosensitizer such as camphorquinone.

**Acute toxicity:** Adverse response to a substance that causes ill effects relatively soon after a single exposure or after multiple exposures over a relatively short time (usually less than 2 weeks).

**Adaptation:** The act of purposefully adapting two surfaces to provide intimate contact.

**Addition reaction:** A polymerization reaction in which each polymer chain grows to a maximal length in sequence.

**Adhesion:** The property of remaining in close proximity, as that resulting from the physical attraction of molecules to a substance or molecular attraction existing between the surfaces of bodies in contact.

**Adhesive failure:** Failure of bond between interface of two materials due to tensile or shear force.

**Adsorption:** The adhesion, in an extremely thin layer, of molecules to the surfaces of liquids or solids with which they are in contact.

**Adherend:** A material substrate that is bonded to another material by means of an adhesive.

**Adhesive:** Substance that promotes adhesion of one substance or material to another.

**Adhesive bonding:** Process of joining two materials by means of an adhesive agent that solidifies during the bonding process.

**Adverse reaction:** Any unintended, unexpected, and harmful response of an individual to a dental treatment or biomaterial.

**Age hardening:** Process of hardening certain alloys by controlled heating and cooling, which usually is associated with a phase change.

**Air-particle abrasion:** Process of removing material, contaminants, stain, or carious tissue by use of air pressure and abrasive particles appropriate for the substrate being treated.

**Allergy:** Abnormal antigen-antibody reaction to a substance that is harmless to most individuals.

**Alloplastic:** Related to implantation of an inert foreign body.

**Alloy:** A crystalline solid with metallic properties that is composed of two or more chemical elements at least one of which is a metal and all of which are mutually soluble in the molten state.

**Alloy system:** All possible alloyed combinations of two or more elements at least one of which is a metal. For example, the binary gold-silver system includes all possible alloys of gold and silver, varying from 100% gold and 0% silver to 100% silver and 0% gold.

**Agar:** A complex sulfated polymer of galactose units, extracted from red algae which is a mucilaginous substance that melts at approximately 100° C and solidifies into a gel at approximately 40° C.

**Amalgam:** Dental amalgam is an alloy of mercury, silver, copper, and tin, which may also contain palladium, zinc, and other elements to improve handling characteristics and clinical performance.

**Amorphous:** Without crystalline structure; having random arrangement of atoms in space.

**Anneal:** To heat a material, such as metal or glass, followed by controlled cooling to remove internal stresses and create a desired degree of toughness, temper, or softness to a material.

**Antiflux:** Material which prevent or confine flow of flux.

**Apatite:** calcium phosphate of the composition $Ca_5(PO_4)_3OH$; one of the mineral constituents of teeth and bones.

**Age hardening:** Process of hardening certain alloys by controlled heating and cooling, which usually is associated with a phase change.

**Amalgamation:** The process of mixing liquid mercury with one or more metals or alloys to form an amalgam.

**Ankylosis:** A condition of joint or tooth immobility resulting from oral pathology, surgery, or direct contact with bone.

**Annealing:** The process of controlled heating and cooling that is designed to produce desired properties in a metal. Typically, the annealing process is intended to soften metals, to increase their ductility, stabilize shape, and increase machinability.

**Anodization:** An oxidation process in which a film is produced on the surface of a metal by electrolytic treatment at the anode.

**Anticariogenic:** Capable of inhibiting or preventing dental caries.

**Appliance:** A dental device that is made extraorally and affixed intraorally, such as a crown, a fixed prosthesis, or an orthodontic bracket.

**Atraumatic restorative treatment (ART):** A clinical procedure performed without dental burs, air/water spray, or anesthesia that consists of manual excavation of carious tissue in a cavitated lesion and restoration of the tooth cavity with a fluoride-releasing cement.

**Attrition:** The act of wearing or grinding down by friction e.g. the mechanical wear resulting from mastication or parafunction, limited to contacting surfaces of the teeth.

**Augmentation:** To increase in size beyond the existing size. In alveolar ridge augmentation, bone grafts or alloplastic materials are used to increase the size of an atrophic alveolar ridge.

**Autogenous graft:** A graft taken from the patient's own body.

**Auto glaze:** The production of a glazed surface by raising the temperature of a ceramic material to create surface flow.

**Autograft:** A graft or tissue derived from another site in or on the body of the organism receiving it.

**Auto polymer:** A material that polymerizes by chemical reaction without external heat as a result of the addition of an activator and a catalyst.

**Autopolymerization:** In resins, the chemical reaction of smaller molecular chain molecules with an activator to form a larger molecular chain; e.g. a tertiary amine activates the benzoyl peroxide, an initiator, which will react with the methylmethacrylate monomer to form polymethylmethacrylate.

**Autopolymerizing resin:** A resin formed when polymerization occurs as a result of a chemical activator.

**Auxiliary dental material:** Substance that is used in the construction of a dental prosthesis but that does not become a part of the structure.

B

**Backbone:** The main chain of a polymer.

**Base:** The portion of a denture that supports the artificial dentition and replaces the deficient alveolar anatomy and gingival tissues (Denture base).

**Back pressure porosity:** Porosity produced in dental castings thought to be the result of the inability of gases in the mold to escape during the casting procedure.

**Backing:** A metal support that attaches a veneer to a prosthesis.

**Base:** A material that is used to protect the pulp in a prepared cavity by providing thermal insulation; a base may also serve as a medicament.

**Base material:** Any substance of which a denture base may be made, such as acrylic resin, vulcanite, poly-styrene, or metal.

**Base metal:** A metal that readily oxidizes or corrodes.

**Base metal alloy:** An alloy composed of metals that are not noble.

**Baseplate:** A rigid, relatively thin layer of wax, shellac, or thermoplastic (heat-, chemically-, or light-activated) polymer adapted over edentulous surfaces of a definitive cast to form a base which, together with an attached occlusion rim made of wax or similar material, serves as the record base.

**Baseplate wax:** A hard wax used for making occlusion rims, waxing dentures, and other dental procedures.

**Basket endosteal dental implant:** A perforated, cylindrical endosteal dental implant, the implant body of which is designed in the form of single, double, and/or triple contiguous cylinder(s).

**Bees' wax:** A low-melting wax obtained from honeycomb and used as an ingredient of many dental impression waxes.

**Beilby layer:** The molecular disorganized surface layer of a highly polished metal; a relatively scratch-free microcrystalline surface produced by a series of abrasives of decreasing coarseness.

**Binary metal alloy:** An alloy that contains two chemical elements at least one of which is a metal.

**Bioacceptance:** The ability to be tolerated in a biological environment inspite of adverse effects.

**Bioactive:** Having an effect on or eliciting a response from living tissue, organism, or cell, such as inducing the formation of hydroxyapatite.

**Bioactivity:** Reactive potential of implant material that allows interaction and bond formation with living tissues; active potential depends on material composition, topography, and chemical or physical surface variations.

**Bioadhesion:** A chemical reactivity that results in attachment between biologic and other materials.

**Biocompatibility:** The ability of a biomaterial to perform its desired function with respect to a medical (or dental) therapy, without eliciting any undesirable local or systemic effects in the recipient or beneficiary of that therapy, but generating the most appropriate beneficial cellular or tissue response in that specific situation, and optimizing the clinically relevant performance of that therapy.

**Bioinductive:** Capable of inducing a response in a biological system.

**Biointegration:** The process by which bone or other living tissue becomes integrated with an implanted material with no intervening space.

**Biomaterial:** Any matter, surface, or construct that interacts with biological systems.

**Biomimetics:** Study of the formation, structure, or function of biologically produced substances and materials (such as silk or conch shells) and biological mechanisms and processes (such as protein synthesis or mineralization) for the purpose of synthesizing similar products by artificial mechanisms that mimic natural structures.

**Bite wax:** A wax form used to record the occlusal surfaces of teeth as an aid in establishing maxillo·mandibular relationships.

**Block copolymer:** Polymer made of two or more monomer species and identical monomer units ("mers") occurring in relatively long sequences along the main polymer chain.

**Bonding:** An adhesive technique in dentistry involving the acid etching of tooth enamel and/or dentin so as to create tags of resin within the tooth structure that results in mechanical retention of the restorative material.

**Bonding agent:** A material used to promote adhesion or cohesion between two different substances, or between a material and natural tooth structures.

**Boxing wax:** A wax sheet form used as a border at the perimeter of an impression to provide an enclosed boundary for the base of the cast to be made from a poured material such as gypsum or resin.

**Brazing investment:** An investment having a binding system consisting of acidic phosphate, such as monoammonium phosphate, and a basic oxide, such as magnesium oxide

**Brittleness:** Relative inability of a material to deform plastically before it fractures.

**Buffing:** Process of producing a lustrous surface through the abrading action of fine abrasives bound to a nonabrasive carrier with or without a liquid or paste medium.

**Bulk reduction:** Process of removing excess material (natural tooth or synthetic structure) by cutting or grinding with rotary instruments to provide a desired anatomic form.

**Burnout:** Process of heating an invested mold to eliminate the embedded wax or plastic pattern.

**Bur:** A steel or tungsten carbide rotary cutting instrument.

# C

**C-factor configuration factor:** This represents the ratio between the bonded surface area of a resin-based composite restoration to the non - bonded or free surface area. The greater the C-factor, the greater the stress that develops at the restoration margin, which can lead to gap formation, marginal breakdown and leakage, and other problems, such as secondary caries.

**CAD-CAM:** The term *CAD* refers to computer-aided design technology, which is based on the use of computer software and systems to assist in the creation, modification, analysis, and optimization of two-dimensional or three-dimensional models of objects. The term *CAM* refers to computer-aided manufacturing of a restorative device using the CAD input file. CAM may be additive (buildup) or subtractive (machining of a device from a larger starting piece of material).

**CAD-CAM ceramic:** A partially or fully sintered ceramic blank that is used to produce a dental core or veneer structure using a computer-aided design (CAD) and computer-aided manufacturing or milling (CAM) process.

**Calcination:** The process of heating a solid material to drive off volatile chemically combined components such as water and carbon dioxide.

**Calcium phosphate cement:** A cement used for bone regeneration usually comprising a powder (di-, tri-, or tetra-calcium phosphate) that dissolves in an aqueous solution from which hydroxyapatite is precipitated.

**Cast:** A dimensionally accurate reproduction of a part of the oral cavity or extraoral facial structures that is produced in a durable hard material from an impression.

**Castable ceramic:** A glass especially formulated to be cast into a mold and converted by heating to a glass-ceramic as a core coping or framework for a ceramic prosthesis.

**Camphoroquinone:** A visible-light-sensitive chemical responsible for initiating free-radical polymerization.

**Carbon fiber:** Filaments made by high temperature carbonizing of acrylic fiber; used in the production of high strength composite materials.

**Castable ceramic:** A glass especially formulated to be cast into a refractory mold and converted by heating to a glass-ceramic as a core coping or framework for a ceramic prosthesis.

**Casting ring:** A metal or silicone tube in which a refractory mold is made for casting dental restorations.

**Casting wax:** A composition containing various waxes with desired properties for making wax patterns to be formed into metal castings.

**Catalyst:** A substance that accelerates a chemical reaction without affecting the properties of the materials involved.

**Catalyst paste (catalyst putty):** A component of a polymerization reaction that decreases the energy required for the reaction and usually does not become part of the final product; however, the term *catalyst* has been used for the structural component of dental materials that initiates the polymerization reaction.

**Cathode:** The negative pole in electrolysis.

**Cavity varnish:** A combination of copal resin or other synthetic resins dissolved in an organic solvent such as chloroform or ether

**Cellulose acetate:** An ester of acetic acid; used as clear prefabricated crown forms for making interim restorations.

**Cavity liner:** A material that coats the bottom of a prepared cavity to protect the pulp; it is applied in a thin layer and usually contains calcium hydroxide or mineral trioxide aggregate (MTA); also includes certain glass ionomer cements used as intermediate layers between tooth structure and composite restorative material.

**Cement thickness:** Distance between the abutment tooth and cemented prosthesis. This dimension is influenced by the design of the prosthesis and the viscosity of the cement during seating.

**Cement/Cementing:** Substance that hardens from a viscous state to a solid union between two surfaces. For dental applications, cements act as a base, liner, restorative filling material, or adhesive to bond devices and prostheses to tooth structure or to each other.

**Cement:** A material that, on hardening, will fill a space or bind adjacent objects.

**Ceramic:** Inorganic, nonmetallic material composed of metallic or semi-metallic oxides, phosphates, sulfates, or other nonorganic compounds. Glass, which is amorphous, is a subset of ceramics.

**Ceramic frits:** Powdered ceramic material fired in a dental laboratory to produce a dental porcelain veneer layer over a core material (metal or ceramic). Frits may be glass or a mixture of glass and crystalline particles, which commonly contain inorganic pigments.

**Ceramic, glaze:** Fine glass powder that can be fired on a dental ceramic core or dental porcelain to form a smooth, glassy surface.

**Ceramic, pressable (hot-pressed ceramic):** Ceramic with a high glass content that can be heated to a temperature and forced to flow under uniaxial pressure to fill a cavity in a refractory mold.

**Ceramic, stain:** A fine glass powder containing one or more pigments (colored metal oxides) that is applied superficially to a ceramic restoration.

**Cermet:** A glass ionomer cement that is reinforced with filler particles prepared by fusing silver particles to glass.

**Chain transfer:** Stage of polymerization in which the free radical on the growing end of one polymer chain is transferred to either a monomer or a second polymer chain.

**Chemically activated resin:** Resin system consisting of two pastes—one containing an initiator (e.g. benzoyl peroxide) and the other an activator (e.g. an aromatic tertiary amine)—which, when mixed together, release free radicals that initiate polymerization.

**Chemically cured composite:** Particle-reinforced resin that is polymerized through a chemical activation process wherein two components are blended together just prior to placement of the composite. Also known as self-cure composite.

**Chondrogenesis:** The development of cartilage.

**Chroma:** Degree of saturation of a particular hue (dominant color).

**Chronic exposure:** The contact with a substance that occurs over a long time (more than 1 year).

**Cinefluoroscopy:** Dynamic fluoroscopic images recorded as a movie file.

**Cobalt chromium alloy:** A low-density, large-grained base metal dental casting alloy with prominent dendritic structure, composed from 60% to 75% cobalt and up to 30% chromium with trace elements that may include small amounts of Mo, Mn, Si, and N; chromium, by its passivation effect, ensures corrosion resistance of the alloy.

**Coefficient of thermal expansion (linear coefficient of expansion):** Change in length per unit of the original length of a material when its temperature is raised by 1 K (1 °C).

**Cohesive strength:** Force of molecular attraction between molecules or atoms of the same species.

**Cohesive:** Molecular attraction between molecules or atoms of the same species.

**Cold welding:** The process of joining metals by metallic bonding. The metal-joining process does not occur by heating or fusion but by pressure applied to the interface between the two parts to be joined; no liquid or molten phase is produced within the interface joint.

**Cold working:** The process of plastically deforming metal at room temperature.

**Colloid:** A solid, liquid, or gaseous substance made up of large molecules or masses of smaller molecules that remain in suspension in a surrounding continuous medium of different matter.

**Color:** Sensation induced from light of varying wavelengths reaching the eye.

**Compaction (condensation):** The process of increasing the density of metal foil, pellets, or powder through compressive pressure.

**Compomer:** Resin-based composite consisting of a silicate glass filler phase and a methacrylate-based matrix with carboxylic acid functional groups; also known as polyacid-modified glass ionomer cement, a term derived from composite and ionomer; a secondary setting mechanism is related to acid-base reactions of the glass filler.

**Composite:** In materials science, a solid formed from two or more distinct phases (e.g. filler particles dispersed in a polymer matrix) that have been combined to produce properties superior to or intermediate to those of the individual constituents; also a term used in dentistry to describe a dental composite or resin-based composite.

**Compressive strength:** Maximum stress a material can sustain under crush loading.

**Color blindness:** Abnormal color vision or the inability to discriminate certain colors, most commonly along the red-green axis.

**Color constancy:** Relative independence of perceived color to changes in color of the light source.

**Color deficiency:** A general term for all forms of color vision that yield chromaticity discrimination below normal limits, such as monochromatism, dichromatism, and anomalous trichromatism.

**Color difference:** Magnitude and character of the difference between two colors under specified conditions; referred to as delta E.

**Color difference equations:** equations that transform Commission Internationals d'Eclairage (CIE) coordinates into a more uniform matrix such that a specified distance between two colors is more nearly proportional to the magnitude of an observed difference between them regardless of their hue.

**Compressive stress:** Compressive force per unit area perpendicular to the direction of applied force.

**Compomer:** A poly-acid modified composite resin, composed of non-reactive glass filler, acid-modified dimethacrylate resin, and an initiator; compomers do not have the capacity to chemically bond to tooth surfaces, therefore, they need primer/bonding resin agents for tooth bonding applications;

**Concentration cell:** Electrochemical corrosion cell in which the potential difference is associated with the difference in concentration of a dissolved species, such as oxygen, in solution along different areas of a metal surface. Pitting corrosion and crevice corrosion are types of concentration cell corrosion.

**Condensation reaction:** A polymerization process in which bifunctional or multifunctional monomers react to form first dimers first, then trimers, and eventually long-chain polymers; the reactions may or may not yield by-products; the preferred term is *step-growth polymerization.* All condensation impression materials yield by-products.

**Contact angle:** Angle of intersection between a liquid and a surface of a solid that is measured from the solid surface through the liquid to the liquid/vapor tangent line originating at the terminus of the liquid/solid interface; used as a measure of wettability, whereby no wetting occurs at a contact angle of 180° and complete wetting occurs at an angle of 0°.

**Contouring:** Process of producing a desired anatomic form by cutting or grinding away excess material.

**Coping:** Metal substructure for a cast-metal or veneered metal prosthesis.

**Copy milling:** Process of cutting or grinding a desired shape to the same dimensions as a master pattern in a manner similar to that used for cutting a key blank from a master key.

**Core ceramic:** An opaque or semi-translucent dental ceramic having sufficient strength, toughness, and stiffness to withstand masticatory forces. Core materials can be glazed or layered with a veneering ceramic to obtain the desired shade, form and function, and/or esthetics.

**Coring:** A microstructure in which a composition gradient exists between the center and the surface of cast dendrites, grains, or particles.

**Corrective wax (dental impression wax):** A thermoplastic wax that is used to make a type of dental impression.

**Corrosion Chemical or electrochemical process:** in which a solid usually a metal, is attacked by an environmental agent, resulting in partial or complete dissolution.

**Coupling agent:** A bonding agent applied to the surfaces of reinforcing particles (filler) to ensure that they are chemically bonded to the resin matrix. Organosilane compounds are the more common class of dental composite coupling agents.

**Craze:** A network of fine cracks or craze lines that are formed in the surface of aqueous-based cements because of rapid dehydration.

**Creep time:** Dependent plastic strain of a solid under a static load or constant stress.

**Crevice corrosion:** Accelerated corrosion in narrow spaces caused by localized electrochemical processes and chemistry changes, such as acidification and depletion in oxygen content. Crevice corrosion commonly occurs when microleakage takes place between a restoration and the tooth.

**Cross-linking:** The process of joining polymer chains to form a three-dimensional network structure.

**Curing chemical reaction:** In which low-molecular-weight monomers (or small polymers) are converted into higher·molecular-weight materials to attain desired properties.

**Crucible:** A vessel or container made of any refractory material (frequently ceramics) used for melting or calcining any substance that requires a high degree of heat.

**Crucible former:** The base to which a sprue former is attached while the wax pattern is being invested in refractory investment; a convex rubber, plastic, or metal base that forms a concave depression or crucible in the refractory investment.

**Cutting:** Process of removing material from the substrate by use of a bladed bur or an abrasive embedded in a binding matrix on a bur or disc.

## D

**Degassing:** The process of removing gases (or other impurities) from the surface of a solid or liquid, usually by heating.

**Devitrification:** To eliminate vitreous characteristics partly or wholly; to crystallize.

**Die:** The positive reproduction of the form of a prepared tooth in any suitable substance.

**Direct metal laser sintering (DMLS):** An additive CAM technique which uses a sintering of metal alloy powder to develop 3D objects.

**Degree of conversion (DC):** Percentage of carbon-carbon double bonds (- C=C-) converted to single bonds (-CC-) during curing to form a polymeric resin. Also known as degree of cure and degree of monomer-to-polymer. conversion.

**Delayed expansion:** The gradual expansion of a zinc containing amalgam over a period of weeks to months. This expansion is associated with the development of hydrogen gas, which is caused by the incorporation of moisture in the plastic mass during its manipulation in a cavity preparation.

**Demineralization:** The loss of mineral, typically calcium and phosphate ions, from tooth structure caused by exposure to organic acids produced by oral microorganisms.

**Dendritic microstructure:** A cast alloy structure of highly elongated crystals with a branched morphology.

**Dental amalgam:** An alloy that is formed by reacting mercury with silver, copper, and tin, and which may also contain palladium, zinc, and other elements to improve handling characteristics and clinical performance.

**Dental ceramic:** A especially formulated ceramic material that exhibits adequate strength, durability, and color that is used intraorally to restore anatomic form and function, and or esthetics. Many formulations are available depending on whether the indication is for a crown, a bridge, an endodontic post or core, an orthodontic bracket, or a veneer. Ceramic products that are used primarily for crowns and bridges include alumina, ceria-stabilized zirconia, glass infiltrated alumina, glass-infiltrated magnesia-alumina spinel, glass-infiltrated alumina/zirconia, lithium disilicate glass-ceramic, yttria-slabilized zirconia, and various glasses and glazes.

**Dental composite:** Highly cross-linked polymeric materials reinforced by a dispersion of amorphous silica, glass, crystalline, mineral, or organic resin filler particles and/ or short fibers bonded to the matrix by a coupling agent.

**Dental plaster (plaster of Paris):** The beta form of calcium sulfate hemihydrate.

**Dental stone:** The alpha form of calcium sulfate hemihydrate.

**Dental wax:** A low-molecular-weight ester of fatty acids derived from natural or synthetic components, such as petroleum derivatives, that soften to a plastic state at a relatively low temperature.

**Dentin bonding:** The process of bonding a resin to conditioned dentin.

**Dentin bonding agent:** A thin layer of resin between conditioned dentin and the resin matrix of a resin composite restorative material.

**Dentin conditioner:** An acidic agent that dissolves the inorganic structure in dentin, resulting in a collagen mesh that allows infiltration of an adhesive resin.

**Denture base:** The part of the denture that rests on the soft tissues overlying the maxillary and mandibular jawbone and that anchors the artificial teeth.

**Denture soft liner:** A polymeric material that is placed on the tissue-contacting surface of a denture base to absorb some of the mastication impact energy by acting as a type of "shock absorber" between the occlusal surfaces of a denture and the underlying oral tissues. A denture soft liner also may be used to engage natural or prosthetic undercuts so as to provide retention, stability, and support.

**Depth of cure:** Depth or thickness of a light-cured resin that can be converted from a monomer to a polymer when exposed to a light source under a specific set of conditions.

**Desorption:** The process of removing molecules that have attached to the surface of a solid by a physical or chemical action; it is a broader term than degassing.

**Dew point:** The temperature at which moisture in air begins to condense such as the temperature at which dew condenses on a cool glass mixing slab.

**Di-and tricalcium silicate:** The main phases present in MTA cement, which are hydraulically active (set with water).

**Die:** A reproduction of a prepared tooth made from a gypsum product, epoxy resin, a metal, or a refractory material.

**Diffusion:** Represents the rate at which a substance is transported through a unit area and a unit thickness under the influence of a unit concentration gradient at a given temperature.

**Dilatant:** Resistance to flow increases as the rate of deformation (shear strain rate) increases. The faster the fluids are stirred or forced through a syringe, the more viscous and more resistant to flow they become.

**Direct restorative material:** A cement, metal, or resin based composite that is placed and formed intraorally to restore teeth and/or to enhance esthetics.

**Direct wax technique:** A process whereby a wax pattern is prepared in the mouth directly on prepared teeth.

**Dislocation:** An imperfection in the crystalline arrangement of atoms consisting of either an extra partial plane of atoms (edge dislocation), a spiral distortion of normally parallel atom planes (screw dislocation), or a combination of the two types.

**Divesting:** Process of removing investment from a cast metal or hot-pressed ceramic.

**Dual-cure resin:** Dental composite that contains both chemically activated and light-activated components to initiate polymerization and potentially overcome the limitations of either the chemical-and light-cure systems when used alone.

**Ductile fracture:** The rupture of a solid structure resulting in measurable plastic deformation.

**Ductility:** Ability of the material to sustain large permanent deformation under tensile load before it fractures.

# E

**Elastic limit:** The greatest stress to which a material may be subjected and still be capable of returning to its original dimensions when such forces are released.

**Elastic modulus:** The stiffness or flexibility of a material within the elastic range; within the elastic range, the material deforms in direct proportion to the force applied as represented by Hooke's law.

**Elastomer:** A polymer that has a glass transition temperature that is below its service temperature (usually room temperature); these materials are characterized by low stiffness and extremely large elastic strains.

**Elastomeric impression material:** A group of flexible chemical polymers that are either chemically or physically cross-linked; generally, they can be easily stretched and rapidly recover their original dimensions when applied stresses are released.

**Electroplating:** The process of covering the surface of an object with a thin coating of metal by means of electrolysis.

**Elongation:** 1. deformation as a result of tensile force application; 2. the degree to which a material will stretch before breaking; 3. the overeruption of a tooth.

**Etchant:** A chemical agent that is capable of selective dissolution of a surface.

**Elastic memory:** Tendency of a solid wax form to partially return to its original shape when it is stored at a higher temperature than that to which it was cooled.

**Elastic modulus (also modulus of elasticity and Young's modulus):** Stiffness of a material that is calculated as the ratio of elastic stress to elastic strain.

**Elastic strain:** Amount of deformation that is recovered instantaneously when an externally applied force or pressure is reduced or eliminated.

**Elastomer:** Any of various polymers having the elastic properties of natural rubber.

**Electromotive series:** Arrangement of metals by their equilibrium values of electrode oxidation potential. Used to judge the tendency of metals and alloys to undergo electrochemical (galvanic) corrosion.

**Endosteal implant:** A device placed into the alveolar and / or basal bone of the mandible or maxilla that transects only one cortical plate.

**Epithelial implant:** A device placed within the oral mucosa.

**Equiaxed grain microstructure:** A cast alloy microstructure with crystal (grain) dimensions that are similar along all crystal axis.

**Esthetics:** Principles and techniques associated with development of the color and appearance required to produce a natural, pleasing effect in the dentition.

**Estrogenicity:** Potential of synthetic chemicals with a binding affinity for estrogen receptors to cause reproductive alterations. Bisphenol-A, a precursor of certain monomers such as Bis-GMA, is a known estrogenic compound that is considered to have possible effects on foetal and infant brain development and behavior.

# F

**Filler:** Inorganic, glass, and/or organic-resin particles that are dispersed in a resin matrix to increase rigidity, strength, and wear resistance, to decrease thermal expansion, due to water sorption, and reduce polymerization shrinkage.

**Feldspathic porcelain:** porcelain fabricated from the natural mineral group feldspar; the material is composed of compounds of oxygen with lighter metals and nonmetals and is predominantly an amorphous (non-crystalline) matrix with one or more crystalline phases (such as leucite $K_2O \cdot Al_2O_3 \cdot 4SiO_2$).

**Fiber-reinforced composite resin:** Composite resin impregnated with glass, carbon, or polyethylene fiber; fibers may be composite resin impregnated by the provider or pre-impregnated by the manufacturer; dental application includes resin-bonded prostheses and posts.

**Flasking:** The process of investing the cast and a wax replica of the desired form in a flask preparatory to molding the restorative material into the desired product.

**Flexible resin removable partial denture:** A metal-free removable partial denture constructed by using one or more thermoplastic resins classified according to ISO 1567 including acetal resins, polycarbonates (polyesters), acrylic resins, and polyamides (nylons) and polyaryletherketones, including polyetherketone.

**Flowable composite resin:** Composite resin that is less highly filled than conventional composite resin and has improved wettability.

**Fluorescence:** A process by which a material absorbs radiant energy and emits it in the form of radiant energy of a different wavelength band, all or most of whose wavelengths exceed that of the absorbed energy; fluorescence, as distinguished from phosphorescence, does not persist for an appreciable time after the termination of the excitation process.

**Film thickness:** The thickness in micrometers of set cement 10 minutes after a load of 150 N has been applied by a flat plate against another flat surface. The thickness should be less than 25 microns for luting cements.

**Final set stage:** At which the curing process is complete.

**Finished and polished restoration:** A prosthesis or direct restoration whose outer surface has been progressively refined to a desired state of surface finish.

**Finishing:** Process of removing surface defects or scratches created during the contouring process through the use of cutting or grinding instruments or both.

**Fracture strength:** Stress required for material failure; represented by a line plotted on a stress-versus-strain graph; this strain may be less than the ultimate strength; i.e. the maximal strain on a sample prior to material failure.

**Fracture toughness:** A mechanical characteristic of a material with cracks as a measure of the resistance and the amount of energy required for fracture.

**Flexural strength (bending strength or modulus of rupture):** Force per unit area at the instant of fracture in a test specimen subjected to flexural loading.

**Flow:** Relative ability of wax to plastically deform when it is heated slightly above body temperature.

**Fluoride recharging:** The process by which a restorative material, specifically glass ionomer cement, absorbs fluoride from a solution with a high fluoride concentration.

**Flux:** Compound applied to metal surfaces that dissolves or prevents the formation of oxides and other undesirable substances that may reduce the quality or strength of a soldered or brazed area.

**Formocresol:** A compound consisting of formaldehyde, cresol, glycerine, and water.

**Fracture toughness:** The critical stress intensity factor at the point of rapid crack propagation in a solid containing a crack of known shape and size.

**Free radical:** An atom or group of atoms (R) with an unpaired electron (-). R--producing reactions that initiate and propagate polymerization and eventually lead to a final set.

**Fusion temperature:** The temperature below which a definite reduction in plasticity occurs during cooling of an impression compound.

**G**

**Galvanic corrosion (electrogalvanism):** Accelerated attack occurring on a less noble metal when electrochemically dissimilar metals are in electrical contact within a liquid corrosive environment.

**Galvanic shock:** Pain sensation caused by the electrical current generated when two dissimilar metals are brought into contact in the oral environment.

**Gel:** A network of fibrils forming a weak, slightly elastic brush-heap structure of hydrocolloid; also the solid network structure of a cross-linked polymer.

**Gelation:** The process of transforming a hydrocolloid from a sol to a gel.

**Glass:** A hard, stiff, amorphous material made by fusing silicates with one or more types of metal oxides, usually an alkali or alkaline earth oxide, boron oxide, or alumina. Radiopaque glass contains strontium oxide, barium oxide, or other high-atomic mass metal oxides that are dissolved in the silicate glass. Fluoride or phosphate compounds may also be incorporated in a glass matrix.

**Glass ionomer cement (conventional GIC):** A cement that hardens following an acid-base reaction between fluoroaluminosilicate glass powder and an aqueous-based polyacrylic acid solution.

**Glass transition temperature (Tg):** Temperature above which a sharp increase in the thermal expansion coefficient occurs, indicating increased molecular mobility.

**Glass-ceramic:** A ceramic that is formed to shape in the glassy state and subsequently heat treated to partially or completely crystallize the object. Glass-ceramic blanks are also available for CAD-CAM processes.

**Glass-infiltrated ceramic:** A crystalline core (framework) ceramic whose interconnected pore network is infiltrated during heating by the capillary inflow of a low-viscosity highly wetting glass. These infiltrated core materials are veneered with porcelain. Alumina, magnesia-alumina spinel, or alumina/zirconia core ceramics can be used for this process.

**Glaze ceramic:** A especially formulated ceramic powder that is mixed with a liquid, applied to a ceramic surface, and heated to an appropriate temperature for a sufficient time to form a smooth glassy layer.

**Graft or branched copolymer:** Polymer in which a sequence of one type of mer unit is attached as a graft (branched) onto the backbone of a second type of mer unit.

**Grain:** Individual crystal in the microstructure of a metal.

**Grain boundary:** The interface between adjacent grains in a polycrystalline metal. Dental alloys are polycrystal line solids consisting of many individual grains (crystals) separated by grain boundaries.

**Grain growth:** The increase in the mean crystal size of a polycrystalline metal produced by a heat-treatment process.

**Grain refinement:** The process of reducing the crystal (grain) size in a solid metal through the action of specific alloying elements or compounds.

**Green state:** The semi-hard, pre-fired condition of a ceramic object. A green ceramic may be wet, as produced by slip-casting, or it may be isostatically pressed to shape prior to firing. Green ceramics are always porous. They are too fragile for use intraorally. Grinding process of removing material from a substrate by abrasion with relatively coarse particles.

**Gutta-percha:** A material composed of trans-polyisoprene rubber with various additives, usually including zinc oxide powder, barium sulfate, and modifiers to adjust the rheology for filling (obturating) a root canal after pulp extirpation and canal preparation; gutta-percha must be used with a root canal sealer to seal the canal from bacterial penetration.

**Gypsum-based investment:** A refractory material consisting of silica and gypsum as a binder used to produce a mold for the metal casting process.

**H**

**Healing abutment:** Any dental implant abutment used for a limited time to assist in healing or modification of the adjacent tissues.

**Heat-activated polymerization:** In resins, a thermal activation of smaller molecular chain molecules to form a larger molecular chain; heat activates the benzoyl peroxide, an initiator, which will react with the methylmethacrylate monomer to form poly-methyl methacrylate.

**Heat-pressed ceramics:** a ceramic material used to cast, in a molten phase, into a refractory mold.

**Hydroxyethyl methacrylate (HEMA):** With the addition of glutaraldehyde, it is one of the agents used in dentin-bonding; polymerizes to form the polymer polyhydroxyethylmethacrylate.

**High fusing ceramics:** A ceramic material with a maturation or fusion range of 1315° to 1370° C (2350 to 2500 F).

**High fusing solder:** Any soldering alloy formulated to melt at approximately 1100° C (2012 F) used to form connectors before ceramic application.

**High noble metal alloy:** As classified by the American Dental Association (1984), any dental casting alloy with at least 60% noble metal (Au, Pt, Pd, Rh, Ru, Ir, Os) by weight with at least 40% gold.

**Hybrid ionomer:** A conventional glass ionomer that has been modified to include methacrylate groups in the liquid component; may contain light-activated initiators; setting is by an acid-base reaction with light and dual polymerization. Also called as resin modified glass ionomer.

**Hydrocolloid:** A colloid system in which water is the dispersion medium; those materials described as a colloid sol with water that are used in dentistry as elastic impression materials.

**Hydroxyapatite ceramics:** A composition of calcium and phosphate in physiologic ratios to provide a dense, non-resorbable, biocompatible ceramic material used for dental implants and residual ridge augmentation.

**Hygroscopic expansion:** Expansion as a result of the absorption of moisture.

**Haptics technology:** That is based on the sense of touch to facilitate computer interactions and control of virtual objects such as the remote control of devices.

**Hardness:** Resistance of a material to plastic deformation, which is typically produced by an indentation force.

**Heat of vaporization:** Thermal energy required to convert a solid to a vapor.

**Heterogeneous nucleation:** Formation of solid nuclei on the mold walls or on particles within a solidifying molten metal.

**High-viscosity glass ionomer cement:** A conventional GIC that contains finer glass particles and a higher powder/liquid ratio for increased packability and strength.

**Homogeneous nucleation:** Formation of nuclei that occur at random locations within a supercooled molten metal in a clean, inert container.

**Hue:** Dominant color of an object; for example, red, green, or blue.

**Hybrid composite:** A particle-filled resin that contains a graded blend of two or more size ranges of filler particles to achieve an optimal balance among the following properties: ease of manipulation, strength, modulus (relative rigidity), polymerization shrinkage, wear resistance, appearance and polishability. Nanohybrids contain at least one dispersed filler with particle sizes of 100 nm or less.

**Hygroscopic setting expansion:** The expansion that occurs when gypsum or a gypsum-bonded investment sets while immersed in water [usually heated to approximately 38 °C (100 °F)].

**Hypersensitivity:** Abnormal clinical reaction or exaggerated immune response to a foreign substance that is manifested by one or more signs and symptoms, such as breathing difficulty, erythema, itching, sneezing, swelling, and vesicles.

# I

**Imbibition:** The act or process of imbibing or absorbing; in dentistry, an example is the absorption of water in hydrocolloid impression materials when stored in water and the resultant dimensional change that occurs.

**Implant:** Any object or material, such as an alloplastic substance or other tissue, which is partially or completely inserted or grafted into the body for therapeutic, diagnostic, prosthetic, or experimental purposes.

**Impression material:** Any substance or combination of substances used for making an impression or negative reproduction

**Indirect pulp capping:** A procedure that seeks to stimulate formation of reparative dentin by placing a material over sound or carious dentin.

**Infrared soldering:** Joining the components of a fixed dental prosthesis (between retainers or retainer and pontic) with a especially designed unit that uses infrared light as its heat source.

**Injection molding:** The adaptation of a plastic material to the negative form of a closed mold by forcing the material into the mold through appropriate gateways.

**Investing:** The process of covering or enveloping, wholly or in part, an object such as a denture, tooth, wax form, crown, etc., with a suitable investment material before processing, soldering, or casting.

**Irreversible hydrocolloid:** A hydrocolloid consisting of a sol of alginic acid having a physical state that is changed by an irreversible chemical reaction forming insoluble calcium alginate.

**Ion exchange strengthening:** The chemical process whereby the surface of a glass is placed in compression by the replacement of a small ion by a larger one while maintaining chemical neutrality.

**Indirect restorative material:** A ceramic, metal, metal-ceramic, or resin-based composite used extraorally to produce prostheses, which replace missing teeth, enhance esthetics, and/or restore damaged teeth.

**Indirect wax technique:** Procedure in which a wax pattern is prepared on a die.

**Induction:** Activation of free radicals, which in turn initiates growing polymer chains.

**Inelastic:** Incapable of sustaining significant elastic deformation without fracturing under stress.

**Inhibitor:** A component that prevents or inhibits undesirable polymerization of the monomeric liquid during storage, in order to prolong shelf-life. An unintended positive effect of inhibiting or preventing premature polymerization is the increase in working time.

**Initial set (of a polymer):** The stage of polymerization during which the polymer retains its shape.

**Initiator:** The component that starts a polymerization reaction; types include photoinitiators, chemical initiators, and heat initiators.

**Inlay wax:** A specialized dental wax that can be applied to dies to form direct or indirect patterns for the lost-wax technique, which is used for the casting of metals or hot pressing of ceramics.

**Intermediate restoration:** A tooth filling placed or prosthesis that is cemented for a limited time, from several days to months, which is designed to seal a tooth and maintain its position until a long-term restoration is produced; also called a temporary restoration.

**Intermediate duration exposure:** The contact with a substance that occurs for more than 14 days and less than I year (compare with acute toxicity and chronic exposure).

**Interstitial atom:** An imperfection in a crystal lattice consisting of an extra atom located between the adjacent atoms in normal lattice sites.

**Ion implantation:** The process of altering the surface of a metal with desirable ionic species.

## K

**Kaolin:** Fine, usually white, clay that is used in ceramics and refractory materials as a filler or extender.

**Knoop hardness tests:** Eponym for a surface hardness test that uses a diamond stylus; used for harder materials and characterized by the diamond- or rhomboid-shaped indentation; the indentation micro-hardness test uses a rhombic-based pyramidal diamond indenter; the long diagonal of the resulting indentation is measured to determine the hardness; this test is suitable for most classes of materials including brittle and elastomeric.

## L

**Latent heat of fusion:** Thermal energy required to convert a solid to a liquid.

**Lethal dose fifty (LDso):** The calculated dose of a substance that is expected to cause the death of 50% of the entire population of specific experimental animals.

**Light-cured/photocured/photoinitiated composite:** Particle-filled resin consisting of a single paste that becomes polymerized through the use of a photosensitive initiator system (typically camphorquinone and an amine) and a light-source activator (typically visible blue light).

**Liner:** The polymeric material used to replace the tissue contacting (intaglio) surface of an existing denture.

**Long-term soft liner:** A resilient polymeric material that is bonded to the tissue-contacting surface of a denture for cushioning and or improved retention. Intended for up to a year of service, they are typically heat-processed, and thus, they are more durable than chemically cured, short-term soft liners and tissue conditioners.

**Lost wax technique:** Process in which a wax pattern, prepared in the shape of missing tooth structure, is embedded in a casting investment and burned out to produce a mold cavity into which molten metal is cast.

**Luting/cementing agent:** Viscous material placed between two components, such as tooth structure and a restoration, that hardens to bind the two components together primarily through micromechanical interlocking, similar to the way mortar holds bricks together.

**Luting agent:** A viscous cement-like material that also fills a gap between the bonded materials.

## M

**Metal collar:** A narrow band of highly polished metal immediately adjacent to the margin on a metal-ceramic restoration.

**Methyl methacrylate resin:** A transparent, thermoplastic acrylic resin that is used in dentistry by mixing liquid methyl methacrylate monomer with the polymer powder; the resultant mixture forms a pliable plastic mass termed dough, which is packed into a mold prior to initiation of polymerization.

**Metal base:** The metallic portion of a denture base forming a part or the entire basal surface of the denture; it serves as a base for the attachment of the resin portion of the denture base and the teeth

**Metal-ceramic restoration:** An artificial crown or fixed complete or partial denture that uses a metal substructure and porcelain veneer.

**Milled ceramics:** a desired form made by subtractive CAM of a homogeneous ceramic block

**Milling:** The procedure of refining or perfecting the occlusion of teeth by the use of abrasives between their occluding surfaces while the dentures are rubbed together in the mouth or on the articulator.

**Modeling plastic impression compound:** S thermoplastic dental impression material composed of wax, rosin, resins, and colorants.

**Modeling wax:** A wax suitable for making patterns in the fabrication of restorations.

**Modulus of elasticity:** In metallurgy, it is the ratio of stress to strain. As the modulus of elasticity rises, the material becomes more rigid.

**Modulus of resilience:** The work or energy required to stress a cubic inch of material (in one direction only) from zero up to the proportional limit of the material, measured by the ability of the material to withstand the momentary effect of an impact load while stresses remain within the proportional limit.

**Monochromatic vision:** Vision in which there is no color discrimination.

**Monolithic:** An object with the same chemical and physical properties throughout its thickness.

**Mucostatic:** The state of the oral mucosa when not displaced by external forces.

**Muffle:** The portion of a furnace, usually removable or replaceable, in which material may be placed for processing without direct exposure to a heating element.

**Munsell color order system:** A color order system, developed in 1905, which places colors in an orderly arrangement encompassing the three attributes of hue, value, and chroma.

**Macromolecule:** A large high-molecular-weight compound usually consisting of repeating units in a chain-like configuration.

**Magnet:** Metallic material in which the component atoms are so ordered that it can attract iron-containing objects or align itself in an external magnetic field.

**Malleability:** The ability of the material to withstand sustained plastic deformation under compressive loads without fracture. Such material can be hammered into thin sheets without fracturing.

**Marginal breakdown:** The gradual fracture of the perimeter or margin of a dental amalgam filling, which leads to the formation of gaps between the amalgam and the tooth.

**Matrix:** A plastic resin material that forms a continuous phase upon curing and binds the reinforcing filler particles.

**Matrix metalloproteinase (MMP):** Any member of a family of at least 19 structurally related zinc-dependent neutral endopeptidases collectively capable of degrading essentially all components of the extracellular matrix.

**Maturation (cement):** The process of hardening a cement matrix through hydration with oral fluids to achieve greater mechanical strength.

**Melting temperature (melting point):** Equilibrium temperature at which heating of a pure metal, compound, or eutectic alloy produces a change from a solid to a liquid.

**Metal-reinforced glass ionomer cement:** A glass ionomer cement that incorporates metal particles to improve certain mechanical properties.

**Metallic bond:** Primary bond between metal atoms.

**Metamerism:** Phenomenon in which the color of an object under one type of light source appears to change when illuminated by a different light source.

**Micelle:** An aggregate of surfactant molecules or ions in solution.

**Microfilled composite:** Composite reinforced with colloidal silica filler particles, approximately 40 nm in size, which can be polished to a highly smooth surface. Microfillers are nondiscrete nanometer-sized particles that are agglomerated into large three-dimensional chainlike networks that drastically increase monomer viscosity.

**Microleakage:** The flow of oral fluid and bacteria into the microscopic gap between a prepared tooth surface and a restorative material.

**Micromechanical bonding:** The mechanical interlocking that is associated with bonding of an adhesive to a roughened adherend surface.

**Microstructure:** Structural features of a metal, including grains, grain boundaries, phases, and defects such as porosity, revealed by microscopic imaging of the chemically or electrolytically etched surface of a flat, polished specimen.

**Mineral trioxide aggregate (MTA):** A tri-and dicalcium silicate-based cement used for vital pulp therapy and endodontic indications including apexification, iatrogenic perforation repair, resorption repair, root-end filling, and sealing.

**Model:** A positive likeness of an object.

# N

**Nano:** The prefix nano refers to one billionth or $10^{-9}$ of a specific unit. A nanometer (nm) is one billionth of a meter ($10^{-9}$ meter) or one thousandth of a micron ($10^{-3}$ m).

**Nanofilled composite/nanocomposite:** Composites with the same-size particles as microfilled composites but the particles have been surface-treated to form isolated and/or loosely bound spheroidal agglomerates (called clusters) of primary nanoparticles. All of the nanocomposites currently being marketed have average primary particle sizes in the 40-nm range and so are of the same size as microfilled composites.

**Nanotechnology:** The branch of technology that focuses on the atomic and molecular scale of matter (below 100 nm), including materials, devices, and other structures.

**Natural glaze:** A superficial layer on a ceramic-ceramic or metal-ceramic prosthesis formed by heating a dental porcelain to form a smooth glassy layer.

**Noble metal:** Gold and platinum group metals (platinum, palladium, rhodium, ruthenium, iridium and osmium), which are highly resistant to oxidation and dissolution in inorganic acids.

**Normal setting expansion:** The expansion that occurs when gypsum or a gypsum-bonded investment sets in ambient air.

**Nucleus:** A stable cluster of atoms in a new phase that forms within a parent matrix phase during the solidification of a microstructure.

**Nickel-chromium alloy:** A low-density, large-grained base metal dental casting alloy with prominent dendritic structure, composed of up to 30% Cr and 70% Ni with trace elements that may include small amounts of Mo, Mn, Si, C, and Al; chromium, by its passivation effect, ensures corrosion resistance of the alloy; increased nickel content tends to result in reduced strength, hardness, modulus of elasticity, and fusion temperature while ductility may increase.

# O

**Obtundent:** An agent or remedy that lessens or relieves pain or sensibility.

**Occlusal wear:** Loss of substance on opposing occlusal units or surfaces as the result of attrition or abrasion.

**Opacity:** The quality or state of a body that makes it impervious to light

**Opaque:** The property of a material that absorbs and/or reflects all light and prevents any transmission of light.

**Opaque dentin:** Modified body porcelain with increased opacity, used where fewer translucencies are required, such as in the gingival area of a pontic or incisal mamelon to mimic existing anatomic features of adjacent natural teeth.

**Opaque modifier:** Colored dental porcelain formulated to be selectively mixed with opaque porcelain to increase the saturation of the desired pigment.

**Opaque porcelain:** The first porcelain layer applied in the metal-ceramic technique to the underlying metal framework to establish the bond between the porcelain and metal while simultaneously masking the dark color of the metallic oxide layer; opaque porcelain provides the primary source of color for the completed restoration.

**ORganically MOdified CERamic (ORMOCER):** A three-dimensionally cross-linked copolymer with polymerizing side chains resulting in low volumetric polymerization shrinkage and less residual monomer.

**Osseointegration:** 1. The apparent direct attachment or connection of osseous tissue to an inert, alloplastic material without intervening fibrous connective tissue; 2. The process and resultant apparent direct connection of an exogenous.

**Oven soldering:** Any soldering procedure that uses heat from a furnace to melt and fuse the solder as opposed to using a gas-air torch, gas-oxygen torch, or laser as the heat source.

**Overglaze:** The production of a glazed surface by the addition of a fluxed glass that usually vitrifies at a lower temperature

**Osseointegration:** The process of forming a direct structural and functional interface between live bone and an artificial implant surface without any intervening fibrous connective tissue.

**Osteoconductivity:** Property of a material that describes its ability to act as a matrix or scaffold and facilitate new bone growth on its surface.

**Osteoinductive:** The ability of a material to form new bone.

**Overglaze:** Thin surface coating of glass formed by fusing a thin layer of glass powder that becomes a viscous liquid at a lower temperature than that associated with the ceramic substrate.

**Oxygen-inhibited layer:** The thin surface region of a polymerized resin containing unreacted methacrylate groups arising from dissolved oxygen, which acts to inhibit the free-radical polymerization curing reaction; also known as the air-inhibited layer.

# P

**P L ratio:** Powder-to-liquid ratio by weight or volume.

**Passivation:** A process whereby metals and alloys are made more corrosion resistant through surface treatment; this process produces a thin and stable inert oxide layer on the external surfaces.

**Phosphorescence:** A form of photoluminescence based on the properties of certain molecules to absorb energy (either near ultraviolet or visible) and emit it in the form of visible radiation at a higher wavelength; distinguished from fluorescence in that light continues to be emitted for some time after the exciting energy has ceased.

**Photoactive:** Reacting chemically to visible light or ultraviolet radiation.

**Photometer:** An instrument for the measurement of emitted, reflected, or transmitted light; for the measurement of luminous intensity, a visual receptor element (the eye) may be used as the measuring device, or a physical receptor element may be used that can be related to the calculated response of a standard observer.

**Physical photometer:** A photometer in which the measurement is made by some physical or chemical effect instead of by visual methods.

**Pink porcelain:** A term for the porcelain that replaces gingival tissues.

**Polishing:** To make surface smooth and glossy, usually by friction; to give luster.

**Polishing agent:** Any material used to impart luster to a surface.

**Polyether:** An elastomeric impression material of ethylene oxide and tetra-hydrofluro copolymers that polymerizes under the influence of an aromatic ester.

**Poly(etheretherketone):** Acronym is PEEK; a highly ordered, flexible, strong, shape-stable, biocompatible polymer machined to final shape, used for removable partial denture frameworks and dental implant components.

**Polymer:** A chemical compound consisting of large organic molecules built by repetition of smaller monomeric units.

**Polysulfide:** An elastomeric impression material of polysulfide polymer (mercaptan) that cross-links under the influence of oxidizing agents such as lead peroxide.

**Poly(vinyl siloxane):** An addition reaction silicone elastomeric impression material of silicone polymers having terminal vinyl groups that cross-link with silanes on activation by a platinum or palladium salt catalyst.

**Porcelain margin:** The extension of ceramic material to the finish line of the preparation without visible metal substructure in the marginal area.

**Porcelain laminate veneer:** A thin, bonded ceramic restoration that restores the facial, incisal, and part of the proximal surfaces of teeth requiring esthetic restoration.

**Post-ceramic solder:** A soldering procedure to join metal-ceramic restorations after final shaping and glazing of the ceramic veneer; also used to join Type III or Type IV gold castings to metal-ceramic units; an alloy formulated for post-ceramic soldering.

**Pre-ceramic soldering:** a soldering procedure joining framework components of a metal-ceramic prosthesis prior to application of the ceramic veneer.

**Precious metal alloy:** An alloy predominantly composed of elements considered precious, such as gold, the six metals of the platinum group (platinum, osmium, iridium, palladium, ruthenium, and rhodium), and silver.

**Pressed ceramics:** A technique designed to produce a desired form by injecting a molten homogeneous ceramic material into a mold.

**Pressed-on-metal ceramics:** A technique designed to produce a desired form by injecting a molten homogeneous ceramic material into a mold containing a metal framework that is veneered with opaque porcelain.

**Pressed-on-zirconia ceramics:** A technique designed to produce a desired form by injecting a molten homogeneous ceramic material into a mold containing a zirconia framework that may be veneered with porcelain.

**Pressure welding:** Bonding of two metals together by sufficiently large force applied perpendicular to the surfaces; such force must be of magnitude to produce permanent distortions that expose a film-free metal contact.

**Packable composite:** A hybrid resin composite designed for use in posterior areas where a stiffer consistency facilitates condensation into a cavity form in a manner similar to that used for lathe-cut amalgams. Also known as condensable composite.

**Passivation:** The process of transforming a chemically active surface of a metal to a less active surface.

**Percent elongation:** Amount of plastic strain, expressed as percent of the original length, which a tensile test specimen sustains at the point of fracture (Ductility).

**Perimplantitis:** An inflammation that develops in and around the area surrounding a dental implant.

**Phase diagram (constitution diagram):** A graph of equilibrium phases and solubility limits for an alloy system as a function of composition and temperature.

**Pitting corrosion:** Highly localized corrosion occurring at metal surface defects such as pits, scratches, and cracks in which the region at the bottom is oxygen-deprived and becomes the anode while the surface around it becomes the cathode. Thus, metal at the base preferentially ionizes and goes into solution, causing the defects to enlarge.

**Plastic flow (of a polymer):** Irreversible deformation that occurs when polymer chains slide over one another and become relocated within the material.

**Plastic strain:** Irreversible deformation that remains when the externally applied force is reduced or eliminated.

**Point defect A:** lattice imperfection of atomic size in three dimensions, such as a vacancy, divacancy, trivacancy, or interstitial atom.

**Polyhedral oligomeric silsesquioxane (POSS):** A molecular-sized hybrid, organic-inorganic resin containing 12-sided silicate cage structures that impart nanoparticle like reinforcement.

**Porcelain, aluminous:** A dental porcelain whose thermal expansion coefficient is suitable for use as a veneer over an alumina core. This porcelain creates the anatomy of the crown and improves the esthetics of the alumina based prostheses.

**Porcelain, dental:** A ceramic produced by sintering a mixture of feldspar, silica, alumina, other metal oxides, pigments, and opacifying agents. Except for porcelain denture teeth, dental porcelain is not made from kaolin.

**Porcelain, feldspathic:** A especially formulated dental porcelain that contains leucite crystals (KAISi,0 6) in a glass matrix that is used for veneering the metal framework of metal-ceramic prostheses. Leucite crystals have high thermal expansion, which makes the porcelain thermally compatible with the high-expansion noble and nickel-base alloys used in fixed prosthodontics. The leucite crystals are often formed by heat-treating potassium feldspar.

**Precipitation hardening:** The process of strengthening and hardening a metal by precipitating a phase or constituent from a saturated solid solution.

**Pressure:** Force per unit area acting on the surface of a material (compare with stress).

**Preventive dental material:** Cement, coating. or restorative material that either seals pits and fissures or releases a therapeutic agent such as Fluoride and/or mineralizing ions to prevent or arrest the demineralization of tooth structure.

**Preventive-resin restoration (PRR):** A conservative, sealed, resin-based composite restoration, usually placed in a minimally prepared occlusal fissure area, with the sealant extending into contiguous uncut fissures.

**Primer:** A hydrophilic, low-viscosity resin that promotes bonding to an adherend substrate, such as dentin.

**Propagation:** Stage of polymerization during which polymer chains continue to grow to high molecular weights.

**Proportional limit:** Magnitude of elastic stress above which plastic deformation occurs.

**Pseudoplastic:** Viscous character that is opposite from dilatant behavior in which the rate of flow decreases with increasing strain rate until it reaches a nearly constant value. Thus, the more rapidly the pseudoplastic fluids are stained or forced through a syringe, the more easily they flow.

**Pseudoplasticity:** The tendency of a material to become less viscous as the shear rate increases and to recover viscosity immediately upon the elimination of shear stress.

**Pulp capping:** A procedure for treating a pulp that has been exposed through carious tissue removal by the application of a medicament.

## Q

**Quaternary alloy:** An alloy that contains four elements at least one of which is a metal.

**Quartz:** An allotropic form of silica; the mineral SiO2 consisting of hexagonal crystals of colorless, transparent silicon dioxide

## R

**Rapid prototyping:** A general term used for several additive layer manufacturing techniques like stereolithography, fused deposition modeling, selective deposition modeling, selective laser melting, selective laser sintering.

**Reflection:** The return of light or sound waves from a surface.

**Refraction:** The deflection of light or energy waves from a straight path that occurs when passing obliquely from one medium into another in which its velocity is different.

**Refractory:** Difficult to fuse or corrode; capable of enduring high temperatures.

**Refractory cast:** A cast made of a material that will withstand high temperatures without disintegrating.

**Refractory die:** Any die material that is capable of enduring the high temperatures that occur during firing or casting procedures; the die is an integral part of the mold; the restoration is directly cast, molded, or fired onto the refractory die.

**Refractory investment:** An investment material that can withstand the high temperatures used in soldering or casting.

**Refractory mold:** A refractory cavity into which a substance is shaped or cast.

**Rebasing:** The process of replacing the entire denture base of an existing complete or partial denture.

**Reline:** The procedures used to resurface the intaglio of a removable dental prosthesis with new base material, thus producing an accurate adaptation to the denture foundation area.

**Remodel:** The morphologic change in bone as an adaptive response to altered environmental demands. The bone will progressively remodel where there is a proliferation of tissue with regressive remodeling when osteoclastic resorption is evident.

**Remount cast:** A cast formed inside the intaglio of a prosthesis for the purpose of mounting the prosthesis on an articulator.

**Resilient:** Characterized or noted by resilience, as capable of withstanding shock without permanent deformation or rupture.

**Resin:** A broad term used to describe natural or synthetic substances that form plastic materials after polymerization; they are named according to their chemical composition, physical structure, and means for activation of polymerization.

**Refractory die:** Any die material that is capable of enduring the high temperatures that occur during firing or casting procedures; the die is an integral part of the mold; the restoration is directly cast, molded, or fired onto the refractory die.

**Reversible hydrocolloid:** Colloidal gels in which the gelation is brought about by cooling and can be returned to the sol condition when the temperature is sufficiently increased.

**Rockwell hardness number:** A hardness measurement obtained from the depth of an indentation after use of either a steel ball or conical diamond point; the Rockwell hardness number is designated to the particular indenter and load used.

**Rouge:** A compound composed of ferric oxide and binders used for imparting a high luster to a polished surface of glass, metal, or gems.

**Recovery:** A stage of heat treatment that results in the partial restoration of properties of a work-hardened metal without a change in the grain structure.

**Recrystallization:** The process of forming new stress-free crystals in a work-hardened metal through a controlled heat-treatment process.

**Refract/Refraction:** The degree to which light is bent when it passes from one medium to another. This makes a spoon appear bent in a glass of drinking water when light passes from air through glass into water. The index of refraction is a measure of this effect.

**Remineralization:** Process of restoring mineral content (calcium phosphate) in demineralized tooth structure.

**Replantation:** Reinsertion of a tooth back into its jaw socket soon after intentional extraction or accidental removal.

**Resin cement:** A resin-based material containing fillers that are cured to form a composite material used for attaching orthodontic brackets and fixed prostheses. Such cements are applied following the application of an etchant and an enamel or a dentin bonding agent to bond to tooth structure. Generally, these cements are less viscous than resin-based composite restorative materials.

**Resin tag:** Extension of resin that has penetrated into etched enamel or dentin.

**Resin-based composite:** A highly cross-linked resin reinforced by a dispersion of amorphous silica, glass, crystalline, or organic resin filler particles and/or fibers bonded to the polymer matrix by a coupling agent.

**Restorative:** Metallic, ceramic, metal-ceramic, or resin-based substance used to replace, repair, or rebuild teeth and/or to enhance esthetics.

**Rheology:** Study of the deformation and flow characteristics of matter (see also viscosity).

**Root canal sealer:** A material used in conjunction with an obturation material for root canal therapy such as guttapercha, to prevent the ingress of fluid or bacteria within the tooth root.

## S

**Sandwich technique:** A restorative technique when applying a glass ionomer to dentin and then overlaying it with composite resin; the synergy of the two materials provides a physiomechanical and esthetic property.

**Saturation:** The attribute of color perception that expresses the degree of color (hue) intensity.

**Scaffold:** A supporting surface, either natural or prosthetic, which maintains the contour of tissue; a supporting framework.

**Semiprecious metal alloy:** An alloy composed of precious and base metals; there is no distinct ratio of components separating semiprecious alloys from another group.

**Separating medium:** A coating applied to a surface and serving to prevent a second surface from adhering to the first.

**Shade:** A term used to describe a particular hue, or variation of a primary hue, such as a greenish shade of yellow.

**Shellac base:** A record base constructed by using a shellac-based wafer that has been adapted to the cast with heat.

**Silica:** Silicon dioxide occurring in crystalline, amorphous, and usually impure forms (as quartz, opal, and sand).

**Silica-bonded investment:** A casting investment with ethyl silicate or a silica gel as a binder, the latter reverting to silica upon heating; this is combined with cristobalite or quartz as the refractory material; such investments exhibit considerable thermal expansion and can be used when casting higher fusing chromium alloys.

**Sinter:** To cause to become a coherent mass by heating without melting.

**Slip-cast ceramics:** A fine-grain ceramic material that is partially sintered to form a porous substructure; the ceramic material can be either aluminum oxide, magnesium aluminum oxide, or a combination of aluminum oxide and zirconium oxide; the porous substructure is subsequently infused with a molten glass to form a strong framework for a fixed dental prosthesis.

**Solder:** The act of uniting two pieces of metal by the proper alloy.

**Soldering antiflux:** A material, such as iron oxide (rouge) dissolved in a suitable solvent, such as turpentine, placed on a metal surface to confine the flow of molten solder.

**Soldering flux:** A material such as borax glass ($Na_2B_4O_7$) applied to a metal surface to remove oxides or prevent their formation to facilitate the flow of solder.

**Soldering index:** (1) a mold used to record the relative position of multiple cast restorations prior to investing for a soldering procedure; (2) a rigid resin connection between multiple cast restorations fixing their relative position prior to a soldering procedure.

**Solidification porosity:** An area of porosity in cast metal that is caused by shrinkage of a portion of the metal as it solidifies from the molten state without flow of additional molten metal from surrounding areas.

**Spatula:** A flat-bladed instrument used for mixing or spreading materials.

**Spatulation:** The manipulation of material with a spatula to produce a homogenous mass.

**Stereolithography (SLA):** A computer numerical control (CNC) additive fabrication of an object; in dentistry, it relates to the laser initiation of light-reactive resin layering to make replicas of casts and devices.

**Subperiosteal dental implant abutment:** That portion of the implant that protrudes through the mucosa into the oral cavity for the retention or support of a crown, a fixed partial denture, or an overdenture.

**Suck-back porosity:** A shrinkage void in a solidified casting opposite the location of the sprue attachment, resulting from a heat swell and localized lingering of molten metal after the casting, as a whole, has solidified.

**Sag:** Irreversible (plastic) deformation of metal frameworks of fixed dental prostheses in the firing temperature range of ceramic veneers.

**Sandwich technique:** Of placing glass ionomer cement as an intermediate layer between the tooth structure and a resin-based composite restorative material; this restoration design combines the adhesion and fluoride-releasing nature of a glass ionomer cement with the esthetic quality and durability of a resin-based composite.

**Self-adhesive:** Ability of a material to adhere to tooth structure without the aid of a dentin or enamel bonding agent.

**Self-assembling materials:** Material systems that automatically transform into prespecified assemblies.

**Self-diffusion:** Thermally driven transfer of an atom to an adjacent lattice site in a crystal composed of the same atomic species.

**Sensitization:** The process by which an allergy antibody is produced, which reacts specifically to the causative foreign substance.

**Set:** The state of being sufficiently rigid or elastic to permit removal from the mouth without plastic deformation.

**Setting time:** The time from the start of mixing to the point where the material loses its flow potential or plasticity.

**Shear strength:** Shear stress at the point of fracture.

**Shear stress:** Ratio of shear force to the original cross-sectional area parallel to the direction of the applied force.

**Shear thinning:** The tendency for viscosity to decrease as the shearing rate increases.

**Short-term soft liner (tissue conditioner):** A resilient polymeric material that is employed for brief periods (up to 14 days) to absorb masticatory impact and adapt to changing ridge contours (e.g. following the extraction of teeth or surgical alteration of an edentulous or partially edentulous ridge). Such materials are typically chemically activated polymers that contain plasticizers.

**Silicate cement (silicophosphate):** Traditional restorative material made from the mixture of a liquid (phosphoric acid) and a fluoride-containing silicate glass powder.

**Silorane:** A tetrafunctional epoxy siloxane monomer that cures via ring-opening polymerization. When the rings open, they lengthen and occupy more space; the resulting expansion offsets a portion of the polymerization shrinkage.

**Sintering:** Process of heating closely packed particles below their melting temperature to promote atomic diffusion across particle boundaries and densification of the mass.

**Slip casting:** Process of forming ceramic shapes by applying an aqueous slurry of ceramic particles to a porous substrate (such as a die material), and removing the water by capillary action. This densifies the deposited ceramic powder into a "green body," which is subsequently sintered to achieve higher density and strength.

**Smart materials:** Synthetic materials that interact with external stimuli such as light, temperature, stress, moisture, pH, and electric/magnetic fields in such a way as to alter specific properties in a controlled fashion. A key feature of smart behavior is the ability of a material to return to its original state after the stimulus has been removed.

**Smear layer:** Poorly adherent layer of ground dentin produced by cutting a dentin surface; also, a tenacious deposit of microscopic debris that covers enamel and dentin surfaces that have been prepared for a restoration.

**Soldering:** Process of building up a localized metal area with a molten filler metal or joining two or more metal components by heating them to a temperature below their solidus temperature and filling the gap between them using a molten metal with a liquidus temperature below 450 °C. In dentistry, many metals are joined by brazing, although the term soldering is commonly used. If the process is conducted above 450 °C, it is called brazing.

**Solid solution (metallic):** A solid crystalline phase containing two or more elements at least one of which is a metal and whose atoms share the same crystal lattice.

**Spinel or spinell:** A porous slip-cast ceramic, $MgAl_2O_4$ ($MgO \cdot Al_2O_3$), that is glass-infiltrated to produce a core ceramic.

**Spring back:** The amount of elastic strain that a metal can recover when loaded to and unloaded from its yield strength; an important property of orthodontic wires.

**Sprue:** The mold channel through which molten metal or ceramic flows into a mold cavity.

**Sprued wax pattern:** A wax form consisting of the prosthesis pattern and the attached sprue network.

**Static mixing:** A technique of transforming two fluid (or paste-like) materials into a homogeneous mixture without mechanical stirring; it requires a device that forces two streams of material into a mixer cylinder, such that as the stream move through the mixer, while the stationary elements in the mixer continuously blend the materials.

**Stem cells:** Biological cells in multicellular organisms that can divide by mitosis and differentiate into anyone of the 200 or more possible cell types in humans and continuously divide to yield more stem cells of the same type.

**Sticky wax:** A type of dental wax that exhibits high adhesion to dry, clean surfaces when it is heated to a plastic condition.

**Strain:** Change in dimension per unit initial dimension. For tensile and compressive strain, a change in length is measured relative to the initial reference length.

**Strain hardening (work hardening):** The increase in strength and hardness and decrease in ductility of a metal that is caused by plastic deformation below its recrystallization temperature; also called work hardening.

**Strain rate:** Change in strain per unit time during loading of a structure.

**Strength:** Maximum stress that a structure can withstand without sustaining a specific amount of plastic strain (yield strength).

**Stress:** Force per unit area within a structure subjected to a force or pressure.

**Stress concentration:** State of elevated stress in a solid caused by surface or internal defects or by marked changes in contour.

**Stress corrosion:** Degradation caused by the combined effects of mechanical stress and a corrosive environment, usually exhibited as cracking.

**Stress intensity (stress intensity factor):** Relative increase in stress at the tip of a crack of given shape and size when the crack surfaces are displaced in the opening mode (also fracture toughness).

**Stress relief:** The reduction of residual stress by heat treatment.

**Subperiosteal implant:** A dental device that is placed beneath the periosteum and overlies cortical bone.

**Supercooled liquid:** A liquid that has been cooled at a sufficiently rapid rate to a point below the temperature at which an equilibrium phase change can occur.

**Superelasticity:** The ability of certain nickel-titanium alloys to undergo extensive deformation resulting from a stress-assisted phase transformation, with the reverse transformation occurring on unloading; sometimes called pseudoelasticity.

**Surface energy:** The excess energy of molecules at the surfaces of materials above that of molecules found in the interior of a material.

**Surface tension:** A measurement of the cohesive energy present at an interface; in the case of a liquid, it is the liquid/air interface. This energy is the result of molecules on the surface of a liquid experiencing an imbalance of attraction between molecules. It has units of mN/m.

**Syneresis:** The expression of fluid onto the surface of gel structures.

# T

**Tarnish:** Process by which a metal surface is dulled or discolored when a reaction with a sulfide, oxide, chloride, or other chemical causes surface discoloration through formation of a thin oxidized film.

**Tensile stress:** The internal induced force that resists the elongation of a material in a direction parallel to the direction of the stresses.

**Thermoplastic:** A characteristic or property of a material that allows it to be softened by heating and then return to the hardened state on cooling.

**Thermal expansion:** Expansion of a material caused by heat.

**Thermal tempering:** Creating a differential in cooling rate between the external and interior of a glass-ceramic resulting in a surface compressive layer and increased flexural strength.

**Tissue conditioner:** A resilient denture liner resin placed into a removable prosthesis for a short duration to allow time for tissue healing.

**Tissue engineering:** A field of research for the growth of tissues or organs used as therapeutic placement in the human body.

**Tissue-integrated prosthesis:** Any dental implant-supported fixed complete or partial denture supported by osseointegrated dental implants.

**Tissue integration:** As clinically observed, the apparent direct and healthy attachment of living tissue to an alloplastic material, i.e. a dental implant.

**Temporary restorative material:** Cement-or resin-based composite used for a period of a few days to several months to restore or replace missing teeth or tooth structure until a more long-lasting prosthesis or restoration can be placed.

**Temporomandibular joint (TMJ):** The junction between the head of the mandible and the temporal bone of the skull.

**Tensile stress:** Ratio of tensile force to the original cross-sectional area perpendicular to the direction of applied force.

**Termination:** Stage of polymerization during which polymer chains no longer grow.

**Ternary alloy:** An alloy that contains three elements at least one of which is a metal.

**Tesla:** Unit of flux density (T) of the magnetic field produced by a magnet.

**Texturing:** The process of increasing roughness of the implant surface area to which bone can bond.

**Thermal compatibility:** Ability of veneering ceramics in metal-ceramic or ceramic-ceramic structures to contract in a manner similar to that of the core metal or ceramic structure during cooling from temperatures above Tg such that transient or residual tensile stress in the veneer is minimized and a protective compressive stress is produced.

**Thermal conductivity (coefficient of thermal conductivity):** Property that describes the thermal energy transport in watts per second through a specimen I cm thick with a cross-sectional area of $1cm^2$ when the temperature differential between the surfaces of the specimen perpendicular to the heat flow is I K (1 °C).

**Thermal diffusivity:** Measure of the speed with which a temperature change will proceed through an object when one surface is heated.

**Thermal expansion coefficient:** Relative linear change in length per unit of initial length during heating of a solid per K within a specified temperature range.

**Thermoplastic polymer:** Macromolecule material made of linear and/or branched chains that softens when heated above the glass-transition temperature (Tg), at which molecular motion begins to force the chains apart and soften the polymer.

**Thermosetting polymer:** Polymeric material that becomes permanently hard when heated above the temperature at which polymerization occurs and that does not soften again on reheating to the same temperature.

**Thixotropic:** Property of gels and other fluids to become less viscous and flow when subjected to steady shear forces through being shaken, stirred, squeezed, patted, or vibrated. When the shear force is decreased to zero, the viscosity increases to the original value. Also known as shear thinning, in which the greater the applied shear force, the less the resistance to flow.

**Toughness:** Ability of a material to absorb elastic energy and to deform plastically before fracturing; measured as the total area under a plot of tensile stress versus strain.

**Toxic:** Capable of causing injury or death, typically by a chemical agent.

**Toxicity:** The relative ability (dose-related effect) of a material to cause injury to biological tissues, ranging from improper biochemical function, organ damage, and cell destruction, to death.

**Translucency:** The quality of light passing through an object in a diffuse manner, only to reveal a distorted image that can be viewed through the material.

**Transmit/Transmittance:** The amount of light passing through an object.

**Transosteal implant:** A device that penetrates both cortical plates and the thickness of the alveolar bone.

**Transparency:** The extent to which light passes through a material and to which an undistorted image can be seen through it.

**Trituration:** The mixing of amalgam alloy particles with mercury in a device called a triturator; the term is also used to describe the reduction of a solid to fine particles by grinding or friction.

## U

**UCLA abutment:** A colloquial term used to describe a dental abutment that is attached directly to the implant body by means of a screw.

**Undercuts:** The recessed areas on dental structures, including teeth, edentulous ridges, prostheses, and restorations.

## V

**Vacancy:** Unoccupied atom lattice site in a crystalline solid.

**Value:** Relative lightness or darkness of a color. Also known as the gray scale.

**Vacuum thermomolding:** Softened sheet of vinyl acetate-ethylene copolymer (PVAc-PE) material can be adapted to the surface of a refractory cast by using vacuum, air, or mechanical pressure (sponge or putty).

**Vickers hardness number (VHN):** A measure of hardness obtained with a diamond pyramidal indenter with a square base and an angle of 136 degrees; VHN is proportional to the ratio of the applied load to the area of the indentation.

**Vitrification:** In ceramics, the progressive fusing of porcelain at high temperatures into an amorphous, more glassy material.

**vander Waals forces:** Short-range force of physical attraction that promotes adhesion between molecules of liquids or molecular crystals.

**Varnish:** A material for application to the floor of a prepared cavity; a solution of natural gum, synthetic resins, or resins dissolved in volatile solvent, such as acetone, ether, or chloroform; not necessarily a cement.

**Viscoelastic:** Term describing a polymer that combines the spring-like behaviour of an elastic solid (such as a rubber band) with that of the putty like behavior of a viscous, flowable fluid (such as honey).

**Viscoelasticity:** The ability of a material to strain instantaneously like an elastic solid during rapid stretching or to resist shear flow and to strain linearly over time (like honey) when a stress is applied slowly.

**Viscosity:** Resistance of a fluid to flow (see also rheology).

**Vital pulp therapy:** The placement of a material in a prepared tooth over an injured pulp to induce the formation of secondary dentin. Pulp capping, cavity lining, and pulpotomies are all vital pulp therapy treatments. Mineral trioxide aggregate (MTA) and calcium hydroxide have been used for this therapy.

**Voxel:** Volumetric picture element that represents a single sample, or data point on a regularly spaced three-dimensional grid.

## W

**Welding:** Process of fusing two or more metal parts through the application of heat, pressure, or both, with or without a filler metal, to produce a localized union across an interface between the workpieces.

**Wettability:** The relative affinity of a liquid for the surface of a solid.

**Wetting:** Relative interfacial tension between a liquid and a solid substrate that results in a contact angle of less than 90°.

**Wetting agent:** A surface-active substance that reduces the surface tension of a liquid to promote wetting or adhesion.

**Working range:** The maximum amount of elastic strain that an orthodontic wire can sustain before it plastically deforms.

**Working time:** Elapsed time from the start of mixing to the time at which the consistency of a material is no longer suitable for its intended use or a rapid rise in viscosity occurs.

**Wrought metal:** A metal that has been plastically deformed to alter the shape of the structure and certain mechanical properties, such as strength, hardness, and ductility.

## X

**Xenoestrogen:** A chemical that is not indigenous to the body but which acts in a manner similar to that estrogen.

## Y

**Yield strength:** The stress at which a test specimen exhibits a specific amount of plastic strain.

## Z

**Zirconia:** A partially stabilized zirconium oxide, usually in the tetragonal phase (t-Zr02), that is used primarily as a core (framework) for dental prostheses. It has also been introduced as a monolithic ceramic to be used without a veneering ceramic.

**Zirconia core:** A partially stabilized tetragonal zirconia (stabilized either by ceria or yttria) that is used for producing the core veneered framework or substructure for crowns or bridges.

**Zinc oxide eugenol cement:** A cement or luting agent resulting by mixing zinc oxide powder with eugenol liquid to form paste used for temporary luting material (Type I), long-term luting agent (Type II), temporary filling material (Type III) or intermediate restoration (Type IV).

**Zinc phosphate cement:** A cement or luting agent resulting from mixing zinc oxide (powder component) with phosphoric acid, water, aluminum phosphate, and zinc phosphate (liquid component); magnesium oxide is often used as a cavity base or as a luting agent.

**Zinc polycarboxylate cement:** A cement or luting agent resulting from mixing zinc oxide, magnesium oxide, (powder component) with an aqueous solution of polyacrylic acid and copolymers.

**Zirconia ceramic post:** A ceramic post used in the restoration of endodontically treated teeth, especially when a metal post may compromise esthetics. It can be used with composite resin or pressed-on-ceramics to form the core.

# Index

Page numbers followed by *f* refer to figure, *fc* refer to flowchart, and *t* refer to table